ESSENTIALS OF
NURSING
PRACTICE
2ND EDITION

EDITED BY
CATHERINE DELVES-YATES

~~JET LIBRARY~~

ADVISORY EDITORS:
KAREN ELCOCK, FIONA EVERETT, CAROL HALL, ROBERT JENKINS,
RUTH NORTHWAY, STEVE TRENOWETH AND WENDY WRIGHT

SAGE

Los Angeles | London | New Delhi
Singapore | Washington DC | Melbourne

Los Angeles | London | New Delhi
Singapore | Washington DC | Melbourne

SAGE Publications Ltd
1 Oliver's Yard
55 City Road
London EC1Y 1SP

SAGE Publications Inc.
2455 Teller Road
Thousand Oaks, California 91320

SAGE Publications India Pvt Ltd
B 1/I 1 Mohan Cooperative Industrial Area
Mathura Road
New Delhi 110 044

SAGE Publications Asia-Pacific Pte Ltd
3 Church Street
#10-04 Samsung Hub
Singapore 049483

Editor: Becky Taylor
Development editor: Christofere Fila
Editorial assistant: Jade Grogan
Assistant editor, digital: Chloe Statham
Production editor: Katie Forsythe
Copyeditor: Sharon Cawood
Proofreader: Thea Watson
Indexer: Adam Pozner
Marketing manager: Tamara Navaratnam
Cover design: Wendy Scott
Typeset by: C&M Digitals (P) Ltd, Chennai, India
Printed in the UK

Editorial arrangement and
Chapters 2, 12, 32 and 40 © Catherine
Delves-Yates 2018
Chapter 1 © Catherine Delves-Yates,
Karen Elcock, Carol Hall, Ruth Northway
and Steve Trenoweth 2018
Chapter 3 © Gabrielle Thorpe and
Catherine Delves-Yates 2018
Chapter 4 © Gabrielle Thorpe 2018
Chapter 5 © Ruth Northway and Ian
Beech 2018
Chapter 6 © Graham Avery 2018
Chapter 7 © Karen Elcock 2018
Chapter 8 © E. Jane Blowers 2018
Chapter 9 © Jacqueline Phipps 2018
Chapter 10 © Fiona Everett and Wendy
Wright 2018
Chapter 11 © Carol Hall 2018
Chapter 13 © Katrina Emerson and Ruth
Northway 2018
Chapter 14 © Rebekah Hill 2018
Chapter 15 © Karen Elcock and Jean
Shapcott 2018
Chapter 16 © Steve Trenoweth and
Wasiim Allymamod 2018
Chapter 17 © Melanie Fisher, Margaret
Scott and Karen Elcock 2018

Chapter 18 © Jill Barnes and Robert
Jenkins 2018
Chapter 19 © Gemma Hurley 2018
Chapter 20 © Robert Jenkins and Jill
Barnes 2018
Chapter 21 © Charlene Lobo, Daryl
Evans and Helen Walker 2018
Chapters 22 and 23 © Rose
Gallagher 2018
Chapter 24 © Valerie Foley 2018
Chapter 25 © Ann Kettyle 2018
Chapter 26 © Irene Anderson 2018
Chapter 27 © Dianne Steele 2018
Chapter 28 © Chris Mulryan 2018
Chapter 29 © Carol Hall 2018
Chapter 30 © Kate Goodhand and Jane
Ewen 2018
Chapter 31 © Mairead Collie and David J.
Hunter 2018
Chapter 33 © Jean Shapcott 2018
Chapters 34 and 39 © Siobhan
McCullough 2018
Chapter 35 © Adele Atkinson 2018
Chapter 36 © Janet Ramjeet 2018
Chapter 37 © Ruth Northway 2018
Chapter 38 © Charlene Lobo 2018

First edition published 2015
This second edition first published 2018

Library of Congress Control Number: 2017958134

British Library Cataloguing in Publication data

A catalogue record for this book is available from the British Library

ISBN 978-1-5264-2405-1
ISBN 978-1-5264-6242-8 (pbk)
ISBN 978-1-5264-4715-9 (pbk and ebook)

At SAGE we take sustainability seriously. Most of our products are printed in the UK using responsibly sourced papers and boards. When
we print overseas we ensure sustainable papers are used as measured by the PREPS grading system. We undertake an annual audit to
monitor our sustainability.

CONTENTS

GUIDE TO YOUR BOOK

"We are the student panel for this book and we are all currently second and third year nursing students. We've road tested the features in this book and the additional exercises online to make sure they work for you – wherever you are in your journey to becoming a nurse. We hope you enjoy the book and the online resources, and that it helps you succeed in your degree and your future career. Good luck!"

ALICE, COURTNEY, EMILY, DAVID, SAPALE AND KAREN.

'The **case studies** are a great tool that puts theory into practice. They provide good examples from different fields of nursing and really make you think. The **additional web** and **video links** and the recommended books and journal articles are great for delving more deeply into each subject. Having additional references all in one place is invaluable and great for assignments.'
- **Karen Halvey**

'**Voices** from patients and students nurses appear throughout the book. They will help you relate to some of the challenges you might face during placements and hear how fellow students have managed to overcome similar situations.'
- Sapana Ghale

'The **chapter summaries** break down the information covered in the chapter. I found them particularly helpful and used them to make revision cards. They are handy if you need information quickly without having to go into all of the detail.'
- Courtney Rees

'The **step-by-step boxes** give new students a head-start before starting clinical skills training in the first year. They are clear and easy to read. I use them as cheat cards to revise for the module assessments. You will find it helpful to go through them before the course starts.'
- Emily Aprile

'The **Activity boxes** help you with moving on to level 5 writing, so great for improving writing skills. The 'Critical reflection' help with developing your analytic and questioning skills and the 'What's the evidence' boxes help you identify relevant evidence which feeds into writing evidence-based assignments.'

- Alice Clement

Don't forget – you can find great online resources at **https://study.sagepub.com/essentialnursing2e** for more help with your learning, whether you are revising, doing assignments or preparing for placement. We've found these really helpful when you want a break from reading and to reinforce your learning in a different way – from reading a case study to taking a quiz. The icons throughout the book will remind you where there is a resource available on the website.

Ace your assessment: When you see this icon, you'll be able to find an answer or guidance to an activity online so you can be sure you are on the right track.

Further reading and useful websites can be found online whenever you see this icon. The articles and links will help you when researching for assignments or if you are interested in exploring a topic further.

Preparing for placement can be nerve racking. The extra case studies online will help you to think through real-life scenarios and feel prepared.

Get to grips: Take a break from the text and watch suggested videos to help you revise and understand.

NOTES ON THE EDITOR AND CONTRIBUTORS

EDITOR

Catherine Delves-Yates is an experienced nurse and a lecturer at the School of Health Sciences, University of East Anglia, UK. She started her nursing career as a student at the Nightingale School of Nursing, London and has worked clinically in adult and paediatric critical care in the UK, and has taught and nursed in America, Africa and Nepal. Her passion is to ensure all nurses have the knowledge, skills and professionalism to deliver effective compassionate care to each of their patients. Catherine is an honorary lecturer at the University of Buea and the Higher Institute of Applied Medical Sciences, Cameroon and an international advisor to the Patan Academy of Health Sciences, Nepal. Currently, she is researching whether nursing students' views of health and illness alter during their pre-registration nursing programme.

ADVISORY EDITORS

The following advisory editors helped work to ensure this book contained accurate and equal coverage of all fields of nursing in a variety of settings:

Learning disabilities: Robert Jenkins and Ruth Northway, University of South Wales

Child nursing: Carol Hall, University of Nottingham

Mental health: Steven Trenoweth, University of Bournemouth

Adult nursing: Karen Elcock, Kingston University and St George's University of London

Clinical skills: Fiona Everett and Wendy Wright, University of the West of Scotland

CONTRIBUTORS

Wasiim Allymamod is a qualified nurse working in an acute service of a London mental health trust. He qualified from the University of West London with first class honours in Mental Health Nursing in 2008. His interests are cognitive behavioural therapy, positive health and mental wellbeing and psychosocial interventions.

Irene Anderson is a principal lecturer in tissue viability and a reader in learning and teaching in healthcare practice at the University of Hertfordshire. Irene has published widely on tissue viability practice and, as well as running and teaching on undergraduate and postgraduate tissue viability courses, she has also run many bespoke projects in healthcare trusts to enhance the management of patients with, and at risk of, wounds. Irene has a degree in tissue viability and a masters degree in nursing. In 2011 she was awarded a national fellowship in teaching by the Higher Education Academy. She is currently engaged in doctoral research exploring the concept of competence in leg ulcer management practice.

Adele Atkinson is an associate professor, learning and teaching, in the School of Nursing, Faculty of Health, Social Care and Education, Kingston University and St George's University of London. She has written and presented widely in interprofessional arenas and is a reviewer for the Journal of Interprofessional Care. Her main interests are exploring ways of exploiting the use of digital media for learning and teaching within healthcare.

Graham Avery is a lecturer in the School of Health and Social Care at the University of Essex. He has been a nurse in a variety of settings within the adult acute sector, but specialised in general surgery, where he was a ward manager and later a practice development nurse. He has also written a book on law and ethics in nursing and healthcare, published several articles on this subject, and has conducted research into non-medical prescribing.

Jill Barnes is an Academic Manager and Head of Professional Regulation at the University of South Wales and senior fellow of the Higher Education Academy. She has had extensive experience in the development of pre-registration nursing curricula, quality enhancement and placement learning. Jill also represents the university on the All Wales Nursing and Midwifery Group, who have been pivotal in working collaboratively with service users, students and placement providers to develop a common assessment of competence tool for nursing students throughout Wales. Jill is currently involved in the development of the extensive work around the implementation of the new NMC Standards relating to nursing, practice supervision and prescribing programmes.

Ian Beech has held clinical posts in drug and alcohol abuse, general surgery, an elderly mentally ill assessment unit, and in community psychiatry. As subject lead for mental health, he combines management with teaching philosophy of nursing, interpersonal relationships in mental health nursing, qualitative research methodology, the empowerment of people in mental healthcare and recovery-based approaches, psychosocial interventions, history of mental health services and spirituality in mental healthcare.

E. Jane Blowers began her career as a registered general nurse (RGN) at Addenbrookes, Cambridge, in 1985. Later, she moved to Nottingham to complete her mental health nurse education and worked in acute mental health services, where she developed a wide range of skills and gained rich experience in mental health practice and team management. During this time, she also completed a BSc (Hons) in Health Studies at Nottingham Trent University. In 2001 she took a post at UEA in the School of Nursing Science, where she has fulfilled a number of exciting roles and completed an MA (Higher Education) and achieved recordable teacher status with the Nursing and Midwifery Council (NMC). She is currently Professional Lead Mental Health. Jane also completed a Doctorate in Education with the School of Education and Lifelong Learning (EDU UEA), which investigated professional integrity in pre-registration nursing.

Mairead Collie has been a registered nurse for almost 30 years, specialising in intensive care. With a passion for teaching and supporting others, Mairead worked for ten years as a practice education facilitator, supporting and advising mentors on their teaching and learning abilities within the practice learning environment. More recently, Mairead joined Glasgow Caledonian University as a lecturer in adult nursing.

Karen Elcock is head of programmes for pre-registration nursing and deputy head of school at Kingston University and St George's, University of London. By background an adult critical care nurse, she has worked in nurse education for over 30 years. Her publications in journals and books cover a wide range of nursing topics with a particular focus on practice education and she is a seasoned speaker at national conferences. She is on the international editorial panel for *Nurse Education in Practice* and a reviewer for the *Journal of Advanced Nursing*. Karen is also a role model for women in higher education as part of the Aurora Leadership Foundation for Higher Education and a mentor on the university Equality Mentoring Scheme for female staff.

Katrina Emerson joined Nursing Sciences in the School of Health Sciences at the University of East Anglia in 2002, having worked for a number of years in sexual health and HIV. Katrina is involved in teaching reproductive and sexual health across pre- and post-registration programmes. In addition, she maintains her interest in sexual health by continuing to practise in reproductive and sexual health. Katrina's research interests include the construction of the homosexual identity in nurse education, early recognition of cognitive impairment in patients with late HIV and the psychological impact of termination of pregnancy. Katrina is Associate Director of Teaching and Learning (pre-registration admissions).

Daryl Evans has been a nurse for over 30 years and is an associate professor at Middlesex University. She has held a variety of positions as a nurse, nurse teacher and health-promotion specialist. She qualified in health promotion after developing an interest in educating patients with long-term conditions. In her role as nurse teacher, she combines teaching health promotion and nursing with practising health improvement for students and staff at the university.

Fiona Everett is currently a nurse lecturer within pre-registration and masters-level nursing programmes with teaching, coordination and research supervision responsibilities. Fiona is also a mentor for the Postgraduate Certificate in Teaching and Learning in Higher Education. She has a wide range of clinical experience, including midwifery, district nursing and research project management within primary care. She has particular interests in clinical skills, dementia care and developing contemporary, supportive approaches to nurse education. She has published in these areas in nursing journals.

Jane Ewen is a chief nurse for professional practice, workforce and education in NHS Grampian providing leadership and management of professional and practice development service and nurse consultant (nutritional care) for the board. Her role involved working across disciplines, and strategically leading and influencing national and local policy related to nutritional care. She practised in a wide variety of acute clinical settings before taking up a facilitator post in a professional and practice development unit. As part of this role, Jane led on a number of practice development initiatives locally and nationally, and works strategically with local higher and further education institutes in both under- and post-registration nurse education and holds a senior associate lecturer position with Robert Gordon University.

Melanie Fisher is senior lecturer and programme lead at Northumbria University, Newcastle upon Tyne, Faculty of Health and Life Sciences. Prior to working in higher education, she held a variety of nursing posts specialising in orthopaedics and trauma. Melanie has a keen research interest in risk management, patient safety, human factors and healthcare law. Melanie recently co-authored a book on patient safety and works collaboratively with partnership healthcare trusts promoting the human factors approach to safer care.

Val Foley is a Clinical Lecturer for undergraduate and postgraduate medical education at The James Cook University Hospital, Middlesbrough. Before moving into medical education, Val specialised in critical care nursing in the UK and abroad for a number of years, with a focus on improving care for the deteriorating hospital patient. During a recent sabbatical in New Zealand to gain exposure to working in other healthcare systems, Val worked as a Critical Care Outreach Nurse Specialist at North Shore Hospital in Auckland. Her varied career includes periods in midwifery, community, research (implementing an EWSS into a UK hospital) and as a an honorary lecturer at the University of East Anglia.

Rose Gallagher is the professional lead at the Royal College of Nursing for infection prevention and control. A varied and at times challenging career in nursing has led to a specific interest in the application of research and guidance to nursing practice. Her role is diverse and she works closely with parliamentarians and nurses in practice. She contributes to scientific work through groups such as the Rapid Review Panel and is currently leading RCN activity on antimicrobial resistance and contributes to infection prevention activity at local, national and international levels.

Kate Goodhand is an adult nursing lecturer at the School of Nursing and Midwifery, Robert Gordon University, Aberdeen. Kate's nursing background was in medical care of the elderly wards, moving on to the role of night coordinator, covering the hospital during out-of-hours. The last 18 years have been in nurse education. Currently, she leads the return to nursing practice course and is involved in clinical skills teaching and simulation. At present she is undertaking a doctorate of professional practice focussed on the use of simulation in nurse education. Her other main interest is staff development and mentoring new colleagues.

Carol Hall is an associate professor in the School of Health Sciences at the University of Nottingham, as well as being a nurse registered to work with children and with adults. She currently directs the pre-registration nursing programmes, and also manages modules and provides teaching in clinical skills, nursing theory and practice. Carol's PhD study explored nurse preparation and practice in administering medicines for children, and subsequent post-doctoral research included work with a national team to develop a benchmark standard for calculation assessment at the point of nursing registration. Carol is very interested in the internationalisation of nursing and nursing education.

Rebekah Hill is a lecturer in adult nursing at the University of East Anglia. She qualified as a registered nurse (adult) in 1990 and worked in a variety of clinical settings, including cardiology, intensive care, medicine and gastroenterology. In 1998 she completed a BSc (Hons) in Nursing Practice, followed by an MSc in Health Sciences in 2000 and an MA in Higher Education in 2003. She completed a PhD in 2011 focused on the experience of those living with hepatitis C.

David J. Hunter is a lecturer in adult health and deputy programme leader for the BSc Adult Nursing programme at the University of the West of Scotland. Before moving into education, David spent nearly ten years as an emergency department nurse and two as a practice education facilitator. He has published articles in both *Emergency Nurse* and *Nursing Standard*. His Professional Doctorate thesis explored student nurses' experiences of compassionate care within the emergency department.

Gemma Hurley is a registered nurse and registered midwife. She joined Kingston University and St George's University as a senior lecturer-practitioner in 2006. Her concurrent clinical work as a nurse practitioner involves clinical assessment, diagnostic reasoning and management of a wide range of presenting illnesses in walk-in centres and general practice. Within the School of Nursing, she currently leads or co-leads a number of modules, including Clinical Reasoning in Physical Assessment and Work Based Learning for Long Term Conditions. She is also pathway leader for Long Term Conditions and teaches on various additional modules such as minor health and non-medical prescribing. Gemma is a peer reviewer for the journal Primary Health Care and has published clinical articles in journals such as Practice Nursing and Practice Nurse. She has presented at several conferences on topics such as nurse-led clinics, advanced nursing practice and contraception and sexual health. She is also now the representative for the School of Nursing on the Faculty Organisational and Staff Development Group.

Robert Jenkins is currently an independent trainer, examiner and consultant after spending 22 years in higher education as an academic manager and subject specialist for learning disability. He has led and taught across a number of undergraduate and postgraduate programmes and modules. He continues to act as an external examiner and is also a senior fellow for the Higher Education Academy. He has undertaken a number of research studies regarding people with learning disabilities, particularly safeguarding, and has published widely in this area. He is a registered learning disability nurse by background and proud grandfather of a young man with autism who is challenging his established views about this condition. His two passions in life still remain – Cardiff City AFC and fighting happiness.

Ann Kettyle is a senior lecturer in adult nursing at Kingston University and St George's University of London. She has been a nurse in adult and mental health for 35 years and has occupied a range of positions in clinical practice and nurse education. In her role as a nurse educator, she has developed the student nurse experience and learning to enhance the delivery of holistic care to service users and their families/carers in any setting.

Charlene Lobo currently works as a consultant in healthcare education and training and also as a Trustee to a voluntary organisation adopting public health approaches to refugee and asylum seeker wellbeing. Prior to this she was a senior lecturer and academic lead for practice education at the School of Health Sciences, University of East Anglia. She has been working in nurse education nearly two decades and as academic lead for practice education has developed innovative solutions to practice learning. Prior to that worked as a health visitor predominantly, expanding her role in public health practice. She has been actively involved in pre-registration curriculum development, taking the lead role in teaching health promotion and public health.

Jonathan Mason has qualifications in learning disabilities and adult nursing, education and management. He was, until his recent retirement, a lecturer at the University of East Anglia. He has a particular interest in educational assessment, and has extensive experience of managing assessment processes and of promoting and facilitating good assessment practices for both students and teachers.

Siobhan McCullough is a lecturer in adult nursing in the School of Nursing and Midwifery at Queen's University Belfast. Her research focuses on nursing and politics, health policy and nursing and care in the community. In her research, she has explored nurses' political participation and how nurses interact with the political system. She is a passionate advocate for political education for nurses to enable and equip them to contribute to and influence healthcare policy making.

Chris Mulryan is senior lecturer in healthcare studies at the University of Bolton, where he teaches the acute illness management module. Chris established the first clinical skills lab and designed the first purpose-built clinical simulation suite at the University of Bolton, which he used to teach the inaugural clinical examinations skills module, which he also designed. Chris is currently researching the impact of supra glottic airway devices on carotid blood flow during cardiac arrest. Alongside this, he is studying for further postgraduate qualifications in infectious diseases and anatomy.

Ruth Northway is professor of learning disability nursing at the University of South Wales. Prior to working in nurse education, she worked with people with learning disabilities in both residential and community settings. Her current post combines teaching and research, and her key interests are the health and wellbeing of people with learning disabilities, safeguarding, and working with people who use services to plan and undertake research. She is editor in chief of the Journal of Intellectual Disabilities, has co-authored a book regarding safeguarding and has authored a number of articles in professional and academic journals.

Jacqueline Phipps began her student nurse training at the Broadland School of Nursing in 1977, qualifying as an SRN in 1980. She completed a Sick Children's Nurse Qualification at Queen Mary's Hospital for Sick Children, Carshalton, in 1983. She has worked in a wide variety of acute children's settings within the Norfolk and Norwich University Hospital, as a staff nurse, ward sister, paediatric development nurse and senior nurse before joining the child branch team of lecturers at the University of East Anglia in 2005. She completed a BA (Hons) degree in Policy, Planning and Leadership for Health Care Professionals in 2006, and an MA in Interprofessional Health Care Education in 2010. She is also course director for the BA (Hons) and MA programmes – Leading Innovation for Clinical Practitioners.

Janet Ramjeet was a lecturer in nursing for over 30 years, teaching psychology to undergraduate and postgraduate nurses and allied health professionals. Her background is in adult and mental health nursing. She taught health psychology and undertook research at the University of East Anglia and was awarded a PhD in coping with inflammatory arthritis. She has published research in nursing and rheumatology journals that examine the roles of coping and social support.

Margaret Scott is a senior lecturer and acting programme leader in Pre-registration Health Studies, in the Faculty of Health and Life Sciences at Northumbria University. She has recently been accepted as a Fellow of the Higher Education Academy. Margaret has 29 years' nursing experience, having worked predominantly in operating departments and anaesthetics prior to moving into nurse education. She is very safety focused due to working for many years in a high-risk work environment and is committed to raising awareness and making a difference in providing safer care.

Jean Shapcott was a senior lecturer in children's nursing at Kingston University and St George's University of London. Prior to entering nurse education, she worked in neonatal intensive care and had a keen interest in supporting students, e-learning and palliative care for children and young people.

Dianne Steele is a lecturer in midwifery in the School of Health Sciences at the University of East Anglia. She has a keen interest in preparing and developing students' skills in safer handling of people techniques and has 24 years of experience. Teaching student nurses and midwives has developed her knowledge of the variety of skills required to ensure safe working practices for staff and the people they care for. Dianne works alongside a team of manual handling trainers within the school as well as integrating health ergonomics across the midwifery programmes.

Gabrielle Thorpe is a lecturer in the School of Health Sciences at the University of East Anglia (UEA) in Norwich and has a clinical and research background in colorectal and stoma care nursing. She has worked as an academic writing mentor at UEA and coordinates and teaches academic skill development on the BSc Nursing curriculum.

Steve Trenoweth has been a nurse in mental health for 23 years. He worked in a wide variety of mental health settings before entering higher education in 2003. He is currently a senior lecturer at Bournemouth University. He has authored several books, chapters and articles on nursing and healthcare, and is an editorial board member of the British Journal of Mental Health Nursing.

Helen Walker is a senior lecturer at the University of the West of Scotland (UWS). She works part time at UWS and part time as a consultant nurse with the Forensic Network. She has over 20 years' experience in clinical practice, the last 13 in forensic mental health and the majority in joint posts with a half-time remit for research. Her main interests are psychological interventions, research methodology, clinical supervision and practice development. Helen has published nearly 20 peer-reviewed journal articles, four book chapters, and regularly presents at conferences.

Wendy Wright is currently the BSc Adult Nursing programme leader and is a lecturer in pre-registration and masters-level nursing programmes at the University of the West of Scotland. Wendy has a wide range of acute clinical experience, including infectious diseases, stroke and elderly admissions. Wendy has particular interests that include clinical skills education for student nurses and the student experience, as well as dementia. She has a Postgraduate Certificate in Professional Education/Teaching and Learning in Higher Education and is a Fellow of the Higher Education Academy.

STUDENT AND NEWLY QUALIFIED CONTRIBUTORS

Throughout the book, you will see thoughts and views from student and newly qualified nurses working with a variety of types of patients:

I have always had an interest in caring for people. After caring for my elderly grandmother who has recently been diagnosed with Alzheimer's disease I realised that nursing was what I wanted to do.

Hannah Boyd, adult nursing student

I became a nurse after working as a support worker with disabled adults for a number of years. I love working with and helping people, I felt nursing would be a great opportunity to develop a career in areas that I feel passionate about.

Charlie Clisby, newly qualified adult nurse working in gastroenterology in a hospital ward

I worked as a support worker 16 years ago and always felt frustrated I did not understand why medication was given or why strategies were put in place. I brought up my two children and decided to come back to this field and combine my need for answers and my desire to help people by becoming a learning disabilities nurse.

Julie Davies, learning disabilities nursing student

I decided to become a nurse after a conversation with a friend who was in nursing training. She made me realise that all the things I wanted in a career could be found in nursing. I wanted the opportunity to help people and communicate with them in a meaningful way and nursing is the perfect way to do this.

Laura Grimley, adult nursing student

I wanted to become an RNLD to promote inclusion and equality for people with learning disabilities. I aim to support people to live as independently as possible, meet their full potential, and achieve their goals, while addressing their healthcare needs.

Michelle Hill, newly qualified RNLD working in a residential setting for people with profound and multiple learning disabilities

My inspiration to train as a nurse initially came from the nursing care my husband received as a multiple sclerosis sufferer. However, I chose to study children's nursing as I have always enjoyed caring for children, their families, and been interested in their healthcare, diet, development and overall wellbeing. Experiencing the dedication, skill, support and professional care nurses have given to my own children in the past also inspired me to train as a children's nurse and one day make a difference to a child and their family's life.

Siân Hunter, child student nurse

Working in nursing is all about people. I really enjoy meeting new people and talking to them, listening to their life experiences and sharing their hopes and dreams. Nursing combines all of these alongside the technical skills and knowledge to help people through some of their most vulnerable moments.

Ben Jones, adult nursing student

I came into mental health nursing after a variety of jobs from medical secretary, to science teaching and group fitness instructing. I had enjoyed the pastoral side of teaching and instructing – talking, engaging with people and wanting to help with their problems. I had also worked within mental health in the NHS and enjoyed the admin side as well as talking with service users. The main aspect of the course I find challenging is that as a mature student who has already had funding, I find the financial aspect and personal responsibilities I have difficult. I have to tackle part-time jobs in addition to the course, to help me through.

Rebecca Kidman, mental health nursing student

I chose to study nursing because I enjoy helping others and love working with people. I also wanted to pursue a career which I have always had a lot of admiration for, making a positive difference to people's lives.

Sophie Lane, learning disability nursing student

It has always been an ambition of mine to become a nurse. Every day is different and it is a career that is constantly changing and progressing. This means that nursing is an ongoing learning process which is something that I thrive on. The most enjoyable part of the course for me is the practice learning experiences. This is where skills and theory fall into place for me when carrying them out daily in a practical environment. The advice I would give to any student nurses is to take all experiences by both hands and get involved in everything that they possibly can.

Karen Millar, adult nursing student

I met my friend who had learning disabilities at a club when I was at school. I learnt so much from her and her friends. This encouraged me to decide to pursue nursing as a career. I decided that working with people with learning disabilities was the way forward for me. Training has had its up's and down's but I never regretted retraining and I am looking forward to help others reach their full potential.

Sarah Parkes, learning disability nursing student

I decided to become a nurse because I wanted a career that was both hard work and also rewarding.

Alice Rowe, newly qualified mental health nurse working in in patient forensic psychiatry

I see individuals that are at a point of crisis with their mental health and being able to work with them to overcome these issues and seeing them leave hospital well and with a sense of hope for the future is very satisfying. My top piece of advice for anyone studying nursing is to organise your time well. Managing the pressures of academic work, placements and personal life can be very challenging.

Samantha Vanes, newly qualified mental health nurse working with acute male inpatients

ACKNOWLEDGEMENTS

The editors and SAGE would like to thank all the students, patients/service users and nurses who contributed their stories to the book and online resources. The book is much richer for your contribution.

We would also like to thank all the students, lecturers and practitioners who helped to review this book's content, design and online resources to ensure it is as useful as possible.

PRACTITIONERS

Ashley Brooks, staff nurse, Stroke Care, Essex

Rachel Hauser, breastfeeding coordinator, Mid Yorkshire Hospitals NHS Trust

Victoria Lynne, children's nurse

Orla McAlinden, lecturer in Nursing (Children and Young People), Queens University Belfast

Joanna Moyle, staff nurse, Learning Disabilities, Abertawe Bro Morgannwgy University Health Board

Jessica Partington, substance misuse nurse, Offender Care

Jillian Pawlyn, senior lecturer, Learning Disabilities, De Montford University

Katie Potter, community adult staff nurse, NHS

Pamela Shaw, health visitor/ practice educator, Queen's Nurse 2014, Health Visitor of the Year 2012

Jackie Summers, community nurse, Learning Disability

Emma Tate, health visitor, Mid Yorkshire Hospitals NHS Trust

Francis Thompson, head of nursing education and standards, West London Mental Health NHS Trust

Lesley, nurse care manager, Learning Disability Team

Special thanks to:

NHS Employers and NHS England for connecting us to the Care Makers network for various student and practitioner voices. www.nhsemployers.org/case-studies-and-resources/2014/11/guidance-on-the-prevention-and-management-of-stress-in-the-workplace

Pamela Shaw, health visitor/ practice educator, Queen's Nurse 2014, Health Visitor of the Year 2012, for connecting us with numerous nurses for voices within the text

PATIENTS, SERVICE USERS, CARERS AND FAMILIES

The stories have been anonymised or first names only used to protect privacy. We wish to thank all of you and give special thanks to the following organisations for working with us to provide some of the voices:

Thanks to Mencap for helping us gather various learning disability voices. If you'd like to find out more about their work, visit the Mencap website at www.mencap.org.uk. If you'd like to donate to Mencap go to: www.mencap.org.uk/donate

certitude Thanks to Teresa Clark at Certitude for helping us gather various mental health service user voices. To learn more about Certitude or to donate, please visit www.certitude.org.uk

Thanks to Joe Way's family for contributing Joe's story. To learn more about Joe's story or donate, go to www.joeway.co.uk

STUDENTS

Rebecca Cavanagh

Gary Clark

Katy Dunn

Rebecca Fleming

Lisa Gray

Evelyn Kyei-Baffour

Brian Smith

Katie Smith

Gemma Vale

Francis Young

LECTURERS

Liz Allibone, Royal Brompton specialist hospital

Liz Aston, Nottingham

Jim Blair, Kingston University

Mary Brady, Kingston University

Paul Buka, University of West London

Dianne Burns, University of Manchester

Angelina Chadwick, University of Salford

Sarah Connor, Kingston Hospital

Sandra Fender, Cardiff University

Joseph Ferris, Ulster University

Ganapathy Ganesalingam, University of West London

Mitchell Gordon, Teesside University

Marie Gressman, Teesside University

Mike Gretton, University of Hull

Margaret Harris, University of the West of Scotland

Christopher D. Hart, Kingston University

Pippa Hillen, University of Brighton

Lorna Innes, NHS Lanarkshire

Sian Jones, University of South Wales

Joann Kiernan, Edge Hill University

Kate Killagon, Teesside University

John Lee, University of Dundee

Orla McAlinden, Queens University, Belfast

Isabel McLatchie, NHS Lanarkshire

Kevin Moore, University of Ulster

Jillian Pawlyn, De Montfort University

Nigel Plant, The University of Nottingham

Steven Pryjmachuk, University of Manchester

Sharon Riddell, Nottingham University Hospitals NHS Trust

Stephen Tee, Kings College London

Vicky Thornton, University of Liverpool

Vanessa Waller, Anglia Ruskin University

Kerry Welch, The University of Nottingham

Rachel Williams, University of the West of England

Swapna Williamson, University of West London

Lastly, the editors and SAGE would like to extend special thanks to the University of the West of Scotland, specifically Fiona Everett and Wendy Wright for working in partnership with SAGE to create the clinical skills videos to support this book.

PUBLISHER'S ACKNOWLEDGEMENTS

The authors and publisher are grateful to the following parties for permission to reproduce their material below.

We are also grateful to Jonathan Mason, who, as co-author of Chapter 3 in the 1st edition of the *Essentials of Nursing Practice,* provided the base for updates made in this edition.

Figure 3.1 An evidence-based practice (EBP) triad, Florida State University (2013) Definition of Evidence-based Medicine. Available at: http://med.fsu.edu/index.cfm?page=medicalinformatics. ebmTutorial (accessed 22 November 2013).

Table 7.2 Types of allegations made as new referrals to the NMC in 2014–15, Nursing and Midwifery Council (2016a) Nursing and Midwifery Council Annual Fitness to Practise Report 2015–16. London: The Stationery Office.

Figure 9.2 Healthcare leadership model, NHS Leadership Academy (2013) Healthcare Leadership Model: The Nine Dimensions of Leadership Behaviour. Leeds: NHS Leadership Academy. Available at: www.leadershipacademy.nhs.uk/wp-content/uploads/2013/10/NHSLeadership-LeadershipMode110-BW-Print.pdf (accessed February 2015).

Table 19.1 Types of decisions nurses make. Thompson, C. and Stapley, S. (2011) 'Do educational interventions improve nurses' clinical decision-making and judgement? A systematic review', *International Journal of Nursing Studies,* 48(7): 881–93.

Figure 19.3 The two poles of decision-making Source. Hamm (1988) 'Clinical intuition and clinical analysis: expertise and the cognitive continuum', in Dowie, J. and Elstein, A. (eds), *Professional Judgement: A Reader in Clinical Decision-Making* (pp. 78–105). Cambridge: Cambridge University Press.

Figure 20.1 Department of Health's (2011) six principles of safeguarding. © Crown copyright.

Figure 21.1 Prochaska and DiClemente's (1982) Transtheoretical Stages of Change model. Prochaska, J.O. and DiClemente, C. (1982) 'Transtheoretical therapy: Toward a more integrative model of change', *Psychotherapy: Theory, Research and Practice,* 20: 161–73.

Table 21.3 Applying Prochaska and DiClemente's (1982) model. Prochaska, J.O. and DiClemente, C. (1982) 'Transtheoretical therapy: Toward a more integrative model of change', *Psychotherapy: Theory, Research and Practice,* 20: 161–73.

Figure 21.3 Tannahill's (2009) model 'The Tannahill model revisited', *Public Health,* 123(5): 396–99.

Table 22.1 Contamination of nurses' hands by different Klebsiella spp following care procedures. Casewell, M.W. and Phillips, I. (1977) 'Hands as a route of transmission for Klebsiella species', *British Medical Journal,* 2: 1315–17.

Figure 22.1 Ayliffe's six-step hand hygiene technique (Adapted from Ayliffe, 1978) Ayliffe, G.A.J., et al (1988) 'Hand disinfection: A comparison of various agents in laboratory studies and ward studies', *Journal of Hospital Infection,* 11: 226–243.

Figure 22.3 Dermatitis and reddening of skin, Health and Safety Executive, available at: http://www.hse.gov.uk/skin/imagelibrary.htm (accessed December 2017).

Table 24.10 Daily fluids Source: Clancy and McVicar (2009) *Physiology and Anatomy for Nurses and Healthcare Practitioners: A Homeostatic Approach,* 3rd ed. London: Hodder Arnold.

Figure 31.1 Bristol Stool Chart. Lewis, S.J. and Heaton, K.W. (1997) 'Stool form scale as a useful guide to intenstinal transit time', *Scandinavian Journal of Gastroenterology,* 32: 920–4.

Figure 32.1 CLEAN, Department of Health (DH) (2010) Essence of Care Benchmarks for Personal Hygiene. London: DH.

Table 36.1 Transtheoretical model including the Stages of Change. Prochaska, J.O. and DiClemente, C.C. (1984) *The Transtheoretical Approach: Crossing Traditional Boundaries of Therapy.* Homeward, IL: Dow Jones Irwin.

INTRODUCTION

This book has been written for nursing students undertaking a degree, no matter what area of nursing practice you are thinking of going into. While the book is primarily aimed at nursing students in the first year of their studies, it presents a solid foundation of relevant material for any nursing student. It serves as an excellent source of reference material throughout your degree and beyond.

This book was developed by a dedicated team of lecturers, practitioners, students, patients and carers to support your study and give you the fullest picture of nursing possible. All have been keen to be involved because they know how important good nursing care is and are aware of the challenges you may face in providing quality care. You may have experienced good care first hand and this may have inspired you to start your own journey to become a nurse. You will probably be aware of news reports highlighting failures in care, and wonder how this can happen. Everyone involved in this book is passionate about providing you with the knowledge, skills and confidence to be the type of nurse who inspires you and to create an environment for practice that prevents the situations you see on the news.

To further help you be the best nurse you can be, we have threaded four fundamental principles throughout the book, which are integral to good nursing care. These are:

Holistic, person-centered care: good nurses don't care for symptoms, they care for patients. That is why a deeper understanding of the whole person you are looking after – physically, psychologically and socially – is key to providing the best nursing care.

Awareness of the needs of all types of patient: no matter what area of nursing you are thinking of specialising in, to provide excellent care you need to be able to respond to the needs of all those you may be working with. The person in your care may be a child or an adult, but they may also have mental health problems or learning disabilities, have a family or others they care for with problems which may affect their own physical or mental health. The world does not operate in compartments – or distinct pieces on a production line – and nor should you. An ability to care for patients across the lifespan with varying health needs, and knowing when and how to refer to other professionals, will make you a better nurse and ultimately contribute to a better healthcare system that truly responds to the needs of the individuals and communities it serves.

Understanding yourself: being kind to yourself and developing yourself is key to achieving the first principle of holistic person-centred care. Good communication and compassion come when you understand yourself and your own motivations as well as the person/people you are communicating with, and part of that is valuing your own mental and physical health. This is why we involved so many students in developing the book – so that you know you are not alone in fear of your first placement, or in worrying that you do not know how to give a bed-bath, or how you will fit everything in.

It is not an easy journey – the challenges of understanding theory, applying it to practice in those first scary moments when you are faced with a patient, deepening your knowledge through wider reading and essay assignments, and demonstrating what you have learnt in exams, are big ones. That is why we have developed this book with a structure that recognises these challenges and gives you the tools you need at each stage of your study to make your learning journey a successful one.

Learning can be fun: it may not feel like it at times, but we hope that you will find, as with most things in life, that the hardest things to learn are often the most rewarding when you finally come to understand them or are able to perform them. We have made the book as interactive as possible, with lots of different forms of learning to keep you excited and interested.

BOOK STRUCTURE

The key element of this book is simplicity. The book focuses specifically on helping you to understand the important information you will cover in the first year of your course, and make it relevant to the care you will deliver to patients. This is done in a range of ways, all of which introduce the essential information you need to understand as a 'skeleton' for you to 'flesh out' with further knowledge. To assist you to do this, you will find sources of further information clearly identified.

In order to assist you to gain the essential foundation knowledge that you as a year one nursing student will need, the book is split into the following themes, each of which forms a part of the book:

Part A. Learning to be a Nurse

Part B. Professional Practice

Part C. Fundamentals of Nursing Care

Part D. Skills for Nursing Care

Part E. Context of Nursing Care

Each of these parts is further divided into chapters, to enable you to develop your knowledge of the important aspects of the theme.

The book presents you with information relating to each of the four fields of nursing practice – learning disability, mental health, child and adult, in an integrated fashion that will assist you to apply it to all of the patients you care for. The knowledge and skills you will be focusing on can be thought of as being 'like an onion', because it is made up of many layers. Each of these layers is separate but depends on the others to form the whole. Just like an onion, when you peel back one layer you are faced with another, and then another, and yet another. It is by gaining an understanding of each layer that you add to the depth of your knowledge and increase your ability to be a good nurse. To support you in this development, you will see that the chapters refer you to other relevant chapters, enabling you to recognise how all the different layers fit together.

REQUIREMENTS FOR NURSE EDUCATION

In the UK, the Nursing and Midwifery Council (NMC) sets educational standards to ensure that your course of study provides you with high-quality nursing education. These standards outline how nursing students must be educated and the competencies and skills you must be able to demonstrate, in order to deliver and manage the current and future needs of all patients. The format of this book is designed to assist you to gain the knowledge and skills required to meet the NMC Standards.

A NOTE ON TERMINOLOGY

During the course of your nursing studies, you will find those who receive care being referred to by a number of different terms, for example service user, client, patient, person or individual. The use of these terms is frequently discussed and you are likely to be involved in contributing to this debate during your course. This topic and the relevant research are considered in greater detail in Chapter 13, with the term patient being identified as the most popular by both those who receive care and those who deliver it. Therefore, while it is recognised that many of the people nurses care for are not unwell, throughout this book, for simplicity and consistency, any person who receives any form of care will be referred to by the term 'patient'.

LEARNING TO BE A NURSE

A

WHAT IS NURSING AND WHAT IS A NURSE?

CATHERINE DELVES-YATES, KAREN ELCOCK, CAROL HALL, RUTH NORTHWAY AND STEVE TRENOWETH

THIS CHAPTER COVERS

- What is nursing and what is a nurse?
- A very brief history of nursing
- An introduction to the fields of nursing practice

- Professionalism and nursing
- The attributes of good nursing

> " Nurses are caring and knowledgeable. They explain what you need to know and treat you as an individual. Nurses support you and your family, physically, psychologically, spiritually and emotionally, but their greatest value is helping you to live the best life possible.
>
> **Martin Yates, patient** "

> " I want nurses to be respected for the care they deliver and the difference they make to every patient they meet. That's why I went into nursing – I wanted to make a difference. It is a privilege to be a nurse.
>
> **Jane Cummings, Chief Nursing Officer for England (2012a)** "

Visit https://study.sagepub.com/essentialnursing2e to access a wealth of online resources for this chapter – watch out for the margin icons throughout the chapter. If you are using the interactive eBook, simply click on the margin icon to go straight to the resource.

INTRODUCTION

Nursing is best described as a professional clinical and caring role focusing on the care of adults, children, families and/or whole communities. So, this means that a registered nurse works with individuals and their carers, families or whole communities, providing nursing care and support. As Martin tells us in the patient's voice at the start of the chapter, a nurse's ability to help patients live the best possible life is of great value and, as Jane Cummings points out, to be a nurse is a privileged status.

This chapter will help you understand what nursing is, and what the role of a nurse is. It will outline how nursing has developed into a modern evidence-based profession, and the fundamental importance of acting in a professional manner at all times will be stressed. The chapter focuses on the many attributes required to make a good nurse; throughout your nursing course, you will realise that good nurses come in a variety of different forms. With the help of lecturers, practice educators, patients, their families and colleagues on your course, you will identify which of these attributes you already possess and which ones you need to develop to enable you to successfully complete your course.

WHAT IS NURSING AND WHAT IS A NURSE?

The essence of nursing is delivering effective care to adults, children, families and/or whole communities. In doing this, nurses work in partnership with individual people, groups of people or the families and carers of those people, helping them to achieve or maintain the best health, independence and quality of life possible.

Nurses work, or practise, in a wide range of settings, in four different fields of nursing practice – mental health, child, learning disability and adult – undertaking a wide variety of roles. While there are many roles which reflect the speciality of each field, there are also core elements which underpin the profession as a whole. These include:

- assisting patients with physical needs
- making autonomous clinical decisions to ensure patients receive appropriate and effective care
- being accountable for providing, leading and coordinating nursing care
- using counselling skills in caring for a patient or group of patients
- supporting and empowering patients to recover or to cope with their needs more effectively
- advocating for patients and communities
- helping children, young people and adults to manage their health by developing partnerships in care with the individual and their families
- delivering education to promote the health of a community
- supporting an individual with a long-term condition to manage their health and live independently
- working in partnership with other healthcare professionals
- playing a proactive and equal role in interdisciplinary teams.

Nurses work with individuals of all ages and cultural backgrounds at all stages of healthcare, from preventing ill health and maintaining good health through to managing acute ill health. No matter where or with whom they practise, nurses always work in a holistic way. The holistic approach is an important theme that we will frequently return to throughout this book: this means we will consider the individual's physical, psychological, social, emotional, intellectual and spiritual needs, as Martin mentioned in the patient's voice at the beginning of the chapter. As well as taking a holistic approach, nurses ensure the care they provide is of the highest quality by applying knowledge from physical and social science, nursing, legal and ethical theory, and technology.

Many nurses will say to you that they are passionate about nursing, as sharing in a patient's achievements – and setbacks – is hugely rewarding. But, as with all intense emotions, nurses may occasionally wonder whether the role is for them. If you ever feel like this, mention it to a registered nurse. It is likely that they will recognise your experience and reassure you that you are not alone in occasionally feeling this way. Becoming a registered nurse is a challenging journey, but your choice to join the nursing profession is probably the best decision you will ever make. Don't expect your nursing course to be easy – becoming a nurse is academically, physically and emotionally demanding. Remember, your course team is available to support you during your student experience. Your journey to becoming a registered nurse will involve experiences you may never have realised existed, and you will discover abilities you did not know you had.

ACTIVITY 1.1: CRITICAL THINKING

Before reading this chapter any further, if you were asked, 'What is nursing and what is a nurse?', what would you say?

✓

ANSWER:
ACTIVITY 1.1

A VERY BRIEF HISTORY OF NURSING

Nursing has its origins in religious orders, domestic servitude, Victorian asylum attendants and the military services. It is still possible today to see the religious and military roots of nursing; you only have to visit a hospital ward to find that the most senior female nurse will often be referred to as 'Sister'.

Mental health and learning disability share much of their history and it was not until the late 1950s that a clear distinction between the two fields emerged, in part due to the 1959 Mental Health Act. Up until the 1970s, learning disability was regarded as an illness requiring medical treatment. Following the NHS and Community Care Act 1990, the social care and medical support of people with a learning disability increasingly moved from institutional settings to the community.

The study of psychiatric disorders can be traced back to ancient philosophers, and although psychiatric hospitals were a feature of thirteenth-century Europe, treatment was severely limited and the patients were not cared for by nurses.

One of the most notable figures in nursing history is an English nurse, Florence Nightingale. Although she is probably the best known figure, she was not the sole founder of the nursing profession: others with just as important an influence were Mary Seacole, a Jamaican nurse, and Betsi Cadwaladr, a Welsh nurse, both of whom cared for patients in the Crimean War alongside Nightingale. Other significant figures include Linda Richards, an American nurse who opened the first nursing school offering psychiatric nursing in 1882 (Boyd and Nihart, 1998), and Charles West and Catherine Wood, the first nurses to specialise in caring for children (Glasper and Coyne, 2002).

Today, to protect the public, in many countries what a nurse is allowed to do is governed by law. Nursing students must achieve set standards to be admitted to the profession and the conduct of registered nurses is regulated. These standards are monitored nationally by regulators such as the UK Nursing and Midwifery Council (NMC). Such careful vetting and monitoring of nursing is not novel: New Zealand was the first country to legislate (in 1901) that nurses must be regulated and other countries quickly followed, with compulsory registration for UK nurses since 1919.

The need for all nurse education courses to be degree-level has been recognised (NMC, 2010) and nursing research is providing an evidence base for the profession (Burns and Grove, 2011). Nursing has always been thought of as honourable and worthy, but is frequently described as having a lowly status.

A graduate-level qualification brings nurses into line with other healthcare professionals and equips them with the necessary skills to deliver, lead and manage high-quality nursing care and contribute to the research profile of the profession.

Nursing today

The aim of the nursing community worldwide is to ensure high-quality nursing care for all patients, with nurses upholding their professional code of ethics and maintaining their individual competence. While there is not a standardised nurse education course worldwide, the national nursing organisational goals are brought together under the watchful oversight of the International Council of Nurses and the existing courses have similarities. In all countries, nursing students study nursing theory and practise their clinical skills before successfully completing their course.

To practise legally as a nurse in the UK, you must hold valid and current registration with the NMC. This shows that you have achieved a standard of nursing education and skill competence which enables you to deliver safe and effective care. Only those achieving this can call themselves a registered nurse (RN).

Nursing today is more challenging than ever, with patients now presenting with far more complex healthcare needs. Healthcare reforms have aimed to put patients at the heart of the health service and there has been a move away from all care being delivered in hospitals; patients are hospitalised for shorter periods and more care is delivered within the community, with many care services delivered outside the NHS by charity, voluntary and independent sector organisations. Such changes have resulted in developments within the nurse's role: the nurse can now provide care and interventions previously delivered by a doctor; or can choose to specialise in a particular area of nursing practice; or can develop, commission or externally audit specialist services; or can become a consultant nurse, researcher or lecturer. Change within healthcare will continue throughout your nursing career; a career which may last more than 40 years. During this time, the role of the nurse will continue to alter and you will constantly develop your skills in order to meet the changing needs of patients.

Changes in healthcare and the nurse's role have also necessitated changes in nurse education, with one of the most recent strengthening the care of patients across the fields of nursing. Examples of patients needing care across fields are people with mental health needs or learning disabilities who develop a long-term condition such as diabetes. Therefore, nursing students currently study a nursing course with generic elements – essential skills which are fundamental to all fields of nursing – as well as elements which are field-specific. This enables them to become competent in a variety of healthcare skills, deliver a wide range of nursing care to all patients and have an integrated, holistic and flexible approach. This approach leads to a more satisfactory and collaborative experience for patients and is why the NMC is currently considering a fully generic degree. This book highlights essential generic skills across the fields and assists you in applying them to each patient in your care, helping you to deliver the best care for all patients.

Nursing across the world

Across the world, nurses have traditionally been female, and despite the existence of equal opportunity legislation in many developed countries since the 1960s and 1970s, nursing continues to be a female-dominated profession. In the UK, for instance, fewer than one in ten nurses are male (NMC, 2016). Within developing countries, however, there are some notable differences: in many African countries, there is an equal or higher proportion of male nurses than female ones; however, to be accepted into a nursing school in Nepal you must be female.

WHAT'S THE EVIDENCE?

Conforming to and resisting dominant gender norms: How male and female nursing students do and undo gender

McDonald (2013) interviews 12 nursing students to find out what makes a good nurse and how gender and gender roles influence this.

Reflection

- Reflect on the aspirations and expectations you have as you begin your nursing career.
- To what extent do you think your gender influences these?

This study was undertaken in the USA. Do you think the findings will be relevant to your country?

- Now read the article and consider how the findings of the study might apply to your views.

Nursing, worldwide, focuses on delivering safe and effective care which enables a patient to achieve the best quality of life possible. However, Virginia Henderson (1897–1996), an American nurse, researcher and theorist, provided the most widely acknowledged summary of the role of the nurse:

> The unique function of the nurse is to assist the individual, sick or well, in the performance of those activities contributing to health or its recovery (or to peaceful death) that he would perform unaided if he had the necessary strength, will or knowledge. (Henderson, 1966: 15)

Nursing is the use of clinical judgement in the provision of care to enable people to improve, maintain, or recover health, to cope with health problems, and to achieve the best possible quality of life, whatever their disease or disability, until death.

RCN (UK) (2014)

Nursing is an autonomous, self-governing profession, a distinct scientific discipline with many autonomous practice features.

Cameroon Nurses Association (2010)

Nursing is the protection, promotion, and optimization of health and abilities; prevention of illness and injury; alleviation of suffering through the diagnosis and treatment of human responses; and advocacy in healthcare for individuals, families, communities, and populations.

American Nurses Association (2012)

A 'nurse' is a person who has a degree in nursing and has passed an examination to be allowed to work in Nepal.

Nepal Nursing Council (2012)

Nurses utilise nursing knowledge and nursing judgement to assess health needs and provide care, and to advise and support people to manage their health. They practise in a range of settings in partnership with individuals, families, whānau and communities. Nurses may practise in a variety of clinical contexts depending on their educational preparation and scope of practice experience.

New Zealand National Nursing Organisations (2011)

Figure 1.1   Nursing across the world

AN INTRODUCTION TO THE FIELDS OF NURSING PRACTICE

In the UK, there are currently four fields of nursing practice – learning disability, mental health, child and adult – each being named after the patients for whom nurses in these fields most frequently care. It is important for nurses to care effectively for all a patient's needs, which may arise from one or more of the fields of nursing practice. Therefore, you will learn about all of these fields.

Learning disability

Learning disability nurses work in partnership with people with learning disabilities and their families and carers in a range of community, residential and healthcare settings. As the needs of people with learning disabilities are diverse, learning disability nurses require a range of knowledge and skills that includes good communication skills (including use of alternative communication approaches), assessment skills, person-centred planning skills and values grounded in equality, inclusion and human rights. The central roles include identifying and meeting health needs, reducing health inequalities and promoting better health outcomes (Department of Health [hereafter DH] et al., 2012). These may be achieved through working as a community learning disability nurse, a primary care liaison nurse, a practice nurse or a school nurse; as a nurse within an assessment and treatment unit, a secure unit or a rehabilitation centre; as a nurse therapist; or as an acute care hospital liaison nurse. As senior and consultant nurses, auditors, researchers or lecturers, learning disability nurses lead and manage services and inform and influence service development. Learning disability nurses work with people of any age, across the lifespan, providing physical and mental healthcare as part of a wider multi-agency and multi-disciplinary team.

Mental health

Mental health nurses' practice involves people of all ages with mental health problems. They care for patients with a wide range of mental health problems (such as schizophrenia, depression and alcohol or drug addiction), using supportive methods to promote positive and therapeutic relationships which focus on social inclusion, human rights and recovery. This aims to enable a patient to develop the ability to live a self-directed life, with or without symptoms, which the patient feels is personally meaningful and satisfying. Nurses who choose to specialise in mental health nursing form part of an interdisciplinary team including occupational therapists, social workers, therapists, psychiatrists and psychologists. Increasingly, care is provided in the community. Many people with severe and enduring mental health problems live alone or with their families at home. There are also facilities such as supported accommodation for people who find independent living particularly challenging. Mental health nurses offer a wide range of services within both the community and hospital settings, including crisis intervention, early intervention, community adult mental health services, community teams, criminal justice teams and drug and alcohol services. The rates of mental health problems in prisons or in other secure services are much higher than in the general population, so mental health nurses are often employed to provide direct care or to advise prison officers or other staff on how to respond to mental distress. Working alongside learning disability specialists, the mental health nurse will also support people with learning disabilities, whether at home or within specialist health or forensic services.

Why learning disability nursing? It covers all fields of nursing; people with learning disabilities are individuals having other conditions which prevent them from being able to carry out tasks on their own. It requires thinking outside the box, the desire to empower people to reach their full potential while problem-solving and enabling choice. I would like to think by supporting people I can make a positive change in their lives.

Sarah Parkes, LD nursing student

I'm not really sure why I chose mental health nursing! I think it is human nature to want to make a difference to someone else's life, and I have an intrinsic compassion for quality care for those who require it most. I have seen the power of kindness and time, and how they can assist people living with mental illness work towards recovery. Furthermore, I enjoy being a part of a collective of people aiming to tackle stigma and ignorance and promoting inclusion and wellbeing.

Alice Rowe, NQ RNMH

In 2009 I spent eight months volunteering as a primary school teacher with young disabled children suffering the genetic effects of the Vietnam War. This experience ignited my passion for caring for people as I became increasingly aware of the issue of mental health and the long-term physical and psychological effects war can have.

Fiona I'Anson, MH nursing student

Children

Children's nurses care for individuals usually between the ages of birth and 19, as well as for their families, in a range of different settings. They care for well children – promoting their health in the school nurse role, for example – and for children with special physical or learning needs, mental health concerns or physical illnesses. These needs can be short or long term, or even lifelong. Children react to illness differently from adults and can develop life-threatening illnesses quickly, so an essential skill for a children's nurse is to recognise this and act immediately.

Children's nursing occurs in many settings – in hospital, the community or the child's home – and children's nurses may work shifts, including nights and weekends, or a more usual working week.

Maintaining the normal daily routine is important, because children find being away from their usual environment distressing and disruptive to the life of their entire family. So, working in partnership with a family and empowering them to care for their child is central, as this enables independence and a return to normal routines.

Children's nurses require a wide range of skills to understand the care needs of babies, children, adolescents and young adults within different settings. Being a children's nurse is both rewarding and challenging, especially when caring for children with a learning disability, or with complex health needs, or those who are terminally ill or die.

Adult

Adult nurses normally work with patients from the age of 16–19 upwards. They aim to promote good health both in healthy individuals and in times of illness, whether that be acute or long term. Given the ageing population, adult nurses are finding their patient population is increasingly the elderly, with complex multiple health problems and the added challenge of dementia. As with the other fields of practice, adult nurses need to be able to prioritise the care they deliver, using a range of skills to achieve this while working in partnership with the patient, the patient's family, carer or friends and other healthcare professionals. Adult nurses provide a wide range of care to improve the quality of patients' lives, sometimes in difficult situations. It is possible to specialise within adult nursing in areas such as cancer care, intensive care nursing, community nursing, surgical nursing or the care of older people. Adult nurses are usually based in hospitals, clinics or community settings and frequently work shifts in order to deliver 24-hour patient care. Adult nurses work with all patients who present to their service, working closely with acute health liaison nurses to meet the nursing needs of people with learning disabilities.

Although it is possible to see both similarities and differences in the care delivered within each of the fields of nursing, one aspect common to all fields is professionalism.

Apply what you have learned about caring for different types of patients by reading the case study on Ngozi, Faith and their children, at https://study.sagepub.com/essentialnursing2e.

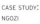
CASE STUDY:
NGOZI

> My inspiration to become a nurse initially came from the care my husband receives for his long-term illness. However, I chose to study children's nursing as I have always enjoyed caring for children and their families, and been interested in their healthcare, diet, development and overall wellbeing. Experiencing the dedication, skill, support and professional care nurses have given to my own children was also inspirational, so one day I will make a difference to a child and their family's life.
>
> **Siân Hunter, child nursing student**
>
> My passion for adult nursing developed when my Nan became terminally ill. The palliative care nurses expressed kindness, compassion and love towards her, attributes that I wanted to possess and utilise myself one day. My interest further increased when I became a carer at a residential home, helping to make a difference to the lives of older people. I enjoy watching medical dramas, but it wasn't until I started my course that I realised adult nursing isn't like it is on television – it's so much better in real life.
>
> **Ali Chapman, adult nursing student**

PROFESSIONALISM AND NURSING

Behaving in a professional manner is fundamental to being a nurse, and this is one expectation that commences at the very start of your course. Before considering this further, however, it is necessary to understand what a profession is and how a professional behaves.

What is a profession?

The term 'profession' is frequently used to describe an activity that is undertaken to earn a living. A more accurate definition, however, is an occupation requiring specific and extensive education, where a code of ethics exists and standards are set which those working in the profession are expected to achieve and maintain at all times. While those who work in a profession receive payment for what they do, their job is hugely important to them and may be described as their vocation. So, 'profession' describes the occupation of individuals with high ethical standards plus specialist knowledge and skills, who are accountable for their actions and behave in the ways described in Figure 1.2.

How do I behave professionally as a nursing student?

As soon as you become a nursing student, you are required to maintain the standards set by the NMC for nurses and midwives (NMC, 2015). The NMC is the UK regulator for the nursing and midwifery professions, safeguarding the health and wellbeing of the public. It achieves this by identifying the personal and professional conduct expected of nursing students and registered nurses within a document that will become fundamentally important to you, called the Code (NMC, 2015). This identifies

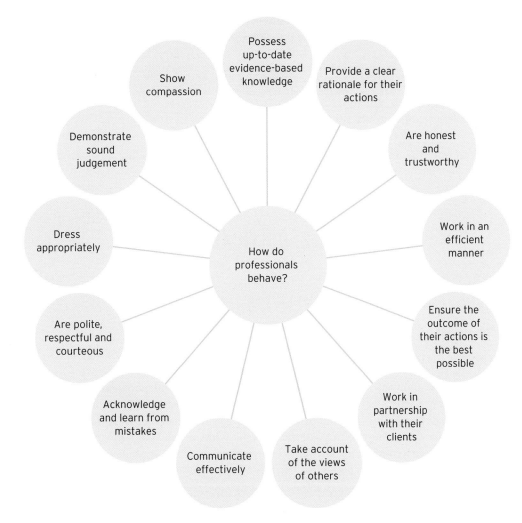

Figure 1.2 How professionals behave

standards which relate to how you must behave as a nurse. These standards apply whether you are in a practice environment or in class, as well as during your personal life, to ensure you uphold the reputation of the nursing profession. Ensuring these standards are upheld in everything you do is an important aspect of being a nursing student, first because members of the public will see you as a nurse, even though you are still learning, and second in preparation for upholding the strict professional standards you will be subject to when you complete your course.

Maintaining professional boundaries is crucial – I always inform anyone I am caring for, and colleagues, that I am a student nurse so they have a clear understanding that I am still learning. I am also much more aware of how the public view nurses, so am conscious of my actions all the time. Whether it be writing a social media status or going out for the evening with friends, nursing is always at the front of my mind, and I think how I would feel if I saw a nurse caring for me behaving inappropriately the night before.

Siân Hunter, child nursing student

The NMC (2015) identifies four core principles which, if you uphold them, will ensure you behave professionally as a nursing student. The core principles are:

- Prioritise people.
- Practice effectively.
- Preserve safety.
- Promote professionalism and trust.

If you are ever uncertain whether your actions or those of others are upholding these standards, make sure you ask your lecturers and/or a registered nurse for advice.

ANSWER:
ACTIVITY 1.2

ACTIVITY 1.2: CRITICAL THINKING

- List ten behaviours expected of a nurse.
- Which three of those on your list do you think are the most important for a nurse?

How should a nurse behave?

All nursing students and registered nurses must follow the standards and guidance of the Nursing and Midwifery Council (NMC, 2015) and be fit to practise, so that patients and the public can trust them with their health and wellbeing. It is impossible to outline exactly how a nurse should behave during every second of the day, because nurses will interpret the standards and guidance in slightly different ways, but it is possible to outline the attributes of a good nurse. These attributes could be considered as the ingredients which make a good nurse – so it is up to you, under the guidance of your lecturers, practice educators and patients, to decide the exact recipe you will use to ensure your actions always uphold the NMC standards.

Patients' voices: what is a good nurse?

Read the patient voices below to find out what patients think a good nurse is and does:

... your blanket, your medicine and your mum all wrapped into one.

Sharon David, patient

... gives time to a patient, gets to know them, goes beyond what brings them into hospital. Is flexible and possesses compassion.

Simon Weston OBE

... cares for the sick, injured and dying, promoting health and preventing disease through education and nursing knowledge, helping patients and their families to cope with illness, making a difference.

Lizzie Evans, patient

Works with those who are ill and their families, supporting them emotionally.

Charles Allen, patient

... my superhero nurse ... because he is thoughtful, caring, and patient.

Lloyd Page, inclusion advisor with Mencap

As a nursing student it wasn't until I became a patient that this made me fully appreciate the value of 'little things'. Getting to know you, sitting with you when you're scared and making you feel nothing is too much trouble. I'll never underestimate the value of spending just a few extra moments with a patient now, because it's that which makes all the difference.

Libbie Bulmer, nursing student

THE ATTRIBUTES OF GOOD NURSING

As Jane Cummings (2012b), Chief Nursing Officer for England, reminds us, good nurses show care and compassion in how they look after patients, finding the courage to do the right thing and acting as the patient advocate, even when this means standing up to people with greater authority, peers, a patient's family members or other healthcare professionals. It is fundamentally important to demonstrate commitment to patients and our profession and ensure we communicate well at all times.

The attributes evident within this definition of a good nurse have been developed further to produce the 6Cs of nursing (DH, 2012). These principles, in combination with the NHS values, reinforce holistic nursing, wherever it takes place.

ACTIVITY 1.3: CRITICAL THINKING

The four countries of the United Kingdom each have their own set of NHS values. Find those that are relevant for your country. Are there any other values you think should be included?

CONCLUSION

In listening to the patient voices in this chapter, it becomes clear that patients value nurses who care for them as individuals, making them feel more comfortable and less afraid. As Libbie says, the 'little things' make a difference. The essence of nursing is delivering effective holistic care to adults, children, families and/or whole communities. In doing this, nurses work in partnership with individuals, groups of people or the families and carers of these people, helping them to achieve or maintain the best possible health, independence and quality of life. It is possible to see both similarities and differences in the care delivered within each of the fields of nursing, but one aspect of nursing common to all fields is professionalism, and behaving in a professional manner is fundamental to being a nurse.

CARE
COURAGE
COMPASSION
COMMITMENT
COMPETENCE
COMMUNICATION

HOLISTIC NURSING

NHS Values

Putting quality and safety above all else	Care and compassion	Equality and inclusion	Working together for patients
Integrating improvement into everyday working	Dignity and respect	Confidentiality	Respect and dignity
Focusing on prevention, health improvement and inequality	Openness, honesty and responsibility	Person-centred approaches	Commitment to quality of care
Working in true partnerships	Quality and teamwork	Risk assessment	Compassion
(NHS Wales, 2011)	(Scottish Government, 2016)	(Social Care Institute for Excellence, 2013)	Improving lives
			Everyone counts
			(Department of Health, 2015)

Figure 1.3   Principles reinforcing holistic care

CHAPTER SUMMARY

- Caring for a patient in a professional manner is fundamental to effective nursing care.
- The role of the nurse has developed from its origins and is constantly evolving to enable the delivery of evidence-based care within a wide range of settings.
- The four fields of nursing within the UK enable nurses to develop specialised skills to ensure patients receive the best care possible.
- Recent changes in nurse education have enabled nurses to continue to develop the skills specific to their field of nursing, but also to develop competency in a range of generic skills.
- There are more similarities than differences in nursing across the globe.
- Good nurses share a range of professional attributes, including the 6Cs and the NHS values.
- Working in partnership with the patient is a fundamental part of good nursing care.

CRITICAL REFLECTION

Holistic care

This chapter has highlighted the importance of the 6Cs and the NHS values in providing holistic care for your patient. Review the chapter and note down all the instances where you think using the 6Cs and the NHS values will help meet the patient's physical, psychological, social, economic and spiritual needs. Think of a variety of different patients across the fields, not just within your own field. You may find it helpful to make a list and refer back to it next time you are in practice, and then write your own reflection after your practice experience.

GO FURTHER

Books

Canfield, S., Hansen, M., Mitchell-Auto, N. and Thieman, L. (2012) *Chicken Soup for the Nursing Soul: Stories to Celebrate, Honor and Inspire the Nursing Profession*. Cos Cob, CT: Backlist. A collection of anecdotes illustrating the difference nurses can make in patients' lives.

Fox, M.J. (2010) *Always Looking Up*. New York: Hyperion. An account, from the patient's perspective, of the difficulties and unexpected changes that accompany Parkinson's disease.

Siviter, B. (2018) *The Student Nurse Handbook*, 4th edition. London: Elsevier. A useful text which is helpful when you are commencing a pre-registration nursing course, as it will help you to understand what is expected from you, how to plan work, and cope with stress.

SAGE journal article

Go to https://study.sagepub.com/essentialnursing2e for free online journal articles for this chapter. If you are using the interactive ebook, simply click on the book icon in the margin to go straight to the resource.

FURTHER
READING:
JOURNAL
ARTICLE

Akhtar-Danesh, N., Baumann, A., Kolotylo, C., Lawlor, Y., Tompkins, C. and Lee, R. (2013) 'Perceptions of professionalism among nursing faculty and nursing students', *Western Journal Nursing Research*, 35(2): 248-271. A study identifying nursing students' and lecturers' views of professionalism in nursing.

Suggested further reading

King's College London (2008) What Matters to Patients: The Nursing Contribution. Policy+ paper, April, Issue 9. Available at: www.kcl.ac.uk/nursing/research/nnru/policy/Policy-Plus-Issues-by-Theme/hownursingcareisdelivered/PolicyIssue9.pdf.

Parliamentary and Health Service Ombudsman (2011) *Care and Compassion?* Available at: www.ombudsman.org.uk/publications/care-and-compassion. A report of the Health Service Ombudsman on ten investigations into the NHS care of older people.

Royal College of Nursing (RCN) (2014) *Defining Nursing*. London: RCN. A Royal College of Nursing publication which defines the essence of nursing, describing what nursing is and clarifying the role of the nurse.

Weblinks

FURTHER
READING:
WEBLINKS

Go to https://study.sagepub.com/essentialnursing2e for weblinks related to this chapter. If you are using the interactive ebook, simply click on the book icon in the margin to go straight to the resource.

www.nmc-uk.org/globalassets/sitedocuments/other-publications/enabling-professionalism.pdf – enabling professionalism describes and demonstrates what professionalism looks like in everyday nursing practice. This will help you to think about how you act as a professional during your daily activities.

www.patients-association.com – the voices of those who use health services.

www.healthcareers.nhs.uk/explore-roles/nursing – information relating to nursing.

www.rcn.org.uk – the Royal College of Nursing offers a range of resources relating to key issues in nursing and specialist advice for learning disability, child, mental health and adult nurses.

www.learningdisabilities.org.uk/our-work/changing-service-delivery/an-ordinary-life – a foundation for people with learning disabilities – 'An Ordinary Life'. This project aims to improve the quality of life for children with complex health needs and/or who are dependent on medical technology.

www.mencap.org.uk/learning-disability-explained – Mencap pages for professionals. Advice and good practice for professionals working with people with a learning disability.

Video links

VIDEO
LINKS

Have a break from the text and go to https://study.sagepub.com/essentialnursing2e for useful videos related to this chapter. If you are using the interactive ebook, simply click on the lightbulb icon in the margin to go straight to the resource.

GREAT FOR
REVISION!

ONLINE
QUIZZES

ACE YOUR ASSESSMENT

Review what you have learned by visiting the book's online resources at: https://study.sagepub.com/essential nursing2e If using your interactive ebook, just click on the icon in the margin to go straight there.

- Test yourself with multiple-choice and short-answer questions.
- Revise key terms with the interactive flash cards.

REFERENCES

American Nurses Association (2012) Home page. Available at: www.nursingworld.org (accessed 9 September 2012).

Boyd, M. and Nihart, M. (1998) *Psychiatric Nursing: Contemporary Practice*. Philadelphia, PA: Lippincott.

Burns, N. and Grove, S. (2011) *Understanding Nursing Research*, 5th edn. Maryland Heights, MO: Elsevier.

Cameroon Nurses Association (2010) 'Safe Care, Safe Practice'. Conference presentation, 5–6 July, Yaounde, Cameroon.

Cummings, J. (2012a) *The Leaders of the Student Pack: Our Winners Revealed*. Available at: www. nursingtimes.net/students/the-leaders-of-the-student-pack-our-winners-revealed/5044817.article (accessed 7 December 2017).

Cummings, J. (2012b) *Chief Nursing Officer Bulletin (August)*. London: DH.

Department of Health (DH) (2012) *Compassion in Practice*. London: DH.

Department of Health (DH) (2015) *The NHS Constitution*. London: DH.

Department of Health, Department of Health, Social Services and Public Safety, Welsh Government and Scottish Government (2012) *Strengthening the Commitment: The Report of the UK Modernising Learning Disabilities Nursing Review*. Edinburgh: Scottish Government.

Glasper, E.A. and Coyne, I. (2002) 'Children first and always: The history of children's nursing – Part one', *Paediatric Nursing*, 14(4): 38–42.

Henderson, V. (1966) *The Nature of Nursing*. New York: Macmillan.

McDonald, J. (2013) 'Conforming to and resisting dominant gender norms: How male and female nursing students do and undo gender', *Gender, Work and Organization*, 20(5): 561–79.

NHS Wales (2011) Governance E-manual Values and Standards of Behaviour Framework. Available at: www.wales.nhs.uk/governance-emanual/values-and-standards-of-behaviour-framew (accessed 5 June 2017).

Nepal Nursing Council (2012) *NNC Licensure Examination Guidelines*. Nepal: Nursing Council.

New Zealand National Nursing Organisations (2011) Glossary of Terms. Available at: www.nursingcouncil.org.nz/Nurses (accessed 13 August 2014).

Nursing and Midwifery Council (NMC) (2010) Nurse Education: Now and in the future. London: NMC.

Nursing and Midwifery Council (2015) *The Code: Professional Standards of Practice and Behaviour for Nurses and Midwives*. London: NMC.

Nursing and Midwifery Council (2016) *Annual Equality and Diversity Report 2015–2016*. London: NMC.

Royal College of Nursing (RCN) (2014) *Defining Nursing*. London: RCN.

Scottish Government (2016) *Everyone Matters: 2020 Workforce Vision*. Edinburgh: Scottish Government.

Social Care Institute for Excellence (SCIE) (2013) Principles of Care. Available at: www.scie.org.uk/workforce/inductionnorthernireland/principlesofcare/confidentiality.asp (accessed 18 June 2017).

BEING A NURSING STUDENT

CATHERINE DELVES-YATES

--- **THIS CHAPTER COVERS** ---

- Studying for a nursing degree
- NMC standards
- Learning about all fields of nursing
- What is expected of you as an independent and professional learner

- Learning in a placement
- The challenges you might meet

> [T]he most important thing to learn as a nursing student is how to communicate effectively. Not just with patients and their families, but also with all healthcare professionals and those teaching you.
>
> **Siân Hunter, child nursing student**

> The most important practical lesson that can be given to nurses is to teach them what to observe – how to observe … this is what ought to make part, an essential part, of the training of every nurse.
>
> **Florence Nightingale (1859)**

Visit https://study.sagepub.com/essentialnursing2e to access a wealth of online resources for this chapter – watch out for the margin icons throughout the chapter. If you are using the interactive eBook, simply click on the margin icon to go straight to the resource.

INTRODUCTION

The time you spend as a nursing student is likely to provide you with a range of new and exciting experiences: making new friends, possibly living away from home for the first time, studying at university, but most importantly being involved in caring for patients. As Florence Nightingale stated more than 150 years ago, observing patients, experiencing how to care for them, is a fundamentally important aspect of your course, and, as Siân tells us, effective communication is vital.

As already outlined in Chapter 1, a nursing course is not like many other university courses. Although you will be encouraged to become involved in the activities available at your university, while you are on placement you will be expected to work full days, evenings, nights, weekends and bank holidays, unlike most other students. You will also have a professional code of behaviour to uphold; behaving in a professional manner is fundamental to being a nurse. As a nursing student, you are required to maintain the standards set by the NMC (NMC, 2015), whether you are in class, in practice or spending an evening socialising.

This chapter will help you understand what it will be like to be a nursing student. It will outline how your course is likely to be structured and will discuss the expectations of you that will be held by lecturers, practice supervisors, practice assessors, patients, their families and the public. The importance of confidentiality is introduced and it is made evident that the principles of behaving in a professional manner are integral to your role as a nursing student. The wide range of support available to you during your course is highlighted, as are strategies you can use to make sure you manage your time effectively; in addition, ways in which you can work to positively influence others are set out.

The principles of behaving in a professional manner are outlined in Chapter 1, so it would be helpful to read this before continuing with this chapter. The theme of professionalism is discussed further in Chapter 7, so when you have finished reading this chapter, read Chapter 7 too.

STUDYING FOR A NURSING DEGREE

Wherever you study your nursing course in the UK, there will be similarities in the courses. It takes three years' full-time study to become a registered nurse. During this time, you will be a university student; you will spend 50 per cent of your course studying on campus and the other 50 per cent in practice learning (or on placement), involved in caring for patients.

Your nursing course is likely to be divided into modules or semesters which will focus on the aspects of nursing you need to understand. Even though your course will have a field specialism (learning disability, mental health, child or adult), for the first year of the course you may well be taught with students studying the other fields of nursing. This will enable you to gain a solid generic foundation of nursing procedures and knowledge common to all patients, and you may even have a placement in a field outside your chosen one. During the second and third years, you will continue to study generic issues and may still be taught with nursing students studying other fields, but there will be an increasing focus on learning the important aspects of patient care and management in your chosen field.

Your course will contain a mixture of theoretical and practical sessions. You will have lectures, seminars, online learning activities and tutorials, but you will also have practical sessions where you will practise nursing procedures in a simulation centre or a 'skills lab' which replicates placement. You may also undertake computer-based simulation exercises. Many universities use patient scenarios as a central aspect of learning, enabling you to investigate how to care for the patient in the scenario given and then present this information to other students.

Part of being a student is demonstrating what you have learned, so you can expect to undertake a wide range of assessments such as presentations, exams, essays, numeracy tests, portfolios, nursing procedure tests and, towards the end of your course, a dissertation. You will also be assessed while you are on placement, to demonstrate that you can care effectively for patients and function safely in practice.

You will be expected to attend sessions and to actively participate in learning. You will work 37.5 hours per week while you are on placement, which will be a mixture of days, evenings, weekends and nights. While some nurses do work 9–5 'office hours', many work shifts, often starting early in the morning and finishing late at night. Sometimes these shifts are 12 hours long. Patients need care throughout the whole 24-hour period every day, including weekends, so you will be expected to attend your placement during all of these times and maybe even on bank holidays. You may have to consider how much time it will take you to travel to and from your placement, as it may be further afield than you might expect. The time taken to commute to and from placement is considered by your university when making placement allocations, but this time is not part of your working day. When you are attending campus-based learning, once again you should expect to be busy each day, for a full day. Although you may not be in taught classes for all of this time, you will be required to undertake a mixture of directed and self-directed study, in addition to attending lectures and other activities.

As I waited to start university I anticipated that on my first day I would be told a mistake had been made, I should not be there! As time went by I realised that I was there for the duration, the good, bad and the ugly, how that scared me. I kept thinking about the negatives, have I made a mistake, do I have what it takes?

At times I felt lonely, as I live with my children without any other personal support network, a considerable distance away from the university. Travelling meant early mornings and late nights. I was prepared to be committed to the course, but not for it to take over my life! What kept me going was [thinking] 'it will be worth it in the end'.

To succeed I devised a strategy – concentrate on one module at a time. I felt totally out of my depth, so being organised seemed the best idea. Make sure you are prepared: consider the time you will need to put in outside university hours. Break everything down, travelling time, university days, placements, extra study hours, and remember time for your family and friends.

Sarah Parkes, LD nursing student

NMC STANDARDS

CASE STUDY:
ACTING
PROFESSIONALLY

Throughout your nursing course, you are likely to see reference made to the *NMC Standards for Proficiency for Registered Nurses* (NMC, 2018a), the *NMC Education Framework: Standards for Education and Training* (NMC, 2018b) and the *NMC Requirements for Pre-registration Nursing Education Programmes* (NMC, 2018c). These publications are designed to ensure that your course provides you with high-quality nursing education, so you can care effectively for patients. More specifically, they outline how nursing students must be educated and the competencies they must achieve in order to deliver and manage the current and future needs of their patients. So, your university has to ensure your course abides by these standards and that you achieve the required competencies.

The format of this textbook is designed to assist you in gathering the knowledge required to meet the NMC Standards. The relevant NMC Standards can be found at: www.nmc.org.uk/standards/, enabling you to focus on the knowledge you require to reach the year-one progression point.

LEARNING ABOUT ALL FIELDS OF NURSING

As already mentioned, during your course you will gain both field-specific and generic knowledge and nursing procedures. This is because some knowledge and nursing procedures are integral to all fields, but also because some patients may require the support of nurses from all fields of nursing at some time in their lives. An example of such a situation is that of people with learning disabilities. It is therefore important that all nurses feel confident in meeting their needs.

Unfortunately, there are many examples indicating that people with learning disabilities often do not receive good healthcare (see Table 2.1). This has been a focus of numerous reports, including *Six Lives* (Michael, 2009), *Death by Indifference* (Mencap, 2007) and the *Confidential Inquiry into Premature Deaths of People with Learning Disabilities* (Heslop et al., 2013), to name just a few. These reports all identify recurring issues.

While the life expectancy of people with learning disabilities is rising, the mortality rate for people with moderate to severe learning disabilities is three times that of the general population, and is particularly high for young adults, women and people with Down's syndrome (Tyrer and McGrother, 2009).

Table 2.1   Issues identified relating to poor care of patients with learning disabilities

Signs and symptoms of illness attributed to the presence of learning disabilities rather than physical illness
Poor communication with people with learning disabilities, their families/carers and other professionals
Treatment options influenced by negative views about the quality of life of individuals with learning disabilities
Interventions not delivered in a timely manner

To overcome some of these issues, it is important to understand what we mean by 'learning disabilities', since this will help us to provide care that meets the needs of the people to whom this label is applied. Many definitions have been put forward, but most comprise three main elements:

- impairment of cognitive functioning
- impairment of social functioning
- the above two are apparent within the developmental period (before the age of 16–18).

All three of these elements must be present for an individual to be viewed as having learning disabilities.

This is significant when considering the provision of healthcare. The impairment of cognitive functioning may mean that people who have a learning disability can find it difficult to understand and retain complex information. This does not mean that they are unable to understand such information; rather, you may have to present it more slowly, avoid 'jargon' and use an easily readable format.

> I am [in the] child field, and learned so much about the importance of communication and listening to the 'voice' of those with learning disabilities. Finding out as much as you can when they come in to your care is vital. Many could not communicate verbally but used eye pointing and facial expressions, and this enabled staff to hear them and respond to their needs appropriately. Some people are not always able to ask for a drink, or monitor what they eat. Some need support with personal hygiene and all aspects of daily living, yet some just need support doing social activities – being taken bowling for example. I feel learning disabilities is a complex area but incredibly rewarding.
>
> **Siân Hunter, child nursing student**

The impairment of social functioning can mean that the person has difficulties with such things as attending to their hygiene and nutritional needs, while also perhaps having very limited verbal communication. In such situations, it is important to gather information from both the individual and their family/carers, to ensure that you understand their usual way of doing things and how, for example, they usually communicate pain and discomfort.

It is not possible here to provide a detailed overview of the nature of learning disabilities, but one final point you need to remember is that the term 'learning disabilities' encompasses a wide range of ability and disability: some people with learning disabilities are married and are bringing up their own families, while others have complex physical and learning disabilities and require a high level of support to meet all of their needs. What this means for nurses is that when you see the term 'learning disabilities', you must not make assumptions. Instead, you need to get to know the individual you are caring for and be aware that additional support may be required to ensure they receive the appropriate healthcare.

WHAT IS EXPECTED OF YOU AS AN INDEPENDENT AND PROFESSIONAL LEARNER

As a nursing student, you are expected to act in a professional manner at all times, following the NMC Code (2015), whether in your university, at your placement or in any other public setting. Becoming a member of a professional community involves respecting all those you meet, as what you say and do and how you present yourself all have a potential influence on how nurses are viewed.

All the hard work you put in to get your university place was just the start – to be successful, you need to continue to work hard. While there are many individuals in your university and placement who will support you in this, it is important to realise that you are responsible for your own learning. This is an approach shared by successful students, so make sure you adopt this way of managing your studies too. Simple strategies will work best. While you are in class, concentrate on what you are being taught, even if those around you are talking. Such conversations are distracting to others and infringe on their learning as well as your own. Help yourself and other students by having private conversations only outside the classroom. Mobile devices open up learning opportunities in the classroom: ensure you are attentive and only use your devices for classroom-related learning activities. It is both disrespectful and unprofessional to use your device to engage in text messaging or other online social activities while in class. Actions such as this in no way uphold professional standards. Respect those who are teaching you, no matter whether they are patients, classmates, nurses or lecturers. As soon as you don't understand something, ask for help – plenty is available, but unless you ask, no one will know you need it. Get into the habit of checking your timetable for the forthcoming week and reading up on what you are going to be taught. Attending a session with some knowledge makes it easier to keep up with what is being discussed and ask questions, rather than desperately trying to write down what is being said and feeling confused.

Throughout your course, make sure you get into the habit of seeking feedback on your performance, whether this is during a placement, in class or on your assignments. Additional help is available from your personal advisor and your university's learning support services.

How do you learn?

When you learn, you depend on three senses to process information. We all have a particular preference for learning using one of these three senses, or a specific combination of them. The three senses used to learn are the visual, auditory and kinaesthetic (body movement) ones, so your preferred way of learning makes you a visual, auditory or kinaesthetic learner (see Table 2.2) – those who use more than one sense have a personal combination of these.

Table 2.2   Learning styles

Visual learners	**Auditory learners**	**Kinaesthetic learners**
Writing notes and colourful illustrations help learning	Reading aloud and listening to information help learning	Being active and tasks that involve action help learning
Prefer to sit at the front of class	Sit in class where they can hear what is being taught	Like to sit in class where they can move around
Remember things by visualising them	Remember things by verbalising them	Remember things by doing them

During your course, lecturers and practice supervisors will present information for you in a range of ways to accommodate different learning styles. However, if you are aware of your preferred learning style, you will be able to learn information in the way you like most. Chapter 23 provides further information on the theory of learning, and you will find personal learning style questionnaires available online for you to investigate your preferred style.

WEBLINK:
ACTIVITY 2.1

ACTIVITY 2.1: REFLECTIVE PRACTICE

You can find a variety of learning style quizzes available for free online. Find out what your learning style is by visiting SAGE edge, or log into your interactive eBook and take the Learning Style quiz.

The fundamental importance of confidentiality

Clearly, understanding the importance of confidentiality occupies a pivotal role in acting professionally as a nursing student. The discussion here aims to highlight its fundamental importance.

A 'duty of confidence' arises when one person tells or discloses information to another in a situation where it is reasonable to expect that the information will not be disclosed. So, if a patient you are caring for tells you something important relating to their illness, you owe them a duty of confidence – a duty placed on you under the terms of the law.

The law of confidentiality means that individuals have the right to expect that any information they provide is used only for the purpose for which it was given and not disclosed without their permission. The nurse must keep this information confidential, no matter whether the patient has given the information or if the information was obtained from someone else – a family member, for example. The exception to this would be if you believed someone may be at risk of harm.

So, you must not only respect a patient's right to confidentiality, but also ensure that patients are informed about how and why information is shared by those who will be providing their care. In summary, this means that you do not share information about a patient unless it is as part of their care; when you are working with patients, you inform them that anything they tell you will be shared between all members of their healthcare team; and, if you find out a patient is at risk for any reason, you tell an appropriate person. Always remember that if you are unsure about disclosing information about a patient or if you think a patient could be at risk, you should ask for advice from your practice supervisor or another suitably qualified person before taking action. The guidelines on confidentiality (NMC, 2015) must be adhered to, so if you include information in your assignments or elsewhere relating to patients, their relatives, staff, lecturers or placement areas, it must be anonymised. It is never acceptable to discuss matters related to the patients in your care outside the clinical setting, or to discuss a patient with colleagues in public where you may be overheard. Never leave information unattended where it may be read by unauthorised people. This also includes ensuring you do not disclose information gained within your professional role to others on social networking sites such as Twitter or Facebook, etc., or mention it in a blog, email or similar. The NMC, your university and all placement areas will have policies on social media – make sure you adhere to these at all times.

ACTIVITY 2.2: LEADERSHIP

Sameer is on placement, helping his practice supervisor to care for a group of six children. The mother of one of Sameer's patients is concerned about the child in the bed opposite and asks: 'Is he very sick, nurse? What is wrong with him? Will he get better?'

- How should Sameer answer these questions?

CHECK YOUR ANSWERS!

ANSWER: ACTIVITY 2.2

LEARNING IN A PLACEMENT

Acting as a professional and independent learner is even more important when you are on placement. Here, professionalism is of the utmost importance as you are working directly with patients and their families, representing your university, nursing students and the nursing profession as a whole. You never know who may be listening to your conversations in the staff canteen or lift, or observing your interactions with patients, other healthcare professionals and the public. Maintaining confidentiality is crucial.

Acting in a professional manner is not something you turn off and on; it is a way of life, a personal standard of excellence whereby you constantly strive to be the best you can be. You will find that patients and the public are unlikely to realise that you are a student and not a registered nurse, so they will anticipate the same standard of professionalism from you as they do from a qualified nurse. You will be expected to be on time on all occasions, arriving prepared for whatever is ahead, whether this is a placement or a classroom session; you will be expected to stay for the full shift in a placement or the entire duration of the lecture.

While on placement, you will be required to dress appropriately. In some areas, this will be uniform; in others, you may wear your own clothes, adhering to the relevant dress code. Once again, it is important to remember that you are representing the nursing profession; you must look smart and clean, and if the placement has a uniform policy you must abide by it.

During your course, you may find that, at times, you disagree with the views put forward by lecturers, qualified nurses or other students. Disagreement, in the form of discussion, is an excellent way to learn and a key part of education. It is also important for nurses to be able to challenge others, otherwise poor nursing practice may be allowed to continue. However, your actions must always uphold the principles involved in being a professional. There are appropriate and positive ways to raise concerns and handle disagreements – by outlining what your concern or disagreement is and describing how you feel about it, thus making it possible to discuss the issue objectively while listening to the other person's view. If after doing this you remain concerned and unable to resolve the disagreement, there are other sources of support available, such as your lecturer or practice supervisor, to help resolve the situation. Always remember that a positive attitude and an optimistic outlook are helpful in all situations, and remaining courteous at all times is imperative. To successfully complete your course and practise as a registered nurse, you are required to abide by the NMC Fitness to Practise regulations, so it is essential to ensure, even when you are worried or stressed, that your conduct is professional.

Apply your knowledge of professional practice by reading case study 2.1 on acting professionally.

CASE STUDY 2.1: AMINA AND DAVE

During Fresher's Week, Amina and Dave attend the 'dress as what you want to be when you finish your course' party. They had collected their nursing uniforms a few days before the party, so they wore them to the party. It was great - meeting other students, making the most of the cut-price drinks in the bar and putting red dye and washing-up liquid in the fountain in the university square.

ANSWER:
CASE STUDY 2.1

- Do Amina and Dave's actions uphold the NMC (2015) Code? If not, why not?

The placements you attend during your course are specifically designed to assist you to achieve the NMC requirements which enable you to become a registered nurse. While on placement, you will be supported and supervised by a qualified nurse, who is called a practice supervisor. Under the guidance of your practice supervisor, you will be able to participate in the care of patients, experience the unpredictable and dynamic nature of the placement environment, and develop your knowledge and nursing procedures by receiving feedback about what you are doing well and where you need to develop further (RCN, 2006).

You will attend placements within a range of different settings, ranging from NHS authorities and trusts providing acute hospital services and community health services (for all patients – mental health, learning disability, child and adult) to the private, voluntary and independent sector (PVI), often called 'third sector organisations' (TSOs). In recent years, changes in the delivery of healthcare have moved many aspects of care away from large acute hospitals to community and PVI third-sector settings, which means that, whatever your field of practice, you may have very few placements in a traditional inpatient or acute hospital. Nursing care for people with learning disabilities is mainly community-based; however, where health needs indicate, the person may be admitted to an acute general hospital or mental health services for inpatient assessment and treatment and, where necessary, individuals may be admitted to forensic services for treatment and rehabilitation.

> At times placement can be overwhelming and challenging. For that reason it is important that we have a person to support us and act as a positive role model. Ultimately my practice supervisors have modelled the nursing procedures and approaches that I now use as a newly qualified nurse, thus it is important that as a student you utilise your practice supervisor while on placement to help you harness attributes that you will go on to use as a qualified nurse.
>
> **Alice Rowe, NQ RNMH**

Support on placement

Typically, you will attend a placement for a number of weeks in order to experience a wide range of aspects of the care delivered to patients. During this time, there will be a number of key individuals available to support you and ensure that you experience well-planned learning opportunities during your placement. Your practice supervisor will offer you support and act as a guide and your practice assessor will complete any assessment that needs to be undertaken during your placement. You may find that some placement areas, especially those where the nurses work shifts, will provide you with two or more practice supervisors. While you are a first-year student, your practice supervisor will supervise you very closely, remaining with you during all of the patient care activities you undertake, but you will find as you progress into the second and third years that they will expect you to undertake patient care activities more independently. You and your practice supervisor are jointly responsible for ensuring that your learning needs are met and that your practice assessor is aware of the assessments you need to complete. Your practice supervisor is hugely valuable in your practice learning. They will be your support – they can explain in simple terms what is happening and why; your translator of unknown terminology and unaccustomed practice; your role model, who can assist you to develop from nursing novice to successful student and then to registered nurse. They want you to succeed and will give their time to ensure your placement is a positive experience. However, in return they will expect you to be active in the learning process, not only being physically involved in patient care but also asking and answering questions, investigating the best ways to deliver care and acting professionally at all times: this includes proactively arranging meetings with both them and your practice assessor to plan and document your learning experience. While you are an important person in the placement area, there are others who are more important: the patients, whose needs must always come first. So, you may find that at times your practice supervisor asks you to undertake nursing procedures you have done many times before to assist them in delivering care, rather than always being able to show you how to perform a new nursing procedure, and sometimes they may be too busy to answer your questions. Make sure you have a notebook in your pocket to write these questions down and ask them at a more appropriate time. Remember that it is by practising nursing procedures that they become perfect. Observe your practice supervisor carefully to see how they manage busy and stressful situations so you can develop these skills yourself, as it will not be long before you are the practice supervisor teaching a new student.

My practice supervisors have all been brilliant and supportive; I have been very lucky. They are the first person you turn to for guidance. Each one has had a different learning style and at times we may not have always gelled at the start. One practice supervisor was very unsure why I was there – by working together, we got through it and I had a wonderful placement where I believe that we both learned something at the end.

Sarah Parkes, LD nursing student

Your practice supervisor is not the only source of support during your placement – you will find many of the other registered nurses, the patients and their carers, healthcare assistants and other nursing students will be keen to teach you and explain things. There are also other qualified healthcare professionals and students, such as doctors, dieticians, pharmacists and therapists, as well as social care professionals such as social workers, who will be very happy to contribute to your knowledge. Learning from and with other health and social care professionals is known as interprofessional learning – an important learning opportunity.

In addition to this wide range of staff willing to assist your learning, you will still have all the support offered by your university, with lecturers who are interested in your experiences and available to offer advice. You will find that each placement is likely to feature one particular lecturer who offers support and guidance to the registered nurses and the students in that area; they may visit you to discuss your progress and assist you and your practice assessor to complete your placement assessment documentation.

ANSWER:
ACTIVITY 2.3

ACTIVITY 2.3: CRITICAL THINKING

Connie is worried about starting her new placement. She is managing her studies well but, due to her dyslexia, finds it difficult to remember all of the information relating to the patients she is caring for. When it is very busy, she worries about forgetting what she has been asked to do.

- How can Connie help her specific learning needs to be met?

THE CHALLENGES YOU MIGHT MEET

While being a nurse is a privilege, there are also challenges. It is possible that you may experience some of these as a nursing student; additionally, being a nursing student brings challenges of its own.

Many nursing students find travelling to placements difficult, as a placement may be some distance from where you live, transport links can be poor and you may need to travel early in the morning or late at night. Finances can also be a cause of stress. Although there are sources of support for which you may qualify, even those who budget carefully can find student life a financial struggle. Then there is the need to manage your studies, work shifts and spend time with friends and family. Most nursing students will tell you that there just aren't enough hours in the day.

Students of learning disability, mental health and child nursing can find it challenging to understand the relevance of the generic elements, especially nursing procedures, within their course. These generic nursing procedures and knowledge are often felt to be adult-related, and their application to other fields is not always immediately clear. However, the equipment used in each of the fields can differ, and the clinical values of, for example, blood pressure, pulse rate or blood test results can vary greatly across age ranges. Nurses need to care for all patients effectively, and are required to ensure their skills remain up to date. Returning to the example of taking blood pressure, this is a fundamental nursing procedure that has to be carried out in a competent manner, but it is not just a case of carrying out everyday nursing actions: an important aspect of the interaction involves talking with the patient, assessing them and developing a therapeutic relationship, and taking opportunities to **empower** and **safeguard** them.

Learning disability nursing students can experience negativity towards their field. This has been described as 'parallel stigma' (Mitchell, 2000), where the stigma attached to people with learning disabilities is transferred to the nurses caring for them. Further to this, learning disability nursing students find it hugely difficult when their actions are met by discrimination, negative expectations and occasional hostility from some members of the public, or even other members of the healthcare team. The increase in placement provision in PVI third-sector services adds further challenges in field and role identity. Despite valuing the holistic practice, knowledge and skills of the learning disability nurses they employ, these services may not identify as healthcare services. A further challenge is the myth that 'people with a learning disability' require nursing care from a learning disability nurse when they are ill. During their lifetime, depending on the health need, a person with a learning disability will require nursing care from a nurse in each field of nursing. Nursing care is no longer the domain of the learning disability nurse. It is important as nursing students that the roles and contributions of each field are recognised early in the first year, so that you can work effectively in partnership with colleagues across all fields to meet the person's individual needs.

Mental health students can find working with patients who are unable to take responsibility for their own behaviour very frustrating. It can be hard to understand this and to appreciate that when things become difficult, it is not the patients' fault. Other healthcare practitioners may express negativity towards this field of practice, and both patients and nurses can experience discrimination and stigma, in a similar fashion to those caring for patients with a learning disability.

Mental health nursing frequently occurs within a highly stressful environment due to the nature of caring for patients with complex mental health needs.

Children's nursing students can find caring for seriously ill children very stressful. Caring for well children, or those with minor illnesses, is very different from being able to cope with, for example, the emotions involved in caring for a pre-term baby or terminally ill children while supporting their family members, who may well be angry and will certainly be hugely stressed themselves.

Adult-nursing students may find it very challenging that many of the patients for whom they are caring are older people – a large number of whom will have dementia – or adults with mental health problems, and feel that this is not what they expected adult nursing to entail. The diverse needs of patients and their general expectations can be difficult to manage, especially in community settings, where nurses have very large caseloads.

If you find these or any other aspects of your course concerning, it is important to discuss your feelings with a lecturer or your practice supervisor, who will be able to support you and help you identify the actions you should take.

It is also essential to ensure that, throughout your course, you remain healthy. While it may be tempting to spend all of your time focused on your studies, remember that you need to apply a holistic approach to yourself. Nurses, including nursing students, are renowned for being poor at taking their own advice when it comes to adopting a healthy lifestyle.

WHAT'S THE EVIDENCE?

'Do as I say, but not as I do': Are next-generation nurses role models for health?

Blake, Malik, Mo and Pisano (2011) investigate whether nursing students live the same healthy lives they promote to their patients.

Reflect on how healthy your lifestyle is. For example, do you:

- participate in at least 2.5 hours of moderate-intensity aerobic activity per week?
- eat five portions of fruit or vegetables daily?
- drink fewer than 3-4 units of alcohol each day if you are male or 2-3 if you are female?
- smoke?

Now read case study 2.2 and consider whether your lifestyle is similar to that of the students within the study.

CASE STUDY 2.2: BILLIE

Billie is at the end of the first year of her nursing course and is doing very well, enjoying attending placements and university sessions. On Saturday night, she drove home after spending an evening socialising with friends and was stopped by the police and breathalysed. To her horror, the result of the breathalyser put her over the limit and the police intend to take her to court for 'driving under the influence of alcohol'.

- Is it necessary for Billie to tell her university what has happened?

ANSWER:
CASE STUDY 2.2

> It is now your job as a nursing student to set an example to other students and patients in order to succeed in your role as a valued healthcare professional. A nursing course not only requires you to act professionally within practice; it also involves you acting in a professional manner at all times.
>
> **Ali Chapman, adult nursing student**

Manage yourself in order to manage others

The ability to effectively manage yourself and others is a skill needed by nursing students and registered nurses alike. While many nurses will tell you that their main problem is not having sufficient time, your professional life will run much more smoothly and you will be far less stressed if you can master the important skill of managing the time you do have.

The key to successfully managing yourself is actually simple: be organised. This will make it very much easier to manage others such as patients and other members of the healthcare team.

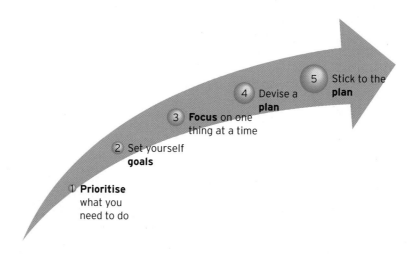

Figure 2.1 Five steps to effective self-management

By following the steps in Figure 2.1, you will not only keep up to date with the requirements of your course but also, if you include time for socialising in your timetable, it will still be possible to see your family and friends. The most difficult step of the five, however, is the last – sticking to the plan. No matter how carefully considered your plan is, if you don't actually carry it out, it will not work!

The role of the nurse is one that is central to all healthcare settings. To undertake this role successfully, nurses need the ability to manage others, whether these 'others' are patients, relatives or members of the healthcare team. Starting to learn how to manage effectively from the beginning of your course makes it far easier to cope with complex situations when you are more senior, but from your very first placement it is important for you to effectively manage situations in which either patient care or the conduct of others in the healthcare team is unacceptable.

Recent reports, such as the Francis Report (2013), provide clear evidence that patient care is not always of the highest quality, and you need to be able to recognise this and act appropriately. Determining whether care is good, however, is actually a more complex issue than it at first seems.

While in university you will learn the most up-to-date way of moving patients, for example, but if patients are not moved in this way when you are on placement, does it necessarily mean that their care is bad – or are they being moved in a different, but just as acceptable, way? To further complicate the situation, just because care isn't good doesn't necessarily mean it is bad. There is a whole range of stages between good and bad care. The key to all of this is to remember the 6Cs and the NHS values, plus the importance of treating all patients with dignity and kindness; then you can ask yourself whether the care you have seen upholds these essential elements. This may help you decide, but if you are still unsure talk to your practice supervisor, lecturer or any other appropriately qualified member of the healthcare team. Ask them to explain why what you have seen is acceptable, and if you are not convinced by their answer, keep asking until you are. Never be afraid to voice your opinion, as long as you do it in a professional manner. Your first responsibility is, at all times, to patients, as they rely on you to protect them from harm. All healthcare settings will have formal procedures whereby concerns can be reported, and your practice supervisor or lecturer will be able to advise you on how to do this.

My nursing course provided insights which enabled me to view challenges positively and made me realise important attributes. One of the key insights is the power of reflection, through which I have learned many lessons. First, if you don't put the hard work in no one else will do it for you. Second, access as many sources of help as you need to attain the standard of work you desire. Third, lecturers do know what they are talking about, and if you pay attention you will learn a lot more. Fourth, no matter what anyone tells you about how exciting, daunting, hard, stressful and rewarding being a nursing student is, until you've experienced it yourself you just won't understand.

On to challenges – you only have to read the news to realise that the NHS is not always great. As a nursing student you may well meet over-worked, stressed nurses with low morale. Do not be deterred, however; recognise that these nurses are unhappy because they care about the patients and want to provide the best treatment for them, but feel unable to do so.

Finally, attributes – the greatest for a nursing student is not knowing. This means you can learn without preconceptions. When I knew nothing, I learned from the patients I worked with about their views of illness. Textbooks have their place, but people experience illness and only they can describe exactly how it feels.

My course tested my resilience to its limit. It challenged me emotionally, physically and academically but I finished the course a far more mature, assertive and self-aware individual.

Alice Rowe, NQ RNMH

The most challenging thing for me has been developing coping strategies to deal with the emotional aspects and impact of the course. The workload, particularly when on placement and needing to complete essays, can be very high and takes a lot of energy and time management to ensure deadlines are met, which can be challenging at the beginning and end of the course. Time management strategies are essential.

Katrina Polfrey, child nursing student

CONCLUSION

Understanding what it means to act as a professional is fundamental to being a successful nursing student, which includes taking responsibility for your own learning and upholding the Code

(NMC, 2015) at all times. As Alice outlines, your journey to becoming a registered nurse is likely to be a rollercoaster ride. There will be lows, but these will be outweighed many times over by the highs. Being able to make a patient's day just slightly better makes everything worthwhile, as the purpose of nursing is to focus on the patient.

CHAPTER SUMMARY

- Throughout your nursing course, you are expected to act as an independent and professional learner.
- The knowledge and nursing procedures you gain will reflect all of the fields of nursing, not just your chosen one.
- Confidentiality is fundamentally important to all aspects of your learning, as well as patient care.
- During your nursing course, there is a wide range of sources of support which you can access.
- Being a nursing student is challenging, but also hugely rewarding.
- Managing yourself effectively is crucial to successfully completing your course.
- You must, at all times, speak out if you witness what you think is bad care.

CRITICAL REFLECTION

Holistic care

This chapter has highlighted the importance of acting as a professional during your nursing course. Review the chapter and note down all the instances in which you think acting professionally will assist you to meet the patient's physical, psychological, social, economic and spiritual needs. Think of a variety of different patients and their families across the fields, not just within your own field. You may find it helpful to make a list and refer back to it next time you are in practice, and then write your own reflection after your practice experience.

GO FURTHER

Book

Sharples, K. (2011) *Successful Practice Learning for Nursing Students*, 2nd edn. Exeter: Learning Matters. An excellent resource to support learning in placements.

SAGE journal articles

FURTHER
READING:
JOURNAL
ARTICLES

Go to https://study.sagepub.com/essentialnursing2e for free online journal articles for this chapter. If you are using the interactive ebook, simply click on the book icon in the margin to go straight to the resource.

Hutchinson, T. and Janiszewski Goodin, H. (2013) 'Nursing student anxiety as a context for teaching/learning', *Journal of Holistic Nursing*, 31(1): 19-24. This study investigates the anxiety that skills simulation provokes in nursing students, and the possibilities for lecturers of using this for role modelling.

Lindh, I., Severinsson, E. and Berg, A. (2007) 'Moral responsibility: A relational way of being', *Nursing Ethics*, 14(2): 129-40. The meaning of moral responsibility in nursing practice is explored within a group of nursing students.

Other journal articles

Mitchell, D. (2000) 'Parallel stigma? Nurses and people with learning disabilities', *British Journal of Learning Disabilities*, 28: 78–81. This article discusses the history of learning disability nursing, raising the issue of both patients and nurses being stigmatised.

Weblinks

Go to https://study.sagepub.com/essentialnursing2e for weblinks related to this chapter. If you are using the interactive ebook, simply click on the book icon in the margin to go straight to the resource.

FURTHER
READING:
WEBLINKS

www.nmc-uk.org – the UK Nursing and Midwifery Council website, which has a wealth of information relating to professionalism.

www.rcn.org.uk/development/students – the RCN student community, offering support for your studies.

www.england.nhs.uk/wp-content/uploads/2016/12/confidentiality-policy-v3-1.pdf – this is the confidentiality policy for NHS England, which identifies a number of important issues you must abide by whilst in practice.

www.nursingtimes.net/useful-links-for-student-nurses/5018595.article – the latest news and resources for nursing students.

www.dh.gov.uk – latest news from the Department of Health relating to healthcare and the NHS.

Video links

Have a break from the text and go to https://study.sagepub.com/essentialnursing2e for useful videos related to this chapter. If you are using the interactive ebook, simply click on the lightbulb icon in the margin to go straight to the resource.

VIDEO
LINKS

ACE YOUR ASSESSMENT

Review what you have learned by visiting the book's online resources at: https://study.sagepub.com/essential nursing2e If using your interactive ebook, just click on the icon in the margin to go straight there.

ONLINE
QUIZZES

- Test yourself with multiple-choice and short-answer questions.
- Revise key terms with the interactive flash cards.

REFERENCES

Blake, H., Malik, S., Mo, P.K. and Pisano, C. (2011) '"Do as I say, but not as I do": Are next generation nurses role models for health?', *Perspectives in Public Health*, 131(5): 231–9.

Francis, R. (2013) *Report of the Mid Staffordshire NHS Foundation Trust Inquiry: Executive Summary*. London: The Stationery Office. Available at: www.midstaffspublicinquiry.com/sites/default/files/report/Executive%20summary.pdf (accessed 28 March 2013).

Heslop, H., Blair, P., Fleming, P., Houghton, M., Marriott, A. and Russ, L. (2013) *The Confidential Inquiry into Premature Deaths of People with Learning Disabilities*. Bristol: Norah Fry Research Centre.

Mencap (2007) *Death by Indifference*. London: Mencap.

Michael, J. (2009) *Six Lives: The Provision of Public Services to People with Learning Disability*. London: The Stationery Office.

Mitchell, D. (2000) 'Parallel stigma? Nurses and people with learning disabilities', *British Journal of Learning Disabilities*, 28: 78–81.

Nightingale, F. (1859) *Notes on Nursing: What it is, What it is Not* (1946 reprint). Philadelphia, PA: Lippincott. Available at: www.archive.org/stream/notesnursingwhat00nigh#page/n5/mode/2up (accessed 1 December 2013).

Nursing and Midwifery Council (2015) *The Code: Professional Standards of Practice and Behaviour for Nurses and Midwives*. London: NMC.

Nursing and Midwifery Council (2018a) *NMC Standards for Proficiency for Registered Nurses*. London: NMC.

Nursing and Midwifery Council (2018b) *NMC Education Framework: Standards for Education and Training*. London: NMC.

Nursing and Midwifery Council (2018c) *NMC Requirements for Pre-registration Nursing Education Programmes*. London: NMC.

Royal College of Nursing (RCN) (2006) *Helping Students Get the Most from their Practice Placements: A Royal College of Nursing Toolkit*. London: RCN.

Tyrer, F. and McGrother, C. (2009) 'Cause-specific mortality and death certificate reporting in adults with moderate to profound intellectual disabilities', *Journal of Intellectual Disability Research*, 53: 898–904.

CORE ACADEMIC SKILLS

GABRIELLE THORPE AND CATHERINE DELVES-YATES

THIS CHAPTER COVERS

- The relationship between theory and practice
- An introduction to evidence-based practice
- Reflection
- The relationship between reflection and evidence-based practice

- Strategies for finding and judging the quality of evidence
- The importance of correctly citing sources of evidence

> I always found it really hard to find the evidence for my essays. I spent hours putting different search terms into CINAHL, sometimes on their own and sometimes in combination with others. I would either end up with two hits or several thousand and when I viewed them one by one, half of them were about topics that had nothing to do with my essay question! Being taught a systematic strategy for literature searching revolutionised my approach – suddenly I could find the literature I needed in a quarter of the time.
>
> **Hiroko, child nursing student**

INTRODUCTION

As nursing students are entering the nursing profession from a range of backgrounds, they will bring with them a vast array of education, work and personal experiences. These experiences will shape their ability to engage with the academic requirements of their course. The most gifted academics were not born with the skills required to study at undergraduate or postgraduate level; they worked at and developed these skills over time. Nursing students are no different. Each piece of work you undertake will make the next piece of work easier to tackle. That said, understanding the rules of academic engagement and adhering to them will make that elusive goal of a good honours degree a little easier to attain and help develop transferable skills that can be used throughout your nursing career.

Together, this chapter and the next aim to unpick the core skills needed to achieve the academic requirements of graduate-level nurse education in the UK. This chapter addresses the relationship between theory and practice by considering the use of evidence to underpin nursing practice, reflection and strategies to find and appraise evidence.

THE RELATIONSHIP BETWEEN THEORY AND PRACTICE

The integration of theory and practice in nursing has been a hot topic for many years. In nursing, the term 'theory' can be used to describe the knowledge and understanding required to make informed, evidence-based decisions about the care of individual patients, while 'practice' is the actual nursing care delivered to individual patients. The term best practice is used to describe the most effective nursing care required to address an individual's specific nursing needs/problems, and only evidence can tell us what the most effective nursing care is in each individual case. In order to deliver best practice, care must be underpinned by appropriate theory to provide the evidence upon which to base clinical decision-making. The balance may be translated into specific courses in different ways, as each university delivering nursing education will interpret the educational needs of its students individually. The nurse you become will be shaped more by how you integrate theory and practice in your own academic and practice-based assessments than by these discrete differences. You must do more than produce work of an appropriate academic standard during your degree; you are required to demonstrate how your theoretical knowledge and understanding of the evidence can be applied to your professional practice and contribute to the development of a sound philosophy of care. Ways in which you can demonstrate the fundamental relationship between theory and practice in your academic work will be highlighted throughout this and the next chapter.

> I am a practical type of person so I learn more from doing as I find the theory side of being a nurse difficult; however, without the theory I would not understand nursing as a whole, and why the interventions and care we undertake are necessary. As complex as research can be, without it I would not understand how to find out why we do things and what is best practice, which is why it is so important.
>
> **Sarah Parkes, LD nursing student**

AN INTRODUCTION TO EVIDENCE-BASED PRACTICE

Evidence is the knowledge and information we use to help us to make effective decisions. This is not just the case in nursing; it applies to all decisions we make in life. For example, in deciding where to undertake your nursing course, you may have consulted university brochures, websites and league tables, spoken to other students and attended open days to enable you to gain further insight into which would be the best 'fit' for you. In effect, you consulted a wide range of information sources and made a decision based on this evidence. In both your academic and practice-based work for nursing, the evidence you use will be similarly wide-ranging – as illustrated in Figure 3.1 – composed of theoretical literature (external evidence), reflective pieces and personal observations in practice (individual clinical expertise) and patients' experiences, values and expectations.

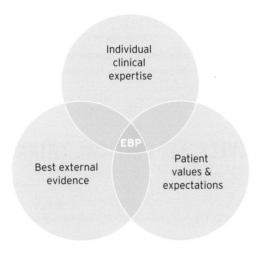

Figure 3.1   An evidence-based practice (EBP) triad

Source: Adapted from Armstrong (2003: 352)

ACTIVITY 3.1: CRITICAL THINKING

What evidence will you use to inform your practice?

Think about the practice-based experiences you have had so far and give examples of evidence that you used to make decisions about patient care in each of the following categories:

- observation
- reflection
- patient experience
- theory/research.

ANSWER:
ACTIVITY 3.1

It is important to understand that there may not be theoretical or research evidence available to inform all of the decisions we need to make, either because the questions are not researchable or because they have not yet been researched. Therefore, using a range of evidence (observation, reflection, patient experience, theory/research) gives us the highest probability that we will deliver the best care for patients.

As we rely on evidence to deliver best practice, it is critical for that evidence to be 'trustworthy'. In order to make a judgement about the trustworthiness of the evidence from your individual nursing expertise, such as through reflection and observation, you need first to take account of the context in which care is being delivered and the professional, moral and ethical considerations that underpin that nursing care. These aspects of the experience should be combined with knowledge of the actual nursing skills being reflected on or observed that is taken from, for example, clinical guidelines or a manual of nursing interventions.

In contemplating the trustworthiness of evidence derived from patient values and expectations, we are not attempting to make judgements about those values and expectations themselves, but about our ability to uncover and understand them. This source of evidence is frequently undervalued but is a fundamental aspect of person-centred care and underpins high-quality nursing practice.

Research (or external evidence) is considered to provide the most reliable source of information to answer the clinical questions we generate. In the simplest terms, research is a systematic way of finding answers to questions. You are encouraged to use research evidence to inform your academic work and clinical practice. This includes both the research studies themselves and any reviews, guidelines or theoretical papers based on research evidence.

ANSWER:
ACTIVITY 3.2

ACTIVITY 3.2: CRITICAL THINKING

Some types of evidence are considered to be more trustworthy than others. Make a list of the sources of evidence you have used in previous academic work. Now rearrange this list, so that those you think most trustworthy are at the top and the least trustworthy are at the bottom.

Critical appraisal

So does it automatically follow that using *any* research will provide the best evidence to inform our practice? Sadly, it is not so simple. Not all research has been conducted in an ethical or rigorous manner, and so the findings of such studies cannot be trusted sufficiently to inform our patient care. Therefore, nurses not only need to find appropriate evidence to answer their questions, but must also have the skills to decide if a piece of research is good enough to be trusted. Judging the quality of research evidence in a systematic way is called critical appraisal and is an essential skill to develop and use, both as a nursing student and after you qualify.

To help you to make a judgement on the quality of evidence, a number of hierarchies of evidence have been devised: lists of different types of evidence that are ranked in order of strength (see Table 3.1). This is similar to the list of evidence you produced in Activity 3.2.

If you look back at the items you listed as evidence in Activity 3.2, it is likely that they will mainly fall into the lower part of this hierarchy, or maybe are not even mentioned at all. This is a common feature of evidence that relates to feelings and experiences. It is very easy to subject a drug, for example, to lots of scientific investigation, finding out how effective it is, but it is very much more difficult to do this when you want to find out how people feel. However, this does not mean that the knowledge gained from reflection or studies investigating the feelings or experiences of groups of patients, or even individual patients, is not valuable; it just means you need to ensure that you don't try to apply this knowledge to every patient experience, or how every patient feels, without first making sure it is trustworthy.

Research

Research is a systematic way of finding answers to questions. Some research generates answers in the form of words and some generates answers in the form of numbers. These answers are known

Table 3.1   Hierarchy of evidence

Strongest	**Type of evidence**	
	Description	Formally called
	The combined results of a number of studies which use a very strict experimental design where there is random allocation of individuals to the treatment they will receive.	Systematic review of randomized controlled trials (RCT).
	The combined results of a number of studies which use a very strict experimental design but individuals are not allocated to treatment by random methods.	Systematic review of non-randomized trials.
	The results of one study which uses a very strict experimental design where there is random allocation of individuals to the treatment they will receive.	A randomized controlled trial (RCT).
	The results of one study which uses a very strict experimental design, but individuals are not allocated to treatment by random methods.	A non-randomized trial.
	The combined results of a number of studies which examine the links between causes and effects.	Systematic reviews of correlational or observational studies.
	The results of one study which examines the links between causes and effects.	A correlational or observational study.
	The combined results of a number of studies that describe an event or experience.	Systematic reviews of descriptive or qualitative studies.
	The results of one study that describes an event or experience.	A descriptive or qualitative study.
Weakest	The understanding and interpretations of a group of people who are experienced in a specific area.	Opinions of authorities or expert committees.

as research data, which are then subjected to more questioning – a process called data analysis. Generally, research that generates answers in the form of words follows a qualitative methodology, and that which generates answers in the form of numbers follows a quantitative methodology. Whether research uses a qualitative or quantitative methodology depends on what sort of question is asked. For example, if you want to investigate how it feels for a patient with a chest infection to take a course of antibiotics, qualitative research would be the most appropriate method, as feelings are best described in words. If you want to investigate which antibiotic is the best at treating a patient's chest infection, quantitative research would be the most appropriate, as numbers allow you to measure effectiveness very precisely. However, it might not be possible to answer some questions with just words or numbers alone. If you wanted to investigate whether the age of a patient with a chest infection altered how they felt while they were taking antibiotics, the question could be best answered by using qualitative research (words) to investigate the patient's feelings, and quantitative research (numbers) to investigate whether the patient's age made any difference. This approach is called mixed methods research.

The research process, whether qualitative or quantitative, follows the same steps, starting with a question and ending in sharing knowledge, as demonstrated in Figure 3.2.

The steps in the research process:

- Identify the question
- Decide which type of research will answer the question in the most rigorous way
- Identify who can help to answer the question and invite them to be involved
- Collect data (answers)
- Analyse the data (find patterns) and establish significance
- See how answers fit with current knowledge and share them

Figure 3.2   Steps in the research process

ACTIVITY 3.3: CRITICAL THINKING

Which type of research methodology – qualitative, quantitative or mixed methods – would best answer these research questions?

- How many jelly babies can a nursing student eat before they are sick?
- What challenges do student nurses experience in their first practice placement?
- Do patients think nurses should wear hats?
- What do nursing students enjoy most in the first year of their course?

ANSWER:
ACTIVITY 3.3

REFLECTION

Reflection can be an important source of evidence, helping us analyse our own observations or actions in a systematic and objective manner in order to produce evidence to underpin future practice.

In its simplest form, reflection is a process that assists you to review a personal experience and then learn from it. As suggested by the word 'reflection', what you are doing is looking carefully at your experience, just as if you were looking in a mirror, and being honest with yourself about what you see.

There can be a difficulty in this approach because whenever we look in a mirror most of us immediately concentrate on our flaws, rather than being objective and appreciating the good things as well as those needing improvement. So, for reflection to be most effective, it needs to follow a set structure.

Using reflection in nursing is an excellent way to develop your skills, increase your knowledge, make sense of challenging situations, review how you interact with others, consider your behaviour and – most importantly – improve patient care. To achieve these outcomes, reflection needs to be an active process, used by nurses to help them understand themselves more effectively and allow them to see how their personal beliefs and values influence their professional behaviour.

Reflection can be undertaken in two ways: reflection-on-action and reflection-in-action (Schön, 1994). It is necessary to understand the differences between these so you can use both types in your personal and professional development:

Reflection-on-action is the most commonly practised form of reflection, which you are likely to use frequently throughout your nursing course. Reflection-on-action is similar to using a video camera to review an experience.

Reflection-in-action involves examining your behaviour and that of others while actually being involved in the experience, thereby reflecting at the same time as being within a situation. Reflection-in-action is a more complex process than reflection-on-action, as you will need to be experienced in a particular situation before you can reflect and act at the same time. However, you may well see your practice educator or another nurse reflecting-in-action and it is something you will undertake at other times. For example, when walking on a slippery pavement you will be subconsciously considering all the available information, assessing where to put your feet and modifying your actions if needed. What you are doing is reflecting-in-action to prevent yourself from falling.

Both types of reflection enable us to critically consider our assumptions about other people, our environment and ourselves. We all have a unique view of our world which previous experience assists us to develop. This view enables us to make sense of and see the world we live in, but only from our personal perspective. Other people, even our closest friends and family, are likely to have a different worldview, so will see things in a different way. Reflection is an important tool to help uncover the values, beliefs and assumptions that our worldview is built on. One of the most important aspects of being a nurse is being able to understand your own behaviour. If you cannot do this, it is very difficult, if not impossible, to consider issues from the perspective of another person – a vital step in developing and maintaining therapeutic relationships with patients.

How do I reflect?

Throughout your nursing course, you will be asked to undertake reflection in the form of reflective writing. Reflective writing will be used as evidence for the achievement of your practice-based learning outcomes, to demonstrate your personal learning and progression in your portfolio and to support your written assessment tasks. If you find it difficult to reflect, you could identify a friend or fellow student to be a 'reflective partner'. Reflecting verbally with a friend or fellow student who is happy to act as a 'reflective partner', can be helpful in two ways. First, and most importantly, it can help you to undertake in-depth reflection on aspects of your developing professional practice or identity that you can later use within a written reflection. Second, in helping your partner to reflect, you will develop an understanding of the kinds of questions and probes that will draw out and explore important thoughts and feelings. As you progress in your course, you can use this understanding to question yourself and improve your own reflective practice.

Because we are human, we frequently focus on the things that go wrong, rather than appreciating what went well. So, if I reflected on walking on a slippery pavement, I might focus on the times I ended up on the ground, rather than considering what I did to stay on my feet. This is far from objective. Although at times it can be useful to focus on things that do not go well, thinking about what you did that was effective or identifying other people's good practice and working out how you can translate this into other situations, is also a constructive approach. To assist you to be objective, a large number of structures, or reflective models, have been devised (de Bono, 1996; Driscoll, 1994; Gibbs, 1988; Johns, 2009; Rolfe, 2010). Each of these reflective models suggests a slightly different approach to help you review both your thinking and your actions. We are going to focus on a model developed by Borton (1970), on which both Driscoll's (1994) and Rolfe's (2010) models are based, focusing on three simple questions: What? So what? Now what? Figure 3.3 shows you how these questions can be expanded to enable you to reflect on a situation in detail.

What? So what? Now what? A model of reflection

What?

- was the experience?
- happened in the experience?
- was my role?
- was I trying to achieve?
- were my actions?
- was the response of others?
- were the consequences, for me/others?
- feelings did the experience evoke in me/others?
- was good/bad about the experience?

So what?

- does this experience teach me about me/others/my patient's care/my attitudes/the attitudes of others?
- was I thinking while I acted?
- did I use as evidence for my actions?
- other knowledge/evidence do I need to consider?
- should I have done to make it more effective?
- is my new understanding of the experience?
- other issues arise from the experience?

Now what?

- should I do in order to make my actions more effective/improve my performance?
- other issues should I consider to make my actions successful?
- are likely to be the consequences of this change in action?

Figure 3.3   Expansion of the Borton (1970) model of reflection

ACTIVITY 3.4: REFLECTIVE WRITING

Using the 'What? So what? Now what?' model (Borton, 1970), reflect on an experience you have had in the past week:

- What were the actions you decided you needed to take as a result of your reflection?
- How are you going to carry these out?

THE RELATIONSHIP BETWEEN REFLECTION AND EVIDENCE-BASED PRACTICE

Both reflection and evidence-based practice are essential in ensuring the care patients receive is of the best possible quality. Reflection, or reflective practice, enables the review of nursing care by questioning how and why decisions are made and care is provided, in order to facilitate better clinical practice. Evidence-based practice ensures that the best evidence is used to make sound and effective decisions. So, it becomes clear that reflection and evidence-based practice are processes that share the same aims.

> Before starting uni, people said I was quite a considered and thoughtful person, so I think I must be naturally reflective. I like to ask lots of questions on placement to understand the reasons why something has or has not happened, reading about the issues or skills involved and thinking how I might act if I were in a similar situation again.. Putting it into words can be difficult; however, I have got better with time and using a model to structure my thinking helps. Writing it down gives me something to look back on too, to see how I have developed and changed since I started and to provide evidence of reflective practice.
>
> **Sarah Parkes, LD nursing student**

When further considering evidence-based practice, particularly the evidence applicable to the daily nursing care of patients, exactly what comprises evidence requires careful thought. It can often be difficult to apply research-based evidence directly to daily patient care, as all patients are individuals with different needs, which may not match those identified in research. In addition to this, the daily decisions a nurse needs to make may not be those considered by research studies and are likely to be based on different ways of knowing, such as experiential, personal, aesthetic and practical knowledge. Nursing knowledge is strongly linked with action, or more specifically action that is effective, so for all nursing care to be evidence-based, the evidence needs to include descriptions of effective practice experiences and nursing actions. Reflection is ideal in providing this evidence, enabling reflection to be both informed by evidence and evidence in itself, as is demonstrated in Figure 3.4.

Figure 3.4   The relationship between reflection and evidence

Evidence, be it observation, reflection, patient experience or theory/research, is central to the provision of high-quality, compassionate nursing care because it tells us which nursing interventions are most likely to address patients' needs. These forms of evidence provide an alternative perspective from our own, which is essential in helping us to question our own understanding and behaviour in a particular situation, increase self-awareness and recognise limitations in our practice that need to be addressed.

STRATEGIES FOR FINDING AND JUDGING THE QUALITY OF EVIDENCE

There is an expectation that, as a nursing student, you will support your academic and practice-based work with current best evidence. However, it is not always easy to find good quality evidence in the first place, let alone make judgements about its suitability to inform practice.

The obvious place for most students to look for information is the internet – it is easy to access and seems to offer a wealth of material at the touch of a button. Indeed, the ability to access information and guidelines from the Department of Health, NICE, the NMC and other 'official' sources opens up a huge resource. However, it is important to remember that the vast majority of online health information is aimed at lay people and patients. It can provide a clear and understandable introduction to complex medical conditions and procedures, but this level of detail is rarely enough to support academic work or to develop clinical understanding. Furthermore, it may be very difficult to tell if this information is based on accurate and up-to-date evidence. Therefore, you need to use databases of current healthcare literature, books written in the required breadth and depth, guidelines for practice and other high-quality sources. A good academic library is essential, with at least an assortment of information sources, access to appropriate databases of health literature and librarian support to facilitate their use.

Searching for literature to support your academic work mirrors the way in which evidence is sought to support clinical decision-making in practice: it is *question-led*. Understanding this symmetry can help you to find, appraise and use a wide variety of evidence to support all your assessment tasks throughout your degree, most of which will require an application of theory to practice. It can also help you to consider, through your own reflection, the extent to which you have witnessed evidence-based practice or can use the evidence to inform your own developing practice. In a bid to save time, many students will focus on one narrow question or use search terms that seem to relate broadly to the topic area, but very few assessment tasks can be addressed by adopting such a limited approach. Start by writing down the questions you wish to answer – making sure they are the right questions for your assessment task – and then consider the most likely sources of information to help answer them. This will help you to develop a systematic search strategy that is not only more likely to prove successful, but will also take the least amount of time.

Understanding the value of different **genres** of literature and how they inform your academic writing will help you to select sources that are appropriate to the questions you seek to answer. Common sources of information include books, journal articles, clinical guidelines and pathways, web-based sources of information and other documents such as Department of Health papers, Care Quality Commission (CQC) standards, etc. Books can provide valuable insight into theoretical principles and concepts underpinning all aspects of nursing care, from clinical skill development to legal and ethical issues. Clinical guidelines and pathways, available through the Department of Health, NICE or other 'official' websites for healthcare practice, will provide the most current evidence-based guidance on best practice and explicit information regarding the sources of evidence on which this guidance is based. However, journal literature is more likely to offer meaningful insights into the application of this knowledge in relation to actual patients or an evaluation of the effectiveness of practice based on these underpinning principles or guidelines (refer back to Table 3.1). Good quality journals will also provide original reports of primary research or systematic reviews of several research studies.

Database searching

Your academic library will provide links to databases of journal literature that can be used to inform your academic work and clinical practice. Retrieving journal citations in this way is more systematic and trustworthy than using the internet directly to source information. Which database(s) you use will depend on the question(s) you are seeking to answer. For example, the most comprehensive evidence base regarding interventions to manage hypertension may be found on a different database from that relating to psychological factors involved in the development of hypertension or treatment concordance in individuals with hypertension, all of which could be issues you wish to address in your assignment exploring adaptation theory in relation to a patient with newly diagnosed hypertension. The databases most likely to provide useful citations and access to journal literature to support your academic work are outlined in Table 3.2.

Table 3.2   Databases of health-related literature

British Nursing Index (BNI): A UK nursing and midwifery database, including articles from medical, allied health and management titles. For core UK nursing and midwifery, it is the most up-to-date resource available.

CINAHL (Cumulative Index to Nursing and Allied Health): The most commonly used database in nursing, providing access to a wide range of general nursing and allied health literature and indexing almost all English-language publications in these fields.

MEDLINE: A database created by the National Library of Medicine providing medical information on medicine, nursing, the healthcare system and other fields from more than 4,800 journals. A good source of information relating to treatment evaluation and explanation.

EMBASE: A biomedical and pharmaceutical database indexing over 3,500 international journals with selective coverage for nursing. A further good source of information relating to treatment evaluation and explanation.

AMED: A database created by the Health Care Information Service of the British Library covering journals in complementary medicine, palliative care and the allied health professions. Citations can help to inform work relating to rehabilitation and interprofessional working.

ASSIA (Applied Social Sciences Index and Abstracts): An indexing and abstracting tool covering health, social services, psychology, sociology and providing an inclusive source of social science and health information from more than 500 journals. Good for finding literature related to social issues, sociology and social care.

PsycInfo: A database of literature predominantly in psychology but also in the related disciplines of medicine, nursing, psychiatry, sociology, pharmacology and physiology. An excellent source of citations relating to psychological adaptation, mental health issues and communication.

The Cochrane Library: An electronic publication providing high quality evidence to inform care from all perspectives and at all levels. Papers bring together research findings from different research studies with similar research aims to explore the strength of evidence for specific interventions.

Developing a search strategy

Accessing an appropriate database is just the beginning of your literature search. Many students (and lecturers!) find that retrieving the most relevant citations to inform their academic work is quite a challenge, as Hiroko says at the start of the chapter. Two things will help you here: the tools available in the database to help you target your search and a clear, objective strategy. At the start of your course, you are likely to have an opportunity to attend a session on database searching at the library. Make sure you go, as this will at least introduce you to the database tools that can facilitate your literature search.

Table 3.3   Developing a search strategy for database searching

DO NOT GO NEAR THE COMPUTER YET!

STEP 1   Refine your search question – be as specific as possible. For example, 'How can a nurse communicate effectively with an adult with learning disabilities?'

STEP 2   Divide your question into three (or more) distinct areas if possible. For example: nursing, communication, learning disability.

STEP 3   Find all the words that could mean the same thing (synonyms) that may be used in the literature – truncate where necessary. It can help to use a thesaurus or dictionary to do this, or to use the subject heading facility when you choose your database, to see how these terms are classified within the database. For example:

1. Nursing: Nurs*/Clinical /Profession*/Healthcare
2. Communication: Communicat*/talk*/speak*/verbal/nonverbal
3. Learning disability: Learning disab*/intellectual disab*/developmental disab*/mental handicap/ cognitive impairment

NOW YOU CAN GO TO THE COMPUTER!

STEP 4   Choose your database – you will usually get more accurate results by searching the database directly rather than using an option to test your search terms in a number of databases at the same time.

STEP 5   a. Take your first set of search terms and enter each one in the search box one at a time. Although you have the option to search for the search term in just the title or abstract of possible papers, it is better to keep it on the default setting when you are starting a new search so you don't miss a paper that uses your search term in one area but not another. Each search term may produce thousands of hits – this is meant to happen. Don't panic.
   b. When you have put them all in and gained a search for each, go to 'search history.' Make sure the search box is clear and combine them all using 'OR'. This will add all the citations together and take out any duplicates – it will usually give you a huge number, especially if you are using broad terms such as care or management.
   c. Leave this search and move on to the second set of search terms. Repeat what you did with the first box of search terms.
   d. When you have combined all the terms for the second search with OR, make sure the search box is clear and in 'search history' select the combined box for search one and the combined box for search two. Combine these with AND – this will find only the papers that have been identified in both searches and will give you a much smaller number, although this may still be too large to search by hand.
   e. Repeat steps a. and b. above for your third set of search terms. When you have a combined number, make sure your search box is clear and select combined search c. and combined searches a. and b. (when you combined with AND and got the smaller number). Combine these with AND. You will now hopefully have a number small enough to search through by hand (e.g. less than 150).
   f. If you have a fourth set of search terms and the number of citations you have after step 'e.' is too large to search by hand, then repeat steps a. and b. Then combine using AND with the results of stage e. If you already have less than 150 citations following step e., consider searching by hand anyway as adding in the fourth set of search terms may remove papers that could inform your search question – this is always a risk when limiting your search.
   g. If, after all that, the number of citations is still too large to hand-search, you could consider refining the search further, either by adding another search term and combining with AND, or by using the 'limit your search' tool. The example used here could be limited by selecting the following limitations: academic (peer-reviewed) journals, papers published in the past ten years, or adults.

Judging the quality of literature

Finding literature to support your academic work and clinical practice is one thing, but knowing if it constitutes good evidence is another. How can you make this judgement and how can you demonstrate that you have considered it in your work? Judging sources of information is a skill that you will develop not just in your nurse education but throughout your career, so don't expect too much too soon – the academics marking your work will be looking for confirmation that you are considering the nature and quality of the evidence you are citing, but will not expect a full critical appraisal of every paper you include. Some useful but simple ways to judge the quality of literature include:

- What question were you originally trying to answer? If a recently published article is broadly related to the topic under exploration but does not actually help to answer your specific question(s), it is likely to be less useful as a piece of evidence than an older paper that does help to answer your questions.
- If a research study is reported in a high-quality, peer-reviewed journal, it is likely to be a better quality study than one reported in a non-peer-reviewed journal. When a paper has been peer-reviewed, someone else has already made a judgement about its quality.
- An article or a chapter is more likely to provide good quality evidence if it is written by someone who is a key writer or researcher in that field, or if it uses what you know to be key pieces of evidence to support the arguments presented.
- Look at the reference list. Is the article or chapter supported by appropriate and varied sources of information?
- When was it published? Other than seminal texts that you will have seen widely cited in other literature in the same area, try to use literature that has been published in the past ten years. However, a word of caution here – current best practice may still be based on robust research findings from 20 or 30 years ago.
- How many articles published since this one have cited it in their reference list? The facility to answer this question is available on some databases of health literature. If a paper was published ten years ago and very few people have used it to support more recent publications in that area, then it may not be of a high standard.
- You may be introduced to appraisal tools for primary research in the research component of your nurse education or nursing programme, e.g. those freely available from the Critical Appraisal Skills Programme (CASP) or the Equator Network. These can help you to work through and appraise the quality of different types of published research. It is unusual for institutions to expect this level of appraisal in the first year, and you should be supported to develop research appraisal skills during the second and third years.

THE IMPORTANCE OF CORRECTLY CITING SOURCES OF EVIDENCE

Once you have found the information you require to answer your question(s) and/or support your academic and practice-based work, make sure it is correctly cited and accessible.

Referencing

A good piece of academic work will provide enough information about sources for the reader of the work to retrieve those sources. Don't think that the person marking your work won't do this – they will, both to ensure that the argument you are developing can really be supported by the literature and to check that you haven't copied any of it directly, if the tone of your work suddenly changes. Different methods are available for academic referencing and your institution is likely to have a preferred method, most often the Harvard system. Your institution will inform you of its preferred method in your course handbook and provide examples of how to cite different sources of information using this method. If you require further guidance, the Palgrave study guide *Cite them Right: The Essential Referencing Guide* (Pears and Shields, 2016) provides a clear and detailed account of the most common referencing methods.

Whatever referencing system is used, you should make sure that the sources of literature are appropriate. Much of your reading should have been completed before you start any detailed written work, so that your work is guided and informed by the ideas and evidence that you have been reading about. This will help your discussion to be based more securely on, and grow more naturally out of, your reading. Key points to remember are:

- Make sure your references are up to date. With the exception of certain 'seminal' texts, your references to clinical knowledge and skills should be drawn from literature published during the previous 5–10 years.
- Avoid using too many direct quotations. A direct (verbatim) quotation indicates that you have read something, but does not, by itself, provide evidence of understanding or application. Try to use your own words and weave references to supporting literature into the fabric of your discussion.
- Place direct quotations (possibly for a key definition) within 'quotation marks' and provide a page number at the end of the reference citation, e.g. 'Harris and Hall (2010: 24)'.
- Have a sufficient number of relevant references. If you use only six different sources in your 3,000-word essay, you are unlikely to satisfy your assessor that you have undertaken an adequate quantity and range of background reading.
- Avoid using too many references. This is a less obvious point, but if your essay becomes a 'patchwork' of references, then it will be difficult for you to demonstrate depth of knowledge, critical analysis and application. Moreover, your own 'voice' will be lost.
- Watch out for any tendency to use 'tagged-on' references – that is to say, references that are simply added on to the end of a paragraph. Rather, integrate your references into the flow of your discussion.

While you are expected to provide references when you use others' work to support your writing, you can – indeed, are encouraged to – use your own logic and rationale to support the connections you make. This does not require a reference, just a clear explanation of your reasoning. However, you are not encouraged to overtly state your own opinion without support.

Reference management systems

Reference management systems are software packages designed to manage the bibliographic particulars of journal articles, reports or other information or documents. There are various referencing systems and your university will probably have specific ones to which they subscribe. Reference management systems are especially useful for downloading citations from database literature searches, for storing electronic copies of papers and for automatically compiling a reference list in a specified style at the end of a piece of writing. However, do consider how you will use this type of system and whether it is compatible with/available on all the computers you use before you sign up. It can be frustrating to start working on a document in the library with the reference management software active and find that the references in any extra work you do at home are not recognised when you open it again in the library the next day.

Plagiarism and collusion

It is fundamentally important to accurately acknowledge your sources in order to demonstrate breadth and depth of reading, knowledge and understanding of evidence-based practice, and to avoid any suspicion of plagiarism. 'Plagiarism' is using other people's work in your own writing without proper acknowledgement. Sometimes it is deliberate and blatant, but in many cases it is due to poor academic practice, rather than deliberate cheating.

'Collusion' means unauthorised cooperation between a student and another person (who might be a fellow student) in producing an assignment. You may find that some assessments actually require you to collaborate with your fellow students. On most occasions, however, there will be a clear expectation that the work is your own, and that you have not colluded with others. The simplest way to avoid any suspicion of collusion is to never show a draft of your written work to a fellow student before you hand it in.

CASE STUDY 3.1: ALEX

Alex had intended to start work on her nursing care study in good time, but ended up leaving it rather late. She found some relevant material on various websites, and then cut and pasted this into her essay. She intended to go back and put this material into her own words, discuss and apply it in the light of her chosen patient and tidy up the references. But the submission deadline loomed and she handed it in as it was.

- Why is this poor academic practice?
- How would a marker detect that there was a problem with Alex's work?
- What can Alex do to improve the quality of her work and avoid the risk of being accused of plagiarism a second time?

If a student is found to have plagiarised or colluded, the penalty is likely to depend on the nature and degree of the problem and the experience and intention of the student. In the case of some muddled referencing with an inexperienced student where there is no evidence of intent to deceive, the student may be given guidance and an opportunity to rectify the problem. But the most serious cases may jeopardise the student's place on the course.

ANSWER:
CASE STUDY 3.1

E-learning

Many institutions are increasingly using a range of technologies – including digital media and internet-based tools and applications to support and inform learning – broadly referred to as e-learning. These technologies may comprise wikis, blogs, online learning tools, apps or survey instruments and/or educational software geared to support and enhance the learning experience.

Examples of these include medications management (information about the medication is presented together with dose calculation software) or anatomy and physiology (where powerful 3D animation and sound are combined). These technologies are usually presented to students within a university 'online/virtual learning environment' to ensure they have a safe, private and secure area in which to learn: this is sometimes called a 'virtual classroom'. Some universities will also invite you to use online tools and technologies which are freely and publicly available and can be seen and commented on by the general public. Students should refer to local and professional guidelines and policies in relation to these open tools and technologies to ensure they use them in the correct context, and also to ensure they are upholding professional communication and behaviour online. Depending on the nature of your engagement with e-learning, you may be required to add your own writing or to view the writing of others. Tools such as wikis or blogs are often unstructured, potentially leading to users adopting an informal writing style. Remember that any writing you post in this way can be widely scrutinised, so it is essential to maintain a professional voice at all times. Likewise, writing that is posted under such circumstances is likely to be the opinion of individual students or lecturers, so would not normally constitute evidence upon which to base academic argument without supplementary evidence derived from the wider literature.

CONCLUSION

It is essential for nursing students to understand the importance of recognising, retrieving and using high-quality evidence to underpin their clinical decision-making. This chapter introduces the notion of evidence-based practice, with specific reference to research and reflection as important sources of evidence. It offers clear strategies for finding and judging the quality of your evidence base and highlights the importance of correctly citing sources of evidence derived from the published literature.

CHAPTER SUMMARY

- Only evidence can tell us what is the most effective nursing care for each individual patient.
- There may not be theoretical or research evidence available to inform all of the decisions we need to make as nurses, either because the questions are not researchable or because they have not yet been researched.
- Using a range of evidence (observation, reflection, patient experience, theory/research) gives us the highest probability that we will deliver the best care for patients.
- As we rely on evidence to deliver best practice, it is critical for that evidence to be 'trustworthy'.
- Research is a systematic way of finding answers to questions. It is considered to provide the most reliable source of information to answer the clinical questions we generate.
- Reflection helps us to analyse our own observations or actions in a systematic and objective manner in order to produce evidence to underpin future practice.
- Understanding the value of different genres of literature and how they can inform academic writing will help you to select sources of information that are appropriate to the questions you seek to answer.
- Using databases of journal literature that can inform your academic work and clinical practice is more systematic and trustworthy than using the internet directly to source information.
- A good piece of academic work will provide enough information about sources of theoretical or research evidence for the reader of the work to retrieve those sources and check them against what has been submitted.

CRITICAL REFLECTION

Holistic care

- Consider which combined sources of evidence will help you to deliver the most effective holistic, person-centred nursing care or to demonstrate this approach in your academic work. What does each source contribute that is not addressed by the others?
- Reflect on your own approach to searching for information. How can the guidance provided in this chapter help you to improve the way you search for evidence to support your practice and written work?

GO FURTHER

Books

Ellis, P. (2016) *Evidence-based Practice in Nursing*, 3rd edn. Exeter: Learning Matters. This book provides a comprehensive overview of evidence-based practice in nursing, making it a valuable resource for students and registered nurses.

Harvey, M. and Land, L. (2017) *Research Methods for Nurses and Midwives: Theory and Practice*. London: SAGE. An excellent book, which provides a comprehensive and understandable introduction to research.

Howatson-Jones, L. (2016) *Reflective Practice in Nursing*, 3rd edn. London: SAGE/Learning Matters. This book will help you to understand the important role of reflective practice in nursing and provide guidance on how you can use reflection to inform and develop your own nursing practice.

SAGE journal articles

Go to https://study.sagepub.com/essentialnursing2e for free online journal articles for this chapter. If you are using the interactive ebook, simply click on the book icon in the margin to go straight to the resource.

FURTHER READING: JOURNAL ARTICLES

Lee, K. (2013) 'Student and infection prevention and control nurses' hand hygiene decision making in simulated clinical scenarios', *Journal of Infection Prevention*, 14(3): 96–103. A research paper investigating how student and registered nurses apply research findings in their clinical decision-making.

Moule, P., Ward, R. and Lockyer, L. (2011) 'Issues with e-learning in nusing and health education in the UK: Are new technologies being embraced in the teaching and learning environments?', *Journal of Research in Nursing*, 16(1): 77–90. An article highlighting a study focusing on the implementation of e-learning in nursing and health science disciplines throughout the UK.

Rew, L. (2012) 'From course assignment paper to publishable manuscript', *Journal of Holistic Nursing*, 30(4): 270–6. This article provides invaluable advice on how the papers you produce during your nursing course could also be published in nursing journals.

Solum, E., Maluwa, V. and Severinsson, E. (2012) 'Ethical problems in practice as experienced by Malawian student nurses', *Journal of Nursing Ethics*, 19(1): 128–38. An interesting article which uses nursing students' reflections on their experiences in practice as a focus for research.

Other journal articles

Armstrong, E.C. (2003) 'Harnessing new technologies while preserving basic values', *Families, Systems and Health*, 21(4): 35–55.

Farrington, N. and Townsend, K. (2014) 'Enhancing nurse–patient communication: a critical reflection', *British Journal of Nursing*, 23(14): 771–775. This article provides insight into how to write a critical reflection and the value of using critical reflection to consider practice problems faced in clinical practice.

Weblinks

FURTHER
READING:
WEBLINKS

Go to https://study.sagepub.com/essentialnursing2e for weblinks related to this chapter. If you are using the interactive ebook, simply click on the book icon in the margin to go straight to the resource.

www.nmc-uk.org/Documents/NMC-Publications/revised-new-NMC-Code.pdf – a direct link to the part of the UK Nursing and Midwifery Council Code of Conduct that highlights the importance of evidence-based nursing practice.

www.rcn.org.uk/professional-development/quality-and-safety/evidence-based-practice – an RCN evidence-based practice resource, providing links to valuable information and including regular evidence-based practice updates.

www.cochrane.org – an international network dedicated to providing high-quality evidence about the effectiveness of care interventions for all those involved in healthcare, through 'Cochrane Reviews'.

www.evidence.nhs.uk – NICE Evidence Services provide internet access to high-quality evidence and guidance for the delivery of best practice in health and social care.

http://rcni.com – *Nursing Standard* section on reflective practice, with links to related articles.

Video links

VIDEO
LINK

Have a break from the text and go to https://study.sagepub.com/essentialnursing2e for useful videos related to this chapter. If you are using the interactive ebook, simply click on the lightbulb icon in the margin to go straight to the resource.

ACE YOUR ASSESSMENT

ONLINE
QUIZZES

Review what you have learned by visiting the book's online resources at: https://study.sagepub.com/essential nursing2e If using your interactive ebook, just click on the icon in the margin to go straight there.

- Test yourself with multiple-choice and short-answer questions.
- Revise key terms with the interactive flash cards.

REFERENCES

Borton, T. (1970) *Reach, Touch and Teach*. London: Hutchinson.

De Bono, E. (1996) *Teach Yourself to Think*. London: Penguin.

Driscoll J. (1994) 'Reflective practice for practise', *Senior Nurse*. 13(Jan/Feb): 47–50.

Florida State University (2013) Definition of Evidence-based Medicine. Available at: http://med.fsu.edu/index.cfm?page=medicalinformatics.ebmTutorial (accessed 22 November 2013).

Gibbs, G. (1988) *Learning by Doing: A Guide to Teaching and Learning Methods*. Oxford: Further Education Unit, Oxford Polytechnic.

Johns, C. (2009) *Becoming a Reflective Practitioner*, 3rd edn. Chichester: Wiley Blackwell.

Pears, R. and Shields, G. (2016) *Cite them Right: The Essential Referencing Guide*, 10th edn. Newcastle-upon-Tyne: Pear Tree Books.

Rolfe, G. (2010) 'Models and frameworks for critical reflection', in G. Rolfe, M. Jasper and D. Freshwater (eds), *Critical Reflection in Practice: Generating Knowledge for Care*, 2nd edn. Basingstoke: Palgrave Macmillan.

Rolfe, G., Jasper, M. and Freshwater, D. (eds) (2010) *Critical Reflection in Practice: Generating Knowledge for Care*, 2nd edn. Basingstoke: Palgrave Macmillan.

Schön, D. (1994) *The Reflective Practitioner: How Professionals Think in Action*. London: Ashgate.

ACADEMIC WRITING AND ASSESSMENT SKILLS

4

GABRIELLE THORPE

--- **THIS CHAPTER COVERS** ---

- Academic writing
- Assessment skills

- Academic support

> I suppose I had always viewed writing as something I did to pass my course. I didn't realise how much I would continue to use the writing skills I have developed in my work as a registered nurse. Since I qualified, I have been involved in writing patient information, the annual report for our service, a student workbook on diabetes and a number of letters to other healthcare professionals. It's good to know that this is a skill that I will carry on developing as I practise.
>
> **Rachel, registered nurse, LD community services**

> Proofreading will prevent you losing marks. After you have read over your essay a hundred times, and you will, I think the small things get missed. Sometimes leaving it a few days and going back with fresh eyes or getting someone else to read it for you will pick up silly mistakes. Adhering to the word limit keeps you focused and ensures you bring together the important elements of your essay. The word count prevents you 'waffling on' and helps you to cut out what is irrelevant. I think it is always best to be organised and in front than behind. It will prevent your work being panicked and rushed.
>
> **Siân Hunter, child nursing student**

Visit https://study.sagepub.com/essentialnursing2e to access a wealth of online resources for this chapter – watch out for the margin icons throughout the chapter. If you are using the interactive eBook, simply click on the margin icon to go straight to the resource.

INTRODUCTION

Achieving a style and tone of writing that convey your knowledge, professionalism, experience and understanding, and demonstrate your ability to apply evidence appropriately is critical to effective nursing practice. The style and content of any piece of writing will depend on its aim and intended readership. For example, we have written this chapter in a style that addresses you, the student, directly. We have used a limited number of references and have aimed to give you a basic understanding of the subjects covered. In most of your own academic work, however, you will be expected to take a more formal and analytical approach. Like Rachel, over the course of your studies you will develop a range of writing skills that you will continue to use throughout your nursing career.

ACADEMIC WRITING

Good academic writing does not need to include long words and complicated sentences; the most important aspects are logical flow, clear discussion and the thoughtful selection of vocabulary to convey exact meaning. In nursing, academic writing is not just about demonstrating understanding; it must also demonstrate an ability to reflect on, and apply theory to, practice.

You will be expected to submit written assignments in a number of different formats. These might include reflective pieces, essay assignments, problem-based learning, practice-based assessments, presentations and dissertations. The mode of submission may vary from hard copy submission through to entirely online submission, making use of the technologies briefly mentioned in the previous chapter. Making an effort to master academic writing early in your nursing education will both make your assessment tasks easier and more successful, and facilitate your transition from student to qualified nurse. Academic writing is a skill to be developed and practice makes perfect. What follows in this chapter lends itself to essay writing or reflective writing, which together will form the majority of the assessed writing tasks you will be required to undertake.

ACTIVITY 4.1: REFLECTIVE PRACTICE

Look at various types of writing (for example, newspaper, magazine, journal, textbook) and reflect on how they are written. Are they written in the first person or do they use a style that is more removed? Are they formal or informal in tone? Why are they adopting a specific style? Who are they writing for? Where are they being published: hard copy, online or both?

What difference does this make to how you read them? It is important to understand that different styles are needed in different circumstances and to consider this in your own writing.

Preparation

The key to preparing for a written assignment is to read and understand the assessment guidelines. Take time to consider how you can best meet the aims and objectives of the work in light of the experiences you may have had in practice and any other guidance provided. If you are clear right at the outset about how to tackle the task successfully, there is less risk of having to change your tactics later. This is also a good time to reflect on any feedback that you may have received from previous assessments – consider how you can emulate a successful writing approach, or avoid making mistakes that cost you marks previously. Reading around the subject and reflecting on the care you have delivered to patients with similar nursing needs will help you to decide on the key areas to be explored and will probably form the basis for the content of the main body of the assignment. Having decided what you wish to write about and sourced appropriate evidence to support your work, it is time to start putting pen to paper, but not to write the whole thing – rather, to write a 'plan'. Planning your work can help to ensure that you address the key learning outcomes and arrange them in a way that flows logically from one paragraph to the next. Planning should also include consideration of the time frame for the assignment: be aware of, and work to, the deadline.

Writing is a very important skill needed in nursing, as well as attention to detail – when writing notes and care plans, all vital information needs to be recorded; however, all nursing documents need to remain factual and truthful. You must make your writing clear so that others can read it and it has to be logical and follow a path. I always found jotting things down on handover sheets helpful to make sure I didn't miss anything when I completed their daily care plan at the end of a shift. Bullet-point what you want to write, then expand at a later date when you have more time.

Sarah Parkes, LD nursing student

Finding your voice

A common misunderstanding is that the most important part of academic writing in nursing is the evidence used to support your developing discussion and arguments. It is not. What your markers or examiners wish to hear in your writing is *your* voice: that is, your arguments that are *supported by* appropriate evidence. This is an important distinction. Owning your arguments and incorporating personal reflection on how your understanding of theory can inform your practice will not only demonstrate to your reader that you understand the important issues at stake and are familiar with the evidence relating to them, but also show that you can use this knowledge to inform your own clinical decision-making.

For this reason, you are discouraged from using large sections of quoted text or listing everything that each article you have read says about a topic. Putting what you have learned into your own words (this is called paraphrasing) and integrating evidence and reflections into your own arguments demonstrate a depth of understanding and an ownership of your work, highlighting your ability to apply theory to your own practice. Incorporating personal reflections on your care experiences will also address issues of applying theory to practice. However, your personal reflections and experiences should be relevant to the issues you are exploring – there is a big difference between critical reflection on practice and writing that has a merely narrative or anecdotal flavour. Consider carefully when to use 'I', and only use it when you can see it is appropriate, as too much 'I' and 'my' will detract from the academic tone of your work. Finding this balance can take time, so try to start reflective writing early in the course – this will help you to develop a reflective style of your own that is effective in helping you to learn from your experiences. Your personal advisor can provide valuable feedback, suggesting improvements to structure and technique.

Some types of writing do not require first-person expression. For example, in critiquing a research study, compiling a service improvement report, writing up patient documentation or discussing anatomy and physiology. Your own feelings and experiences are not relevant, and so you should avoid writing in the first person.

Introducing your work

Before you start, be clear about the aim or purpose of your essay. For some essay assignments, you might be given a very clear question or topic that you are expected to address, but for others (especially longer pieces of work, including dissertations) you may be given more scope to choose your own focus. In this case, it is helpful to ask: 'What is the question I am trying to answer in this essay?' or 'What is the problem I am trying to solve?'

A good introduction to any theoretical or practice-based assignment or reflection will contain some common features:

- Provide the aim or purpose of your assignment in your own words.
- If your assignment is focused on a specific patient, outline the characteristics and circumstances of that person, along with their clinical presentation and context of care.
- Introduce and explain any theoretical model, concept or framework that is going to underpin your assignment.
- Define any key terms that will be used.
- State how you have dealt with any ethical issues, including consent from, and the confidentiality of, your patient.
- Outline the structure of your assignment.
- Use reflection when introducing your work to explain your personal rationale for choosing to focus on a particular topic or patient.

Logical flow

A strong piece of written work starts by clearly setting out its intentions and then takes the reader on a 'journey' through the work in a logical and coherent way. It is difficult to read a piece of work if it is not clear why something is being discussed, or how it relates either to the original aims set out in the introduction or to the paragraphs around it. There are a number of useful tricks that can help you to achieve logical flow in your writing:

Structure – Presenting your ideas in a logical sequence is central to achieving logical flow. Making decisions about when you introduce certain parts of your discussion should start with your plan, although allow yourself the option to change your mind as you write!

Even though you may not use many (or any) headings in your finished work, it can be helpful to use them in drafts to help with structure. For example, in a piece of reflective writing, using headings such as 'What?', 'So what?' and 'Now what?' (Borton, 1970) helps to ensure that your experience has been 'thought through', not merely described.

Remember that accurate punctuation and grammar are essential to achieving flow in the structure of your writing.

Signposting – This refers to summarising distinct features of what you are about to say or what you have just said and drawing attention to how they relate to each other, the whole assignment's aim or the next section of work. Signposting helps the reader to understand the reasons behind the structure of your work, to gain a picture of the work as a whole and to know where you are taking them. It should start in the introduction and continue throughout the work (see Figures 4.1 and 4.2).

This passage comes at the end of the introduction to the paper, where the aims, objectives and contextual information about the patient and their condition have already been discussed.

Stoma-forming surgery for ulcerative colitis during childhood involves physical changes to appearance and bodily function, the development of competence in self-care, psychological adjustment, social adaptation and potential challenges in family relationships and friendship groups.

The purpose of this sentence is to signpost the issues the literature says patients are likely to experience.

These issues will be explored in relation to James' experience, current best evidence and the nursing care he required.

The purpose of this part-sentence is to tell the reader what is going to be discussed.

Starting with bodily change as the 'lynch pin' of the whole experience.

The purpose of this is to say what is coming next and that it is the most important issue.

Figure 4.1   An example of effective signposting

Firstly... secondly... thirdly... moving on now to...

as stated previously... similarly... Furthermore... in contrast... Therefore... To summarise... In conclusion...

Figure 4.2   Good words to use when ... signposting

Shape

Consider the shape of an hourglass: broad at the top, narrow in the middle and broad at the bottom (Figure 4.3). This can be a useful analogy for achieving logical flow in your writing. Start with a broad introduction, providing an overview of the overall aim of the work and contextual information about the area or experience to be explored and any theoretical frameworks to be used. Then provide a detailed (narrow) exploration of the issue or patient care you seek to explore. Re-widening your discussion in your conclusion demonstrates how the work you have done can inform both your clinical practice with other patients and your understanding of the wider context of nursing as a profession.

Using and constructing paragraphs – Paragraphs are the backbone of any piece of writing and central to achieving logical flow. As a rule of thumb, you should use one paragraph to discuss one point, although it may take several paragraphs to develop a central argument in your work. Consider starting a paragraph with a 'theme sentence' that indicates what that paragraph is going to be all about. Use signposting or 'linking' between paragraphs to help highlight how the points you are exploring relate to each other. See the worked example in Table 4.1 to gain an idea of how this could be done.

Breadth versus depth – When faced with a mountain of literature about your broad topic area, it can be difficult to decide whether you should use your word limit to show how much you know about the whole subject or focus on fewer points in more detail. This really depends on the aims and objectives of the assessment or work. Sometimes students can address both by demonstrating their understanding of the breadth of a subject in their introductory contextual overview, and then selecting (with justification) a smaller number of key areas to focus on in the main body. Your personal advisor will be able to guide you regarding this.

Critical analysis – The word 'analysis' means breaking ideas, concepts or problems down into their component parts, clearly distinguishing between things that differ, setting out the logical steps in an argument or identifying the key elements in a complex concept or problem. The word 'critical' has to do with exercising informed judgement and perceiving the strengths and weaknesses of an argument or a piece of evidence.

Figure 4.3 An hourglass

Table 4.1 Using PEAN to structure paragraph writing

A useful acronym to bear in mind when writing paragraphs relating to practice, as in a case study, is PEAN: Point – Evidence – Apply – Nursing. For example, the following is a paragraph discussing how your patient, Michael, developed acute depression following stroke.

POINT	State the point you wish to make clearly and succinctly at the start of the paragraph.
	Depression can progress from an acute problem following stroke into a longer-term issue and attempting to minimise the possibility of this was an important part of Michael's community nursing care plan.
EVIDENCE	Explore the point using appropriate evidence:
	Depression lasting longer than x weeks is classed as chronic or long-term depression (ref). Two recent studies found that up to x% of people following cerebral infarction of this nature can experience depression for longer than x weeks following their initial presentation (refs), highlighting this as a significant risk for Michael.
APPLY	Demonstrate how the evidence can be applied to the individual patient you are discussing:
	Key pre-disposing factors for chronic depression following stroke are a, b and c (ref) and as Michael had experienced a and c during the time I was caring for him, addressing this was an essential part of his care at that time, as was seen in his attempts to … while c became evident when he discussed his feelings about …
NURSING	Show what evidence-based nursing care is indicated for this person as a result of the information presented and why, and evaluate any care that was actually undertaken:
	A number of nursing interventions could address this potential problem. 'Ref' identified the positive impact of x intervention to reduce the risk of chronic depression in people already experiencing acute depression following a stroke. This could be incorporated easily into Michael's care. Encouragement to incorporate x and y activities could also benefit Michael, as participants with a similar presentation were shown to respond positively to these activities in a large study of psychological adaptation following a stroke in 158 men aged 40-70 (ref). As Michael had already responded well to x intervention, this could be continued with the consent of his GP and reviewed again in one month. I was mindful that routine nursing support was to reduce for Michael and felt that these interventions would provide both alternative avenues of support and regular contact with the healthcare system if required.

Table 4.2   Good words to use for …
critical analysis

'the main purpose was to …'

'the reason for this is …'

'this is important/relevant because …'

'one strength/weakness of this study is …'

'comparing this with …'

'it follows/this suggests that …'

'the effectiveness could be evaluated by …'

'Critical analysis', then, is the ability to show in your writing how the evidence you have considered and evaluated in preparing for your written work has informed or challenged your understanding of the issues under discussion and can (or cannot) be applied to the nursing care of a given individual/patient group. It is much easier to include critical analysis in your writing if you adopt critical thinking and reasoning in your engagement with nursing theory and academic and professional practice. Price and Harrington (2016: 13) explore critical thinking as a process 'where different information is gathered, sifted, synthesised and evaluated in order to understand a subject or issue', highlighting the importance of this skill at all stages of the nursing process and in interprofessional team working. See Table 4.2 for good words to use when using critical analysis.

Synthesis – This is the skill – or art! – of putting ideas together and making interpretations. It is relatively simple to demonstrate that you have read well around the topic area of your assignment. It is more difficult to show explicitly through your writing how the literature you cite informs your knowledge and understanding of the patient in your case study or the nursing care you implemented or suggest for them. More difficult still is to explain how you have compared and contrasted different strands of literature to *build* your understanding of your patient and their care and to make new interpretations drawn from your considerations of the evidence. Accomplishing this advanced academic writing skill will not only drastically improve the logical flow of your work, but will also demonstrate your ability to critically explore and analyse the evidence to inform your clinical practice. You must master the art of synthesis if you are aiming for a first-class honours degree.

Written expression

An additional aspect of academic writing to consider is written expression. In addition to the advice already given, further areas for you to consider are:

Precision – Precision refers to finding exactly the right word(s) to convey meaning. Common errors include using a word that sounds similar to the one you want but means something completely different ('papillary' instead of 'pupillary', for example) and using a word that means something similar but misses the exact meaning you wish to express. Listen to the voice in your head that says 'that doesn't sound quite right' or 'I'm not really sure what that word means', and always have a dictionary and thesaurus nearby to help you find the words you need.

Clarity – While it is important to find the right words to convey meaning, persistently choosing long and complex words when there is a simpler way to express meaning will make your work difficult to read and understand. It is hard enough to write an assignment; trying to write it in a voice that is not your own because it sounds 'more academic' will confuse both you and your reader. Keep it simple. Your assessors will readily detect when you are being 'pseudo-intellectual'!

Writing style – Students are often told that their writing is 'too descriptive'. But what does this mean? Defined simply, descriptive writing answers the question 'what?' but neglects other questions such as 'how?', 'why?', 'so what?' and 'now what?' In academic work, descriptive writing not only uses more words than is necessary, but also makes it more difficult to see the point being made. Here are some useful tips for avoiding descriptive writing:

- Express the point you wish to make succinctly in the first line of each paragraph.
- Write with an active rather than a passive voice. In active writing, the subject is near the start of the sentence, closely followed by a strong verb; in passive writing, the subject is often 'buried' and the verb tends to be weaker. For example, compare 'Mark complained that the compression stockings were uncomfortable' (active) with 'the compression stockings made Mark feel uncomfortable' (passive).
- Compare and contrast the different sources you are using.
- Avoid repetition – have you made the same point twice using different words? Can you combine these sentences?
- Keep sentences to two lines long or fewer – three lines at the most.
- Ask someone to proofread your work and leave sufficient time to refine it.
- Look at the balance of your work. Is one section longer than the others? This might suggest descriptive writing and/or that you have drifted away from the point!
- Are you still answering the assignment question? Use your assignment plan to keep to the point. Ensure any new material is relevant to the assignment's aim.

Nuanced expression – When evaluating evidence, be sparing in your use of strong expressions such as 'proof'. It is much more likely that research provides 'some evidence', 'strong evidence' or even 'convincing evidence'. When discussing your patient, be careful with words such as 'must', 'should', 'ought'. These words suggest little flexibility in either care decisions or patient experience. Try to use more subtle expression in your writing with words, such as 'could'/'can', 'might'/'may', 'suggests', 'it is likely that', and so on. And be careful to distinguish between *fact* and *interpretation*: don't just say 'the patient was very upset'; explain what the patient said or did that led you to believe that she was 'very upset'.

Concluding your work

Your conclusion has the power to leave your reader either with an emphatic understanding of the importance and meaning of your critical discussion *or* feeling underwhelmed by the inadequate drawing together of the strands of the arguments you have been presenting. Don't just re-describe what you have covered without any deeper analysis of the meaning or consideration of the application to practice. Use reflection in your conclusion to summarise what you have personally learned from studying this particular topic or patient. Nowhere must the theory/practice relationship be more explicit than in your conclusion.

ACTIVITY 4.2: REFLECTIVE PRACTICE

Reflect on the best way to write a conclusion. Take a step back from a piece of written work you have recently produced and ask yourself: What is the meaning of this work? How has it helped me to understand this patient or subject better? What can I take from this to inform my nursing practice? How does this impact on my understanding of nursing as a profession? What other questions does it compel me to ask and to answer?

These are the issues you need to include in your conclusion.

Before submission

Proofreading

Planning your writing to incorporate time to refine your work could be the difference between an adequate and an excellent mark. Here are some suggestions for how you can do this:

- Proofread your work carefully: read and re-read it to identify and correct typographic errors, long and convoluted sentences, ill-defined terms, lack of logical flow and poor written expression. A simple spelling or grammar check on your computer will not do all this work for you (it will not, for example, distinguish between 'there' and 'their').
- Students often ask whether it is permissible to get someone else to proofread their work. You should check your own university's policy on this. Typically, you will find that you are permitted to have someone else (but not a fellow student) check your work's spelling, grammar and punctuation, but not make or suggest substantive changes to the content.
- Read your work out loud to yourself to identify any sentences or paragraphs that do not make sense. If you stumble over sentences or lose the sense of what you are saying, then you may need to refine your writing.
- If you find it difficult to focus on more than one thing, then read your work through several times with a different 'hat' on each time: for example, looking at punctuation, spelling, long sentences, logical flow and written expression separately.

Word allowances

You may be given a word limit for a written piece of work, probably including everything in the body of your essay, but excluding your list of references and appendices. If you exceed this limit, you may be penalised. It is easy to check the number of words you have written using your computer: simply highlight the text that you wish to measure and the computer will give you the word count. Most universities will expect you to state the word count on your submission sheet and/or submit an electronic copy of the assessment, so they can check this easily.

There is more to academic writing than words on paper. There has to be a theme, structure and plan; there is a word count that has to be considered and a deadline. I work best when I write a plan, factoring in the deadline and make sure I allow time for proofreading. Feedback from my personal advisor about how my writing is coming on and advice on whether any changes need to be made can be really useful.
I allow plenty of time for proofreading and printing before handing it in.

Sarah Parkes, LD nursing student

Timing

If you don't adhere to the published submission deadline, you can expect to be penalised. However, most universities have processes in place for applying for an extension under certain (limited) circumstances. If you realise that there is a significant reason why you might not meet the deadline, for example due to ill health or personal crisis, arrange as early as possible to apply for an extension to the submission deadline.

ASSESSMENT SKILLS

We have focused so far on academic writing skills for tasks such as essay assignments. However, you will probably be set a wider range of assessment tasks, such as exams, Objective Structured Clinical Examinations (OSCE's), presentations and assessments of practice. If you understand the nature and purpose of each of these, you will increase your chances of success, so it is essential that you are familiar with and understand the guidance provided for you, both at the start of your degree programme and in preparation for specific assessment tasks.

ACTIVITY 4.3: REFLECTIVE PRACTICE

Familiarise yourself with your own module, field and course handbooks to ensure that you understand how assessments are planned and undertaken at your own university. What different types of assessment will you be required to undertake over the duration of your course?

Rules and criteria underpinning assessment

Formative and summative assessments

You will experience both **formative** and **summative** assessments on your course.

Formative assessments are those that give you and your lecturer feedback on your progress. Examples would include: a quiz set at the end of a lecture; a workbook that you complete over a period of time and then receive feedback on from the lecturer; feedback from a facilitator on your contribution to a problem-based learning session; and a meeting with your practice educator part way through a period of practice-based learning in order to determine if you are 'on target' to meet the required learning outcomes.

Summative assessments are those that have to be passed in order for you to progress on the course and complete it successfully. Examples include written exams, essay assignments, dissertations, Objective Structured Clinical Examinations (OSCEs), portfolios and assessments of practice.

Pass marks; number of attempts; marking criteria

Some of your work may be assessed on a pass/fail basis. Other work will be given a grade. Familiarise yourself with the criteria against which your work will be assessed, and with the marking schemes that will be used for grading purposes, to understand how your university translates these grades into the classification of your final award (see Table 4.3).

Your university will have regulations governing various aspects of your course, including the number of assessment attempts you will be allowed. You may find that you are allowed up to two attempts at any given piece of work. If you do need to prepare for reassessment, make sure that you take careful note of the marker's feedback and contact your personal advisor in order to agree an action plan.

Table 4.3   What you need to know for any summative assessment

Will the work be graded, or assessed on a pass/fail basis?

What are the criteria against which the work will be assessed?

How many attempts are allowed?

What are the method and timescale for receiving feedback on my work?

Submitting your work

Your work may need to be submitted electronically or handed in as a hard copy. Make sure you find out both how you should submit your work and when it is due to be submitted by. Universities are increasingly moving to electronic submission for assessment, so they are able to use text-matching software to ensure that the work you hand in is your own and has not been copied from other sources.

Portfolios

A portfolio is a record of your academic and clinical progress, and a compilation of your evidence of learning and achievement. Compiling a comprehensive portfolio is more than an assessment task, it is a lifelong learning skill that your degree programme enables you to develop as you begin your professional career pathway. Your professional portfolio may or may not be formally assessed during your degree programme, but it will provide the vast majority of material required to complete your sign-off assessment at the end of the course. Keeping your portfolio(s) organised and up-to-date, therefore, will make the sign-off process far more straightforward and stress-free than it might otherwise be. Nurses must also go through a process of 'revalidation' with the NMC every three years, which requires a portfolio of evidence to be assessed by a second qualified nurse and confirmed by them that it meets the NMC standards. Understanding what is involved in compiling a portfolio during your degree programme will make the process of revalidation much easier when you become a registered nurse. See Table 4.4 for what you might include in a portfolio.

When arranging the material in your portfolio, remember **CORE** (below) and make sure that you read and follow the portfolio guidelines you are given by your university:

- **C**omplete – all the required elements are present.
- **O**rganised – with a contents page, and logical arrangement of the material (each of the main entries should have a title and a date).
- **R**elevant – not containing redundant or surplus material.
- **E**vidence-based – you are linking theory and practice on a regular basis and referencing appropriately.

In the first year I did not compile my portfolio until the last term. It was a big mistake! Keep your portfolio up to date as you go along, adding anything that has been pertinent to your learning experience. I found it particularly helpful reviewing my portfolio at the end of each term to reflect on what I had learned over the term.

Alice Rowe, NQ RNMH

Table 4.4   Portfolio content

A portfolio may include ...

- Critical incident analyses – structured reflective pieces on situations or experiences that have had particular significance for you
- Copies of the written work you have submitted for summative assessment, along with the markers' feedback
- Copies of your practice assessments, together with any written supporting evidence
- Reflection on your overall progress during the course
- A record of contact with your personal advisor, along with a summary of the main issues discussed and the main decisions agreed
- A record of your attendance, together with plans to address any shortfalls or other concerns

ACADEMIC SUPPORT

You will be allocated a member of the teaching staff from your university who can offer you support and advice. Different universities use slightly different names to refer to this person: they may be known as your personal tutor, personal advisor or academic advisor, for example. Issues you might discuss with them could include academic work, sharing practice experiences and reflecting on them and understanding the student support systems available in the university. It would be useful to find out about the additional information and help that are available in areas such as note taking, essay writing, revision technique, referencing and plagiarism awareness. Other help will be available to specific groups, for instance students with specific learning difficulties – such as dyslexia – and students for whom English is an additional language.

Mitigating factors

From time to time, a student's progress can be adversely affected by circumstances outside their control, such as illness (your own or that of a close relative) or bereavement. Your university is likely to have a process whereby such circumstances can be declared by the student (along with supporting evidence) and then considered in conjunction with any assessed work that was being undertaken at the time. Although it is unlikely that the actual result of the assessment would be changed, one possible outcome might be that the assessment attempt is 'voided', allowing you to re-take the assessment as if it were your first attempt.

Academic appeals

Your university will also have a policy and procedure whereby any concerns you may have about the assessment of your work can be investigated. Those concerns may be to do with mitigating circumstances, inadequate assessment or even possible prejudice or bias. If your appeal is upheld, this may lead to a change in the mark or grade or to a 'voiding' of that assessment attempt, enabling you to make a further attempt.

If you were considering submitting an appeal, you would need to think about: the nature of your concerns; what information or evidence you can provide to support these concerns; who you might approach for support and advice; and the timescale for submitting an appeal.

Apply what you have learned about submitting assignments and academic support by reading the case study on Josh's assignment at https://study.sagepub.com/essentialnursing2e.

CASE STUDY:
JOSH'S
ASSIGNMENT

CONCLUSION

Developing a clear and professional style of academic writing is not only the cornerstone of good academic practice, it can also help develop skills to use after you qualify. Nursing requires a wide range of written communication tasks, all with a different voice and style: record-keeping, letter-writing and report-writing tend to require an objective, formal style; written patient information needs to be more friendly and direct; presentations, handovers and patient documentation require a clear, evidence-based approach to articulate the rationale behind your clinical decision-making. Continuous professional development (CPD) and lifelong learning are an integral part of nursing practice today; having mastered academic writing, you can face them with confidence and the expectation of further academic and professional progression.

CHAPTER SUMMARY

- Academic writing is not just about demonstrating understanding; it must also demonstrate an ability to reflect on, and apply theory to, practice.
- Owning your arguments and incorporating personal reflection into how your understanding of theory can inform your practice demonstrate that you understand the important issues at stake, are familiar with the evidence relating to them and can use this knowledge to inform your decision-making in practice.
- A strong piece of written work starts by clearly setting out its intentions and then takes the reader on a 'journey' through the work in a logical and coherent way.
- A useful acronym to bear in mind when writing paragraphs relating to practice, as in a case study, is PEAN: Point – Evidence – Apply – Nursing.
- Familiarise yourself with the criteria against which your work will be assessed, and with the marking schemes that will be used for grading purposes.
- Ensure you understand the sources of support available to you and use these to help you during your course.

CRITICAL REFLECTION

Holistic care

- How will you demonstrate a holistic, person-centred approach to care in your academic writing?
- Reflect on your own writing style. How many of the features of academic writing highlighted throughout the chapter do you incorporate into your writing? Which would be easy to do and which might take a bit more thought and practice?

GO FURTHER

Books

Price, B. and Harrington, A. (2016) *Critical Thinking and Writing for Nursing Students*, 3rd edn. Exeter: Learning Matters. This book will assist you to think critically and reflect on experience, and translate this into your written assessments.

Reed, S. (2015) *Successful Professional Portfolios for Nursing Students*, 2nd edn. Exeter: Learning Matters. This book not only provides a comprehensive overview of portfolios for nursing students but is also a valuable resource for registered nurses.

Journal articles

Bailey, A., Zanchetta, M., Velasco, D., Pon, G., & Hassan, A. (2015) 'Building a scholar in writing (BSW): a model for developing students' critical writing skills', *Nurse Education in Practice*, 15:524–529. This article outlines a model for developing academic writing skills in nursing, breaking down the individual skills of critical thinking and writing into understandable steps applicable to health sciences students.

Hunker, D.F., Gazza, E. A. and Shellenbarger, T. (2014) 'Evidence-based knowledge, skills, and attitudes for scholarly writing development across all levels of nursing education', *Journal of Professional Nursing*, 30(4): 341–346. This paper provides a comparison of the knowledge, skills and attitudes required for academic success at different levels of nursing education.

Jeffries, D., McNally, S., Roberts, K., Wallace, A., Stunden, A. D'Souza, S. and Glew, P. (2018) 'The importance of academic literacy for undergraduate nursing students and its relationship to future professional clinical practice: a systematic review', *Nurse Education Today*, 60: 84–91. This research study highlights some key factors that influence academic success in nursing students and the relationship between academic writing and critical thinking in clinical practice.

Weblinks

FURTHER
READING:
WEBLINKS

Go to https://study.sagepub.com/essentialnursing2e for weblinks related to this chapter. If you are using the interactive ebook, simply click on the book icon in the margin to go straight to the resource.

Royal College of Nursing: www.rcn.org.uk/students
The RCN student community, offering support for your studies.

Nursing Standard journal website: https://rcni.com/nursing-standard/students/nursing-studies
Advice and information for student nurses on a range of academic skills.

Nursing Times journal website: www.nursingtimes.net/students
Links and guidance for students on a range of academic issues, among others.

All Nurses student support pages: http://allnurses.com/nursing-student/
Links and guidance for nursing students on a range of issues, some academic.

Video links

VIDEO
LINKS

Have a break from the text and go to https://study.sagepub.com/essentialnursing2e for useful videos related to this chapter. If you are using the interactive ebook, simply click on the lightbulb icon in the margin to go straight to the resource.

ACE YOUR ASSESSMENT

Review what you have learned by visiting the book's online resources at: https://study.sagepub.com/essential nursing2e If using your interactive ebook, just click on the icon in the margin to go straight there.

ONLINE
QUIZZES

- Test yourself with multiple-choice and short-answer questions.
- Revise key terms with the interactive flash cards.

REFERENCES

Borton, T. (1970) *Reach, Touch and Teach*. London: Hutchinson.

Price, B. and Harrington, A. (2016) *Critical Thinking and Writing for Nursing Students*, 3rd edn. Exeter: Learning Matters.

PROFESSIONAL PRACTICE

B

The aim of this part of the book is to introduce you to the fundamental professional skills you will need to develop during your time as a nursing student. These skills are extremely important and will underpin all aspects of your life, not only when you are caring for patients but also when you are at home, socialising with friends or shopping at the local supermarket.

In nursing, professional skills lie under the surface of all aspects of the care we deliver, whether this is giving an injection, talking through a person's history or care plan or supporting a parent to provide the special care their child needs. Some of these professional skills are quite rightly enshrined in law or in professional documents such as the NMC standards or Code, and therefore knowing and abiding by them is an essential, and often legal, requirement for practice. Failure to abide by a professional code or the law could result in a fitness to practise hearing or a court case, and while this thought is scary, it is more important to make sure you think about why these professional and legal requirements exist.

This part of the book covers law, ethics, accountability and professionalism; highlighting why legal, ethical and professional requirements are so important. Many of the qualities that patients value most highly relate to these fundamental areas, so you need to understand them. As Karl reminds us, we need to ensure we are professional in all our actions, and as Julie points out, 'switching off' is not an effective coping strategy. This is why it is important to have a clear understanding of how you can become a resilient nurse, to ensure you are able to fully engage in the care you deliver.

In nursing, the emphasis is on not just following rules, but also on thinking about why those rules need to be followed. This is a crucial factor in ensuring patients always receive the best care possible, as are being resilient and understanding not only how to change practice but also why the process of changing practice is everybody's responsibility. The voices in this part opener highlight the importance of these issues – read them and keep them in mind as you work through the chapters in this second part of the book.

ETHICS

RUTH NORTHWAY AND IAN BEECH

5

--- THIS CHAPTER COVERS ---

- What do we mean by ethics?
- The importance of values
- Ethical theories

- Ethical principles
- Ethical decision-making

I am John, I am 18 years old and I have been told I have a moderate learning disability and I am on the autistic spectrum. This means that I can find it difficult to relate to other people and often get disturbed by busy places with a lot of noise. Last week I fell and broke my wrist, which meant I had to go to hospital, but when I got there it was really noisy and people were rushing about all over the place. My dad asked them if there was somewhere quiet I could wait and explained about my autism but they said I would have to go to the waiting area with everyone else. By the time it was my turn to be seen I couldn't cope anymore, I was in a lot of pain and I hit out at the doctor when he tried to look at my wrist. He said that unless I could cooperate he couldn't do anything. My dad mentioned that if it had been possible for me to wait in a quiet area I would have been OK. The doctor said that they couldn't give one patient preferential treatment.

John, patient

Over the past week I have built up a really good relationship with one of the patients on the ward. She is in hospital due to depression and was very withdrawn but over the past week her mood has lifted. This afternoon she confided in me that she feels she wants to kill herself as she can see no purpose in her life, but she then went on to say that she had told me in confidence and that I must not tell anyone. I wanted to respect her confidentiality but I know there are times when this is not possible: this seemed to be one of them. However, I worried that if I told someone it would ruin the relationship I had with her. I decided that I had to tell her I would have to discuss what she had told me with the nurse in charge. She became very angry with me and I still feel unsure as to whether I did the right thing or not.

Jocelyn, second-year MH nursing student

INTRODUCTION

In our day-to-day lives, we are often confronted with questions about what is right and wrong, good and bad. The same is true in our professional lives: as nurses, we question whether we are doing the 'right' thing for the people we support and whether the care we provide is 'good' or 'bad'. We may have made the decision to become a nurse as we felt the values that underpin the profession reflect our personal value base and yet find that the reality of practice challenges those values. Ethics is concerned with such issues and, by providing us with frameworks to help us analyse situations, it helps us to examine different explanations, consider different courses of action and provide a rationale for our decision-making and subsequent behaviour.

The importance of ethics to nursing can be seen in the fact that the NMC Code (2015) is a code of professional standards and ethics are integral to this. This chapter will therefore introduce you to some key ethical principles and approaches, helping you to recognise ethical dilemmas, and provide you with a framework to help you in ethical decision-making.

WHAT DO WE MEAN BY ETHICS?

People face dilemmas throughout their lives. However, dilemmas such as what to have for lunch are not ethical dilemmas. An ethical dilemma is one in which a person is faced with a decision about how to act based on what is considered to be right or wrong, or, as Rowson (2006) puts it, where a number of ethical principles apply, yet the principles make conflicting demands upon decision-makers. In both John's and Jocelyn's stories at the start of the chapter, a number of ethical questions arise:

- Is taking a particular approach to the care of one person giving that person some sort of preferential treatment?
- What balance should we try to achieve between following a policy and looking at the context?
- Should we act to try to bring about a good outcome, even if it means people other than John not having access to a quiet area?
- Is patient confidentiality more important than patient safety?

Seedhouse (2009) suggests that if we want to understand what ethics is, it is important to first understand what it is not. Although a strange starting point, this alerts us to the fact that ethics does not provide us with a single perspective as to what is right and what is wrong; instead, it involves considering issues from different perspectives. Indeed, it helps us to identify the questions we need to ask rather than providing clear answers. Weaver et al. (2008) regard nurses as needing to develop a sense of 'ethical sensitivity', which means acting with intelligence and compassion in situations of clinical uncertainty. Such sensitivity is based in the ability to draw on clinical experience, formal learning and ethical codes to anticipate the consequences of action, and to act.

Some might find the process of attaining ethical sensitivity difficult because they want clear rules as to what is 'right' or 'wrong'. Such rules would be neither possible nor desirable, as the 'best' decisions and actions will vary according to context. As a nursing student, it is not possible to learn exactly what to do in all situations, but it is possible to develop the knowledge and skills to be able to assess a situation, consider alternatives, weigh up the most appropriate course of action and evaluate the impact. Such an approach would help Jocelyn, in the student voice at the start of the chapter, decide whether she had taken the best possible course of action. Even the most experienced nurse is regularly challenged by ethical issues and continues to learn from them. Reading this chapter will be the first step of a journey that should continue throughout your career as a nurse.

Developing ethical sensitivity challenged the way I view people and helped me to break down social stereotypes I previously possessed. For instance as a nurse you may have to care for people who misuse drugs; developing ethical sensitivity will help you see past your own ethical opinions on drug use and aid you in seeing other perspectives, and this will ultimately improve the care provided to individual patients.

Charlie Clisby, NQN

There are different approaches to the study of ethics. For example, there is a field of study known as meta-ethics devoted to such problems as whether good, bad, right and wrong can even exist (Fisher, 2011). In the context of this chapter, however, we are concerned with what is sometimes referred to as 'applied ethics'. Thompson et al. (2006: 384) suggest that, in the context of nursing, this means 'being able to act responsibly, appropriately and effectively in various situations, and it also means being able to provide a clear, coherent and reasoned justification for one's decisions and actions with reference to commonly accepted standards'.

This definition reinforces the point made above, in that it highlights that nurses practise in a range of different situations but our behaviour is expected to be responsible, appropriate and effective, irrespective of the setting. Second, it introduces the importance of being able to provide a sound rationale for our decisions and actions (or non-actions). Finally, it suggests that in making our decisions we refer to 'commonly accepted standards' to decide what is appropriate. To begin your ethical journey, take some time to complete Activity 5.1.

ACTIVITY 5.1: DECISION-MAKING

Where do you think nurses might find the information and resources to tell us the 'commonly accepted standards' for our practice? Try to identify as many sources as possible.

ANSWER:
ACTIVITY 5.1

THE IMPORTANCE OF VALUES

Values are the ideas and beliefs that are important to us as individuals and may come from a variety of sources. Fry and Johnstone (2008: 210) have defined values as:

A standard or quality that is esteemed, desired, considered important or has worth or merit. Values are expressed by behaviours or standards that a person endorses or tries to maintain.

ACTIVITY 5.2: REFLECTIVE PRACTICE

- Take some time to try and identify some values that you feel are important to you and think about where you feel these values may have come from.
- Have your values changed over time? Compare yourself now with when you were 15 years old.

ANSWER:
ACTIVITY 5.2

It is important to recognise that two or more of our values may occasionally clash. For example, nurses working in forensic mental health or forensic learning disability settings who value supporting people with mental health problems, but condemn murder, may find themselves supporting someone who has killed another person. Also, nurses can experience a clash of values, where they feel that their duty is to provide the best possible care but organisational values emphasise financial concerns and remaining within budget. It can sometimes be tempting to sit back when values are challenged and take the path of least resistance. When a child clearly does not want to undergo a procedure but their parents agree it should go ahead, it is possible to think: 'I'll let this piece of practice that concerns me go this time because it hasn't done too much harm.' However, cumulative acts of this nature can easily lead to large-scale neglect or abuse, as seen in reports concerning failures in care (Francis, 2013).

It is important that we are also aware of times at which we may consider we are doing things for the 'right reason' from our perspective and value base, rather than from those of the person we are nursing. The Mental Capacity Act 2005 was enacted to ensure that adults are provided with the necessary support and information to reach their own decisions; where it is deemed they lack the capacity to do so, then a group of people who know them well are able to reach the required decision in the person's 'best interest'.

Reaching and making these decisions may again challenge our own ethical stance, given the need to respect the decisions of people assessed as having capacity, however 'unwise' we may consider them.

As individuals, we come to nursing with our own set of values, which will be a synthesis of the societal, community, religious and family influences that have shaped and socialised us during our developmental period and subsequent life experience. However, nursing brings us into contact with patients and colleagues who also have their own individual value bases. This means that we need to be aware of and regularly re-examine our personal values so that we can develop effective working relationships.

The experience of patients receiving healthcare may not reflect the same standards outlined within a relevant policy. Sometimes patients will still experience poor care despite the existence of up-to-date policies. When you are delivering care, ask patients whether they are happy with the services they are receiving, make sure you are aware of the relevant policies and ensure the care you are providing is evidence-based. This is fundamentally important and something you should always apply to your practice.

CASE STUDY 5.1: HARRY

Harry is 43 years old and is a third-year nursing student specialising in children's nursing. He is a family man and believes very strongly in the importance of children being brought up in a loving home with two parents. His own children have now grown up and he has decided that the time is right to fulfil a long-held dream to study nursing. He has recently commenced a placement working with a community children's nurse.

Today, they are going to see a new patient, 11-year-old Lucy. She has recently been discharged home following abdominal surgery and they are going to check the wound. She is understandably worried about having the dressing removed and Harry tries to involve her in conversation about what she likes doing with Mummy and Daddy. Lucy, however, looks confused and then says she doesn't have a mum, she has two dads. It is then Harry's turn to look confused, until he realises that her parents must be a gay couple. He finds this difficult to respond to, as he has always felt uncomfortable about homosexuality and doesn't really agree with gay couples bringing up children.

- Should Harry disclose his feelings to his practice educator?
- Should Harry be honest with Lucy and her parents about his feelings?

ETHICAL THEORIES

As nurses, we may find ourselves in situations where we have to make judgements when our values conflict. For example, we may value loyalty to colleagues and the care of vulnerable people: how do we then act when we see a colleague giving care that we consider to be below standard? Ethical analysis of situations can help clarify the questions that we should be asking in such situations. Two ethical theories help by asking us either to consider what the consequences of our actions will be or to consider whether the actions are right in themselves, regardless of the consequences (Sandel, 2010).

WHAT'S THE EVIDENCE?

FURTHER READING: RESPECT IN MENTAL HEALTH

Respect is a key part of nursing care. Cutcliffe and Travale (2013), in their article 'Respect in mental health', recognise that there is, unfortunately, occasionally a disconnect between policy and what actually occurs in practice. In their article, they present three case studies – on the use of seclusion, respecting professional boundaries, and horizontal workplace violence – to help present a forum which allows them to write and speak about respect in real-world contexts:

- Read the article and identify the role respect plays in these three cases.
- How is respect reflected in the NMC standards?
- What steps could you take to ensure you are being respectful of your patient's needs?

Consequentialism

The first of the theories we discuss, the consequentialist view, requires us to consider the likely consequences of an action before acting, and then to act in such a way as to produce a positive outcome. The philosopher Jeremy Bentham (1748–1832) believed that all human beings could agree that they desire happiness, and so actions could be judged on whether they maximised pleasure and minimised pain. He called this 'utility', leading to his philosophical approach becoming known as 'utilitarianism'. From a utilitarian perspective, a nurse faced with a dilemma should consider which action would create the greatest pleasure and least amount of pain for the most people, and act accordingly.

Utilitarianism

There are two major objections to utilitarianism. The first is that it does not take individual rights into account and fails to protect minorities (Sandel, 2010). Michael Burleigh (2002), for example, describes the involvement of nurses in the euthanasia of people with mental illnesses and learning disabilities in Germany in the 1930s and 1940s. This policy was promoted based on the argument that such minority groups were draining the resources of society while contributing little or nothing. A second objection is the difficulty of assigning some common numerical value – for example, a unit of happiness or worth – that can allow actions to be held up for comparison. Sandel (2010) offers an example of what happens when an attempt is made to do this by considering the example of the Philip Morris tobacco company, which commissioned a cost-benefit analysis for the Czech government on the effects of smoking. The analysis demonstrated that smoking was more financially beneficial for the government than smoking prevention. While smokers cost more in terms of healthcare for smoking-related diseases, they die at a younger age and so save on state pension payments and care for the elderly. In the face of these two objections, many people would argue that there are times when an action is simply wrong.

John Stuart Mill (1806–1873), Bentham's student, tried to rescue utilitarianism from the sort of objections discussed above. For Bentham, each individual act should be judged on the basis of its consequences. Mill attempted to develop a more rule-based approach in which a person should follow rules that, if kept, would create a greater degree of utility than if they were broken. So, he would encourage people to consider what sort of society would be created if there were a rule allowing nurses to engage in the deliberate killing of minorities, compared with a society that did not allow this. Having created a set of rules, it would be allowable, however, for exceptions to the rule to take place should greater utility be the result. An example of this might be that society benefits on the whole if everybody follows the rule that traffic should stop at a red traffic light; nevertheless, there may be single occasions when it would create a better consequence if that rule were to be broken, such as an ambulance going through a red light in order to help someone who has had a cardiac arrest.

While this later approach to utilitarianism, often referred to as rule utilitarianism, appears to address the flaws in what can be termed act utilitarianism, it can be argued that ultimately there is no difference. Because exceptions can be made to rules in individual circumstances to bring about a favourable outcome, the act always trumps the rule in the final analysis (Taylor, 1975).

Deontology

If we have a problem with the idea that the ends justify the means, then perhaps we have to reject consequences providing the judgement, and find an alternative. One alternative theory would argue that actions are right or wrong in and of themselves. The German philosopher Immanuel Kant (1724–1804) argued that people should act on two considerations: first that, irrespective of desires, we must act according to our duty; second, that we cannot treat any human being as a means to an end. This approach, known as deontology, may seem to be a more satisfactory way of decision-making; when we consider how this might work in practice, it is possibly not so straightforward. Imagine a situation where a community mental health nurse becomes aware that a patient is just about coping at home as long as visits are maintained at the current level, but the nurse is due to take annual leave and fears that during their leave the situation may deteriorate. The nurse may feel that the best course of action would be to arrange admission, but Kant would argue that this would be using the patient to allow the nurse to have a worry-free holiday.

CASE STUDY 5.2: GEMMA

Gemma is a Band 5 nurse working in an acute medical ward within a large hospital. Yesterday, a new patient was admitted due to a severe respiratory infection. This patient, Sarah, is 21 and has severe learning and physical disabilities. She needs assistance with all aspects of personal care and receives her nutrition via a **PEG tube**. As she is currently feeling very ill, she is not very responsive, but her parents have told the ward staff that she is usually very alert, loves music and has a 'wicked' smile. During her shift today, Gemma has become very aware that two of the other patients in the same bay as Sarah are speaking very negatively about her, saying things such as 'I don't know why they are treating her', 'She would be better off dead' and 'It's a waste of money keeping people like that alive'. As a nurse, Gemma finds such views as this very difficult to hear, as she believes that all human life has value and that everyone is entitled to healthcare. Furthermore, Gemma has a younger brother who has severe learning disabilities, and she finds it offensive to hear comments like this that devalue her brother's life as well as Sarah's.

- Should Gemma challenge the assertions made by the other patients at the risk of damaging the nurse/patient relationship that she has with them?
- Is it possible that Gemma is allowing her own personal experiences and values to interfere with her ability to provide care to all of her patients in a professional manner?

ANSWER:
CASE STUDY 5.2

ETHICAL PRINCIPLES

Beneficence

The principle of beneficence can be defined as the desire to do good – that is, to bring about a good outcome – and so might be seen to resonate with utilitarianism. However, Kant also finds room for the concept of beneficence, not because it brings about a good outcome but because it is based on a universal duty to try to do good for others (Hurley, 2003). A nurse in a crisis resolution mental health team who arranges for the admission of a patient who appears to be deteriorating may call upon the principle of beneficence as the rationale. From a theoretical perspective, it may be because of a desire to bring about a good consequence or because of respect for the person who has temporarily lost the ability to act in a rational and autonomous way.

Beneficence is often grouped in discussion with the principle of non-maleficence: the desire to do no harm. Discussions on ethics in healthcare sometimes quote the work of the English poet, Arthur Hugh Clough (Chew, 1987), who, in his poem *The Latest Decalogue*, produced the often-quoted phrase: 'Thou shalt not kill; but need'st not strive officiously to keep alive.' This is often used as a means of encapsulating the principle of non-maleficence.

Non-maleficence

The major difference between non-maleficence and other principles is that this principle can be met by doing nothing, whereas the others require action. This principle might be called upon when, in end-of-life care, nurses decide to withhold certain care and treatment that were previously being given. However, the furore over the Liverpool Care Pathway (LCP) in the media (BBC, 2013) demonstrates that, for many people, the decision to do nothing may be seen as an action in itself.

Thomas Aquinas (1225–1274), the influential Catholic philosopher and theologian, is often given credit for adding a further consideration when considering the rightness and wrongness of actions. Take a situation, for example, in which a health professional who is opposed to abortion has to decide what to do when a pregnant woman who has cancer of the cervix can be treated but will lose the baby as a result. Aquinas' doctrine of double effect holds that if an act has an intended consequence (the treatment of cancer) and an unintended but likely side effect (the abortion of the foetus), the actor cannot be held responsible for the unintended consequence.

Autonomy and justice

Two other ethical principles often explored in relation to nursing and healthcare are autonomy and justice. Autonomy is concerned with respecting the ability of individuals to be self-determining: in other words, they are able to make their own decisions. This is particularly relevant when seeking consent for treatment and interventions. If, for example, an adult decides that they do not wish to undergo chemotherapy for a treatable cancer, so long as they understand what the treatment could offer, the potential consequences of their decision and the implications of their refusal, then health practitioners would need to respect their decision even if they do not agree with it. However, what if the patient was 12 years old and made the same decision? Would their views be respected in the same way? Similarly, what if the adult had a mental health condition as a result of which they had paranoid thoughts that other people were trying to kill them? Would their views be respected? Autonomy is, therefore, a principle that needs to be considered alongside other principles such as non-maleficence (not doing harm), and where an individual's autonomy is limited either due to age or mental capacity, then other people may need to make decisions in their best interests.

Justice is concerned with issues such as equality and fairness. In healthcare, this might lead us to consider issues such as whether it is right that where you live can affect your standard of health. It also makes us consider how we use resources and whether they are used in a fair and just way. For example, we may need to make reasonable adjustments to the way we offer services to ensure that disabled people are able to access health services. This might include providing additional school nursing support within a school setting for a child with complex health needs. Even if such adjustments are expensive, the costs can be justified on the basis that additional support is required to access services on an equal level to other people.

The ethical theories and principles discussed demonstrate that there are many apparent answers to the question of how to act when faced with a dilemma in practice. Consider how the nurse should act in case study 5.3.

CASE STUDY 5.3: PETER

Peter is 39 years old and married with two children. He used to work in a warehouse but was made redundant last year and has found it very difficult to find work since. His wife reports that he has been spending more and more time by himself and tends to spend most of the day in bed. Over the past few months, she has had to remind him to wash and shave. He has been losing weight recently and is uncommunicative for long periods. His wife says she is very worried and thinks he has 'given up'.

Peter has been diagnosed as experiencing a 'moderate depressive episode'. He has never experienced mental health problems before. Recently, Peter has said that he wishes he had never been born and that he would be 'better off dead'. His wife is becoming increasingly distressed, as are his children.

Peter has been prescribed anti-depressants but reports that he does not want to take them. His community psychiatric nurse (CPN) says that if he does not take them, 'he will be taken to hospital and forced to take them'. His CPN says that Peter 'owes it to his family to get better' and that he 'must take the tablets or he will be letting them down'.

- What principles of healthcare ethics has the CPN violated?
- If you were the CPN, how would you support Peter?
- How could the framework identified in Table 5.1 be applied to Peter's case?

CHECK YOUR
ANSWERS!

ANSWER:
CASE STUDY 5.3

ETHICAL DECISION-MAKING

A number of frameworks to assist ethical decision-making are available, and you may find it helpful to look at a few books on ethics in order to find the one that is most useful to you. Rowson (2006) provides one such framework.

Apply your knowledge of using this ethical framework by reading Arthur Sampson's case study, at https://study.sagepub.com/essentialnursing2e.

CASE STUDY:
ARTHUR
SAMPSON

> Ethical dilemmas are difficult; everyone has their own views and principles of what they would do, but as a nurse, we have to be non-judgemental and unbiased. We must support our patients/clients and their families and carers with their choices and decisions even if they are not the choices we would necessary choose.
>
> **Sarah Parkes, LD nursing student**

Table 5.1   Applying an ethical framework

1. Before applying any ethical consideration, first consider whether there are any legal or professional rules that should be applied. If there are no legal or professional imperatives, then consider the situation from an ethical position.
2. Consider which ethical principles might be applicable.
3. Reflect on how you might apply any rules of thumb or guidelines from the profession, or how your own values might influence your interpretation of the ethical principles normally.
4. Reflect on whether the criteria in 3 should be adjusted to this particular situation.
5. If the demands of the various ethical principles conflict, is there an acceptable compromise that meets as many demands of the ethical principles as possible or, if not, which demands do you consider to be the most important?
6. How might any infringement of principles be minimised?
7. Taking 1-6 into account, act accordingly.

> I have found learning about ethics a challenge, because there is no right or wrong answer.
>
> **Siân Hunter, child nursing student**

CONCLUSION

Ethics is concerned with clarifying the questions that should be asked prior to making decisions about how to act and, by providing us with frameworks to help us analyse situations, helps us to examine different explanations, consider different courses of action and provide rationales for our decision-making and subsequent behaviour. The fundamental importance of ethics in nursing is made clear when you read the NMC Code (2015). In your role as a nursing student, you will be involved in a wide range of ethical issues during the everyday care of patients. Reflection on these experiences will enable you to consider your own values and examine situations in a variety of ways by applying different ethical theories and principles. While we all have our own set of personal values, the care we deliver to patients must be non-judgemental at all times.

--- **CHAPTER SUMMARY** ---

- All nurses encounter a range of ethical issues in their day-to-day practice.
- It is important that we develop ethical sensitivity so that we recognise ethical issues.
- Ethics requires us to provide a reasoned, sound rationale for our professional actions.
- Commonly held values inform actions at individual, professional, community and societal levels.
- Different ethical theories and principles encourage us to examine situations in different ways.
- At times, we can be faced with decisions that seem to require us to do two incompatible or undesirable things: these are ethical dilemmas.
- Various frameworks are available to assist nurses with ethical decision-making.

--- **CRITICAL REFLECTION** ---

Holistic care

Identify an example from your own practice when you felt there were ethical issues in delivering holistic care. Having read this chapter, try to identify the nature of the ethical issues and what possible courses of action were open to you. Which option would you take? Why?

- Having read this chapter, think about what further learning you need to do in relation to ethics. How will you achieve this?

--- **GO FURTHER** ---

Books

Brykczynska, G. and Simons, J. (2011) *Ethical and Philosophical Aspects of Nursing Children and Young People*. London: Wiley-Blackwell. An excellent book focusing on issues relating to children and young people.

Chadwick, R., Tadd, W. and Gallagher, A. (eds) (2016) *Ethics and Nursing Practice*, 2nd edn. London: Palgrave Macmillan. A book that explores ethical issues in nursing practice across a range of client groups and care settings, including a chapter on nursing and public health.

Melia, K. (2013) *Ethics for Nursing and Healthcare Practice*. London: SAGE. Provides an overview of ethics specifically applied to nursing. Ethical approaches and principles are also considered.

Royal College of Nursing (RCN) (2013) *Dignity in Health Care for People with Learning Disabilities*, 2nd edn. London: RCN. Available at: www.rcn.org.uk/professional-development/publicatons/pub-004439

Wheeler, H. (2012) *Law, Ethics and Professional Issues for Nursing: A Reflective and Portfolio-Building Approach*. London: Routledge. A useful introduction to ethics which also makes links to legal issues.

SAGE journal articles

FURTHER READING: JOURNAL ARTICLES

Go to https://study.sagepub.com/essentialnursing2e for free online journal articles for this chapter. If you are using the interactive ebook, simply click on the book icon in the margin to go straight to the resource.

Bagnasco, A., Cadorin, L., Barisone, M. (2018) 'Ethical dimensions of paediatric nursing: A rapid evidence assessment', *Nursing Ethics*, 25 (1): 111-122. This paper explores some of the particular ethical issues that arise when nursing children.

Blomberg, K. and Bisholt, B. (2016) 'Clinical group supervision for integrating ethical reasoning: Views from students and supervisors', *Nursing Ethics*, 23(7): 761-9. This article explores the use of group supervision with students as a strategy for enhancing their ethical reasoning.

Burston, A. and Tuckett, A. (2013) 'Moral distress in nursing', *Nursing Ethics*, 20(3): 312-24. This article explores the literature regarding moral distress in nursing and considers the implications at both an individual and an organisational level.

Fernandes, M. and Moreira, I. (2013) 'Ethical issues experienced by intensive care unit nurses in everyday practice', *Nursing Ethics*, 20(1): 72-82. This article seeks to identify ethical issues that intensive care nurses perceive as arising in their practice. Personal and institutional practices are considered both as contributing to these issues and as strategies for addressing them.

Hemm, M.H., Gjerberg, E., Husum, T.L. and Pederson,R. (2018) 'Ethical challenges when using coercion in mental healthcare: a systematic literature review', *Nursing Ethics*, 25 (1): 92-110. This paper explores the evidence relating to ethical issues in the use of coercion within mental health care.

Milliken, A. and Grace, P. (2017) 'Nurse ethical awareness: understanding the nature of everyday practice', *Nursing Ethics*, 24 (5): 517-524. This paper encourages awareness of the ethical issues that arise in everyday nursing practice.

Solvoll, B.A., Hall, E.O.C., Brinchmann, B.S. (2014) 'Ethical challenges in everyday work with adults with learning disabilities', *Nursing Ethics*, 22 (4): 417-427.

Weblinks

Go to https://study.sagepub.com/essentialnursing2e for weblinks related to this chapter. If you are using the interactive ebook, simply click on the book icon in the margin to go straight to the resource.

FURTHER READING: WEBLINKS

www.instituteofmedicalethics.org/website – a website providing information regarding key ethical issues such as capacity, consent and end-of-life care, as well as details of training events and other resources.

www.icn.ch/who-we-are/code-of-ethics-for-nurses – an international code of nursing ethics produced by the International Council of Nurses.

www.nmc-uk.org – the website of the Nursing and Midwifery Council, where the Code and other professional guidance documents can be accessed.

ACE YOUR ASSESSMENT

Review what you have learned by visiting the book's online resources at: https://study.sagepub.com/essential nursing2e If using your interactive ebook, just click on the icon in the margin to go straight there.

ONLINE QUIZZES

- Test yourself with multiple-choice and short-answer questions.
- Revise key terms with the interactive flash cards.

REFERENCES

BBC (2013) Liverpool Care Pathway: They told my family I was dying. Available at: www.bbc.co.uk/news/health-23698071 (accessed 14 May 2017).

Burleigh, M. (2002) *Death and Deliverance: Euthanasia in Germany 1900–1945*. London: Pan.

Chew, S. (1987) *Arthur Hugh Clough: Selected Poems*. Manchester: Carcanet.

Cutcliffe, J. and Travale, R. (2013) 'Respect in mental health', *Nursing Ethics*, 20(3): 273–84.

Fisher, A. (2011) *Metaethics: An Introduction*. Durham: Acumen.

Francis, R. (2013) *Report of the Mid Staffordshire NHS Foundation Trust Public Inquiry*. London: The Stationery Office. Available at: www.midstaffspublicinquiry.com/sites/default/files/report/Executive%20summary.pdf (accessed 14 May 2017).

Fry, S.T. and Johnstone, M. (2008) *Ethics in Nursing Practice: A Guide to Ethical Decision Making*. Oxford: Blackwell Publishing.

Hurley, P. (2003) 'Fairness and beneficence', *Ethics*, 113: 841–64.

Nursing and Midwifery Council (2015) *The Code: Professional Standards of Practice and Behaviour for Nurses and Midwives*. London: NMC.

Rowson, R. (2006) *Working Ethics: How to be Fair in a Culturally Complex World*. London: Jessica Kingsley.

Sandel, M. (2010) *Justice: What's the Right Thing to Do?* London: Penguin.

Seedhouse, D. (2009) *Ethics: the Heart of Health Care*, 3rd edn. Chichester: Wiley-Blackwell.

Taylor, P. (1975) *Principles of Ethics: An Introduction*. Belmont, CA: Wadsworth.

Thompson, I.E., Melia, K., Boyd, K.M. and Horsburgh, D. (2006) *Nursing Ethics*, 5th edn. Edinburgh: Churchill Livingstone.

Weaver, K., Morse, J. and Mitcham, C. (2008) 'Ethical sensitivity in professional practice: Concept analysis', *Journal of Advanced Nursing*, 62(5): 607–6.

LAW

GRAHAM AVERY

THIS CHAPTER COVERS

- Understanding negligence
- Court cases

- The law and providing healthcare
- Confidentiality

My name is George and I am 48 years old. I have been in hospital once or twice before and I have always been looked after very well. The staff are very busy and I could see that occasional mistakes were likely to happen, but it never occurred to me to sue the hospital. However, after having surgery on my hand, I am now unable to move the fingers and have been told that this is a permanent disability. I was never warned that this could happen and it means that I can no longer work as a carpenter.

George, patient

My name is Alisha and I am about to start my first placement as a nursing student on a children's ward. I have heard several horror stories of nurses who have made mistakes on the wards and who have been sacked by their employer. I have also heard that patients are much more likely to sue these days and I am terrified of being put in this position. It is obvious to me that I need to work hard to be competent so that my patients are as safe as possible, but I also need to know something about the law to protect myself and the organisation.

Alisha, nursing student

Visit https://study.sagepub.com/essentialnursing2e to access a wealth of online resources for this chapter – watch out for the margin icons throughout the chapter. If you are using the interactive eBook, simply click on the margin icon to go straight to the resource.

INTRODUCTION

It has been said that the only two certainties in life are death and taxes. We might, however, add a third: that wherever and whenever human beings live in close proximity to each other, a set of rules and legal principles will be established. The more advanced the civilisation, the more sophisticated and complicated these legal principles become. They have a number of purposes, most notably to protect the health and safety of individuals and to protect rightful financial and property interests. Above all, though, the function of the law is to promote justice and fairness for all citizens.

Many nurses, similarly to Alisha, will state that they are frightened by the law, but it should not be seen as a stick with which to beat them. In fact, the law has shown itself to be very protective of healthcare professionals in the past, acknowledging that they have a difficult and demanding job and that society does not benefit from punishing those who serve the interests of others. Nevertheless, the law also recognises that there are standards that should be met when caring for patients, and practice that falls below these standards must inevitably be penalised, particularly if patients are harmed as a result.

It is not possible to provide an outline of all the legal principles affecting nurses in this chapter, and you are advised to look at the suggested texts listed at the end. We can, however, look at three areas of the law that have the most impact on healthcare practice: negligence, consent and confidentiality.

CASE STUDY 6.1: ROSHAN

Roshan is a nursing student on placement in a residential nursing home and is escorting an elderly female resident (Mrs Howe) to the toilet one afternoon. A carpet runs along the floor leading to the toilet and this has become heavily stained. In an effort to clean it, the domestic staff have poured buckets of water onto it, but have not placed any 'wet floor' signs nearby. As Roshan walks with Mrs Howe, she slips and falls to the floor, fracturing her left wrist. In the process, she drags Mrs Howe down with her, and Mrs Howe sustains a fractured left hip.

- Was a **duty of care** owed by the nursing home to the resident and the nursing student?
- Has the nursing home breached a reasonable **standard of care?**

UNDERSTANDING NEGLIGENCE

This scenario is loosely based on the Scottish case of *Dillon v Greater Glasgow Health Board* [2011] CSOH 67, and serves as a useful illustration of how the law operates in such circumstances. The cause of action here is negligence and the claimants (that is, the victims who are bringing the action) are both Roshan and Mrs Howe. The defendants (that is, the people who are being sued in this action) are whoever owns the nursing home: most commonly this will be a private owner, but it may be a National Health Service trust. In order to win this action, both claimants will need to establish three fundamental elements, seeking positive answers to each of the following questions:

1.   Was a *duty of care* owed by the nursing home to the resident and the nursing student?

Duty of care

The simple answer to this question is 'Yes'. By virtue of Mrs Howe's status as a resident in the nursing home, those looking after her automatically have a duty of care. This is a long-held principle of the common law (i.e. the law derived from cases and made by judges), and is generally the easiest hurdle for any claimant to overcome. There may be some circumstances in which it is unclear whether or not a duty exists, but these are rare within healthcare. As soon as an organisation and its individual practitioners accept the responsibility of treating and/or looking after patients or residents, a duty of care is automatically established.

I always believed that negligence in nursing was because of an accident, but after recent press articles I am shocked that anyone could treat someone like that, let alone a nurse. Why would a person go into a job that needed care, compassion and understanding of people's needs and hurt and abuse them? I am just horrified.

Sarah Parkes, LD nursing student

This common law duty extends, of course, to the nursing student. Roshan has a duty of care to Mrs Howe and authority for this position comes from *Caparo Industries v Dickman [1990]* 2AC 605. In this case, the court developed a three-stage test, all three of which needed to be proven by the claimant:

1. There must be foreseeability of damage.
2. There must be proximity between the parties.
3. It must be just and reasonable to impose a duty of care.

Quite clearly, all three apply in our scenario, as they will with all other healthcare interventions. But Roshan is also owed a duty by the owners of the nursing home. In addition, the owners have statutory duties (i.e. that law which has been made by Parliament) to provide a safe system of work for their employees under the Health and Safety at Work Act 1974. There are a variety of other regulations deriving from European law which impose added responsibilities on employers to ensure that the workplace is safe (for example, the Workplace (Health and Safety and Welfare) Regulations 1992, which are concerned with the general state of premises). In consequence, we can state with confidence that the first obstacle standing in the path of a claim for negligence has been successfully negotiated. We must therefore move on to the second question:

2. Has the nursing home breached a reasonable *standard of care*?

Standard of care

In order to answer this question, we must first have an understanding of what we mean by 'reasonable'. The *professional* standard of reasonableness emanates from the medical case of *Bolam v Friern Hospital Management Committee* [1957] All ER 118, where it was found that a doctor would not be negligent 'if he has acted in accordance with a practice accepted as proper by a responsible body of medical men skilled in that particular art' (per McNair, J. at 212). In essence, this *Bolam test*, as it has come to be known, states that a professional's actions and performance will be judged alongside those of his or her peers. Or, to put it another way, what would the reasonable practitioner do in the same or similar circumstances? Clearly, the standard expected of a practitioner rises in proportion with the skills practised by that individual. The actions of a plastic surgeon, for example, would be judged alongside those of another competent plastic surgeon. Similarly, the actions of a staff nurse would be judged alongside those expected of a reasonably competent qualified nurse.

The professional standard, however, does not apply in this case, for neither the domestic staff nor Roshan are qualified. In such circumstances, the 'reasonable man' test is used, which owes its origins to a very old case, *Blyth v Proprietors of the Birmingham Waterworks* [1856] 11 Exch. 781, and which has been defined as the 'man on the street' or 'man on the Clapham omnibus' test (from *Hall v Brooklands Auto-Racing Club* [1933] 1 KB 205). To put it another way, the 'reasonable man' would be expected to respond to circumstances and act in such a manner as any sane, moderately intelligent and sensible individual would. We might call this 'common sense', although it has often been argued that sense is far from common.

Applying this test to our scenario, we must ask whether the domestic staff have acted reasonably by pouring large volumes of water onto the carpet. The possible argument that this was common practice at the home would not, of itself, be a defence if there was an appropriate and practical alternative. In other words, was the action of throwing buckets of water onto the carpet the only way in which it could have been cleaned in the circumstances? Having soaked the carpet, the domestic staff could reasonably have been expected to put up warning signs nearby. They might argue that they were in the process of locating these signs as soon as they had cleaned the carpet, but that Roshan and Mrs Howe came along before they had the chance to erect them. However, this argument would not be considered logical, for the reasonable person would have these signs to hand *before* applying water to the carpet.

Liability

Does Roshan escape **liability** here? If, for example, she had seen the domestics soaking the carpet or it was patently obvious that it was wet, she could reasonably have been expected to take appropriate precautions. For example, she could have transferred Mrs Howe to the toilet in a wheelchair, and/or she might have been able to find a route that bypassed the wet floor. If it can be shown that both the domestic staff and Roshan have acted reasonably, there has been no breach in the standard of care and therefore no action in negligence: the injuries to Mrs Howe and Roshan would consequently be seen as little more than an unfortunate accident. On the assumption that there has been a breach, though, we must now turn to a third question.

3.   Has the breach caused reasonably foreseeable harm?

ACTIVITY 6.1: CRITICAL THINKING

- Would Roshan's liability be increased if she was a third-year nursing student, only a few weeks from qualifying?
- If the healthcare institution looked after small children, people with severe learning disabilities, patients with reading difficulties or blind people, what purpose would be served by a wet floor warning sign? What other measures would one expect to be in place?

ANSWER:
ACTIVITY 6.1

Harm

Essentially, this question asks three things. First, has harm been caused? Compensation is awarded for damage caused, and, if there is no damage, there can therefore be nothing to compensate. In our scenario, however, it is clear that harm has occurred, for both Mrs Howe and Roshan have sustained fractures. Second, is the harm reasonably foreseeable? Could, for example, the domestics have reasonably foreseen that soaking the carpet with water would make it slippery? This is not as simple a question as one might imagine, for a carpet is more absorbent of water than a smooth or polished surface. Nevertheless, the domestics could, at the very least, have tested this hypothesis, and their failure to put up a warning sign meant that anybody walking on the carpet would be blissfully unaware that it constituted a hazard.

Third, has the breach in the standard of care been directly responsible for the harm? This is known as the 'but for' test and would be expressed in this scenario thus: *but for* the domestics' negligence in soaking the carpet with large volumes of water and failing to put up warning signs, this incident would not have happened. It is conceivable, for instance, that Mrs Howe's legs simply gave way, resulting in both she and Roshan falling to the floor. If so, then it is doubtful that the wet carpet made any material difference to the incident, for it was just as likely to happen on a perfectly dry floor.

COURT CASES

In those cases that come before the courts, there is generally a defence made to one or more of these questions, making it difficult for claimants to win. Bear in mind that the burden of proof lies with them (not the defendants), and they must prove their case on the balance of probabilities. Failure to do so will see the case dismissed and no compensation will be awarded. Moreover, even though the nursing home might accept liability for both Mrs Howe's and Roshan's injuries, they might be able to argue that Roshan had been at least partly responsible for this incident. Let us imagine, for example, that Roshan spilt some water herself and failed to clear it up; or that she was fully aware of the hazard created by the domestics, but took no appropriate measures to avoid a fall. In such circumstances, it might be argued that Roshan has contributed to her own injuries, and her compensation may be reduced accordingly.

The above discussion has given a brief overview of the elements of negligence, and these same principles could be applied to a wide range of situations. Where there is an injury, there is usually a claim; but equally there is often a defence, and the history of such claims suggests that the odds are weighted in the defendants' favour. Of course, the most effective method of avoiding such claims is not to do anything that can be perceived as negligent, but this is often a lot easier said than done. However, every individual within the field of healthcare practice (whether they are qualified or unqualified) should acknowledge that any action performed will have an impact on others. The goal of healthcare is to ensure that this impact is a positive rather than a negative one.

Sometimes unwittingly mistakes occur at work. I have learned that no matter how busy work may be it is always best to stop and think to ensure that you are comfortable with the decisions you are making. If you observe negligence at work ensure that you report it in the correct manner to prevent the incident occurring again.

Alice Rowe, NQ RNMH

CASE STUDY 6.2: JOE

Joe is a 24-year-old man who has autism and a severe learning disability. He lives with his mother (aged 56) and requires a high level of care, support and supervision. His mother receives quite a lot of this support from social services, but she has developed a chest infection and is clearly suffering from exhaustion. Joe is taken into a behavioural support unit while his mother recuperates, but he exhibits challenging and aggressive behaviour while there. Even when his mother asks for his return, the unit refuses to discharge him, arguing that his mental state is too unstable.

- What legal authority does the behavioural support unit have to detain Joe against his will?

THE LAW AND PROVIDING HEALTHCARE

Consent

The behavioural support unit will undoubtedly be able to claim that it is making a clinical judgement here and is operating in the best interests of both Joe and his mother. If Joe was below the age of 18, his mother would be able to consent on his behalf; if she refused such consent and the unit felt this was an unwise decision, they would need to refer to the courts for a judgement. Neither of these situations applies here, however: Joe is an adult and his mother no longer has decision-making authority for her son. Therefore, in answering the question of what legal authority the unit has for detaining Joe against his will, we must consider two areas of legislation that deal with issues of **consent**: the Mental Health Act 1983 (amended by the Mental Health Act 2007) and the Mental Capacity Act 2005.

These laws apply to England and Wales, and there is separate provision in Scotland, with the Mental Health (Care and Treatment) (Scotland) Act 2003 and Adults with Incapacity (Scotland) Act 2000, and Northern Ireland, with the Mental Health (Northern Ireland) Order 1986. The Mental Health Act will apply when a patient has been diagnosed as being mentally ill, which is defined as 'any disorder or disability of the mind' (s1 [2]). Learning disability was originally on the list of those conditions that qualify as a mental disorder, but was removed by the Mental Health Act 2007. However, autistic spectrum disorder remains on the list, and learning disability will continue to qualify if it is accompanied by seriously aggressive or irresponsible behaviour.

The process of detaining a patient under the Mental Health Act follows a well-trodden path and usually begins by invoking s2, which authorises admission for assessment. Two doctors and an approved mental health professional (AMHP), who will usually be a social worker but could be a mental health nurse, an occupational therapist or a psychologist, must provide written recommendations that detention is necessary and admission under this section can last for up to 28 days. If the unit believes that Joe needs to remain beyond this time, s3 must then be invoked, which authorises admission for treatment. Once again, two doctors and an AMHP must make this recommendation, and it allows for detention of up to six months. Beyond this time, it is renewable indefinitely for periods of one year, but it must be reviewed on a regular basis by a Mental Health Review Tribunal.

The definition of 'treatment' under the Mental Health Act includes 'nursing, psychological intervention and specialist mental health habilitation, rehabilitation and care' (s145 [1]), and the evidence from our scenario suggests that this might apply to Joe. There is, however, a general reluctance to section patients if at all possible. For one thing, it is still perceived as stigmatising, although it is doubtful that Joe would be affected by this. Second, it may damage efforts to establish a therapeutic relationship with the patient, for there are close similarities here to the situation of a prisoner and his jailer.

Finally, the process of detention is very bureaucratic and requires a lot of resources. For these reasons, it is considered preferable to admit patients informally (s131) if at all possible.

Competence

It is generally assumed that the patient must be competent before agreeing to informal admission and that his or her consent should be given voluntarily. The reality, though, is that there are many patients in hospitals and nursing homes who are informal admissions, but who are unable to consent on their own behalf. Therefore, does admission as an informal patient require active consent or merely the absence of dissent? This was a question addressed by the case of *R v Bournewood Community and Mental Health NHS Trust*, ex parte L [1998] 3 All ER 289 (HL), to which we will return shortly. Suffice it to say at this point that an informal patient should be able to leave the care setting whenever she or he wishes, although a mental health nurse can forcibly detain that person for up to six hours if it is felt that their mental disorder is such that this is necessary for their health or safety or for the protection of others (s5 [4]).

Given the reluctance to avoid detaining patients under the Mental Health Act, perhaps the Mental Capacity Act 2005 could offer some assistance. This Act authorises the deprivation of a person's liberty without recourse to sectioning, providing that certain criteria are established and safeguards are in place. The regulations dealing with these so-called Deprivation of Liberty Safeguards (DoLS) were inserted into the Mental Capacity Act 2005 (Schedule A1) by means of the Mental Health Act 2007 and were implemented in April 2009 in response to a ruling by the European Court of Human Rights on the *Bournewood* case (mentioned earlier). There are a number of assessments that must be made before a DoLS is authorised, some of which are straightforward. For example, the patient must be at least 18 years old, she or he must be an informal admission, and they should not have a valid Advance Decision to refuse treatment. In addition, they must be diagnosed with a mental disorder, and this diagnosis will be made by a suitably qualified doctor. Beyond this, the two main areas of assessment are rather more complex.

Capacity

The first of these is a mental capacity assessment, and it is a fundamental principle of this Act that every adult is presumed to have the capacity to make their own decisions (s1 [2]), even if those decisions appear to us to be unwise or even dangerous (s1 [4]). They can therefore consent to treatment and can refuse treatment, and failure to respect the latter will constitute a Battery (or Trespass to the Person), which is actionable in the courts. The presumption of capacity, however, can be overturned, but the healthcare professionals must demonstrate that the patient has been fully assessed before declaring that they are incompetent to make decisions for themselves. In other words, it is not for the patient to prove their competence; rather, the burden of proof falls on the healthcare team. The test of competence can be found in s3 of the Mental Capacity Act, in which it is said that the patient must fail at least one of the following elements before being declared incompetent:

1. He (or she) must be able to understand the information given to him.
2. He must be able to retain that information.
3. He must be able to weigh the information in the balance to arrive at a decision.
4. He must be able to communicate his decision by any means.

Although everything in our scenario points to the fact that Joe will clearly fail this assessment, there is a requirement in the Mental Capacity Act 2005 that healthcare professionals must do everything within their power to enhance decision-making capacity (s4 [4]) – but the practical difficulties in our scenario are obvious.

WHAT'S THE EVIDENCE?

Decision-making capacity

Gunn, M.J., Wong, J.G., Clare, I.C.H. and Holland, A.J. (1999) 'Decision-making capacity', *Medical Law Review*, 7(3): 269-306 found that people with learning disabilities were often capable of a much higher level of understanding than many gave them credit for, provided that the information was conveyed in a certain manner.

A finding of incompetence does not, by itself, constitute a justification for holding somebody against their wishes, and it must therefore be shown that detention is in the patient's best interests. The assessment of best interests must be undertaken by a different healthcare professional from the person who performed the mental health assessment and it is important that a wide variety of views are considered (including those of Joe and his mother).

ACTIVITY 6.2: CRITICAL THINKING

ANSWER:
ACTIVITY 6.2

What strategies could you use to enhance Joe's understanding of why he was not being allowed to go home?

Independent mental capacity advocate

Moreover, it is also important to secure the services of an **independent mental capacity advocate (IMCA)**, whose role it is to support the patient through this process and to be prepared to challenge any aspect that is not procedurally or morally correct.

Once the best interests assessor is satisfied that a deprivation of liberty is warranted, this recommendation is made to the supervisory body (the Clinical Commissioning Group or local authority) and a standard authorisation is subsequently made. Following this, the managing authority (in our scenario, the behavioural support unit) is entitled to take any measures to restrain Joe that it thinks are necessary, provided that such measures are proportionate (i.e. not excessive) and that there is no less restrictive alternative (MCA s6).

ACTIVITY 6.3: CRITICAL THINKING

ANSWER:
ACTIVITY 6.3

- What forms of physical restraint do you think are acceptable (if any) when dealing with confused, restless or aggressive patients?
- When answering these questions, consider the information in Chapter 5 relating to ethical issues.

The complicated process involved in obtaining a Deprivation of Liberty Safeguards (DoLS) authorisation has inevitably meant that they have not been invoked as often as they should have been. However, the Supreme Court decision in *P v Cheshire West and Chester Council* [2014] UKSC 19 propelled them back into the limelight. In this case, it was held that a person is objectively deprived of his/her liberty if, for more than a non-negligible period of time:

S/he is under continuous supervision and control, and

S/he is not free to leave.

This 'acid test', as it is known, is beautiful in its simplicity and it clearly applies to Joe. It does, however, apply to many other patients in hospitals, care homes and hospices, and the evidence suggests that the system is unsustainable in its present form. It seems reasonable to assume, therefore, that the law will undergo change in the future, but justice dictates that its underlying principles will remain. The courts currently expect health authorities to set the bar very high when authorising DoLS and they need to be convinced that detention of a patient is significantly preferable to returning that person to their family (see *Hillingdon London Borough Council v Neary* [2011] EWHC 1377 (COP)). Anything less than this represents a significant intrusion upon an individual's liberty and is disrespectful of the rights of vulnerable people.

CASE STUDY 6.3: ENTHUSIASTIC STUDENTS

Two nursing students have just completed a shift on a ward for older people with mental infirmity and are travelling home on the bus. They have had a particularly good day, in which they have observed a variety of new therapeutic interventions and feel that they are learning a lot from this placement. They begin to share their experiences with each other and to talk about some of the patients they have cared for. Unfortunately, the wife of one of these patients is sitting immediately behind them and hears every word of their conversation. She makes an official complaint to the hospital.

- Have these students committed a disciplinary offence and does the patient's wife have a cause of action?

CONFIDENTIALITY

It cannot be said that the two students have acted with malice in this scenario. Indeed, their enthusiasm for nursing is laudable, and it is inevitable that they will want to discuss their experiences with each other. There is, however, an appropriate time and place for this discussion, and a bus trip does not fall into this category.

All healthcare professionals are entrusted with the maintenance of patient confidentiality, and any breach of this rule will be taken very seriously. The reasons for this are fairly self-evident: if people cannot trust healthcare professionals to keep their medical details secret, they will be unlikely to divulge information. In consequence, it will be more difficult to reach a diagnosis and initiate appropriate treatment.

Clearly, there is an *ethical* dimension to the upholding of patient confidentiality, and qualified nurses also have a *professional* duty under the Nursing and Midwifery Council's Code of professional conduct (2015), in which it is said that you must (at paragraph 5.1) 'respect a person's right to privacy in all aspects of their care'. In addition, a *contractual* duty binds all personnel who work in the National Health Service (including nursing students) and other providers of care to maintain patient confidentiality (DH, 2003). Finally, a *legal* duty exists, but this is slightly more problematic. There are, indeed, a number of circumstances where confidentiality can be legally breached: for example, where the patient consents to the release of their medical information; where a court orders the information to be disclosed; and when it can be argued that a breach serves the public interest. The last of these is the most controversial and deserves a separate section in its own right, but it has no application in our scenario. Given, therefore, that the nursing students have no defence to the charge that they have breached confidentiality, we must now consider what remedies (if any) are available to the patient's wife.

I always ensure I never, ever talk about any patients, not even to colleagues if outside the workplace. Should I need to discuss a patient with another member of staff/professional, I ensure we are in an area where we cannot be heard by other patients or their families. It can be difficult on a busy ward but it is not impossible. Being aware when talking to patients in a bay should be considered – talking loudly so that everyone can hear breaches their right to confidentiality and can also be incredibly embarrassing and undignifying for them. Always using a pseudonym if you refer to patients/families/colleagues in essays so they cannot be recognised is equally important.

Siân Hunter, child nursing student

She might invoke the common law and her cause of action would be that of negligence. Applying the three elements outlined in our first scenario, we can see that the nursing students had a duty of care to the patient and breached that duty by relating his confidential medical information in a public arena. Whether the wife can be said to have been harmed by this incident, however, is doubtful. She could point to a certain level of psychological distress, but the courts have always been reluctant to allow compensation for such claims. Where they have succeeded, the victim has been left with a debilitating and long-lasting psychiatric injury, requiring medical intervention (see *North Glamorgan NHS Trust v Walters* [2002] EWCA Civ. 1792). With the knowledge that all three elements of negligence must be satisfied, we are forced to come to the conclusion that this is an unlikely route towards success for the patient's wife.

A second possibility is the Data Protection Act 1998, which can award compensation for breaches of confidentiality, not only for physical and economic damage but also for psychological distress (s13 [2]). The problem for the wife, however, is that the Act applies only to information that has been recorded in a written or computerised form. It does not apply to verbal information and cannot therefore be a source of redress in this scenario. A final legal avenue for the wife is the Human Rights Act 1998, which recognises a personal right to privacy (Article 8). Once again, though, the 'rewards' available are unlikely to justify the expense and effort of bringing this case to court.

In consequence, the wife may simply be left with the satisfaction of knowing that the nursing students will inevitably face disciplinary proceedings for this breach of confidentiality. The extent of disciplinary action is impossible to estimate, for it is largely content-specific. For example, if the nature of the conversation between the nursing students was malicious, condescending and disparaging towards the patients, it is likely that the disciplinary panel would seriously question the value of their continuation on the course. In the absence of such malice, one would hope that this incident would be seen as thoughtless behaviour caused by inexperience and the exuberance of youth. An apology to the wife and a solemn undertaking that this error will never be repeated would seem to be an appropriate response here. It is by no means certain, however, that this is how the panel would respond, and they would be entitled to terminate the students' contracts. At the very least, the students will be on a warning, and it is fair to assume that their conduct will be closely monitored for the duration of their studies.

You can apply your knowledge of mental health provision by reading Amelie's case study, at https://study.sagepub.com/essentialnursing2e.

CASE STUDY:
AMELIE

ACTIVITY 6.4: CRITICAL THINKING

- If you felt very strongly that the quality of care on a ward was unacceptably low, to whom should you report this?
- If a patient had severe learning disabilities and no relatives, would a breach of their confidentiality cause that person any harm?

ANSWER:
ACTIVITY 6.4

ACTIVITY 6.5: CRITICAL THINKING

Based on what you have learned in this chapter in relationship to confidentiality and capacity, do you think patient confidentiality is more a myth than a reality?

What can be done to ensure a patient's medical details are kept safe, while ensuring there is good communication between the individual carers involved? How will this promote holistic care of your patient?

ANSWER:
ACTIVITY 6.5

CONCLUSION

This chapter has highlighted some of the main areas of the law that affect healthcare professionals. As mentioned earlier, it is by no means exhaustive and you are encouraged to read more detailed texts. Ignorance of the law is not a defence and those who make no effort to understand it may well be destined to fall foul of it. We live in an increasingly litigious society and patients are now more aware of their rights than has ever previously been the case. Notwithstanding this, however, we should remember that healthcare law has developed to protect the interests of patients. In this, we can see that the law and nursing have a common purpose.

CHAPTER SUMMARY

- Healthcare law has developed to protect the interests of patients, and nurses have a duty to ensure that they abide by its principles.
- For a claimant to win an action on negligence, three elements must be satisfied: that a duty of care was owed to the patient, that there has been a breach in the standard of care and that the breach has caused reasonably foreseeable harm.
- The Mental Health Act 1983 can be invoked to impose treatment upon patients against their will, but this treatment can only be for the mental illness from which the patient suffers.

- There is a presumption that adults have the capacity to make decisions, but this can be overturned if the patient fails the test of competence outlined in the Mental Capacity Act 2005.
- Treatment can be given to an incompetent patient without their consent, provided that it can be shown to be in their best interests.
- The maintenance of patient confidentiality is a sacrosanct principle within healthcare, and those who breach it may face legal, contractual and professional penalties.

CRITICAL REFLECTION

Holistic care

- Reflect on the ways in which you and your organisation can reduce the possibility of errors occuring.
- Think of situations in the workplace where patient consent has been difficult to obtain. Are you satisfied that the correct procedures have been followed, or could these situations have been handled more effectively?

GO FURTHER

Books

Avery, G. (2017) *Law and Ethics in Nursing and Healthcare*, 2nd edn. London: SAGE.

Carr, C. (2015) *Unlocking Medical Law and Ethics*, 2nd edn. London: Hodder Education.

Dimond, B. (2017) *Legal Aspects of Nursing*, 7th edn. Harlow: Pearson Education.

All of these texts are deliberately aimed at those who are new to the subject of healthcare law. They are therefore written in an accessible style, contain a lot of useful information and offer a range of questions for students to consider.

Bartlett, P. and Sandland, R. (2014) *Mental Health Law: Policy and Practice*, 4th. Edn. Oxford: Oxford University Press. This book may not be for the beginner, but it is a comprehensive overview of mental health law in this country and is extremely well-written.

Brazier, M. and Cave, E. (2016) *Medicine, Patients and the Law*, 6th edn. Manchester: Manchester University Press. This is another well-written text, which covers a broad range of areas pertaining to health care law and incorporates ethical analysis.

Griffith, R. and Tengnah, C. (2017) *Law and Professional Issues in Nursing*, 4th edn. London: Sage. This recently updated book is a very good introduction to the law for nursing students. It covers all the important areas of practice and it is written in a very accessible style.

McAlinden, O. (2012) 'Ethical and legal implications when planning care for children and young people', Chapter 4 in D. Corkin, S. Clarke and L. Liggett (eds), *Care Planning in Children & Young People's Nursing*. London: Wiley-Blackwell. This chapter contains very useful advice relating to the legal issues involved in caring for children and young people.

Journal articles

Fullbrook, S. (2007) 'Legal principles of confidentiality and other public interests: Part 1', *British Journal of Nursing*, 16(14): 874-5. This article reviews the case law pertaining to confidentiality and emphasises the importance of this concept to healthcare.

Hodgson, J. (2009) 'Modern negligence law: Contribution of the medical cases', *British Journal of Nursing*, 18(21): 1320-1. This article reviews the medical cases that have shaped the law of negligence and its application to healthcare.

Simpson, O. (2011) 'Consent and assessment of capacity to decide or refuse treatment', *British Journal of Nursing*, 20(8): 510–13. This article gives an overview of the law of consent, making specific reference to patients' rights to be given appropriate information, and considers those occasions when decision-making passes to healthcare professionals.

Annual fitness to Practice Report: www.nmc.org.uk/globalassets/sitedocuments/annual_reports_and_accounts/annual-report-ftp-report-overview-2016-2017.pdf

Weblinks

Go to https://study.sagepub.com/essentialnursing2e for weblinks related to this chapter. If you are using the interactive ebook, simply click on the book icon in the margin to go straight to the resource.

FURTHER
READING:
WEBLINKS

Annual fitness to Practice Report: www.nmc.org.uk/globalassets/sitedocuments/annual_reports_and_accounts/annual-report-ftp-report-overview-2016-2017.pdf

The following resources provide case-law judgments and Acts of Parliament:

British and Irish Legal Information Institute – www.bailii.org

Ministry of Justice: Mental Capacity Act (code of practice and easy read booklet) – www.justice.gov.uk/protecting-the-vulnerable/mental-capacity-act

Office of Public Sector Information – www.legislation.gov.uk/ukpga

Supreme Court – https://supremecourt.uk/decided-cases/index.html

Video links

Have a break from the text and go to https://study.sagepub.com/essentialnursing2e for useful videos related to this chapter. If you are using the interactive ebook, simply click on the lightbulb icon in the margin to go straight to the resource.

VIDEO
LINKS

ACE YOUR ASSESSMENT

GREAT FOR
REVISION!

Review what you have learned by visiting the book's online resources at: https://study.sagepub.com/essentialnursing2e If using your interactive ebook, just click on the icon in the margin to go straight there.

- Test yourself with multiple-choice and short-answer questions.
- Revise key terms with the interactive flash cards.

ONLINE
QUIZZES

Mental Health Act (MHA) 1983 (as amended by Mental Health Act 2007)

Section 1 [2]:   Defines mental disorder as 'any disorder or disability of the mind'.

Section 2:   Covers the criteria necessary for detention of a patient for <u>assessment</u> of his or her mental disorder, which may remain in place for up to 28 days.

Section 3:   Covers the criteria necessary for detention of a patient for <u>treatment</u> of his or her mental disorder.

Section 5 [4]:   Authorises a nurse to detain a patient who wishes to leave a hospital for up to six hours or until a medical practitioner is able to attend the patient.

Section 131:   Covers the informal admission of patients for treatment of mental disorder.

Section 145:   Provides a definition of medical treatment, which includes nursing, psychological intervention, specialist mental health habilitation, rehabilitation and care.

Mental Capacity Act (MCA) 2005

Section 1 [2]:   States the principle that an adult patient is assumed to have capacity unless proven otherwise.

Section 1 [4]:   States the principle that a person is not to be treated as incompetent simply because she or he makes an unwise decision.

Section 3:   Outlines the test of capacity, at least part of which a person must fail if held to be incompetent to make a decision.

Section 4 [4]:   Imposes an obligation on the healthcare professional making an assessment of a patient's best interests to endeavour to encourage that patient to participate in the decision-making process as much as possible.

Section 6:   Authorises the restraint of incapacitated patients, provided that it is a proportionate response.

REFERENCES

Department of Health (DH) (2003) *Confidentiality: NHS Code of Practice*. London: DH. Available at: www.gov.uk/government/uploads/system/uploads/attachment_data/file/200146/Confidentiality_-_NHS_Code_of_Practice.pdf (accessed 18 February 2015).

Gunn, M.J., Wong, J.G., Clare, I.C.H. and Holland, A.J. (1999) 'Decision-making capacity', *Medical Law Review*, 7(3): 269–306.

Nursing and Midwifery Council (NMC) (2015) *The Code: Professional Standards of Practice and Behaviour for Nurses and Midwives*. London: NMC.

Cases

Blyth v Proprietors of the Birmingham Waterworks [1856] 11 Exch. 781

Bolam v Friern Hospital Management Committee [1957] 2 All ER 118

Caparo Industries plc Dickman [1990] 2 AC 605

Dillon v Greater Glasgow Health Board [2011] CSOH 67

Hall v Brooklands Auto-Racing Club [1933] 1 KB 205

Hillingdon London Borough Council v Neary [2011] EWHC 1377 (COP)

North Glamorgan NHS Trust v Walters [2002] EWCA Civ. 1792

P v Cheshire West and Chester Council [2014] UKSC 19

R v Bournewood Community and Mental Health NHS Trust, ex parte L [1998] 3 All ER 289 (HL)

Legislation

Adults with Incapacity (Scotland) Act 2000

Data Protection Act 1998

Health and Safety at Work Act 1974

Human Rights Act 1998

Mental Capacity Act 2005

Mental Health Act 1983

Mental Health Act 2007

Mental Health (Care and Treatment) (Scotland) Act 2003

Mental Health (Northern Ireland) Order 1986

Workplace (Health and Safety and Welfare) Regulations 1992

ACCOUNTABILITY AND PROFESSIONALISM

KAREN ELCOCK

THIS CHAPTER COVERS

- An overview of accountability
- The importance of professionalism in nursing

- Fitness to practise

"

The scariest thing about qualifying as a nurse is realising that you can no longer hide behind your practice educator; you are totally accountable for your actions. During my course I went to see an NMC fitness to practise hearing and it really brought home to me how important it is to understand the Code and abide by it, but more importantly not to be afraid to ask for advice when unsure.

Julie Rogers, registered nurse

"

"

Becoming a qualified LD nurse scares me – to think that in a few months I could be working in a setting as a nurse with lots of responsibility and remembering nothing. I do wake up sometimes and think: can I really do this; do I know enough to meet everyone's expectations?

Sarah Parkes, LD nursing student

"

Visit https://study.sagepub.com/essentialnursing2e to access a wealth of online resources for this chapter – watch out for the margin icons throughout the chapter. If you are using the interactive eBook, simply click on the margin icon to go straight to the resource.

INTRODUCTION

Ask students what they worry about most when they qualify and accountability is often cited. There is little doubt that you will find that accountability and professionalism will be discussed throughout your course – a lot! This is because both are fundamental to becoming a registered nurse and underpin both the NMC *Standards for Registered Nurse Education* (2018) and the Code (NMC, 2015). This chapter explores the concepts of accountability and professionalism, starting with what accountability means and who precisely you are accountable to as a student and later as a registered nurse. Being accountable for your actions (or inactions) is only part of becoming a professional. In this chapter, the reasons why professionalism and trust, as one of the four themes in the NMC Code, are so important in nursing will be looked at and related to the NMC's requirements for fitness for practice, not only at the end of your course so that you can register with them, but also throughout your nursing career. Case studies in which nurses have been found to fall below the expected standard will be used to help you understand the consequences of either failing to follow the NMC Code or bringing the nursing profession into disrepute. The aim of this chapter is to help you understand why the expectations, relating to your behaviour, of your university and the people you will work with in practice are so important. Further to this, the chapter outlines the impact of your conduct falling below expected standards on not only your ability to register as a nurse, but also on the trust the public have in nurses.

Before reading this chapter, you may find it helpful to look at Chapter 1, which introduces you to the concept of professionalism.

AN OVERVIEW OF ACCOUNTABILITY

While 'accountability' is a word that will be used repeatedly throughout your course, you will find that it is often used in the context of being a registered nurse, and so may only appear relevant to you after you have qualified. This, however, is not the case, and so it is important to understand what accountability means for you now as a student, and how this changes when you qualify. You also need to understand its relevance for those healthcare professionals with whom you will come into contact, who will be supporting your learning and delegating care activities to you when you are in practice. Linked closely with accountability is the concept of responsibility; it is important to understand the difference between the two, as they both have relevance to you as a nursing student.

Responsibility relates to the acceptance and carrying out of a task or duty within a person's sphere of competence, whereas accountability can be defined as being required or expected to justify actions or decisions (Sharples and Elcock, 2011). An individual has to 'account' to a person or an organisation for their actions, omissions and decisions in carrying out a duty or task. In nursing, the question of to whom you are accountable will depend on whether you are a registered nurse or a student.

Accountability and the registered nurse

Cornock (2011) suggests that, in order to be accountable, a nurse needs to have the freedom (autonomy) and authority to be able to make a professional judgement on which actions to take, based on their knowledge of the possible options and consequences of each. In making that professional judgement, a registered nurse is accountable to a number of people and organisations:

- their profession (the Nursing and Midwifery Council), through the Standards set out by the NMC in the Code (NMC, 2015) and other standards and guides
- their employer, through their contract of employment
- society, through criminal or civil law
- the individual and public in general, via their duty of care.

Should a registered nurse's conduct – in relation to their behaviour, competence or health – raise concerns about their fitness to practise, they could be called to account to one or more of the above. For example, an employer may invoke their disciplinary process or capability process and, depending on their findings, also refer the nurse to the NMC.

A patient or their family could use the civil courts to sue a nurse if they believe that they have been negligent. Criminal law would be used to prosecute a nurse if they have broken the law. There is a memorandum of agreement between the police and the NMC, so where a nurse is convicted of a recordable offence the police will inform the NMC, who may then convene a fitness-to-practise panel. Equally, the NMC may inform the police where a nurse is found to have committed a serious crime (Sharples and Elcock, 2011).

Invariably, a registered nurse cannot deliver all the care required by patients alone, and in those circumstances they will need to make a decision on which tasks or activities can be appropriately delegated to others – including healthcare assistants, nursing students (RCN, 2015) and lay carers (NMC, 2018).

Accountability and the nursing student

Learning in practice will usually take place under the supervision of a registered nurse, but at times you may be supervised by other health or social care professionals. Initially, this will be close supervision, but as you develop your confidence and competence this supervision will increasingly be carried out at a distance (Hall and Ritchie, 2013). The registered nurse will assess your level of competence, knowledge and understanding before delegating a task or activity to you. It is very important that you inform the nurse if you feel any task delegated to you is beyond your level of competence. While the registered nurse will remain accountable for the overall care to be delivered, if you accept responsibility for the tasks delegated to you, you will then become accountable for your actions, omissions and decisions in performing those tasks (RCN, 2015). As a student, you can be held to account by:

- the university
- the law, through your duty of care.

This may seem quite scary, but what is key here is being clear about what you feel competent to undertake. The registered nurse is accountable for her decision to delegate and is required to ensure that it is appropriate to delegate it to someone else, that they have the required skills and knowledge and that they understand what is required and have accepted responsibility for the activity delegated (RCN, 2015). If you are asked to do something you have not done before, or don't feel that you have yet acquired the required level of competence and confidence, then you are within your rights to say so. However, once you accept the delegated activity, you have a duty of care to the patient to deliver it to a standard that is considered reasonable for a nursing student at your stage of the course. This is known as the Bolam test and is used in courts of law when looking at standards of care in negligence cases (Griffith and Tengnah, 2017).

Activity 7.1 asks you to look at tasks for which you should not accept responsibility as a student.

ANSWER:
ACTIVITY 7.1

ACTIVITY 7.1: LEADERSHIP AND MANAGEMENT

There are certain tasks/activities that nursing students cannot undertake until they are qualified. These may be listed in your course handbook; your practice educator should also be able to tell you. Make a note of what these are.

THE IMPORTANCE OF PROFESSIONALISM IN NURSING

Your ability to demonstrate professionalism is an essential course requirement that will be assessed through theoretical and practical assessments as well as through how you conduct your personal life. This latter part can be quite a challenge to come to terms with, so it is important here to help you appreciate why your conduct has to meet expected standards, both on your course and outside it.

First and foremost, the ability to demonstrate professionalism is essential to ensure public trust in nursing as a profession (NMC, 2015). There have been a number of reports into failings in the quality of care given to patients in recent years, such as *The Report of the Mid Staffordshire NHS Foundation Trust Public Inquiry* (Francis, 2013), a report into the abuse of people with a learning disability at Winterbourne Hospital (DH, 2012) and a series of reports called *Patient Stories* by the Patients Association, each of which have caused damage to the reputation of nursing. Nurses care for people when they are at their most vulnerable; children, young people, the elderly, people with mental health problems and those with a learning disability are seen as most vulnerable (RCN, 2013) and these people in particular therefore need to have confidence that the care that they will receive will be of the highest quality. Reports and media stories that describe poor quality care or abuse of patients can cause additional anxieties for patients and their carers when they are using healthcare services, and impact on their trust in nursing as a profession.

The Code (NMC, 2015: 3) makes clear the importance of trust, that good nursing practice 'promotes trust through professionalism' and that failing to comply with the Code may bring your fitness to practise into question and endanger your registration.

I feel so upset when I hear stories – some are truly horrific and unimaginable, yet it has happened. I do not believe there is any excuse for abuse and poor care. If there is a problem nurses need the courage to stand up and shout out – patients put their trust in us, and we need to protect them, their health and wellbeing.

Siân Hunter, child nursing student

There is no excuse for poor care. Providing good care should be the number one priority of any healthcare professional. If you witness care that you deem as poor raise it with either your practice educator or lecturer. Poor care should not be tolerated by anyone – it is our responsibility to identify areas of poor care and do everything in our power to put a stop to it.

Alice Rowe, NQ RNMH

FITNESS TO PRACTISE

The NMC defines fitness to practise as 'having the skills, knowledge, good health and good character to do their job safely and effectively' (NMC, 2017). The main function of the NMC is to protect the public and ensure that nurses and midwives registered with it maintain the appropriate skills and knowledge to ensure safe and effective practice and uphold the professional standards it sets.

Where a registered nurse's knowledge, skills, good health or good character is impaired, this may result in a referral to the NMC, who investigate allegations of misconduct, lack of competence, criminal behaviour or serious ill health, and will make a judgement on whether a nurse's fitness to practise is impaired.

As a student, you are not accountable to the NMC; however, an ability to demonstrate compliance with the NMC Code throughout your course is essential and this will be monitored by the university. On successful completion of your course, your university will sign a declaration to the NMC that you are of good health and good character sufficient to practise without supervision. This supports your own self-declaration of good health and character when you apply to register with the NMC.

The NMC requires each university to have its own processes to manage concerns regarding a student's fitness to practise (see Activity 7.2). Should any concerns arise regarding your health or professional behaviour (character), the university will use these processes to make a judgement on your fitness to practise. The outcome of these will depend on the seriousness of the concerns raised, the evidence to support them and the student's response to and insight into the concerns raised.

ACTIVITY 7.2: REFLECTIVE PRACTICE

Take a look at your university's fitness-to-practise policy:

- Does it identify the types of concerns that may lead to a student being referred to them?
- What are the penalties should any allegations be upheld?
- Does it identify where you can get support and advice should you ever be called to a fitness-to-practise panel?

ANSWER:
ACTIVITY 7.2

Until 2015, the NMC published a guide for students which listed actions and behaviours which could cause concerns regarding a student's fitness to practise, however this was replaced by the Code (2015) which is now THE guide on professional conduct for students as well as registered nurses and midwives. Table 7.1 offers some examples of the more common reasons why a student may be referred to a fitness-to-practise panel at their univeristy.

Some of the below will very obviously be a cause for concern, but you may feel some are less serious or do not seem to impact directly on patients. However, while some may not relate directly to patient care, they can bring into question a student's honesty, integrity and trustworthiness and therefore raise doubts about how that individual may act when caring for patients.

The idea of a nurse breaching confidentiality and sharing information about me and other patients online is quite scary. What if it went viral and everyone knew private things about my health that I wouldn't even tell my closest friends? I want to feel I can be honest when talking with a nurse, so if I was afraid that I might be mocked on Twitter for something I said, it would definitely affect how openly I would describe issues.

Chris, patient

Table 7.1   Potential areas of concern for 'fitness to practise'

Area of concern	Examples
Cheating or plagiarism	Whilst this may relate primarily to your exams and assignments, it could also include forging a practice educator's or academic's name or signature on your practice assessment document
Unprofessional behaviour	Aggressive, violent or threatening behaviour
	Misuse of the internet or social media/networking sites
	Breaches of confidentiality
Dishonesty	Failure to disclose criminal convictions on your application or after starting your course
	Forging timesheets
	Fraudulent claims for money, e.g. benefits
Health concerns	Drug or alcohol abuse
	Failure to seek medical treatment or other support where there is a risk of harm to other people by not doing so
Criminal convictions or cautions	Whilst not all criminal convictions will necessarily lead to a fitness-to-practise panel, failing to disclose any you receive will

The NMC publishes the outcomes of all investigated cases that lead to actions to ensure that trust of the public in the profession is maintained and to safeguard the public from nurses or midwives whose fitness to practise is found to be impaired. It is important to note that only a very small number of nurses have allegations made against them. During 2015–16, concerns were raised about 0.8 per cent of nurses and midwives on the NMC register (NMC, 2016a). The types of allegations reported to the NMC during 2014–15 are shown in Table 7.2.

WHAT'S THE EVIDENCE?

WEBLINK: TYPES OF ALLEGATIONS

Table 7.2   Types of allegations made as new referrals to the NMC in 2014–15

Types of allegations	Percentage
Misconduct	80%
Lack of competence	5%
Criminal	11%
Health	3%
Fraudulent entry	Less than 1%
Determination by another body (for example, Irish Nursing Board, Health and Care Professions Council)	Less than 1%
Total	**100%**

Source: Nursing and Midwifery Council (2015) *Nursing and Midwifery Council Annual Fitness to Practise Report 2014-15.* Read the full report on the NMC website and read more about how the NMC handles concerns and complaints about nurses and midwives on its web page, 'Concerns about nurses or midwives'.

- Reflect on how the Code provides guidance that clarifies your responsibilities with regard to the examples of misconduct, competence, ill health and criminal behaviour.
- If you had concerns regarding the conduct of a nurse or nursing student, how does the NMC guidance assist you in deciding whether you need to raise your concerns more formally?

As you can see in Table 7.2, misconduct is the most common reason for referral to the NMC. The NMC (2016b) defines misconduct as 'conduct which falls short of what would be proper in the circumstances' and can include the conduct of a nurse or midwife in their personal life as well as at work. Since January 2016, a new area of concern that the NMC will now consider is 'not having the necessary knowledge of English' (NMC, 2016a).

Although the NMC publishes the outcomes of its fitness-to-practise hearings on its website, providing full details of the allegations, the decision-making process and the sanctions decided on, details related to health concerns regarding a nurse or midwife are not made public. The sanctions that the NMC can levy against a registrant are:

- *A caution order* (1–5 years) – the registrant's NMC record will show that they are subject to a caution order and any enquirers about their registration will be informed about the Order.
- *Conditions of practice order* – the NMC sets conditions under which the registrant may continue to practise (e.g. under supervision, restricted from working in certain settings, further training, engaging with occupational health) for up to three years.
- *Suspension order* – registration as a nurse is suspended for up to one year, after which it can be extended, replaced, confirmed or revoked.
- *Striking-off order* – the nurse is removed from the register and cannot apply to be restored for five years. At that point, they would need to demonstrate that they are fit to practise and would usually need to complete a Return to Practice course before being able to register with the NMC again.

Social media is widely used by students and by organisations: your university may have a Facebook page or a Twitter account, for example. If you use a social network, you can adjust the privacy settings so that the public cannot see what is written; however, anything you post or share on a social network that is available to view by a friend or colleague can be easily shared with others and therefore become public.

To uphold your professional 'online' profile as a nurse, it is important you carefully consider what you are uploading and writing online and that you think before you post. Cross (2014: 134) reminds us of the importance of being proactive in managing what we share, stating: 'there's a common belief that once something is on the Internet, it's there forever. The permanence of social media requires you to accept that once data is released online, it may be available forever'. While not necessarily true, it may seem like it, especially if the data is embarrassing. Remember, once it's out there, it's out there. So, if in doubt, don't put it out there!

It is very important that you consider your behaviour when utilising any online form of communication. Your conduct will be judged in the same way whether in the 'real world' or online, and if it is judged to raise concern regarding your fitness to practise or bring the profession into disrepute (NMC, 2016c), your continuance on the course or your ability to join the NMC register could be put at risk.

Use your common sense. Do not discuss anything on a social networking site in terms that could be viewed as derogatory towards your staff members or patients. Maintain confidentiality and professionalism at all times. The easiest method to avoid a tricky situation is to not post anything work-related on a social networking site.

Alice Rowe, NQ RNMH

Social networking sites can be difficult – as much as it is easy to keep in touch with friends and family, I find it is not always easy to monitor what they put on a status. I always make sure that I am careful who I accept as a friend and mindful of what I write so I do not offend anyone.

Sarah Parkes, LD nursing student

CASE STUDY 7.1: SOCIAL NETWORKING

Jenna is not enjoying her placement and posts a series of comments on Twitter about how bored she is and makes some derogatory comments about the staff she is working with. In the final week of her placement, she posts pictures of herself at a party which show her drinking alcohol and looking dishevelled. She then tweets in the morning how she has a major hangover and is going to be late for work but at least it's her last day.

A student at university who is a Facebook 'friend' and Twitter follower is concerned by what she has seen and informs her personal tutor. Following an initial investigation, Jenna is referred to the university fitness-to-practise panel. The panel finds that her fitness to practise is impaired as her actions have failed to uphold the reputation of her profession; however, based on the remorse Jenna shows and her insight into how her actions were not in keeping with the Code, the panel decides to impose a condition rather than discontinue her from the programme. Jenna is also informed that should she request a reference from the university, it may be required to disclose that she has been subject to a fitness-to-practise hearing.

- Read the NMC (2016c) guidance on using social media responsibly.
- Consider what action you might take if a nursing student or other healthcare professional posted something that you felt was inappropriate on a social networking website.
- Reflect on your online persona, your web presence and posts you have made in the past. What information 'about you' is available publicly? What photos have you posted? What does it say to others about you? Consider where there may be areas for improvement.

ANSWER:
CASE STUDY 7.1

As a nurse, you will be involved in both clinical and **therapeutic interventions** for patients. The nature of these interventions, coupled with the patient's dependency on the nurse, mean that patients are seen as vulnerable, as they are less able to protect themselves and may have difficulty recognising appropriate boundaries (Council for Healthcare Regulatory Excellence, 2008). Patients and carers therefore need to be able to trust the nurse to maintain professional boundaries at all times, to prevent exploitation or abuse which can cause them significant harm (Halter et al., 2007). As a student, managing professional relationships can be challenging; therefore, if at any time you find yourself in a difficult situation with a patient, it is important to seek guidance from your practice educator or a member of staff at the university.

CASE STUDY 7.2: SEXUAL BOUNDARIES

This case centred on a registered nurse (LD) and his relationship with a female patient. Following the investigation, he was proven to have:

- inappropriately touched a patient on her bottom
- given the patient his personal telephone number
- suggested to the patient that they should meet socially by offering to accompany her to a parent-and-child group.

Outcome: Fitness to practise impaired.

Sanction: A striking-off order with an interim suspension of 18 months (this allowed the registrant time to appeal if they wished to).

- Consider your experience so far and how you would respond to a patient who wished to cross the professional boundary of the nurse–patient relationship.
- Would you have any additional concerns if the patient had a learning disability?

ANSWER:
CASE STUDY 7.2

CASE STUDY 7.3: SAFEGUARDING AND CONFIDENTIALITY

Sarah is a nursery nurse at a clinic who is concerned that a child, whom we shall call Betty, may have sustained non-accident related injuries, and has referred Betty and her mother to a health visitor. The health visitor met with Betty and her mother, who gave an explanation for Betty's injuries. The mother also mentioned that she had spoken to her social worker (who had been allocated to the family as Betty had been identified as a 'child in need'). The health visitor contacted social services the following day. Social services raised concern that they had not been informed on the day that the health visitor saw Betty. It was revealed that the mother had not actually been in contact with her social worker; as a consequence, Betty had to undergo a more intrusive medical examination than would have been the case if she had been referred on the day she'd been seen by the health visitor.

In the same month, the health visitor was at a case conference with a family, where she mentioned the first names of another family whom they also knew. This constituted a breach of confidentiality. In light of these events, the health visitor referred herself to the NMC.

(Continued)

The charges were that the health visitor:

- did not immediately report the matter to Betty's social worker
- did not establish whether Betty's mother had already contacted Betty's social worker
- did not seek advice from a colleague at the trust
- did not arrange for Betty to receive a medical examination without delay in order to establish the nature of the condition or injury
- on 30 September 2010, disclosed confidential information during a case conference where the name of one family was revealed in the presence of another family.

Outcome: Fitness to practise impaired.

Sanction: Caution order – three years.

ANSWER: CASE
STUDY 7.3

- Look at the NMC Code and identify which sections you believe the health visitor breached and reflect on your responsibility for responding to a safeguarding concern.

There were two issues here: one around the failure of the health visitor to act to safeguard the child concerned; the second around a breach of confidentiality. As a nurse, you will come into contact with children and vulnerable adults where you may have concerns regarding safeguarding issues. What this case identifies is the importance of making your concerns known immediately where you believe a child or an adult may be at risk.

The breach of confidentiality issue is a reminder that you must always be aware that people around you may be familiar with the person you are discussing – particularly on community placements or in community hospitals, which serve the local community.

The common theme in each of the case studies is the issue of trust. The importance of trust is made clear in the NMC Code (2015: 15), with the theme 'promote professionalism and trust'. Trust is essential to the nurse–patient relationship (Feo et al., 2017) – without it, an effective relationship cannot be established, and this can impact on the patient's confidence in sharing information with you that may be important to their care and on their willingness to comply with therapeutic interventions, which could have serious consequences for their wellbeing.

CONCLUSION

This chapter has explored the concepts of accountability, professionalism and fitness to practise as they relate to both the registered nurse and to you as a student. Considering these issues will help you gain a clear understanding of why your university and the people with whom you come into contact in clinical practice constantly talk to you about the importance of your conduct and behaviour both when in practice and at university, as well as in your personal life. Nurses are in a privileged position and the public need to be able to trust that your conduct will always be of the highest standard.

CHAPTER SUMMARY

- Both students and registered nurses can be held accountable for their actions, but whom they are accountable to differs.
- Students who accept a delegated activity are then responsible for their actions.
- As a nursing student, you are part of a profession where your behaviour both at work and in your personal life will be judged against the NMC Code.
- The public need to have confidence and trust in individual nurses and nursing as a profession if effective therapeutic relationships are to be developed.
- It is the role of the NMC to protect the public, and they set clear guidance for students and universities on areas that may cause concern about a student's fitness to practise.
- Students whose character or health raises concerns regarding their fitness to practise may be referred to a fitness-to-practise panel, which could lead to their removal from the course.

CRITICAL REFLECTION

Holistic care

This chapter has highlighted the importance of ensuring you follow the NMC Code and act professionally at all times when providing holistic care for your patient. Think about a patient for whom you have cared recently and consider how you ensured that their trust in you was well founded. Consider how generating trust might be different with patients from different fields of practice. Make a note of your thoughts; refer back to this next time you care for a patient and then write down your own reflections of that experience.

GO FURTHER

Books

Avery, G (2016) *Law and Ethics in Nursing and Healthcare: An Introduction*. London: Sage. Covers key concepts that you need to understand in exercising accountability in your practice.

Griffith, R. and Tengnah, C.A. (2017) *Law and Professional Issues in Nursing* (Transforming Nursing Practice Series), 4th edn. Exeter: Learning Matters. Covers a range of topics that will help you to understand how to deliver safe and effective practice within the law and the NMC Code.

Sellman, D. (2011) *What Makes a Good Nurse: Why the Virtues are Important for Nurses*. London: Jessica Kingsley. A thought-provoking book that explores the importance of the virtues that underpin nursing, many of which also underpin professional practice.

SAGE journal articles

Go to https://study.sagepub.com/essentialnursing2e for free online journal articles for this chapter. If you are using the interactive ebook, simply click on the book icon in the margin to go straight to the resource.

FURTHER READING: JOURNAL ARTICLES

Copeland Smith, G. and Knudson, TK (2016) 'Student nurses' unethical behavior, social media, and year of birth', *Nursing Ethics* 23(8): 910–918. An interesting article that looks at the use of social media by students and how it links with ethical conduct.

Other journal articles

David, T.J. and Lee-Woolf, E. (2010) 'Fitness to practice for nursing students: Principles, standards and procedures', *Nursing Times*, 106(39): 23–6.

Ellis, J., Lee-Woolf, E. and David, T. (2011) 'Supporting nursing students during fitness to practice hearings', *Nursing Standard*, 25(32): 38–43.

Two really useful articles which explain the process and provide guidance for students who may be referred to a fitness-to-practise panel.

Sprinks, J. (2015) 'Updated Code stresses nurses' accountability for delegation of tasks to competent colleagues', *Nursing Children and Young People*, 27(2): 7–8. Explores the NMC Code from the perspective of a children's nurse.

Weblinks

FURTHER READING: WEBLINKS

Go to https://study.sagepub.com/essentialnursing2e for weblinks related to this chapter. If you are using the interactive ebook, simply click on the book icon in the margin to go straight to the resource.

www.nmc-uk.org – the NMC provides a range of guidance documents on good conduct and good character, fitness-to-practise issues, raising concerns, social media guidance and guidance for students.

www.rcn.org.uk/professional-development/accountability-and-delegation – this RCN web page provides guidance on accountability and delegation, a useful guide for you to download and a video to watch.

www.rcn.org.uk – the RCN website provides a range of guidance for registered nurses as well as useful information for students around professional issues.

Video Links

Accountability and Delegation by the Royal College of Nursing – www.rcn.org.uk/professional-development/accountability-and-delegation

A useful guide to understanding these key concepts in nursing.

Professionalism in Practice – www.nmc.org.uk/standards/professionalism/professionalism-in-practice/

You will find three animations on this website to show you how to use the NMC framework *Enabling Professionalism in Nursing and Midwifery Practice*

VIDEO LINKS

Have a break from the text and go to https://study.sagepub.com/essentialnursing2e for useful videos related to this chapter. If you are using the interactive ebook, simply click on the lightbulb icon in the margin to go straight to the resource.

ACE YOUR ASSESSMENT

ONLINE QUIZZES

Review what you have learned by visiting the book's online resources at: https://study.sagepub.com/essentialnursing2e If using your interactive ebook, just click on the icon in the margin to go straight there.

- Test yourself with multiple-choice and short-answer questions.
- Revise key terms with the interactive flash cards.

REFERENCES

Cornock, M. (2011) 'Legal definitions of responsibility, accountability and liability', *Nursing Children and Young People*, 23(3): 25–6.

Council for Healthcare Regulatory Excellence (CHRE) (2008) *Clear Sexual Boundaries between Healthcare Professionals and Patients: Responsibilities of Healthcare Professionals*. London: CHRE.

Cross, M. (2014) *Social Media Security: Leveraging Social Networking While Mitigating Risk*. Rockland, MA: Syngress.

Department of Health (DH) (2012) *Department of Health Review: Winterbourne View Hospital Interim Report*. London: HMSO.

Feo, R., Rasmussen, P., Wiechula, R., Controy, T. and Kitson, A. (2017) 'Developing effective and caring nurse–patient relationships', *Nursing Standard*, 31(28): 54–62.

Francis, R. (2013) *Report of the Mid Staffordshire NHS Foundation Trust Public Inquiry*. London: HMSO. Available at: www.midstaffspublicinquiry.com/report (accessed 21 April 2017).

Griffith, R. and Tengnah, C.A. (2017) *Law and Professional Issues in Nursing*, 4th edn. Exeter: Learning Matters.

Hall, C. and Ritchie, D. (2013) 'The professional nurse: Image and values in nursing'. Chapter 3 in *What is Nursing? Exploring Theory and Practice*, 3rd edn. Exeter: Learning Matters. pp. 37–60.

Halter, M., Brown, H. and Stone, J. (2007) *Sexual Boundary Violations by Health Professionals: An Overview of the Published Empirical Literature*. London: Council for Healthcare Regulatory Excellence. Available at: www.professionalstandards.org.uk/docs/default-source/publications/research-paper/sexual-boundary-violations-2007.pdf?sfvrsn=4 (accessed 21 April 2017).

Nursing and Midwifery Council (NMC) (2015) *The Code: Professional Standards of Practice and Behaviour for Nurses and Midwives*. London: NMC.

Nursing and Midwifery Council (2016a) *Nursing and Midwifery Council Annual Fitness to Practise Report 2015–16*. London: The Stationery Office.

Nursing and Midwifery Council (2016b) *Preliminary Consideration of Allegations Guidance*. London: NMC.

Nursing and Midwifery Council (2016c) Guidance on Using Social Media Responsibly. Available at: www.nmc.org.uk/standards/guidance/social-media-guidance (accessed 21 April 2017).

Nursing and Midwifery Council (2017) What is Fitness to Practise? Available at: www.nmc.org.uk/concerns-nurses-midwives/what-we-do/what-is-fitness-to-practise (accessed 22 March 2017).

Nursing and Midwifery Council (2018) *Standards of Proficiency for Registered Nurses*. London: NMC.

Royal College of Nursing (RCN) (2013) *Rights, Risks and Responsibilities in Service Redesign for Vulnerable Groups*. London: RCN.

Royal College of Nursing (RCN) (2015) *Accountability and Delegation: A Guide for the Nursing Team*. London: RCN. Available at: www.rcn.org.uk/professional-development/accountability-and-delegation (accessed 21 April 2017).

Sharples, K. and Elcock, K. (2011) *Preceptorship for Newly Registered Nurses*. Exeter: Learning Matters.

RESILIENCE

E. JANE BLOWERS

THIS CHAPTER COVERS

- What is professional resilience?
- Professional requirements for good health

- Psychological concepts for resilience

“

Although it isn't possible to predict the challenges you will face as a nurse, during the few months I have been a newly qualified nurse I now realise how important it was to develop my resilience during my nursing course! As a nursing student you have a vast amount of support available to help you develop the skills of bouncing back and taking positive action so you can become resilient. Make the most of this; try out new coping strategies to support your existing ones and ensure you make the most of all the experiences you have.

Alice Rowe, NQ RNMH

”

“

It is very difficult not to get caught up with everyday uni life; it is important that you offload and talk about anything you have found difficult. Not only is it good for your mental health but it will also help you to get through your degree.

Sarah Parkes, LD nursing student

”

Visit https://study.sagepub.com/essentialnursing2e to access a wealth of online resources for this chapter – watch out for the margin icons throughout the chapter. If you are using the interactive eBook, simply click on the margin icon to go straight to the resource.

INTRODUCTION

Are you clear about what professional resilience is, how you can achieve this and how it is significant for holistic patient care? Thinking about your own nursing practice, how resilient are you? As suggested in the student voice above, might you benefit from taking further action to keep psychologically and physically healthy?

All of these issues will be explored within this chapter in order to help you understand what is meant by professional resilience, and its importance in enabling you to meet your professional requirements.

Nursing is both a challenging and highly rewarding career choice. Your three-year nursing course will be an inspirational but also, at times, stressful journey. This chapter will help you put your experiences of being a nursing student in context and recognise that while your individual experiences are highly personal and important, many of the challenges that you encounter will also be shared by your fellow students. Throughout the chapter, the topics discussed will increase your insight into some of the strategies you can adopt to improve your professional resilience by maximising the benefits of your course.

WHAT IS PROFESSIONAL RESILIENCE?

The term 'resilience' is often used to describe a desirable characteristic within nursing, or any profession. It originates from the English word 'resile', which means 'to bounce or spring back' (Agnes, 2005, cited in Smith et al., 2008: 194). Resilience is important for all healthcare professionals, helping them to stay physically and psychologically healthy despite working in an environment in which they frequently deal with stress and adversity. Resilience involves skills that can be learned and developed (McAllister and McKinnon, 2009), just like being able to write an essay, and will be not only relevant to your experiences as a nursing student, but also a fundamental aspect of your practice throughout your entire nursing career.

To be honest I have found it stressful from the start, being a mature student; my husband is disabled and [having] four young children with no family to physically support us has been really tough. The workload, the extra study at the end of the day, every day, research, travelling. Caring for my family or just seeing friends has been a challenge, but I am still here. Talking with other students and giving each other support when days are dark really lifted me up. I spoke to my academic advisor who gave me some great advice. Talking to second and third years was really inspirational. I remind myself what I am doing and the reasons why. It will be the most rewarding thing I will have done since having my children and will be worth it in the end, to make that difference to someone's life.

Siân Hunter, child nursing student

I was never particularly good at essay writing and that was apparent when I first started my nursing training. I wondered how I would ever get through three years of this! But I soon found a wealth of knowledge and support via the university; I attended some private tutorials and did some online learning packages which really helped get my writing skills up to scratch.

Charlie Clisby, NQN

The need to be professionally resilient

Becoming a nursing student involves a period of adjustment from your previous role, such as the one you inhabited at school or college or in employment. Taking on the role of a university student undertaking a professional course such as nursing requires that you become professionally socialised in order to meet the requirements of the Nursing and Midwifery Code (NMC, 2015a) and achieve the standards for entry to the professional register when you complete your course.

During their adjustment to being a university student and becoming a professional, many students experience significant life events, such as changes in their own health or the health of family members and friends, or changes in their personal circumstances. Such changes are stressful and add to the usual stresses experienced by nursing students, such as academic demands, worries regarding placements, the need to meet the emotional demands of nursing, and financial issues.

It has been recognised that it is important to care for the psychological health of university students (IPPR, 2017) and 'Nursing students are … juggling several roles, which demand a high level of commitment and competence' (Evans and Kelly, 2004: 474). This chapter suggests a number of ways you can positively develop your ability to cope during your nursing course.

CASE STUDY 8.1: DARIKA

Darika is six months into her nursing degree. She has been enjoying her course and nursing has been her lifelong ambition. Recently, Darika's parents told her that they are going to end their relationship. She is very shaken by this news, as is her sister, who is a year younger than her. Darika is confused about what has happened at home since she left and feels guilty about being away at university. She is also worried about the financial implications of this, as her parents have been helping her to pay for a car, which she has found very helpful for travel to her placements.

In addition to this, Darika has recently failed the first submission of a summative assessment - an essay focusing on communication. She has always been successful in previous studies, never failing anything else. Darika is beginning to doubt herself, wondering if nursing is for her. Darika's friends on the course all seem to be very successful, which puts her off sharing some of her own doubts. She does not want to discuss the situation with her sister or parents as she feels that they have sufficient worries of their own. Spend ten minutes answering the following questions:

- If Darika was at your university, what sources of support would be available to help her cope with her current situation?
- What personal actions can Darika take to improve her current situation?
- If you were Darika's friend, what would you do?

ANSWER: CASE
STUDY 8.1

For many university students, one of the biggest challenges when they start their course is finding a balance between the many new and exciting social opportunities available to them and spending sufficient time studying. As a student on a nursing course, this is further complicated by the need to abide by health-related professional requirements.

PROFESSIONAL REQUIREMENTS FOR GOOD HEALTH

The Nursing and Midwifery Council (NMC) requires nurses and nursing students to be of 'good health' and provides information about this for students (see www.nmc.org.uk/education/becoming-a-nurse-or-midwife/when-studying-to-be-a-nurse-or-midwife).

WEBLINK:
NMC.ORG

In professional guidance to universities 'good health' has the following definition:

> 'Good health' means that the applicant is capable of safe and effective practice either with or without reasonable adjustments. It does not mean the absence of a health condition or disability. (NMC, 2015b)

When you start your nursing course, a university occupational health assessment will confirm that you are of good health, and throughout your course you are also required to make an annual self-declaration that this remains the case. Before you register as a nurse at the end of your course, the NMC requires that your good health is confirmed by your university.

This means that, first as a nursing student and then as a registered nurse, you need to take the positive action required to promote your own health. As a nurse, you have a responsibility to be a healthy role model to others, which involves maintaining healthy behaviours to maintain your wellbeing and enable you to fulfil your nursing role effectively. This will provide a benefit not only to you, but also to your patients, colleagues and employers.

Your responsibility as a healthy role model to others

Contemporary nursing practice emphasises the proactive promotion of health. As a nursing student and future registered nurse, you are a role model. Key National Health Service (NHS) initiatives, such as Making Every Contact Count (NHS, 2013), emphasise the importance of health promotion at every opportunity. Social learning theory demonstrates the importance of modelling behaviours (Bandura et al., 1961), meaning that for nurses to promote health in patients, they should be demonstrating healthy behaviours themselves. Role-modelling healthy behaviour will have an impact on patients and your fellow nursing students, as well as family and friends. Therefore, taking steps to manage your own health and wellbeing is a vital aspect of professionalism.

I enjoy running and cycling when I have the time because they help clear my mind and are free to do. I find that this makes me more alert throughout the day and helps me to de-stress.

Sarah Parkes, LD nursing student

Identifying actions to achieve professional resilience

Staying healthy and feeling able to cope throughout your nursing course is hugely important. McAllister and McKinnon (2009) and Turner (2014) discuss personal characteristics which can positively influence resilience. These include pro-social behaviour, empathy and a positive self-image.

Cope, Jones and Hendricks (2014) found that nurses' resilience and continued practice could be influenced by social support from family, friends and colleagues, pride in their work and putting patients' needs before their own. Moreover, Evans and Kelly (2004) found that coping and feeling satisfied with their course were important factors in the wellbeing of nursing students. Other important factors were:

- self-efficacy
- dispositional control
- support.

Avoidance coping was found to be a predictor of a reduction in wellbeing (Gibbons et al., 2010), making it clear that avoiding situations is not an effective way to deal with stressful events or to build your resilience. Rather than avoiding situations that you find stressful by 'burying your head in the sand', it is preferable to use positive strategies (see Table 8.1) which relate to your sense of achievement and enable you to positively influence your situation.

Table 8.1   Positive strategies to increase your resilience

Develop your key skills and knowledge	Take advantage of all opportunities on offer at your university and in practice settings, as this will foster a sense of self-growth and achievement.
Adopt good personal organisational skills, including those related to effective time management	Have a plan – this can increase your sense of being in control of your situation. It can also influence others' image of you as a professional and reinforce your own positive self-image as you become professionally socialised.
Develop your self-awareness	Understanding yourself will help you to adopt the most helpful personal strategies and take action related to your development needs. Awareness of the impact you have on others will also help you to seek the most appropriate support and advice.
Recognise your own stress and take responsibility for this	Use positive actions to manage yourself. Recognise any maladaptive coping strategies you may use, such as drinking too much alcohol or comfort eating, rather than potentially more positive ways of relaxing, and build or introduce more positive strategies.
Increase your sense of belonging	This involves understanding how you can contribute to the team-working environments in both your university and practice settings – the more you give, the more rewarding you are likely to find your experiences.
Consider how you can adopt local or national wellbeing policies and strategies	As a way of promoting your personal health and that of patients, family, friends and other students.
Have a voice	Express your views via your university and practice-area systems, such as module and course evaluations. Join your student council and student union, and participate in the university societies you find interesting.

ACTIVITY 8.1: REFLECTIVE PRACTICE

Use the suggestions in Table 8.1 to outline two activities which you could try to increase your resilience.

CASE STUDY 8.2: JACK

Jack is an adult health nursing student on placement in a busy surgical ward. He feels uncomfortable with the dynamics of the ward team and has questions regarding the way in which the work is organised. Jack is unsure if his perceptions are accurate and is conscious that he can have a tendency to externalise his stress rather than considering all perspectives – he has become aware of this through previous feedback and some of his reflective work on the course. Jack has been feeling particularly stressed recently. Three other students are also currently placed on the ward and Jack thinks these individuals are all having a very successful placement. It is his view that they seem to have more access to learning opportunities than he does, and he is wondering why this is. Spend ten minutes answering the following questions:

ANSWER: CASE
STUDY 8.2

- What could be making Jack think that the other students on his placement are having access to more learning opportunities than he is?
- What personal actions would you advise Jack to take to improve his situation?

PSYCHOLOGICAL CONCEPTS FOR RESILIENCE

An understanding of the key psychological concepts you are studying as part of your course will enhance the development of your personal professional resilience. These concepts include self-awareness, self-efficacy, adjustment and coping, factors all positively associated with developing resilience. They are introduced within the following sections of this chapter and their importance in professional resilience is highlighted.

Developing self-awareness to enhance your professional resilience

As is identified and discussed in Chapter 16, self-awareness is related to recognising personal feelings and abilities and having realistic levels of self-confidence. This concept has two key components, both relating to perception:

1. perception of self
2. perception by others.

Table 8.2   Areas to consider in relation to your self-awareness

Thoughts
Feelings
Behaviours and self-management strategies
Beliefs
Attitudes
Values
Aspirations and fears
Goals and motivation
Preferences/dislikes
Past experiences

Source: Barker (2007)

Nursing students have responsibilities in relation to the development and maintenance of their self-awareness. Barker (2007: 42) states: 'Once the nurse starts to develop self-understanding, they are then faced with the need to address issues about themselves.' So increasing your self-awareness is a positive action, which will help you to bounce back when things are challenging. Your nursing course is an opportunity to learn many things about yourself, and Table 8.2 highlights some areas you might decide to consider.

It is also possible that experiences you have with patients, their families or other healthcare professionals may enable you to learn previously unrealised things about yourself.

As a nursing student I learned to be grateful for the small things. Discharging a patient when they have spent a long time in your care, or simply making them smile, outweighs the prospect of a pay packet at the end of the month. We are lucky in that we get to spend time with people from all walks of life. I strongly believe that the conversations we have with individuals greatly impact the way we choose to approach our own challenges and help us become better rounded people.

Alice Rowe, newly qualified MH nurse

Using a Johari window (Luft, 1969, cited in Rana and Upton, 2009) is another way to help you to learn more about yourself. A Johari window is made up of four panes that divide your personal awareness into four different aspects:

Open – what I know about myself that others know too – the public area

Hidden – what I know about myself that others do not know – the private area

Blind – what others know about me, but I am unaware of

Unknown – what no one knows about me

Each of us has our own unique window. So, if I were to complete my Johari window, I would fill in the four panes as in Figure 8.1.

Open - what I know about myself that others know too - the public area

For example, my name, my description and my likes and dislikes. Much of the information in this pane is factual, but my feelings and motives would also be included. The more you get to know me, the bigger this pane will become.

Hidden - what I know about myself that others do not know - the private area

If we do not know each other very well there will be lots of information in here, but as you get to know me some of this information will move to the open pane.

Blind - what others know about me, but I am unaware of

A simple example of this could be that while writing on the wipe-board I smudged marker pen on my chin. You can see this but I cannot. However, if you tell me that I have got ink on my chin, this information would no longer be in my blind spot.

Unknown - what no one knows about me

This pane can be used to explore new understandings. For example, if I shared an experience with you which we then discuss and attempt to understand the significance of, we would both gain new knowledge about me.

Figure 8.1   My Johari window

ACTIVITY 8.2: REFLECTIVE PRACTICE

Draw a Johari window relating to your self-awareness. Include your thoughts and feelings relating to any feedback, formal or informal, that you have received from peers, patients, carers, practice educators and lecturers.

- When you have completed your window, can you see any discrepancies between your view of yourself and those held by others? Where this occurs, what do you think the reasons are?
- How has this activity helped you to develop and learn from your own view of yourself? How might this new knowledge influence your future actions?
- How can being self-aware enhance your resilience as a nursing student?

CASE STUDY 8.3: CARLA

Carla is a learning disabilities nursing student. The recent unexpected death of a service user with whom she had been working has left her feeling emotionally exhausted. Carla is shocked by the impact that this experience has had on her and is beginning to question whether she has the resilience to fulfil a professional role where death may be encountered unexpectedly.

- What type of support do you think Carla needs to seek to answer her questions?
- What advice would you give Carla if she asked you how she could develop her resilience?

ANSWER: CASE
STUDY 8.3

Considering your Johari window will help to increase awareness of your self-knowledge and perceptions, plus the knowledge and perceptions of you that others hold.

Put this activity in your portfolio and discuss it with your personal advisor when you next meet.

Self-efficacy

The concept of self-efficacy is related to a 'belief that you can perform adequately in a particular situation', with your sense of personal competence influencing how you think things are going, your drive to engage and succeed and how you actually perform (Banyard, 1996: 176). Therefore, there is a relationship between your self-belief and the successful completion of your nursing course. While you must not be over-confident – because recognising your limitations and the boundaries of your role makes you a safe practitioner – confidence in your own abilities is important (NMC, 2015a). Using strategies to build your confidence – such as practising skills you find difficult, with support, rather than avoiding them – is important for success. If you believe you are able to engage in certain types of actions successfully, you are much more likely to put effort into carrying them out, and this will make you far more likely to develop the necessary skills to succeed. Bandura (1977) suggested that it is a good thing if people have beliefs about their self-efficacy that are slightly higher than the evidence would suggest, because this encourages them to aim higher and, by doing so, to try harder and so develop their skills and abilities even further.

CASE STUDY:
ABHA

Apply your understanding of self-efficacy by reading Abha's case study, at https://study.sagepub.com/essentialnursing2e.

Adjustment and coping

Adjusting as you move from one role to another is an important aspect of success. During your nursing course, you will go through a process of adjustment in order to successfully perform a professional role in which you have mastered many diverse skills. Coping during this process involves managing situations effectively. Lazarus and Folkman (1984) define coping as constantly changing cognitive and behavioural efforts which enable the individual to manage external and/or internal demands that, at times, seem to exceed their current resources. Therefore, in more simple terms, it is important to recognise that adjustment is a natural psychological process and that it is usual not to feel in full control of new situations.

WHAT'S THE EVIDENCE?

Five ways to mental wellbeing – the Foresight Report

The Foresight Report (2008) investigated the nation's mental health and made five recommendations as to how people can improve their mental wellbeing. We can think of these as the mental health equivalent of 'eating five portions of fruit and vegetables a day'.

1. **Connect...** With the people around you. With family, friends, colleagues and neighbours. At home, work, school or in your local community. Think of these as the cornerstones of your life and invest time in developing them. Building these connections will support and enrich you every day.

2. **Be active...** Go for a walk or run. Step outside. Cycle. Play a game. Garden. Dance. Exercising makes you feel good. Most importantly, discover a physical activity you enjoy and that suits your level of mobility and fitness.

3. **Take notice...** Be curious. Catch sight of the beautiful. Remark on the unusual. Notice the changing seasons. Savour the moment, whether you are walking to work, eating lunch or talking to friends. Be aware of the world around you and what you are feeling. Reflecting on your experiences will help you appreciate what matters to you.

4. **Keep learning...** Try something new. Rediscover an old interest. Sign up for that course. Take on a different responsibility at work. Fix a bike. Learn to play an instrument or how to cook your favourite food. Set a challenge you will enjoy achieving. Learning new things will make you more confident as well as being fun.

(Continued)

5.   Give... Do something nice for a friend, or a stranger. Thank someone. Smile. Volunteer your time. Join a community group. Look out, as well as in. Seeing yourself, and your happiness, as linked to the wider community can be incredibly rewarding and creates connections with the people around you.

Think about all of the activities you have taken part in so far today. Can you identify two instances when you could have integrated one of the above into your activities?

Figure 8.2   The mental equivalent of 'eating five portions of fruit and vegetables a day'
Images © Robin Lupton

As is outlined in the student voice, feeling overwhelmed is a normal response, which you can actually use to help you. When you begin to feel that you are not fully in control in a situation, this feeling is reminding you that you need to further develop your positive coping strategies. This will not only help you to feel in control of the situation when it next arises, it will also increase your professional resilience. For some individuals, change can be exhilarating; others will find it daunting. However, it doesn't actually matter how you feel – you can still increase your chances of a positive outcome via reflection on previous experiences, taking proactive action and tackling a challenging situation with support. Increasing your self-awareness, self-efficacy, adjustment and coping skills will support your mental wellbeing, enabling you to become more professionally resilient.

At times throughout the course, particularly in the past year, I felt incredibly overwhelmed. Initially, shedding a few tears and panicking worked a treat. However, after a short while I realised neither of those coping strategies were helping me gasin control. After the tears and grumpy behaviour, seeking support and advice from peers, lecturers and practice educators enabled me to think clearly and diffuse the situations that were challenging me.

Alice Rowe, NQ RNMH

The role of mental wellbeing in enhancing professional resilience

The health and mental wellbeing of NHS staff are the focus of the Boorman Report (DH, 2009). This report recommends that individual NHS trusts should prioritise a range of health and mental wellbeing services to raise the profile of staff health. The Boorman Report is important because it identifies a relationship between staff health and mental wellbeing and patient satisfaction. The report includes recommendations related to reducing smoking and harmful drinking in staff. The National Institute for Health and Care Excellence (NICE) (2009) and NHS Employers (2014) also offer guidance on promoting staff's mental wellbeing. So, it has been recognised that working in the NHS can be stressful, but also that this stress can be managed effectively and, more importantly, that working keeps you mentally well.

Work is important for mental wellbeing (from NICE, 2009)

Mental wellbeing is a dynamic state in which the individual is able to develop their potential, work productively and creatively, build strong and positive relationships with others and contribute to their community. It is enhanced when an individual is able to fulfil their personal and social goals and achieve a sense of purpose in society.

CASE STUDY 8.4: CHANDRAN

Chandran is a mental health nursing student. He considers himself a hard-working and understand-ing nursing student, and he is dismayed that on several occasions the service users he has met have commented that he could not understand their circumstances. Chandran feels that these perspec-tives are related to his age and is becoming disheartened, as he is juggling the competing demands of his theory and practice assessments and beginning to question his commitment to a profession in which he feels unappreciated.

- What advice would you give Chandran to help him feel more appreciated?

ANSWER: CASE STUDY 8.4

CONCLUSION

Professional resilience is important for your success both during your nursing studies and within your ongoing career as a registered nurse. As a resilient contemporary health professional, there is much for you to be proud of regarding your achievements within the challenging and rewarding profession of nursing. This chapter has encouraged you to make the most of the opportunities – within your pre-registration course and beyond – to develop the skills and knowledge required to bounce back as you face professional challenges. Your understanding of the links between maintaining your own health and wellbeing and the professional requirements of being a nurse is important for your resilience, as is functioning as a reflective, self-aware practitioner with effective coping strategies that enable you to adjust and cope as your exciting professional journey develops.

CHAPTER SUMMARY

- Being a nursing student is both a challenging and rewarding experience. To adjust and cope with the requirements of this, you will benefit from adopting proactive strategies to enhance your personal and professional resilience.
- Professional resilience is the ability to 'bounce back' in stressful situations. It is an important attribute for contemporary healthcare professionals.
- Nurses are expected to proactively promote the health of others. It is important that you fully consider the implications of your health behaviours as a role model.
- Maintaining professional wellbeing can be enhanced by a good understanding of psychological concepts such as coping, adjustment and self-awareness.
- National policy literature such as the Foresight Report (2008) and NICE (2009) guidance offers helpful, evidence-based advice for maintaining wellbeing.
- NHS organisations have a responsibility to promote the health of their employees.
- Nurses have a professional requirement to maintain up-to-date knowledge and be of 'good health'.

CRITICAL REFLECTION

Holistic care

This chapter has highlighted the importance of professional resilience when providing holistic care for patients:

- Think about a person for whom you have cared recently and make a note of how your own health and wellbeing have been important to enable your provision of optimum care.
- Think of a particularly challenging situation you have encountered during your nursing course and make a list of the factors which had a positive effect on your ability to cope with this situation.

GO FURTHER

Books

Nef (2011) Five Ways to Wellbeing: New Applications, New Ways of Thinking. Available at: www.nhsconfed. org/Publications/reports/Pages/Five-ways-to-wellbeing.aspx. A set of evidence-based public mental health messages aimed at improving the mental health and wellbeing of the whole population.

Rana, D. and Upton, D. (2009) *Psychology for Nurses*. Harlow: Pearson. This psychology textbook contains important theory that will enhance your understanding of both your own behaviour and that of others. This knowledge is empowering and reassuring, and will effectively underpin your practice as you build your professional resilience.

SAGE journal article

FURTHER
READING:
JOURNAL
ARTICLE

FIND OUT
MORE!

Go to https://study.sagepub.com/essentialnursing2e for free online journal articles for this chapter. If you are using the interactive ebook, simply click on the book icon in the margin to go straight to the resource.

Zeller, J.M. and Levin, P.F. (2013) 'Mindfulness interventions to reduce stress among nursing personnel: An occupational health perspective', *Workplace Health & Safety*, 61(2): 85–9. An article considering mindfulness training, an evidence-based approach to increase situational awareness and positive responses to stressful situations, as an inexpensive strategy to reduce stress and improve the quality of nurses' work lives.

Other journal articles

Gibbons, C., Dempster, M. and Moutray, M. (2010) 'Stress, coping and satisfaction in nursing students', *Journal of Advanced Nursing*, 67(3): 621-32. This interesting research focuses on pre-registration nursing students. The article provides evidence of the importance of taking control of your situation, and that personal action increases your sense of wellbeing and effectiveness of coping.

Harris, R.C., Rosenberg, L. and O'Rourke, M.E.G. (2014) 'Addressing the challenges of nursing student attrition', *Journal of Nursing Education*, 53(1): 31-7. This article examines the need for more nurses, including those from diverse backgrounds. Attrition rates among schools of nursing are discussed, along with at-risk student characteristics and previous attempts to increase student success.

FURTHER
READING:
WEBLINKS

Weblinks

Go to https://study.sagepub.com/essentialnursing2e for weblinks related to this chapter. If you are using the interactive ebook, simply click on the book icon in the margin to go straight to the resource.

www.makingeverycontactcount.co.uk – the NHS (2013) document Making Every Contact Count: Guide and Toolkit provides useful contemporary NHS resources which focus on health and wellbeing.

www.nhsemployers.org/search-results?q=stress – the NHS Employers (2014) document Guidance on the Management and Prevention of Stress in the Workplace includes guidance on preventing and managing workplace stress.

www.nhs.uk/Tools/Pages/Wellbeing-self-assessment.aspx – a wellbeing self-assessment tool to self-assess your current state of wellbeing.

https://assets.publishing.service.gov.uk/government/uploads/system/uploads/attachment_data/file/480482/NHS-Constitution_WEB.pdf – this website provides access to the NHS Constitution, a vital document for articulating responsibilities and values within our National Health Service.

www.nice.org.uk/nicemedia/pdf/PH22Guidance.pdf – NICE guidance accessed via this web link is an important evidence-based source of information regarding the promotion of mental wellbeing in the workplace.

Video links

Have a break from the text and go to https://study.sagepub.com/essentialnursing2e for useful videos related to this chapter. If you are using the interactive ebook, simply click on the lightbulb icon in the margin to go straight to the resource.

VIDEO
LINKS

ACE YOUR ASSESSMENT

Review what you have learned by visiting the book's online resources at: https://study.sagepub.com/essential nursing2e If using your interactive ebook, just click on the icon in the margin to go straight there.

ONLINE
QUIZZES

- Test yourself with multiple-choice and short-answer questions.
- Revise key terms with the interactive flash cards.

REFERENCES

Bandura, A. (1977) 'Self-efficacy: Toward a unifying theory of behavioural change', *Psychological Review*, 84(2): 191–215.

Bandura, A., Ross, D. and Ross, S.A. (1961) 'Transmission of aggression through imitation of aggressive models', *Journal of Abnormal and Social Psychology*, 63: 575–82.

Banyard, P. (1996) *Applying Psychology to Health*. London: Hodder and Stoughton.

Barker, S. (2007) *Psychology: Vital Notes for Nurses*. Oxford: Blackwell Publishing.

Cope, V., Jones, B. and Hendricks, J. (2014) 'Why nurses choose to remain in the workforce: Portraits of resilience', *Collegian: The Australian Journal of Nursing Practice, Scholarship and Research*, 23(1): 87–95.

Department of Health (DH) (2009) *NHS Health and Wellbeing: The Boorman Report*. London: DH.

Evans, W. and Kelly, B. (2004) 'Pre-registration diploma nursing student stress and coping', *Nurse Education Today*, 24: 473–82.

Foresight Report, The (2008) *Mental Health and Capital: Making the Most of Ourselves in the 21st Century*. London: Government Office for Science.

Gibbons, C., Dempster, M. and Moutray, M. (2010) 'Stress, coping and satisfaction in nursing students', *Journal of Advanced Nursing*, 67(3): 621–32.

Institute for Public Policy Research (IPPR) (2017) *Not by Degrees: Improving Students' Mental Health in the UK's Universities*. London: IPPR.

Lazarus, R.S. and Folkman, S. (1984) *Stress, Appraisal and Coping*. New York: Springer.

McAllister, M. and McKinnon, J. (2009) 'The importance of teaching and learning resilience in the healthcare disciplines: A critical review of the literature', *Nurse Education Today*, 29: 371–9.

National Health Service (NHS) (2013) Making Every Contact Count: Guide and Toolkit. Available at: www.makingeverycontactcount.co.uk (accessed 18 February 2015).

NHS Employers (2014) Guidance on the Management and Prevention of Stress in the Workplace. Available at: www.nhsemployers.org/search-results?q=stress (accessed 8 December 2017).

National Institute for Health and Clinical Excellence (NICE) (2009) *Public Health Guidance 22: Promoting Mental Wellbeing at Work*. London: NICE.

Nursing and Midwifery Council (NMC) (2010) *Standards for Pre-registration Nursing Education*. London: NMC.

Nursing and Midwifery Council (2015a) *The Code: Professional Standards of Practice and Behaviour for Nurses and Midwives*. London: NMC.

Nursing and Midwifery Council (2015b) Character and Health Decision-making Guidance. Available at: www.nmc.org.uk/globalassets/sitedocuments/registration/character-and-health-decision-making-guidance.pdf (accessed 3 May 2017).

Rana, D. and Upton, D. (2009) *Psychology for Nurses*. Harlow: Pearson.

Smith, B., Dalen, J., Wiggins, K., Tooley, E., Christopher, P. and Bernard, J. (2008) 'The brief resilience scale: Assessing the ability to bounce back', *International Journal of Behavioural Medicine*, 15: 194–200.

Turner, S. (2014) 'The resilient nurse: An emerging concept', *Nurse Leader*, 12(6): 71–3.

THE ROLE OF THE NURSING STUDENT IN EFFECTING CHANGE

9

JACQUELINE PHIPPS

THIS CHAPTER COVERS

- The context and nature of change within the NHS
- Being a leader as a student nurse

- A leadership model for nursing students
- Strategies and tools for leading and managing change

My name is Robert. I am 85 and have been admitted to a male medial unit for treatment for a urinary tract infection and pneumonia. I have been so distressed because I have not been able to carry out my own hygiene care and my clothes and body are smelling. Today James, a student nurse, was the first person to listen to me about my worries. James helped me to have a shower and shave and found some clean clothes for me to wear. I feel so much better now.

Robert, patient

Today I worked on a male medical unit and was caring for Robert. He became really distressed because he had not had a wash or shave for three days. He told me that no one had asked him if he needed help. I helped Robert with his hygiene needs and communicated the need for Robert having assistance for washing and shaving in his care plan.

James Greystone, student nurse

INTRODUCTION

What do you feel about Robert and James' story? What do you think might have been the impact for Robert as a result of the change that James made? Change is often described as a process that causes something to be different, or as moving from one state to another. Robert and James, in the patient and student voices at the start of this chapter, clearly demonstrate that small changes can make a difference in the way that patients experience care.

This chapter introduces the concept of NHS change in terms of improving the quality of healthcare. It highlights the importance of leading change for quality improvement when caring for patients and your role within this. It provides some guidance on strategies and tools for managing change.

THE CONTEXT AND NATURE OF CHANGE WITHIN THE NHS

Since the inception of the NHS, it has been characterised by constant change. Successive governments have pursued policies that have set out the case for change in the NHS based on the core principle of improving the quality of care for patients. However, given the subjective nature of quality, quality improvement can be difficult to define. Some of the common concepts generally associated with change, in terms of quality improvement within the NHS, include improving patient outcomes, decreasing risk and improving patient safety, improving the patient experience and reducing waste. The context for change over the years in the NHS has been driven by various elements. These elements are inextricably linked. These can be considered as drivers for change, because they can be used to influence or 'drive' the need for and direction of change in order to improve the quality of care (Department of Health, 2010; Ham et al., 2016; NHS England, 2016).

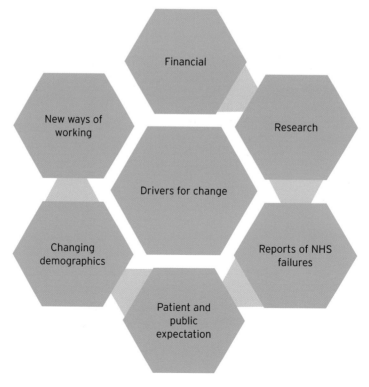

Figure 9.1 Drivers for change

ACTIVITY 9.1: CRITICAL THINKING

Go to the Nuffield Trust interactive timeline at http://nhstimeline.nuffieldtrust.org.uk – this charts the evolution of the NHS from its inception through to 2010. Using the interactive timeline to learn more about particular events which contributed to widescale change in the NHS, think about the drivers for change and the quality improvements associated with the events.

ANSWER:
ACTIVITY 9.1

In common with many health policies which have gone before, Five Year Forward (NHS, 2014) sets out the contextual drivers for why and how the NHS must change. It highlights the fact that people are living longer, and this often results in them having multiple and complex needs. It also alludes to how patients' expectations regarding their choice in where and how their healthcare is delivered have increased greatly since the inception of the NHS. Patients expect to be able to express their views and have them acted on, which was not the case in 1948 when the NHS was introduced. Further drivers for change also include reference to the way that the NHS functions, including the emergence of new ways of working, new care delivery models and new technologies. Five Year Forward also sets out the need for the NHS to ensure that the care delivered is efficient and value for money.

This view not only set out the need for change and for a direction of change in the NHS, it also identified who would be responsible for leading and managing different aspects of the changes. However, there is recognition within the policy that a top-down approach to change alone will not ensure the delivery of high-quality healthcare. Change for the purposes of quality improvement will require the leadership efforts of everyone working at all levels in the NHS.

BEING A LEADER AS A STUDENT NURSE

It may seem hard to think of yourself as a leader when you are new to the role of nursing student. As being an effective leader in the NHS is more about upholding professional values and behaving in a way that demonstrates a commitment to improve quality of healthcare and influence change, it is possible for nursing students to fulfil this role by upholding the principles and values of the NHS Constitution (DH, 2015) and the NMC Code (2015).

CASE STUDY:
JOHN

The NHS Constitution (DH, 2015) sets out the six values that everyone working in the NHS is expected to demonstrate in order to deliver high-quality care:

- working together for patients
- respect and dignity
- commitment to quality of care
- compassion
- improving lives
- everyone counts.

The NMC Code (2015) can help you understand what standards you need to adhere to in order to put the needs of your patients first and to deliver care that is safe and effective. The Compassion in Practice policy (Department of Health and NHS Commissioning Board, 2012) clearly sets out the principles of being a leader and change champion at the point of care. The fundamental values of the 6Cs can help you to understand the leadership behaviours that you should embrace in order to have direct impact on the quality of care for the patients and the people you support every minute of every day.

For example, we can all differentiate between speaking kindly to another person and being sharp and dismissive. We can all recognise when a person is being hurried and not given the time they require. It is clear to see when a decision is being made for a person, rather than someone explaining the options and letting them choose for themselves. While it is important that you spend considerable time and effort during your nursing course developing your skills and knowledge, at the end of your course the nursing care you deliver will still need to demonstrate the leadership values and behaviours that you will use to ensure the delivery of high-quality care.

The Leading Change, Adding Value framework for nursing, midwifery and care staff (NHS England, 2016) builds on Compassion in Practice and sets out the responsibility of nurses for achieving quality care. The framework offers 10 aspirational commitments which can assist you as a student nurse to achieve quality healthcare and implement change, based on improving patient outcomes, improving patient experience and providing value for money.

NHS 10 Commitments

1. We will promote a culture where improving the population's health is a core component of the practice of all nursing, midwifery and care staff.
2. We will increase the visibility of nursing and midwifery leadership and input in prevention.
3. We will work with individuals, families and communities to equip them to make informed choices and manage their own health.
4. We will be centred on individuals experiencing high-value care.
5. We will work in partnership with individuals, their families, carers and others important to them.
6. We will actively respond to what matters most to our staff and colleagues.
7. We will lead and drive research to evidence the impact of what we do.
8. We will have the right education, training and development to enhance our skills, knowledge and understanding.
9. We will have the right staff in the right places and at the right time.
10. We will champion the use of technology and informatics to improve practice, address unwarranted variations and enhance outcomes.

ACTIVITY 9.2: REFLECTIVE PRACTICE

ANSWER:
ACTIVITY 9.2

- Think about a patient for whom you cared during your last placement.
- How did your care reflect the values and principles of the NHS constitution, the NMC Code and the 6Cs?
- How did your care reflect your commitment to delivering high-quality care?

A LEADERSHIP MODEL FOR NURSING STUDENTS

The Healthcare Leadership Model (NHS Leadership Academy, 2013) can also help you understand the types of effective leadership behaviours required for delivering high-quality care and leading quality improvement at the point of care. This model of leadership contrasts with the traditional view of change within the NHS as entirely top-down and highlights the responsibility of everyone in the NHS to become better leaders, whether they have a formal leadership role or not. It describes the things you can see leaders doing at work and is organised in a way that helps everyone to see how they can develop as a leader. It applies equally to the whole variety of roles and care settings that exist within health and care. It reinforces the message that leadership of quality healthcare and quality improvement is everyone's responsibility.

Figure 9.2 Healthcare leadership model

Source: NHS Leadership Academy (2013) at www.leadershipacademy.nhs.uk/resources/healthcare-leadership-model

NHS
LEADERSHIP
ACADEMY

The model is made up of nine dimensions. For each of the dimensions, there is a description of what leadership is and what it is not and why it is important. Leadership behaviours within each of the dimensions are presented on a four-part scale from 'essential' through 'proficient' and 'strong' to 'exemplary'. You can use this model to understand how the way that you behave can demonstrate acts of leadership which focus on a commitment to delivering high-quality care in your day-to-day practice. For example:

- ensuring that you role-model behaviours that reflect the professional values, standards, responsibility and accountability of nurses to delivering high-quality care (NMC, 2015)
- ensuring that you create time to build therapeutic relationships in order to listen and respond to the actual needs of individuals
- ensuring that you work in ways that help to reduce the waste of resources and maximise the value of every nursing intervention
- ensuring that you deliver care to your patient that is based on the best evidence in order to improve their health and wellbeing
- having the courage to speak up when you have concerns, even if it may involve some risk to yourself
- acting as a change agent by making suggestions for small, evidence-based changes to ensure the delivery of quality care.

CASE STUDY 9.1: JANE

My name is Jane and I have an eating disorder. I have just been told that my care is being transferred from the Child and Adolescent Mental Health Service to the Adult Mental Health Service. My key worker, Alex, understands my problems really well – I don't want to talk to

(Continued)

someone new. Alex keeps telling me that it is normal to be anxious and promises that I will be OK, but I don't believe him. I don't think that I can go to the appointment he has arranged to meet the new people who will be caring for me in future. (Jane, patient)

- What values and leadership behaviours could Alex draw on to act as a change agent and help to improve the quality of care during this period of transition of care for Jane?

STRATEGIES AND TOOLS FOR LEADING AND MANAGING CHANGE

Acting as a change agent for quality while you are a nursing student is not necessarily about being responsible for radically redesigning services. It can be as simple as taking opportunities to use your knowledge to communicate the need for a small, evidence-based change to improve the quality of care for your patients. Whatever the context, nature or extent of your involvement as a change agent, it is key that you understand the importance of using effective change management strategies, service improvement tools and evaluation methods for effectively leading and managing change. Change management strategy basically means adopting a systematic and deliberate approach to managing a change project. Service improvement tools are those that can be used to help identify and reduce the risks associated with the change project. Evaluation methods use established data collection and data analysis techniques to measure whether the intended quality outcomes of the change project have been achieved. There are numerous strategic change management frameworks that use defined steps to guide the process of change (Gopee and Galloway, 2013; Iles and Sutherland, 2001).

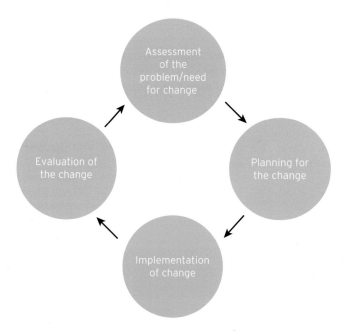

Figure 9.3   Strategic change management model

The strategic change model was designed to help student nurses to understand the process of change and quality improvement. The model presents strategic change management as a cyclical change process similar to the four stages of the nursing process.

Assessment of the problem/need for change

Whenever you are involved in change, it is important to communicate why change is needed. This is the first stage of the change management process which involves making the case for change. This stage of the change requires you to identify what you intend to change, the reason why change may be needed and the intended desired future state at the end of the change process. Within this stage, you should consider how you can communicate the rationale for, and the aims and objectives of, the intended change. This stage of the change process requires you to research the best available evidence associated with the inextricably linked drivers that can support the rationale for change. A robust analysis of the evidence base of the drivers for change will help you to communicate the intended aims and outcomes in terms of quality improvement, based on improving patient outcomes, improving patient experience and providing value for money. Once a case for change has been made, you may have the opportunity to be involved in the planning, implementation and evaluation of the change.

Planning for the change

This stage of the change management process involves defining and scoping the change project. At this stage, you need to consider who will need to be involved, what is possible, how it can be achieved and how the quality outcomes will be measured. It is also the stage at which you need to think about the risks and challenges associated with the change project and how these may be managed, either before or within the implementation stage. The success of this stage of the change management process will be dependent on you selecting the appropriate evidence-based service improvement tools. Your choice will be dependent on their suitability to the context, nature, size and level of the change management project (The Health Foundation, 2013; Iles and Sutherland, 2001; NHS Institute for Innovation and Improvement, 2010).

For example, stakeholder management tools can help you to select the most appropriate people with the right expertise and knowledge to help you to design a robust plan appropriate to the service. Including people who have the authority will help you to understand the governance and approval mechanisms required to implement the change. There are also various tools that you can use to consider creative and innovative solutions for achieving the aims and objectives of the change project. This is the stage where you will need to consider what the emotional response of others will be to the change. There can be a number of factors that will influence people's emotional response and resistance to the proposed change. They may not understand the need for change or feel that they do not have the skills or knowledge to make the transition very well; or they may not understand or value the proposed benefits associated with the change. You can help to reduce the risks of human resistance to change through the development of a robust communication plan for sharing the vision of the change and detailing the support mechanisms that will be available to people prior to and throughout the implementation stage of the change process. Planning for support mechanisms such as large-scale or small-scale meetings and training workshops prior to and during the change and throughout the implementation stage of the change can help people build their confidence, skills and knowledge and help them to overcome their fear of the change (The Health Foundation, 2013; Iles and Sutherland, 2001; NHS, 2011; NHS Institute for Innovation and Improvement, 2010).

WHAT'S THE EVIDENCE?

Selecting the correct tool for the change

The Health Foundation (2013) has produced an excellent document called *Quality Improvement Made Simple* (http://reader.health.org.uk/QualityimprovementMadeSimple).

A range of service improvement tools is also available from the NHS Institute for Innovation and Improvement, which bring together a number of theories and techniques for service improvement which are helpful in managing change.

Review the document and consider how you could apply these tools to implement a change in practice.

This is also the stage where you will need to make plans regarding what data collection and data analysis methods to use. Measurement and gathering data are vital elements of any attempt to improve performance or quality, and are also needed to assess the impact of the change. Developing plans for robust data collection and data analysis methods will help you to ensure rigorous and transparent measurements of the quality outcomes of the change at the evaluation stage. You may need to think about collecting data as a baseline measurement prior to the implementation stage. This could serve as the basis for a comparison measurement, with subsequent data collected at the evaluation stage (Raleigh and Foot, 2010).

Implementation of change

This is the stage at which you actually start making changes. It will be important at this stage that you continue to pay attention to maintaining the motivation for and commitment to the change as well as managing any areas of conflict or resistance to change from people whom the change may effect.

Evaluation of the change

This is the final stage of the change management process, in which you will measure whether the planned quality improvements have been achieved. This stage also includes the development of plans to address any problems or further need for change that may have been identified by the change management process. Evaluating change is a very important stage, which is often missed – but it is this final step which ensures that the change endures and is sustained. By evaluating a change, it is possible to start the change process again – giving it a cyclical nature, as once again the need for further change is considered (Gopee and Galloway, 2013; Raleigh and Foot, 2010).

CASE STUDY 9.2: RAFAL

Rafal, a mental health field student, is thoroughly enjoying his first placement on a surgical ward. He and his practice educator often care for patients in Bay 1, which is next to the emergency admissions bay. Today, Rafal and his practice educator are caring for patients in Bay 1 again. When Rafal asks the patients if they had a good sleep, they all become rather angry and tell him that 'sleep is impossible here because the telephones and call bells in the emergency admissions bay keep ringing all night'.

Rafal can't stop thinking about this during the rest of his shift and decides that something needs to be changed to help the patients get a better night's sleep.

- How can Rafal use the strategic change management model to present a plan to improve the environment and help patients sleep better?
- How could Rafal measure the quality impact of any changes that he will make?

ANSWER:
CASE STUDY 9.2

CONCLUSION

Healthcare policy sets out the case for change within the NHS based on the core principle of improving quality. Everyone working in the NHS must be responsible for improving quality. The healthcare leadership model can help you to understand the leadership behaviours that you can engage in to make small changes which impact on the quality of healthcare that you deliver to your patients. There are various strategic change models on service improvement that you can use to help you manage the process of change. Robust data collection and data analysis methods will help you to measure the quality impact of any changes that you make.

CHAPTER SUMMARY

- The context and nature of change within the NHS focuses on quality improvement.
- Quality improvement and change is the responsibility of everyone working in health and care.
- Effective leadership behaviours can help student nurses to support quality improvement and change at the point of care.
- Utilising effective change management strategies, appropriate service improvement tools, data collection and evaluation methods can help identify the need for change and reduce risks associated with the implementation and evaluation of change.

CRITICAL REFLECTION

- Reflect on how you could use the strategic change model to implement a change in practice.

GO FURTHER

Books

Andriopoulos, C. and Dawson, P. (2009) *Managing Change, Creativity and Innovation*, 2nd edn. London: SAGE. This book brings together comprehensive aspects of change and innovation management, providing an accessible and wide-ranging resource for study, debate and inspiration. Balancing theory with practice, this book considers the human aspects of managing change and creativity.

Gopee, N. and Galloway, J. (2013) *Leadership and Management in Healthcare*, 2nd edn. London: SAGE. This book emphasises how management theory applies to care for all healthcare professionals, regardless of the position they hold, and supports them to develop their skills through action points, case studies and good practice guidelines.

Sullivan, E, J. and Garland, G. (2013) *Practical Leadership and Management in Healthcare: For Nurses and Health Professionals* . Pearson. This chapters within this book reflect some of the important themes and approaches to leading change identified within this chapter. It will be a valuable additional resource to help support your development as a leader and change agent at all stages of your nursing career.

Journal articles

Govier, I. (2009) 'Examining transformational approaches to effective leadership in healthcare settings', *Nursing Times Special Supplement: Leadership Skills for Nurses*, 12–15. Available at: www.nursingtimes. net/Journals/1/Files/2009/12/3/NT%20Leadership%20Supplement.pdf. This article explores how transformational and authentic leadership reflects the core values underpinning nursing and the act of caring. It also discusses how these leadership approaches can be applied by nurses to respond and adapt to change while ensuring the delivery of high-quality care.

Nelson-Brantley, H, V. Ford D, J. (2016) 'Leading change: a concept analysis', *Journal of Advanced Nursing*, 73(4), 834–846. This research used concept analysis to identify descriptions, antecedents, consequences and empirical referents of the concept of leading change at the point of care. A theoretical definition and conceptual model of leading change were developed from the findings. Whilst the authors recommended future studies that use and test the model, the study can provide nurses with a broader understanding of the some of the concepts associated with leading change.

Shanley, C. (2007) 'Management of change for nurses: Lessons from the discipline of organizational studies', *Journal of Nursing Management*, 15: 538–46. This article provides an insight into how much change can be planned and controlled, how top-down and bottom-up approaches to change can be combined, the role of emotions in the change management process and the connection between theory and practice in managing change.

Willcocks, S.G. (2012) 'Exploring leadership effectiveness: Nurses as clinical leaders in the NHS', *Leadership in Health Services*, 25(1): 8–19. This literature-based study explores the history and policy background of nurse leadership. It reviews a range of approaches to leadership and applies its theoretical findings to case studies of nurse leaders.

Weblinks

FURTHER READING: WEBLINKS

Go to https://study.sagepub.com/essentialnursing2e for weblinks related to this chapter. If you are using the interactive ebook, simply click on the book icon in the margin to go straight to the resource.

www.improvinghealthandlives.org.uk – Improving Health and Lives is a partnership between Public Health England (formerly the North East Public Health Observatory), the Centre for Disability Research at Lancaster University (CeDR) and the National Development Team for Inclusion (NDTi), funded by the Department of Health. The organisation aims to provide better, easier to understand information on the health and wellbeing of people with learning disabilities.

www.health.org.uk – the Health Foundation is an independent charity providing a range of resources to help practitioners make improvements to health services.

www.england.nhs.uk/sustainableimprovement – the NHS Improving Quality site is hosted by NHS England and brings together knowledge, expertise and experience to help practitioners transform care within the NHS.

www.kingsfund.org.uk – the King's Fund is an independent charitable organisation that works to improve healthcare in the UK and provides resources for practitioners associated with health policy analysis, health publications and other resources.

www.leadershipacademy.nhs.uk – the NHS Leadership Academy provides a centre of excellence and a beacon of best practice on leadership development for all practitioners working in NHS-funded care. For example, it created the healthcare leadership model (NHS Leadership Academy, 2013). The model is made up of nine dimensions. For each dimension, leadership behaviours are shown on a four-part scale which ranges from 'essential' through 'proficient' and 'strong' to 'exemplary'. The scale is not tied to any particular job roles or levels. This leadership model was designed for the use of anyone who works within a healthcare or other service setting, regardless of whether or not they have a formal leadership responsibility. The model provides a working framework for nursing students to demonstrate the complexity and sophistication of the development of their leadership behaviours as they move up the scale. See www.leadershipacademy.nhs.uk/wp-content/uploads/2013/10/NHSLeadership-LeadershipModel-10-Print.pdf.

Video links

Have a break from the text and go to https://study.sagepub.com/essentialnursing2e for useful videos related to this chapter. If you are using the interactive ebook, simply click on the lightbulb icon in the margin to go straight to the resource.

VIDEO
LINKS

ACE YOUR ASSESSMENT

Review what you have learned by visiting the book's online resources at: https://study.sagepub.com/essential nursing2e If using your interactive ebook, just click on the icon in the margin to go straight there.

ONLINE
QUIZZES

- Test yourself with multiple-choice and short-answer questions.
- Revise key terms with the interactive flash cards.

REFERENCES

Department of Health (DH) (2010) *Equity and Excellence: Liberating the NHS*. London: The Stationery Office.

Department of Health (2015) The NHS Constitution: The NHS belongs to us all. Available at: www.gov.uk/government/uploads/system/uploads/attachment_data/file/480482/NHS_Constitution_WEB.pdf (accessed 5 June 2017).

Department of Health and NHS Commissioning Board (2012) Compassion in Practice: Nursing, midwifery and care staff – Our vision and strategy. Available at: www.england.nhs.uk/wp-content/uploads/2012/12/compassion-in-practice.pdf (accessed 18 February 2015).

Gopee, N. and Galloway, J. (2013) *Leadership and Management in Healthcare*, 2nd edn. London: SAGE.

Ham, C., Berwick, D. and Dixon, J. (2016) Improving Quality in the English NHS. Available at: www.kingsfund.org.uk/sites/files/kf/field/field_publication_file/Improving-quality-Kings-Fund-February-2016.pdf (accessed 5 June 2017).

Health Foundation, The (2013) *Quality Improvement Made Simple: What Everyone Should Know about Healthcare Quality Improvement: Quick Guide*. London: The Health Foundation. Available at: www.health.org.uk/public/cms/75/76/313/594/Quality%20improvement%20made%20simple%202013.pdf?realName=rskqP0.pdf (accessed 18 February 2015).

Iles, V. and Sutherland, K. (2001) *Managing Change in the NHS: Organisational Change – A Review for Health Care Mangers, Professionals and Researchers*. London: National Co-ordinating Centre for NHS Service Delivery and Organisation R & D.

National Health Service (NHS) (2011) First Steps towards Quality Improvement: A simple guide to improving service. Available at: https://qi.elft.nhs.uk/wp-content/uploads/2016/01/nhs-improvement-guide-to-service-redesign.pdf (accessed 5 June 2017).

NHS (2014) *Five Year Forward View*. London: NHS.

NHS England (2016) Leading Change, Adding Value: A framework for nursing, midwifery and care staff. Available at: www.england.nhs.uk/wp-content/uploads/2016/05/nursing-framework.pdf (accessed 5 June 2017).

NHS Institute for Innovation and Improvement (2010) The Handbook of Quality and Service Improvement Tools. Available at: www.miltonkeynesccg.nhs.uk/resources/uploads/files/NHS%20Ill%20Handbook%20serviceimprove.pdf (accessed 18 February 2015).

NHS Leadership Academy (2013) *Healthcare Leadership Model: The Nine Dimensions of Leadership Behaviour.* Leeds: NHS Leadership Academy. Available at: www.leadershipacademy.nhs.uk/wp-content/uploads/2013/10/NHSLeadership-LeadershipMode1-10-BW-Print.pdf (accessed 11 February 2015).

Nursing and Midwifery Council (NMC) (2015) *The Code: Professional Standards Practice and Behaviour for Nurses and Midwives.* London: NMC.

Raleigh, V.S. and Foot, C. (2010) Getting the Measure of Quality Opportunities and Challenges. Available at: www.kingsfund.org.uk/sites/files/kf/Getting-the-measure-of-quality-Veena-Raleigh-Catherine-Foot-The-Kings-Fund-January-2010.pdf (accessed 5 June 2017).

The aim of this part of the book is to highlight the aspects of care you will always need to consider when working with patients. In nursing, there is a range of fundamental issues that are integrated into all aspects of the care we deliver; it is the nurse's skill that enables them to devise the unique mix that is effective for each patient. This is what enables a nurse to deliver the best care possible and this is a skill you will practise frequently during your course.

An important factor in all settings is that the care a patient receives must be based on sound theory. There are also fundamental nursing values that must be upheld at all times, such as respect, compassion and dignity. Upholding these values, in addition to communicating effectively in all situations, is a feature of good nursing, as are a systematic approach to care, the ability to assess and manage risk, and maintaining clear records. These, in combination with an understanding of the importance of safeguarding patients and making sound decisions regarding their care, will form the central core of your nursing knowledge.

While nurses spend a considerable amount of their time considering illness, it is also an important aspect of the nursing role to promote health at every opportunity and to deliver effective patient education. These are the abilities that will enable you to empower patients to become more aware of and adopt healthier behaviours.

This part of the book covers the wide range of important topics that will enable you to fulfil the many demands of a nurse's role. As Francis points out, our role can make a real difference to people's lives, and as Ashley highlights, it is important not to hold back, and to be an advocate for patients. The voices in this part opener highlight the importance of key issues in delivering care – read these and keep them in mind as you work through the chapters in this third part of the book.

DELIVERING EFFECTIVE CARE

FIONA EVERETT AND WENDY WRIGHT

——————————— THIS CHAPTER COVERS ———————————

- What makes good care and what makes care good?
- How you can apply quality care initiatives within your practice

- The role of the Nursing and Midwifery Council (NMC) in making care good
- When care is not good

"

My name is Vijay, I am 67 years old and I recently had a coronary artery bypass graft. I have now been discharged from hospital and I am recuperating at my daughter's home. I have also received a visit from the district nurse, to review my progress, which was arranged before I came out of hospital.

I was extremely happy with the care that I received while in hospital and I have asked my daughter to help me write a letter thanking all of the staff involved. I was cared for by a variety of healthcare professionals: nurses, doctors, physiotherapists, occupational therapists, radiographers, and many more. I was impressed by the professionalism demonstrated by them all. I was treated with dignity and respect and made to feel at ease, as all staff were more than happy to answer any questions. They took the time to explain any procedure before it was carried out. I was really impressed by the level of knowledge demonstrated by staff when providing care.

It was good to be given written information explaining my care – for example, how long my hospital stay was likely to be, what to expect after surgery and what type of diet and exercise would help me recover. I was always involved in making decisions about my care and was impressed by the genuine caring attitudes of all the health professionals I met.

Vijay, patient

"

"

I remember feeling anxious and excited about the prospect of placements when I was a first-year student because I was worried that I did not have enough knowledge or experience, but I also felt excited that I could make a contribution to caring for patients.

During my nursing programme I learned that the provision of patient care is complex and that every care episode brings a new set of challenges. My knowledge, skills, confidence and competence have grown and developed and this has prepared me to become a registered nurse.

One of the most important things I learned is to listen to the patient and their relatives and carers, to make sure that care can be tailored to meet their individual needs, and to always put the patient at the centre of the care provided. It is also important that care is always underpinned by professional, legal and ethical principles and policy.

To help me focus upon this I have composed a word cloud of the things that I think, and that patients have told me, are important [see Figure 10.1].

Harriet, NQ LD nurse

"

Figure 10.1   Harriet's word cloud

INTRODUCTION

Do you feel anxious and excited at the prospect of caring for patients? Would you like to make a meaningful contribution to care provision? How can you make sure your knowledge, skills, confidence and competence all develop in order that you will feel prepared to become a registered nurse? How can you be the best nurse you can be? What can you do that will make a patient's bad day just a little better?

Vijay's story outlines some important elements of care and highlights what patients value. Harriet's comment demonstrates that the provision of effective care involves many issues, some of which are dependent on the individual providing the care – in other words, you.

There are many factors nurses must take into consideration when providing care, such as benchmarking, evidence-based care, the role of the Nursing and Midwifery Council (NMC), the regulation and inspection of care delivery, the utilisation of clinical standards and guidelines, models of care, assessment tools and the application of person-centred care. These are considered throughout this chapter in order to help you find the answers to some of the many questions you will have relating to the care you provide to patients.

WHAT MAKES GOOD CARE AND WHAT MAKES CARE GOOD?

Nursing is often described as a 'caring' profession. Most students enter nursing because they want to 'care' for other people. In order to ensure that the care provided is 'good', benchmarks for good practice are used. Benchmarks are a way to identify best practice and allow the standard of care to be measured. A document called *The Essence of Care* (DH, 2003, revised 2010) provided a range of benchmarks which identified best practice and enabled nurses to improve existing practice by comparing and sharing ways of caring for patients through a recognised framework. Another example of benchmarks is the Scottish Executive (2007) document *Better Health, Better Care*, which advocates that the Institute of Medicine's six dimensions of quality care provision should form the foundations of care and be made evident in all care provided. The six dimensions of quality care provision are:

- person/patient-centred
- safe
- effective
- efficient
- equitable
- timely.

A similar initiative designed to maintain high standards of care is *The High Impact Actions for Nursing and Midwifery* (NHS Institute for Innovation and Improvement, 2009). This initiative involved a group of senior nurses who selected a core number of actions posted on the High Impact website. Eight high-impact actions evolved (see Table 10.1). These actions were deemed to be areas where significant improvement in quality can be achieved for patients, which has been underpinned by contemporary research evidence. You may already have made a contribution to some of these, depending on your placement experience so far.

Table 10.1   High-impact actions for nursing and midwifery

Category of action	Action
Your skin matters	No avoidable pressure sores in the NHS
Staying safe, preventing falls	Demonstrate a year-on-year reduction in the number of falls sustained by older people in NHS-provided care
Keeping nourished, getting better	Stop inappropriate weight loss and dehydration in NHS-provided care
Promoting normal birth	Increase the normal birth rate and eliminate unnecessary caesarean sections through midwives taking the lead role in the care of normal pregnancy and labour, focusing on informing, educating and providing skilled support to first-time mothers and women who have had one previous caesarean section
Important choices – where to die when the time comes	Avoid inappropriate admission to hospital and increase the number of people who are able to die in the place of their choice
Being fit and well to care	Reduce sickness absence in the nursing and midwifery workforce to no more than 3%
Ready to go – no delays	Increase the number of patients in NHS-provided care who have their discharge managed and led by a nurse or midwife where appropriate
Protection from infection	Demonstrate a dramatic reduction in the rate of UTIs for patients in NHS-provided care

Source: NHS Institute for Innovation and Improvement (2009)

Other, more recent examples of initiatives designed to ensure care is of a high quality are the Scottish government's (Scottish Executive, 2010) strategy, *The Healthcare Quality Strategy for NHS Scotland* – which is also underpinned by the views of the Scottish people (see box below) – and the Department of Health's Compassion in Practice (DH and NHS Commissioning Board, 2012), which focuses on the '6Cs': care, compassion, confidence, communication, courage and commitment. You can see that both documents have a very similar focus and use very similar, if not the same, words with regard to the integral elements of the provision of good care.

THE HEALTHCARE QUALITY STRATEGY FOR NHS SCOTLAND

- Caring and compassionate staff and services
- Clear communication and explanation about conditions and treatment
- Effective collaboration between clinicians, patients and others
- A clean and safe care environment
- Continuity of care
- Clinical excellence. (Scottish Executive, 2010)

COMPASSION IN PRACTICE: NURSING, MIDWIFERY AND CARE STAFF – OUR VISION AND STRATEGY

- Care
- Compassion
- Confidence
- Communication
- Courage
- Commitment. (DH and NHS Commissioning Board, 2012)

Both of the documents highlighted in the boxes above resulted from consultation with a wide range of people, which is integral to the formation of realistic policies that ensure care is good. Government legislation therefore plays a major role in defining criteria, the roles of healthcare providers and the expectations of the public in relation to care. As this differs within the four countries that make up the United Kingdom, it is important that you refer to the government legislation and policy which reflect the country in which you are practising.

> Working as a registered nurse, I have provided support and teaching to first-year student nurses bathing patients while promoting dignity and care. I felt proud to contribute to their learning while demonstrating positive nursing care. Currently I am a 6Cs Champion and am using this to influence colleagues in delivery of the six actions of care.
>
> **Katie Potter, staff nurse, adult community hospital**

The Compassion in Practice: One Year On document (DH and NHS Commissioning Board, 2013) reflects a range of qualitative evidence, which includes real examples of good practice and individual comments. These may help you to understand what the 6Cs mean.

HOW YOU CAN APPLY QUALITY CARE INITIATIVES WITHIN YOUR PRACTICE

In order to deliver any care, first, informed consent must be obtained from the patient or the person who holds the legal right to consent, such as a parent. Establishing and building rapport and trust with a patient and their family or carer is a fundamentally important element of care. Respecting the patient's right to consent to or to refuse treatment is a crucial aspect in helping you to deliver care in a manner that is acceptable to the patient.

However, consideration must also be given to the age of the patient and their mental capacity. You should therefore always underpin your practice with the relevant policy – for example, if the patient is a child, what is the legal age of consent? If the patient has a mental health problem, learning disability or degenerative condition which impairs their mental capacity in relation to being able to provide consent, it is important that you are aware of the implications of this. This means therefore that you should always encourage and assist parents and carers to contribute to the care process of assessment, planning, implementation and evaluation (APIE) in order to ensure care is person-centred.

As Harriet highlighted at the start of the chapter, person-centred care is an important ingredient in making care good.

CASE STUDY 10.1: KATIE

Katie is 10 years old and attends her local primary school. She was sent home from school because she was complaining of a sore tummy. Her mum took her to her GP and he advised that Katie should be admitted to hospital. Katie has been diagnosed with appendicitis and you have been asked to help prepare her for theatre.

- Using the information within the patient and student voices at the start of this chapter, what do you think it is important to consider in delivering effective care while you prepare Katie for theatre?

CHECK YOUR ANSWERS!

ANSWER: CASE STUDY 10.1

Care based on evidence

Care provided by nurses should always be based on the best evidence available. However, it is important to understand what is meant by 'evidence' and how it should inform your care. Some examples of sources of evidence utilised in the provision of care may include randomised controlled trials, surveys and case study research.

As a graduate profession, nursing is consistently building a supporting body of knowledge applying the above approaches and others, in order to collect data which can then be used to inform practice. Questioning nursing practice is therefore essential in order to enable this body of knowledge to grow and to be utilised. Craig and Smyth (2012) advocate that it is essential that nurses are able to identify and critically analyse evidence in order to justify their practice. Being able to do this is considered one of the attributes of a graduate. As a nursing student, you are working towards becoming a graduate, so are in an ideal position to question practice in order to develop your knowledge and skills (NMC, 2015).

Evidence-based practice involves using the current best evidence in your patient care, which also takes into consideration patient preference and individual judgement. A range of evidence, such as national guidelines, policies and systematic reviews, was used to develop all of the benchmarks applied in the UK.

Using the best evidence available in all aspects of your nursing practice promotes care delivery that is both safe and effective.

> To deliver evidence-based care, you have to keep your knowledge base up to date by reading research and literature and follow local and national policies and procedures.
>
> Sarah Parkes, LD nursing student

WHAT'S THE EVIDENCE?

A critical analysis of compassion in practice

Dewar and Christley (2013) examine the importance of compassionate practice and how policy should reflect values that are important to healthcare staff.

- What does compassion mean to you?
- How can you contribute to compassionate care?
- Now read the article and consider whether you would draw the same conclusions as the authors.

THE ROLE OF THE NURSING AND MIDWIFERY COUNCIL (NMC) IN MAKING CARE GOOD

The NMC has an important role to play in setting standards for education programmes and in the regulation of the nursing profession. The NMC provides standards and guidelines designed to prepare safe and effective practitioners who will provide high-quality, evidence-based care to their patients. These standards and skills are not only referred to at the start of each chapter in this book, but will also be evident within the documentation you receive from your university and will assist your practice educator in assessing your performance in your placement area.

Being a good nurse also encompasses the ability to deliver safe care which demonstrates skills, knowledge and understanding in tandem with person-centred care. As a nursing student, ultimately, it is extremely important that you work within the limitations of your competence and do not undertake any aspect of care that you are not qualified to carry out. This is not always as easy as it sounds: sometimes you may focus more on the physical aspects of care or the psychological ones, and important areas where care is required may be missed. This may reflect your strengths or your personal or professional areas for development and reinforces an important point made earlier in the chapter: the provision of effective care is dependent on many factors, some of which are dependent on the individual providing the care. It is your responsibility as a nursing student, and ultimately as a registered nurse, to ensure that at all times you provide the patient with the best care you possibly can.

Who decides if care is good?

Within the UK, the Professional Standards Authority for Health and Social Care maintains registers on all of the healthcare professions. All healthcare professionals who practise in any of the four countries that make up the UK must be registered with one of the 12 regulators. There are also designated organisations that regulate and inspect the delivery of care. Again, specific standards or benchmarks have been set, but these vary depending on the type of service being delivered. For example, in England, the Care Quality Commission (CQC) carries out this role. In Scotland, it is carried out by Social Care and Social Work Improvement Scotland (SCSWIS), which is an independent organisation responsible for scrutinising and improving care, social work and child protection services. In Wales, the Care and Social Services Inspectorate Wales (CSSIW) carries out this role, and in Northern Ireland it is undertaken by the Regulation and Quality Improvement Authority (RQIA). Regulation and inspection of the quality of care by an independent body are important in ensuring patients receive the best care.

It is possible that while you are on a placement you may observe care or a clinical skill being carried out in different ways, varying from one setting to another. It is necessary to appreciate that there may be more than one way to deliver care or to carry out a skill correctly. An experience such as this provides you with a valuable learning opportunity to question practice and develop your knowledge and skills.

> CQC inspections can be stressful – no one wants to receive a bad report or criticism – but just remember that they are there to help improve the quality of care your clinical area provides. See any points for improvement made by such inspection as positive as they ultimately ensure that your patients receive the best quality care.
>
> **Charlie Clisby, NQN**

ACTIVITY 10.1: CRITICAL THINKING

Think about your practice learning experiences so far:

- Have you observed care or a skill being carried out in different ways?
- What questions would this prompt you to ask your practice educator?
- Because care or skills are carried out differently by different people, does this necessarily mean they are being done wrongly?
- How can these different experiences help your learning?

ANSWER:
ACTIVITY 10.1

Care regulators and standards

As already mentioned, one of the roles of care regulators is to set standards to ensure that your patients receive the best possible care. It is likely that you will come across standards set by the following bodies, both while you are on placement and when you are relating theory to practice.

NICE

The National Institute for Health and Care Excellence (NICE) is an organisation in England which has devised a set of care standards, in collaboration with NHS and social care professionals, their partners and patients, which are designed to measure improvements in a particular area of care. These standards are also helpful to anyone involved in the delivery, reception or scrutiny of care. NICE quality standards enable:

- health and social care professionals and public health professionals to make decisions about care based on the latest evidence and best practice
- people receiving health and social care services, their families and carers and the public to find information about the quality of services and care they should expect from their health and social care provider
- service providers to quickly and easily examine the performance of their organisation and assess improvement in the standards of care they provide
- commissioners to be confident that the services they are purchasing are high quality and cost-effective and focused on driving up quality.

NICE quality standards are central to supporting the government's vision for an NHS and social care system focused on delivering the best possible outcomes for people who use services, as outlined in the Health and Social Care Act 2012.

SIGN

The Scottish Intercollegiate Guidelines Network (SIGN) was established in 1993 in order to improve healthcare for the people of Scotland through the dissemination and development of guidelines based on the best available evidence. These guidelines were intended to reduce variation in practice and outcomes. In 2005, SIGN became part of Health Improvement Scotland, which has the key responsibility to help NHS Scotland and independent healthcare providers deliver high-quality, evidence-based, safe, effective and person-centred care and to scrutinise services to provide public assurance about the quality and safety of that care. This organisation builds on work previously carried out by the Scottish Health Council, SIGN, the Healthcare Environment Inspectorate and the Guidelines and Audit Implementation Network (GAIN) in Northern Ireland.

NMC

The Nursing and Midwifery Council (NMC) is a statutory body which was established in 2002 by the parliament of the UK, enabled by the Nursing and Midwifery Order (2001). The NMC is the regulatory body for nursing, midwifery and health visiting, with a main aim being to safeguard the health and wellbeing of the public. The NMC maintains a register of eligible practitioners and also sets and reviews the standards for their education, training, conduct and performance. The NMC also investigates claims of substandard practice; these investigations are known as fitness-to-practise hearings.

My name is Sue. My daughter Nicki died two years ago aged 26, after receiving appalling care. She was ill and wasn't going to have a long life but she shouldn't have died the way she did. It's just cruel. Nicki was a happy, sociable and generous girl; she loved making people smile.

It all started when Nicki was 14. She started having fits, sometimes 20 a day. Sometimes she was so weak she could hardly hold her head up. It was a frightening time for us all.

When she was 18 she had a brilliant doctor called Dr Rakshi. At her funeral he said: 'She was just a fantastic girl – an ill girl, but an inspiration to us all.' This great care continued on Damson ward; Nicki only had to press a buzzer and there were nurses at her side. So we knew compassionate and professional care was possible. They were fantastic on Damson ward. We've actually got pictures of Nicki lying in the bed – she's got something like 22 teddy bears around her. And they used to get the blue gloves and they used to blow them up for her – make balloons. And because it was nearing Christmas, we took in a small Christmas tree and put it on her bedside cabinet. The next day we went in and they'd decorated it all. She had a TV in her room that they'd arranged for her. They used to sit in a chair and feed her. The physio was brilliant too; he used to come in every day and even when Nicki didn't feel like doing anything he'd make her laugh and get on her good side.

Just a few months later Nicki was admitted to a different ward, where staff treated her so badly that she rapidly deteriorated. The list of shocking treatment is endless. Sometimes it felt like they just forgot about her. They put Nicki's food, drink and medication out of her reach. Because she hadn't eaten or drunk anything for so long, her veins collapsed, so they couldn't take any blood – for two weeks she was just a pin cushion. Nobody would listen to me, and I knew exactly how my daughter was feeling and what she needed.

I will never forget the Nicki who sat with us, bellowing at the telly when Arsenal were playing. The Nicki who drank tea like it was water and who came home with armfuls of flowers as random presents. That's my Nicky. I will never forget.

Sue, mother of Nicki

WHEN CARE IS NOT GOOD

In the past decade, health and social care staff have witnessed poor standards of care and service failure, staff bullying and abuse and the unnecessary deaths of vulnerable people in their care. Poor standards of care for people with a learning disability were scrutinised by Mencap's reports *Treat Me Right!* (2004), *Death by Indifference* (2007) and Michael's Report (2008), *Healthcare for All*, generating recommendations which will have a lasting impact on learning disability services and general health services in all sectors. Following these, the Confidential Inquiry into Premature Deaths of People with Learning Disabilities (CIPOLD) was established, taking place from 2010 to 2013. In this time, it reviewed the deaths of 247 people with learning disabilities within five primary care trusts in the south-west of England. The study revealed that

> the quality and effectiveness of health and social care given to people with learning dis-
> abilities was deficient in a number of ways. Key recommendations are made which were
> they individually and collectively implemented, would lessen the risk of premature death
> in people with learning disabilities. (Heslop et al., 2013: 129)

In 2011, through televised undercover footage of the criminal actions of staff at Winterbourne View, we witnessed further unacceptable standards of care and abuse. The Department of Health commissioned a Serious Case Review: the reports which followed presented comprehensive recommendations to prevent a reoccurrence of such behaviour and improve services (DH, 2013). Following on from this, Bubb (2014) produced a report, *Winterbourne View: Time for Change*.

Poor standards of care are also evident in other services: a recent inquiry into substandard care within Mid Staffordshire NHS Foundation Trust led to the publication of the Francis Report (2013), which made a number of recommendations in order to prevent reoccurrence. It is therefore important that you understand that healthcare professionals have not only a professional but also a legal duty of care to those they are caring for.

As we have highlighted throughout this chapter, the provision of care abides by legislation, is regulated and inspected and follows professional guidelines. While these elements are all of fundamental importance, none is more important than the recipient of care. So, the decision as to whether care is good or not must therefore encompass the opinions of all those involved in this process – and none are more important than patients.

ACTIVITY 10.2: REFLECTIVE PRACTICE

Reflect on what action you would take if you observed care or a skill being carried out in a sub-standard way:

- Who would you report this to?
- What questions might you be asked?
- What further actions might you need to take?

You may find the information contained within the student handbook provided by your university and the NMC website sections 'What is fitness to practise?' and 'Raising concerns: Guidance for nurses and midwives' particularly helpful in answering these questions.

ANSWER:
ACTIVITY 10.2

The patient experience

The patient is the most important person in the healthcare system. Patient- or, as it is more frequently referred to, person-centred care is very much at the forefront of contemporary policies. The principles of this approach are concerned with the right of individuals to have their values and beliefs respected – their *personhood* – as this is what makes us all unique and authentic individuals. In order to uphold this right, it is necessary to ensure all the care we deliver is person-centred. Remembering the *Ten Essential Shared Capabilities* (NHS Education for Scotland, 2012) while providing care is an ideal way to ensure this. The *Ten Essential Shared Capabilities* are:

- working in partnership
- respecting diversity
- practising ethically
- challenging inequality
- promoting recovery
- identifying people's needs and strengths
- providing service user/patient-centred care
- making a difference
- promoting safety and positive risk taking
- personal development and learning.

Receiving healthcare frequently involves the patient in a wide range of new and possibly difficult experiences, which may well be accompanied by a large degree of uncertainty. Uncertainty can be seen as a challenge to both the patient and those providing care. Person-centred care will help to minimise this uncertainty by ensuring that the patient is involved at all times.

ACTIVITY 10.3: REFLECTIVE PRACTICE

Use the *Ten Essential Shared Capabilities* (listed above) to reflect on the care you have been involved in delivering in practice:

- How have you observed person-centred care being delivered?
- Now write a reflection relating to your experience.

ANSWER:
ACTIVITY 10.3

Apply your knowledge of person-centred care by reading Bruno and Anna's case study, at https://study. sagepub.com/essentialnursing2e.

CASE STUDY:
BRUNO &
ANNA

Involving patients and carers is welcomed in contemporary nursing practice as it promotes person-centred decision-making and partnership work, both of which facilitate the matching of care to patients' needs. The NMC Code (2015) makes specific reference to nurses respecting the contribution that individuals make to their care and wellbeing. Furthermore, it also highlights the role of the nurse as an advocate, aiding those in your care to access relevant care, information and support.

> While on placement in a learning disabilities children's short breaks respite home, one experience that stood out the most was a young girl coming to stay, who was autistic. Upon arrival, Sarah went straight to the videos and I had a conversation with her mother about her stay. She informed me of Sarah's routines, likes and dislikes, one routine being that she liked to take her bag to her room and unpack it herself. Knowing this prevented her becoming anxious or frustrated, and once this was done we could go in later on and log her belongings without causing her any upset or distress, made our care for her effective. In my opinion working alongside Sarah's mum really made a difference to Sarah's visit.
>
> **Siân Hunter, child nursing student**

As the patient is the most important person within any care environment, it is extremely important that there is a mechanism which allows them and their family or carers to provide feedback on the service they receive. Patient satisfaction is often measured against the six dimensions suggested by the Institute of Medicine, highlighted at the start of the chapter: person-centred, safe, effective, efficient, equitable and timely.

CASE STUDY 10.2: JULIE

Julie is 50 years old and is receiving support from a community psychiatric nurse (CPN). You have been accompanying the CPN to visit Julie and her family at their home and have been involved in the ongoing assessment and review of her care and treatment.

- What questions would you ask Julie and her family to ensure that they are happy with the care that you have provided?

ANSWER:
CASE STUDY 10.2

The opinions and expectations of patients, their families and carers on healthcare provision are often based on their own experiences. These experiences can be multiple and varied, relating to a wide range of care settings. Some examples which enable feedback on and monitoring of care provision are patient surveys, waiting list times and hospital-acquired infection rates. This feedback and monitoring of care may be carried out at local or national level.

How can you always deliver good care?

The fundamental role of the nurse is to care. This involves the ability to observe, listen and think holistically about individual patients' needs while maintaining dignity and respect. Interaction with patients should always be carried out in a way that fosters a meaningful relationship which will enable you and the patient to work in partnership to understand that patient's needs from their own perspective, before identifying ways in which those needs can be met.

For care to be effective, a holistic and integrated approach should be used. This approach embraces and is informed by all of the main elements discussed within this chapter so far: evidence-based practice, government legislation, NMC guidance, best practice guidelines and standards, clinical governance and the rights of individuals. So, when assessing, measuring and recording vital signs, you are also incorporating:

- hand hygiene and its importance in infection prevention and control
- effective communication, including language and physical contact
- moving and handling, including positioning patients and your proximity to the patient when measuring vital signs
- use of equipment and ensuring patient safety with this, including infection prevention and calibrating equipment.

The Nursing and Midwifery Council's (2015) code of professional standards also underpins every aspect of care, and reminds us of the relevance of our duty of care, patient consent, confidentiality, communication, feedback and the recording of observations (Everett and Wright, 2011).

It is therefore important that you realise there are a number of important ingredients which will help you in the delivery of good care, which include:

- using the best evidence available to you and ensuring it is from a reliable source
- preparing yourself – attending class, reading notes and related materials, being attentive in class (skills and theory)
- seeking academic support from your university lecturer or practice educator, identifying your learning needs, utilising reflection and gaining as much clinical experience as possible, supervised by your practice educator. This helps to develop your potential and prepare you in a comprehensive and meaningful way for your future career as a graduate and a professional.

You will be provided with many opportunities throughout your nursing programme which will enable you to develop your potential and to recognise your development needs.

Ultimately, it is the little things that make all the difference: think back to Vijay's comments at the start of this chapter and make sure you integrate these into your care. Never underestimate the importance of holding a patient's hand, greeting them with a smile, listening to their story and gaining an understanding of their individuality.

How to demonstrate effective care in clinical skills assessments

As part of your nursing programme, you will undertake clinical skills assessments. This will give you an opportunity to demonstrate that you can perform the skill, that you have the knowledge that underpins the skill and that you can demonstrate the professional attributes associated with the skill. In other words, it will allow you to demonstrate effective care by utilising a holistic integrated approach to care (Everett and Wright, 2011). Hutchfield and Standing (2012) describe this as 'knowing, showing and doing' – the building blocks of competence.

While you will be taught and assessed by your practice educator during your placement experience, many of the fundamental nursing skills you will be taught and assessed on during the first year of your nursing programme can also be achieved through simulation. Examples of these are:

- communication
- hand hygiene
- basic life support
- clinical observations
- administration of medication
- aseptic technique
- moving and handling.

Don't forget the importance of the 'little things that make all the difference' during any simulated skills teaching or assessment. Make sure these are always evident in your practice.

It is natural to get nervous about any exams, and OSCEs are no different – make sure beforehand that you understand what will be required of you. Seek extra support from your personal advisor or similar person, stay off social media sites where everyone is talking about it as it will just confuse and worry you, and finally, if you have completed all the practical revision work, then all you can then do is your best.

Sarah Parkes, LD nursing student

The aim of using simulation to teach skills and assess achievement is to allow you to gain confidence and experience in a safe environment without putting patients at risk. It is also possible that you will be required to undertake an Objective Structured Clinical Assessment (OSCE), which will allow you to demonstrate that you have achieved the requirements of the NMC (2015) and that you are fit for purpose.

When taking an OSCE, in order to be aware of exactly what the examiner requires you to do, you need to understand the examination criteria. Examiners will be looking for underpinning knowledge in relation to the skills being assessed (cognitive domain), the actual performance of the skill (psychomotor domain) and the appropriate attitude and professional approach (affective domain).

ACTIVITY 10.4: CRITICAL THINKING

For your first-year OSCE, you have been asked to assess, measure and record a patient's temperature, pulse and respiratory rate:

- Using the headings 'Psychomotor Domain', 'Cognitive Domain' and 'Affective Domain', identify what you will need to do in order to demonstrate effective care.
- Locate an example of an assessment criterion from your university (ask one of your lecturers). This is a marking tool used by an examiner to make sure that they are focusing on the elements required during an assessment. It may provide a useful template which will help you to complete this activity.

ANSWER:
ACTIVITY 10.4

CONCLUSION

Within the increasingly complex area of contemporary nursing care, there is no doubting the importance of evidence-based practice, benchmarking, regulation of care providers, agreed quality standards and those providing care being held responsible and accountable for their practice. However, nursing is a complex and creative process which relies on you applying your knowledge to the care of your patients in a way that connects them with their world and experiences. The importance of care and compassion in nursing must never be forgotten and you must demonstrate attributes such as authenticity, congruence, respect and warmth at all times. Integrate these attributes into the care you deliver in your own unique manner, developing your personal capabilities for relating to patients. Remember, as Vijay says at the start of the chapter, the importance of patients' values being treated with dignity and respect.

CHAPTER SUMMARY

- In order to ensure that the care provided is 'good', benchmarks for good practice are applied.
- Questioning nursing practice is essential in order to enable the body of knowledge to grow and to be used to provide care of the best quality.
- NMC standards and guidelines are designed to prepare safe and effective nurses capable of providing evidence-based care.
- As a nursing student, you must work within the limitations of your competence and never undertake any aspect of care that you are not qualified to carry out.
- Decisions regarding whether care is good or not must encompass the opinions of everyone involved in this process.
- In order to demonstrate effective care, a holistic, integrated, person-centred approach must be applied.
- The importance of care and compassion in nursing must never be forgotten and you must demonstrate attributes such as authenticity, congruence, respect and warmth at all times.

CRITICAL REFLECTION

Holistic care

Bloomfield et al. (2010) highlight the core principles that underpin safe clinical practice as being:

- infection control
- evidence-based practice
- accurate documentation
- effective communication
- maintaining dignity and respect.

Reflect on how you have seen these integrated into the holistic care you have been involved in delivering to patients:

- How would you apply these in an OSCE?
- How do they relate to the psychomotor, cognitive and affective domains?

GO FURTHER

Books

Aveyard, H. and Sharp, P. (2013) *A Beginner's Guide to Evidence-Based Practice in Health and Social Care*, 2nd edition. Maidenhead: Open University Press. An aid to understanding evidence-based practice utilising a step-by-step approach to using evidence in practice in a practical and straightforward way.

Hutchfield, K. and Standing, M. (2012) *Succeeding in Essays, Exams and OSCEs*. Exeter: Learning Matters. An aid to preparing and succeeding in essays, exams and OSCEs in order to become an NMC-registered graduate nurse.

Liggett, L. (2011) 'Appendicectomy', Chapter 24 in D. Corkin, S. Clarke and L. Liggett (eds) *Care Planning in Children and Young People's Nursing*. London: Wiley-Blackwell. An excellent guide to the best care for children and very useful when planning care such as for Katie in case study 10.1.

Journal articles

Dean, E. (2013) 'Lessons in delivering good care', *Nursing Standard*, 27(44): 16–18. A report on a London hospice's innovative approach to supporting patients and training staff.

Pemberton, S. and Richards, H. (2013) 'A vision of the future for patient experience', *Nursing Times*, 109(33/34): 19–21. A report on a foundation trust that developed a patient experience vision which engaged staff in creating a healthcare model for the future.

Watterson, L. (2013) '6Cs + Principles = Care', *Nursing Standard*, 27(46): 24–6. A useful mapping of the 6Cs and the RCN's Principles of Nursing, which highlights core professional values and behaviours.

Weblinks

Go to https://study.sagepub.com/essentialnursing2e for weblinks related to this chapter. If you are using the interactive ebook, simply click on the book icon in the margin to go straight to the resource.

FURTHER
READING:
WEBLINKS

www.rcn.org.uk/clinical-topics/clinical-governance/professional-resources – the Royal College of Nursing website offers a wealth of information, including a useful section on clinical governance which incorporates the perspectives of the countries that constitute the UK.

www.careinspectorate.com – the Care Inspectorate website offers a wealth of information on service regulation and provides access to inspection reports.

www.cqc.org.uk – the Care Quality Commission website also offers a wealth of information on service regulation and provides access to inspection reports.

www.nice.org.uk/guidance/qualitystandards/qualitystandards.jsp – the National Institute for Health and Care Excellence (NICE) provides access to quality standards in health, social care and public health.

www.knowledge.scot.nhs.uk/making-a-difference/resources/ten-essential-shared-capabilities.aspx – NHS Education for Scotland (2012) *The Ten Essential Shared Capabilities: Supporting Person-centred Approaches – A Learning Resource for Health Care Staff*. This web page is a useful learning resource which supports patient-centred care in line with legislation.

www.sign.ac.uk – the Scottish Intercollegiate Guidelines Network (SIGN) website provides access to national clinical guidelines containing recommendations for effective practice based on current evidence.

Video links

Have a break from the text and go to https://study.sagepub.com/essentialnursing2e for useful videos related to this chapter. If you are using the interactive ebook, simply click on the lightbulb icon in the margin to go straight to the resource.

VIDEO
LINKS

ACE YOUR ASSESSMENT

Review what you have learned by visiting the book's online resources at: https://study.sagepub.com/essential nursing2e If using your interactive ebook, just click on the icon in the margin to go straight there.

ONLINE
QUIZZES

- Test yourself with multiple-choice and short-answer questions.
- Revise key terms with the interactive flash cards.

REFERENCES

Bloomfield, J., Pegram, A. and Jones, C. (2010) *How to Pass your OSCE: A Guide to Success in Nursing and Midwifery*. Harlow: Pearson Education.

Bubb, S. (2014) Winterbourne View: Time for Change. Available at: www.england.nhs.uk/wp-content/uploads/2014/11/transforming-commissioning-services.pdf (accessed 18 April 2018).

Craig, J.V. and Smyth, R.L. (2012) *The Evidence-Based Practice Manual for Nurses*. London: Churchill Livingstone/Elsevier.

Department of Health (DH) (2003) *The Essence of Care: Patient-focused Benchmarking for Health Care Practitioners*. London: The Stationery Office.

Department of Health (2013) *Winterbourne View Hospital: Department of Health Review and Response*. London: TSO. Available at: www.gov.uk/government/publications/winterbourne-view-hospital-department-of-health-review-and-response (accessed 18 April 2018).

Department of Health (DH) and NHS Commissioning Board (2012) Compassion in Practice: Nursing, Midwifery and Care Staff – Our Vision and Strategy. Available at: www.england.nhs.uk/wp-content/uploads/2012/12/compassion-in-practice.pdf (accessed 18 April 2018).

Department of Health (DH) and NHS Commissioning Board (2013) Compassion in Practice: One Year On. Available at: www.england.nhs.uk/wp-content/uploads/2016/05/cip-one-year-on.pdf (accessed 18 April 2018).

Dewar, B. and Christley, Y. (2013) 'A critical analysis of compassion in practice', *Nursing Standard*, 28(10): 46–50.

Everett, F. and Wright, W. (2011) 'Measuring vital signs: An integrated teaching approach', *Nursing Times*, 107(27): 16–17.

Francis, R. (2013) *The Mid Staffordshire NHS Foundation Trust Public Inquiry: The Francis Report*. Available at: www.midstaffspublicinquiry.com/report (accessed 18 April 2018).

Heslop, P., Blair, P., Fleming, P., Hoghton, M., Marriott, A. and Russ, L. (2013) *Confidential Inquiry into Premature Deaths of People with Learning Disabilities (CIPOLD)*. Bristol: Nora Fry Research Centre. Available at: www.bris.ac.uk/cipold (accessed 18 April 2018).

Hutchfield, K. and Standing, M. (2012) *Succeeding in Essays, Exams and OSCEs*. Exeter: Learning Matters.

Mencap (2004) *Treat Me Right!* London: Mencap. Available at: www.mencap.org.uk/sites/default/files/2016-08/treat_me_right.pdf (accessed 18 April 2018).

Mencap (2007) *Death by Indifference: Following up on the Treat Me Right! Report*. London: Mencap. Available at: www.mencap.org.uk/sites/default/files/2016-06/DBIreport.pdf (accessed 18 April 2018).

Michael, Sir J. (2008) *Healthcare for All: Report of the Independent Inquiry into Access to Healthcare for People with Learning Disabilities*. London: Department of Health.

NHS Education for Scotland (NES) (2012) *The Ten Essential Shared Capabilities: Supporting Person-centred Approaches – A Learning Resource for Health Care Staff*. Edinburgh: NES. Available at: www.knowledge.scot.nhs.uk/making-a-difference/resources.aspx (accessed 18 April 2018).

NHS Institute for Innovation and Improvement (2009) *High Impact Actions for Nursing and Midwifery*. London: NHS Institute for Innovation and Improvement.

Nursing and Midwifery Council (2015) *The Code: Professional Standards of Practice and Behaviour for Nurses and Midwives*. London: NMC.

Scottish Executive (2007) *Better Health, Better Care: A Discussion Document*. Edinburgh: Scottish Executive.

Scottish Executive (2010) *The Healthcare Quality Strategy for NHS Scotland*. Edinburgh: Scottish Executive.

INTRODUCTION TO NURSING THEORY

CAROL HALL

THIS CHAPTER COVERS

- A toolbox for nursing
- Nursing theory – how models for nursing practice are constructed
- Using nursing philosophy in the care you deliver
- Nursing theory and nursing evidence: how do they work together?

Hi, my name is Celia, and I am a primary school teacher. I fell over in the sports hall this morning – silly really, I slipped on the floor. It was wet where the caretaker had washed it. He does it every morning and we are not meant to go in until it is dry, but it is a short-cut to the head's office and everyone does it all the time. My own fault, I suppose. Anyway, now I am in A&E and they tell me my wrist is broken in two places and it needs an operation to fix it. It certainly looks a funny shape at the moment. I don't know how I am going to cope. I'm a single mother with two kids, plus I have my job to think about; being busy with a class of 31 children, I am really worried about work and how I am going to pay the bills and the mortgage if I can't go to work. I don't get paid unless I work and my husband does not give us enough for the children as it is.

Celia, patient, ACUTE

At times, your job could involve not only looking after your patient but their families too. A placement in which I worked for children with LD required lots of work with the families – the families are entrusting you with their loved ones and need to know they can visit, approach with problems, ask what's happening and know their ideas, thoughts and feelings are being listened to as well.

Sarah Parkes, LD nursing student

INTRODUCTION

Celia's story demonstrates the complexity and challenge of the nursing care you will be delivering in your practice. Celia's is not an unusual case, and her story shows how one small slip can transform the life of a patient and their family, identifying many complexities for nurses who care in this situation.

Delivering the best nursing care is a priority for nursing as a profession and for those who work as nurses, wherever the care that they give is delivered. In order to be able to give the best care, we must recognise what the best care is and what this means to different people.

At a basic level, this appears simple: those who are cared for should be safe and comfortable and, in essence, the nurse should 'do no harm', to quote Florence Nightingale (Wagner and Whaite, 2010). However, to be sure that this is actually the case, it is critical to look more deeply. This chapter will explore what the nature of nursing is, the core concepts of nursing and the importance of being a skilled nurse. The chapter will draw on all fields of nursing to take examples, and will particularly consider application to two mini case studies. It may be useful to read Chapter 1 before this chapter, so you understand what nursing is about today.

A TOOLBOX FOR NURSING

Throughout this chapter, all the models and processes of nursing we consider are simply part of the toolbox which enables you to ensure effective care as a nurse. As with any tool, the skill of the user and the capability of the tool within the context are important. What reports such as the *Mid Staffordshire NHS Foundation Trust Public Inquiry* (Francis, 2013), *Improving the Safety of Patients in England* (Berwick, 2013), the *Review into the Quality of Care and Treatment Provided by 14 Hospital Trusts in England* (Keogh, 2013) and the report on Winterbourne View Hospital (DH, 2013a) show us is that without such capabilities, no model, tool or benchmark standard alone can create excellent nursing. We will return to Celia later in the chapter, as her story raises many issues, but it is important to remember that despite the complexity of her needs, it is critical that nursing care is always holistic, individualised and person-centred.

Getting the basics right

Today, nursing is a profession which has had to determine the important patient care goals within a target-driven National Health Service (NHS), and this has led to criticism of nurses and those who assist them. 'Surely getting the basics right is most important', the newspapers shout in every article about poor care they identify, and they are correct – basic care is a right for all patients, but it is something which can go wrong, for individuals and for organisations (for instance, NMC fitness-to-practise hearings illuminate poor practice by individuals, while organisations are subject to scrutiny by the Care Quality Commission (CQC)).

The Francis Report (2013) made an important point in recognising that care given in hospitals identified as 'poor' was not uniformly poor, but neither was care given in a 'good' hospital uniformly good, so no one has any room for complacency. The NHS as a whole service has taken these issues seriously, researching why some care is substandard and developing innovative ways to address the issues faced. The 6Cs (DH, 2012), the publication of NHS values in all countries of the UK (e.g. NHS Scotland, 2013; NHS Choices, 2015) and 'caring around the clock' (Hutchings, 2012) are but a few initiatives in which nurses have been encouraged to think about their patients and to ensure the comfort and safety of patients in hospital settings.

In community care, a greater focus on basic care needs and on the individual's capacity to identify and 'whistleblow' on poor care is evident, with the scandals of Winterbourne View (DH, 2012) and Tawel Fan Community Mental Health Hospital raising the alarm about poor care. In light of such issues, new ways of thinking about community and hospital care provision are emerging, linking the health needs of the patient with needs for social care – for instance, new 'integrated services' are enabling nursing and health services to become integrated with social care, promoting better standards and support for both health and social care (e.g. Salford NHS Trust Integrated Care Organisation (ICO)).

While thinking about all of the problems, issues and challenges faced by nursing may not appear the best way to begin, there is also much to be celebrated in nursing today. By appreciating a little more of the philosophy and theory, you will be able to understand the actions taken to ensure that your patients are safe and effectively cared for and to understand their personal and contextual needs. This will also help you to understand your future role more fully wherever you provide nursing care.

NURSING THEORY: HOW MODELS FOR NURSING PRACTICE ARE CONSTRUCTED

To think effectively about nursing, it is important to explore a definition of the actions of those involved – the actors – within the nursing scenario. Like a good play, it is also important to consider the setting and the intended goal of the activity proposed. This takes you further than thinking about what nursing is and how its knowledge is constructed, and on to thinking about what being a nurse means within a wider context of caring for a patient in a given situation. In Chapter 1, you thought about the nurse as someone who is qualified, and also about yourself in terms of becoming a nurse. Now you need to be thinking about what it is that a nurse actually does and how they perform their role in practice. This will vary according to where nursing takes place. If, for example, you explore the role of the nurse in a community mental health setting, you may find that the core focus of the nurse's work with patients may be on empowering and enhancing the patient's self-esteem and improving their capacity to manage their own care and their life, while managing any potential risks. Alternatively, when looking after the needs of a patient in critically ill adult nursing or in a children's intensive care unit, you may see the nurse also acting as an authority, offering skills and expertise to deliver nursing and working in partnership to help ensure that families are informed when making decisions may be particularly difficult.

Let's have a look at a real-life case study (11.1). This time the family are in a community care setting located at home.

CASE STUDY 11.1: SURINDERJIT

Surinderjit is 13 years old and his parents' only child. He has speech, language and communication needs, complex health needs and physical disabilities which mean he must receive his food artificially. He is an expressive boy and tends to be hyperactive. He attends a school for children with special needs, where nurses enable him to be fed using a **percutaneous endoscopic (PEG) tube**, but is at home in the morning and evening, and requires considerable attention. His father owns a business

(Continued)

and works long hours, leaving much of the care to Surinderjit's mother. The family lives in a terraced house on the outskirts of a large city known for its concentration of Sikh families. They live in the home of their extended family, although the only living relative is Surinderjit's paternal grandmother, Mrs Sukhdeep Kaur, who is 79. She speaks little English, although she has lived in England for many years and her sons were born here. The family is bilingual, speaking Punjabi and English. Mrs Kaur's husband died some years ago. She has, until recently, been physically fit and helped to care for her grandson, but was admitted to hospital four weeks ago following a stroke which resulted in right-sided **hemiplegia** and some difficulty with speaking. Mrs Kaur was discharged home two weeks ago with a supportive care package which includes social care morning and night to enable her to wash and dress, and nursing care to dress a small ulcer on her leg which resulted from damage when she fell. It is becoming clear, however, that the family is finding the pressure of caring for Mrs Kaur and Surinderjit challenging. The house is small and the amount of equipment needed to care for Mrs Kaur makes it very cramped. Mrs Kaur's daughter-in-law identifies that Mrs Kaur tried to get up to go to the toilet and fell again yesterday, and she is worried that Mrs Kaur will hurt herself. She is very stressed and says that Mrs Kaur had only just been to the toilet when it happened and surely did not need to go again. She says that Mrs Kaur seems disorientated and confused since she returned home. Mrs Kaur's daughter-in-law doesn't think the family can continue like this.

- How would the nurse's role be different if they were looking after Mrs Kaur, as compared to looking after Celia?
- How would this differ again if you were looking after Surinderjit as a learning disability nurse working as a school nurse at his school?

Imagine that Surinderjit is 19 years old:

- How would this differ if you were looking after Surinderjit as a learning disability nurse working as the nurse at his college?

In thinking about the above scenario, it can be seen that there are differences to Celia's story at the start of the chapter. Celia will have an operation very soon, while Mrs Kaur will need daily care for a long time. You may have thought that Mrs Kaur's nurse is working in the community visiting people at home, while Celia's nurse is in a hospital and the nurse caring for Surinderjit is in a school. In each case, the nursing care offered will be different because the individual patient and their context are different. The next question you may have could be: if the roles of those providing care are so different, how is it that they are all nurses? The answer to this lies in the ways in which these nursing roles are similar or common, rather than in their differences.

Core concepts of nursing

The practice of nursing is dependent on some key elements, and these are of critical importance when understanding nursing. The four core earliest and most commonly identified domains are those of Yura and Torres (1975), and for simplicity they have been adapted to:

- nursing
- patient
- health
- society.

For the purposes of this chapter, it is enough to identify that these core concepts are fundamental in defining any kind of nursing, and to then explore briefly what might be meant within each concept.

More expert theorists who have considered nursing models to try to explain how nursing and nurses function, have examined individual philosophical beliefs in greater detail and the relationships between these and the above nursing concepts. Your personal nursing philosophy relates to the way in which you view nursing, including your beliefs about nursing – and your values. You may consider epistemology – your views about knowledge and logical reasoning about nursing and you may consider your perspectives on acceptable standards of ethical conduct or behaviour. You may also reflect over political thinking about the society which you serve and metaphysical thinking related to worldly existence. This reflection should lead you to a consideration of your concept of 'being' or 'ontological' thought about what nursing 'could' or 'should' be (Hall, 2013, adapted from Chitty and Black, 2011; Gobbi and Brown, 2006). Developing your own philosophy enables your blueprint for nursing practice to emerge. Hall and Ritchie (2013) explore this in more detail, and you are invited to consider how your own philosophy might contribute to the kind of care you feel is professionally concordant for you as a nurse. For you at the moment though, it is important to realise that philosophical approaches to nursing care can be different and this may affect the way in which you deliver care. Perhaps the best example might relate to a philosophical perspective about the nature of the patient. Someone who believes that a 'patient' is someone whose being is dependent on the nurse as a knowledgeable doer may proffer care which reflects a paternalistic approach towards the patient, whilst someone whose philosophy identifies the patient as self-determining and the source of knowledge about their own care may see nursing as being much more about a partnership.

The core concepts of Patient, Nursing, Health and Society have been recognised within most models of nursing since an American Nursing Association survey evidenced them formally. However, if you go back to models outlined as early as Nightingale's 1895 'Nursing, what it is and what it is not' (translated into modern nursing by Fitzpatrick, 1992), it is quite possible to see the interplay of these concepts in creating an environment for nursing to be delivered.

ACTIVITY 11.1: REFLECTIVE PRACTICE

Think about your nursing. How would you define the above concepts in *your* practice? And what would *you* say about the relationship between them? For example, would you *define* yourself as a nurse who works with your patients in an equal way? Do you negotiate care with them *or* do they lead in their care decisions? This is a consideration about the definition of the concepts of 'nurse' and 'patient' and the relationship between these two concepts. It is a starting point to think about the development of a theoretical stance for your nursing, and it is important, when you are giving care, for you to think about who and what may be in control and how this might be changed for better outcomes. It is important for leaders of nursing to be clear about how they want nursing to be delivered, too. A shared belief about nursing can help everyone to work in the same direction and towards the same vision. This discussion will now be considered further in respect of the case studies in this chapter.

Why have a blueprint or model for nursing practice?

As we have seen, just by considering the differences in care required by Celia, Mrs Kaur and Surinderjit, the various ways in which nursing is perceived can be quite different. Having an identified model or blueprint for care can be useful for nurses as it aids nursing thinking, planning of care and communication, plus it represents an ideology and expectations for all who work within a comparable area. While to some extent a core mission statement or philosophy (available in some placements) can do this, a model or framework adds detail by applying the ideas to nursing concepts. A model itself cannot actually deliver nursing care, but it can give clear ideas about how it is to be achieved. It may also cover all the care given and support the development of care pathways or the development of tools related to an aspect of care delivery. The skills and knowledge required for care delivery are the preserve of the nurse and you will need to develop these and use them appropriately, in combination with tools to deliver care. Common process delivery tools you may find in your nursing today include SBAR, APIE and SOAPIER.

USING NURSING PHILOSOPHY IN THE CARE YOU DELIVER

So, how are such tools, models and philosophies relevant to the everyday nursing care you deliver? Considering the theoretical aspects of the core concepts of nursing helps you to appreciate and communicate the care you are giving. Models address care and offer you definitions of the knowledge within the discipline of nursing. They aid communication about what your role as a nurse is; how the patient may be viewed; what the context or environment of nursing might contribute; and what the intended outcome of care might look like, which enables you to make accountable leadership decisions. Tools must be used in addition to any theoretical model in order to enable the process to work in a practical situation. A model relies on concepts which have definitions, are culturally determined and change over time; models are, therefore, dynamic, and the ways in which they are used should change to meet contemporary needs.

ACTIVITY 11.2: RESEARCHING MODELS OF NURSING

- Use your nursing library to identify a classical conceptual model of nursing such as Roper, Logan and Tierney's (RLT) Activities of Living model (RLT, 1980) (you could also choose Roy (1970) or Peplau (1951)).
- Use the search tools to identify a few journal articles about the model and look at book chapters which include descriptions and critiques over the time since the original model was published. Read the articles critically, evaluating their strengths and weaknesses.
- How has the model changed over the years? Is it different when evaluated by more recent writers? Why is this the case?
- If you chose RLT, you can now check your answers with our ideas in the next section.

Exploring the core theoretical concepts of a meta-paradigm of nursing

When considering a meta-paradigm of nursing, which essentially means taking a big view of what nursing is about, the first core concept of nursing is the nurse themselves, and their work. One of the most important considerations relates to what we know as nursing and what nursing knowledge is. Carper's seminal work (1978) defined nursing by the kinds of knowledge the nurse would need, including ethical, empirical, personal and aesthetic knowledge and consideration of the praxis of nursing. Within this, the importance of art and science, the need for critically evaluated best evidence and personal and ethical awareness are all clearly defined. Although dated, these ideas remain valid when considering contemporary nursing and its emphasis on the values of those who deliver care.

The remaining three concepts (identified earlier) will now be investigated. After this, we will look at how one model of nursing, that of Roper, Logan and Tierney (RLT) (1980, 2000), defined the four concepts and how this has been developed and changed to be used in practice today.

Patient

In order to nurse, it is important to have a patient to look after. While this may sound obvious, it is important to think of the role a patient and their family might play in receiving care. In times past, it was entirely acceptable for patients to be cared for by nurses until they were nursed back to health. Indeed, if you look at RLT's original descriptions of the patient and the role of their nurse, the expectation was that the nurse was primarily the doer, making the patient the one who was 'done unto'. Thus, the patient was defined as being on a continuum of dependency to independence in their life activities, relying on the nurse to provide care where they were dependent. In recent years, though, a more contemporary view of the patient has developed. The more modern view has been that founded on the original work of theorists such as Dorothea Orem (1914–2007), an American theorist who identified a need for patients to be empowered and their role of a normally self-caring individual who simply requires nursing to offer support in difficult times geared towards the idea that the self-caring person will re-emerge.

Clearly, when thinking about the patient in this way there are advantages, such as a greater emphasis on returning to independent living. This is also politically helpful in terms of the resources required to finance the NHS, as keeping people in their own homes and communities means a greater likelihood of them retaining their independence for longer, with greater reliance on informal care and supportive nursing than hospital provision. The result of this change means a greater concentration of critically ill patients in the hospital or residential areas provided by the NHS and a changing role for nurses in these areas, moving towards more specialised roles. This takes us on to consider the role of the environment, or society, in care.

Society (or environment)

The society or environment in which nursing takes place influences how and what care may be and what the expectations are. There is even a school of theoretical thought which suggests that the role of the nurse can only ever be to influence the care environment and enable the patient to achieve the optimal situation in which to become healthy or maintain their health. Two theorists who recognised this view are Florence Nightingale (1859, cited in Wagner and Whaite, 2010) and, more recently, Roy (1970). This may seem an odd priority for someone who is nursing patients, but if we relate it to the case studies in this chapter, providing a safe environment for Celia is going to be critical as she prepares for her operation and as she recovers. Much of the initial care given by the nurse will be focused on monitoring and ensuring that Celia's post-operative environment has all that is required (including the provision of oxygen, suction, monitoring equipment and analgesia) to ensure she recovers safely.

The care environment approach is particularly critical where resources are limited and decisions may need to be made about who receives the available treatment. We now return to the case of Surinderjit and consider some further information.

CASE STUDY 11.2: SURINDERJIT REVISITED

Surinderjit's family have explored many avenues for care and treatment. They know there is a facility in another country which treats young people with needs such as his, which could allow him greater independence. Surinderjit's family have been campaigning for support from the NHS to enable him to receive the treatment in the UK; however, the treatment required is expensive and provision of this resource would mean denying treatment to other NHS patients which could allow greater independence, such as hip and knee replacements. Many people across the world are like Surinderjit, because healthcare providers must make difficult choices about who should receive treatment and how much to invest in different care. In the UK, this has been identified as the 'postcode lottery' and there are many examples in the newspapers.

- What other environmental situations can you think of which may influence how and when nursing might be delivered, and to whom?

It is possible to think of situations where resources are very limited – in countries where there are insufficient life-saving resources, for example. Care decisions in these circumstances are influenced by what is not available and resources go to ensuring the fittest survive. Equally, the care setting may also be influenced by what is available and cultural expectations may vary as a result. When Mrs Kaur was admitted to hospital, she expected her family to visit and stay with her. Although Mrs Kaur and her family had lived in the UK for many years, Mrs Kaur's experience of hospitals related to caring for her own mother when she was hospitalised in India, during which time Mrs Kaur had stayed with her mother to care for her throughout her whole hospital stay. Thus, she was quite confused when her family was asked to leave and did not stay to care for her. Mrs Kaur's cultural expectations were different from those of the prevailing culture within which she was being cared for.

The final consideration to explore is that of health.

I am very passionate about effective communication in nursing, talking to your patient, observing their body language and creating an environment where they feel able to talk to you about anything. Doing this will aid you in gauging whether your patients' needs are being met.

Charlie Clisby, NQN

Health

When considering definitions of health, the World Health Organization (1946) and Henderson (1966) offer perhaps the two most well-known and sustained views in respect of a patient's health. Henderson proposed that an outcome of health may not necessarily be defined as a healthy life but that of a peaceful death, while the WHO record that health is not merely reflected in the absence of disease or disability, it also lies in the individual's capacity to manage their circumstances in a healthy manner. These views are important and in the UK they underpin the *NHS Constitution* (DH, 2013b). For Mrs Kaur and her family, a healthy future may involve establishing the ability to continue to work well with Surinderjit as he grows into adolescence, given the change in Mrs Kaur's physical circumstances and mental capacity. For Celia, her health outlook might be very different in the short and longer term: although it would be expected that her arm would heal within a few months, she may undergo serious mental stress as the result of being the sole earner in her family, and having a job which relies on her being available to work. Given Celia's history of depression following her divorce, ensuring a healthy outcome may mean giving consideration to her mental wellbeing and ensuring she has adequate social support as she works out how to support her family during the time she is unable to work. Without this, Celia may need support from mental health services if her anxiety and depression return. She is a single mother and, as working will be difficult, this temporary physical disability will affect her financial commitments. There is evidence that poverty and lack of stability are far more common for individuals who have long-term disability issues or who support family members with disability, than for others in society.

Changing care needs

In real-life situations, theoretical frameworks are useful to aid the care that is given initially, but this often needs to change as the setting the patient is cared for within changes. Thus, theoretical frameworks need to be supplemented to ensure the patient receives the best nursing care throughout their whole experience. To demonstrate how this can be achieved, the template offered by Roper, Logan and Tierney's Twelve Activities of Living Model will now be explored.

Roper, Logan and Tierney

Roper, Logan and Tierney (RLT) first devised their model of nursing in the 1980s as a British model, one of many emerging at that time from the NHS. The model is situated within, or represents, a time of changes in how care was being provided. Care delivery was moving from the task-orientated approach strongly identifiable in the 1960s, where care focused on nurses carrying out the same routinised task for all patients in an area (for example, giving pressure area care or taking temperatures), to the prevalent theme of 1980s care delivery – promoting the benefits of individualised care. Models of care such as RLT enabled nurses to think about providing all the care needed by the individual patients for whom they were responsible. Today, we see that this shift has been successful in enabling holistic care; however, task-based 'intentional rounding' has been implemented in areas where patients are largely independent but where some assistance may be required. This can be considered to be a hybrid approach, as it does continue to focus on individuals rather than the task-based, whole-ward perspective.

I have used different elements of two models in practice so far, Soler and Surety, and it really helped me to develop a therapeutic relationship with a young boy who was admitted and could not speak English. I thought of the way and where I positioned myself, eye contact and spatial awareness.

Siân Hunter, child nursing student

TWELVE ACTIVITIES OF LIVING

In the RLT model, the patient is assessed according to a comparison between their normal activity and the current position. It was reasoned by RLT that, where a gap was identified, nursing would be required until the patient had resumed their usual independence or learned to manage their new circumstances, thus reaching a state of health. In later editions, the 12 activities of daily living were amended to 12 activities of living (see Figure 11.1), since the activities were critiqued as not necessarily occurring on a daily basis.

- Maintaining a safe environment
- Communicating
- Breathing
- Eating and drinking
- Elimination
- Washing and dressing
- Controlling temperature
- Mobilisation
- Working and playing
- Expressing sexuality
- Sleeping
- Death and dying

Figure 11.1   Activities of living

Image © Robin Lupton

The RLT model is part of the toolbox which enables you to ensure effective care. However, it is your ability which is important. Without a nurse who can 'knit' compassion, care, dignity, person-centred and value-based approaches into all they do, using a model alone does not deliver excellent nursing care.

The focus of the nurse in later editions was also widened from that of 'doer' to someone who enabled the patient, and a greater focus on social and psychological elements enhanced the original assessments. For many years, this model formed the basis for documentation used in the assessment of patients, especially in care settings for adults' and children's health. Today, you will see many recognisable elements in the care you offer if you are in the adult or child fields of nursing. In other areas, including mental health, a variety of models are used: Peplau's, Newman's and biopsychosocial models, for example. Increasingly, mental health trusts devise their own models, based on mental, psychological, medical, behavioural, social, physical and forensic areas and encompassing risk. Once again, the Go Further section at the end of this chapter offers additional reading for you to increase your knowledge.

Returning to RLT, this remains a model of nursing which views the patient as a whole person who is nursed in respect of the activities undertaken in normal daily life. RLT is frequently used in the UK, especially in adult nursing. It assesses the patient's ability to undertake 12 activities of daily living (adapted from Henderson's 1966 US model). This was a small step from the medical systems approach which divided patients into their body systems.

Applying RLT to the care of Celia, it would be useful to consider her early needs in respect of her injury and the impact on her usual living activities. If she subsequently required mental health support, a different model or care pathway approach may be more useful in order to empower her. Suggestions might include the TIDAL Model (Buchanan-Barker, 2004) which focuses on empowering individuals.

ACTIVITY 11.3: REFLECTIVE PRACTICE

Reflect on the care you were involved in delivering during a recent placement:

- What model of care was used?
- How did it help you meet the patient's needs?

Assessment tools

While models such as RLT have value in assessment, in today's nursing, where interprofessional care pathways are well developed, assessment tools are now applied much more specifically than ever before and care is planned in light of evidence collated from these. Examples include the use of national early warning scores (NEWS) and assessment using situation background assessment recommendation (SBAR).

These tools have the benefit of being multi-professional in use and enable physical care needs to be communicated rapidly. While the original models of nursing are still in evidence, they have largely made way for care pathways where care is evidenced and written into core requirements used for all patients. The development of care plans for patients now applies a combination of individual assessment, skilled collation and use of the correct evidence-based tools and care pathways to enable the most effective delivery of the best nursing care.

NURSING THEORY AND NURSING EVIDENCE: HOW DO THEY WORK TOGETHER?

Robustly evaluated evidence has changed nursing through providing nurses with justification for the practice they deliver. Changes in practical care, from the management of pressure areas in an older people's home to the positioning of babies in their cots, have changed nursing and improved longevity and life quality. It is clear that evidence must work alongside nursing models and theories in enabling effective nursing to happen and to be justified and effectively evaluated.

WHAT'S THE EVIDENCE?

WEBLINK:
WITHER
NURSING
MODEL

McCrae, N. (2012) 'Whither nursing models? The value of nursing theory in the context of evidence-based practice and multidisciplinary health care', *Journal of Advanced Nursing*, 68(1): 222–9.

McCrae (2012) presents an evidence-based discussion around the role of nursing models and theory in the modern clinical environment.

(Continued)

Reflection

Think about how you can use evidence within your personal philosophy of nursing to add to the quality of your knowledge and the care that you give?

Now read the article and consider how the findings might contribute to your use of models, theories and evidence in the future.

CONCLUSION

Nursing theory and philosophy form an important basis of your everyday nursing practice, combining with evidence used to evaluate and develop the best care to give. It is important to note that models and processes of nursing are simply part of the toolbox which enables you, as a nurse, to ensure effective care. Like any tool, though, it is the skill of the user and the capability of the tool within the context which are important. What the Francis, Berwick and Keogh reports (all 2013) teach us is that without a skilled nurse, no model, tool or benchmark standard has the capability to provide excellent nursing.

CHAPTER SUMMARY

- Delivering the best nursing care is a priority for nursing as a profession. In order to be able to give the best care, we must recognise what best care is and what this means to different people.
- Considering the theoretical aspects of the core concepts of nursing helps you to appreciate and communicate the care you are giving.
- Nursing models address care and aid communication about what your role as a nurse is, how the patient may be viewed, what the context or environment for nursing might contribute and what the intended outcome of care might look like.
- Models and processes of nursing are simply part of the toolbox which enables you to ensure effective care as a nurse.
- Models and processes of nursing can be used within each field of nursing and will be useful to you in delivering patient care.
- There are four core concepts found in the meta-paradigm, or worldview, of nursing theory, and these are linked together in a model in order to enable you to provide holistic care.
- Nursing theories are developed while they are being used and intertwined with interprofessional theories to enrich the effectiveness of care delivery.

CRITICAL REFLECTION

Holistic care

This chapter has highlighted the importance of the use of a blueprint for models of care when determining an appropriate care pathway for your patient. Think about someone you have cared for recently and make a list of ways in which caring for them with an understanding of their personal situation can help meet their wider physical, emotional, social, economic and spiritual needs. Develop a comparison of the care you might plan for the different patients in this chapter. Now add your own patient, comparing the differences in respect of the definitions of their care. What model is your care based on and how is holistic care delivered?

Write your own reflection about your experience.

GO FURTHER

Books

Hall, C. (2013) 'Theory and practice: Understanding the nature of nursing as a caring activity', in C. Hall and D. Ritchie (eds) *What is Nursing?* 3rd edn. Exeter: Learning Matters. pp. 61–84. This chapter develops the theoretical consideration of caring further and reviews some different models for each field of practice. The application of the theoretical considerations to different case situations means that this text is complementary to the chapter you have just read and will further extend your understanding and application of the conceptual elements of nursing theory.

Roper, N., Logan, W. and Tierney, A. (2000) *Activities of Living Model of Nursing*. Edinburgh: Churchill Livingstone. Perhaps the best-known British model of nursing care, but criticised for its perspective on the role of the nurse (as controlling care) and its medical and rather reductionist approach. This model developed dynamically through the 1990s and still forms the basis of many UK frameworks for nursing care today. It is most likely to be taught as a baseline for thinking about the practical application of a nursing philosophy.

Journal articles

Barker, P. (1998) 'It's time to turn the tide', *Nursing Times*, 94(46): 70–2. This short summary of the TIDAL model and its application in mental health nursing enables you to see how a model can benefit client care in the mental health setting.

Moulster, G., Ames, S. and Griffiths, T. (2012) 'A new learning disabilities framework', *Learning Disabilities Practice*, 15(6): 14–18. This summary of a learning disabilities framework enables you to see how a model can benefit client care in the learning disability setting.

Murphy, F., Williams, A. and Pridmore, J. (2010) 'Nursing models and contemporary nursing 1: Their development, uses and limitations', *Nursing Times*, 106: 23. This article continues a discussion about the use of models in nursing and their relative benefits and limitations.

Weblinks

Go to https://study.sagepub.com/essentialnursing2e for weblinks related to this chapter. If you are using the interactive ebook, simply click on the book icon in the margin to go straight to the resource.

FURTHER
READING:
WEBLINKS

http://youtu.be/7_Ncwz5nY2c – this weblink demonstrates cancer patients' satisfaction with their care. Think about this from the perspective of the nurses delivering the care, how the nurses see their own role, the role of their patients and the vision of health as a goal and the impact of society.

www.tidal-model.com/ – this weblink will help you to learn more about the TIDAL model for mental health nursing and think about how this approach might be applied in your care.

www.england.nhs.uk/nursingvision – view this link and think about the underpinning philosophy of the 6Cs. What is being said about the nature of the nurse and the nature of the patient in particular? Also ask yourself – is it a good idea to have a strategic vision for a whole country? The 6Cs apply to the whole of England. What might the limitations of this approach be?

Berwick, D. (2013) *A Promise to Learn: A Commitment to Act – Improving the Safety of Patients in England*. National Advisory Group on the Safety of Patients in England. Available at: www.gov.uk/government/uploads/system/uploads/attachment_data/file/226703/Berwick_Report.pdf. Look at section three of the summary of this report. This identifies the need for patient and public involvement in care. You can also see a vision or model for all professions including nursing, which clearly identifies putting the patient first and including them in decision-making. Think about how you could use these findings and recommendations in your nursing practice to make sure patients remain safe.

───── ACE YOUR ASSESSMENT ─────

ONLINE
QUIZZES

Review what you have learned by visiting the book's online resources at: https://study.sagepub.com/essential nursing2e If using your interactive ebook, just click on the icon in the margin to go straight there.

- Test yourself with multiple-choice and short-answer questions.
- Revise key terms with the interactive flash cards.

REFERENCES

Berwick, D. (2013) *A Promise to Learn – A Commitment to Act – Improving the Safety of Patients in England*. National Advisory Group on the Safety of Patients in England. London: Department of Health. Available at: www.gov.uk/government/uploads/system/uploads/attachment_data/ file/226703/Berwick_Report.pdf (accessed 28 March 2013).

Buchanan-Barker, P. (2004) *The Tidal Model: A Guide for Mental Health Professionals*. London: Brunner-Routledge.

Carper, B.A. (1978) 'Fundamental patterns of knowing in nursing', *Advances in Nursing Science*, 1(1): 13–24.

Chitty, K. and Black, B. (2011) *Professional Nursing Concepts and Challenges*, 6th edn. Missouri: Saunders Elsevier.

Gobbi, M. and Brown, J. (2006) 'Introduction to professional studies in nursing', In J. Brown and P. Libberton (eds) *Principles of Professional Studies in Nursing*. London: Palgrave Macmillan, pp.3–24.

Department of Health (DH) (2012) *Compassion in Practice*. London: DH.

Department of Health (2013a) *Winterbourne View Hospital: Department of Health Review and Response*. London: TSO. Available at: www.gov.uk/government/uploads/system/uploads/attachment_data/ file/213215/final-report.pdf (accessed 18 February 2015).

Department of Health (2013b) *The NHS Constitution: The NHS Belongs to US All*. Available at: https://assets.publishing.service.gov.uk/government/uploads/system/uploads/attachment_data/ file/480482/NHS_Constitution_WEB.pdf (accessed 18 February 2015).

Fitzpatrick, J. (1992) 'Reflections on Nightingale's perspective of nursing', in F. Nightingale, *Notes on Nursing: What it Is, and What it Is Not*. Philadelphia, PA: Lippincott. pp. 18–22.

Francis, R. (2013) *Report of the Mid Staffordshire NHS Foundation Trust Public Inquiry* (The Francis Report). London: The Stationery Office. Available at: www.midstaffspublicinquiry.com/sites/ default/files/report/Executive%20summary.pdf (accessed 28 March 2013).

Hall, C. (2013) 'Theory and practice: Understanding the nature of nursing as a caring activity', in C. Hall and D. Ritchie (eds) *What is Nursing?* 3rd edn. Exeter: Learning Matters. pp. 61–84.

Hall, C. and Ritchie, D. (2013) *What is Nursing*, 3rd edn. Exeter: Learning Matters.

Henderson, V. (1966) *The Nature of Nursing: A Definition and its Implications for Practice, Research and Education*. New York: Macmillan.

Hutchings, M. (2012) 'Caring around the clock: Rounding in practice', *Nursing Times*, 108(49): 12–14.

Keogh, Sir B. (2013) *Review into the Quality of Care and Treatment Provided by 14 Hospital Trusts in England (Keogh Review)*. London: NHS England.

McCrae, N. (2012) 'Whither nursing models? The value of nursing theory in the context of evidence-based practice and multidisciplinary health care', *Journal of Advanced Nursing*, 68(1): 222–9.

NHS Choices (2015) The Principles and Values of the NHS in England. Available at: www.nhs.uk/NHSEngland/thenhs/about/Pages/nhscoreprinciples.aspx (accessed 10 December 2017).

NHS Scotland (2013) *Everyone Matters: 2020 Workforce Vision*. Edinburgh: The Scottish Government.

Peplau, H.E. (1951) 'Toward a new concept in nursing and nurse education', *American Journal of Nursing*, 51(12): 722–4.

Roper, N., Logan, W.W. and Tierney, A.J. (1980) *The Elements of Nursing*. Edinburgh: Churchill Livingstone.

Roper, N., Logan, W. and Tierney, A. (2000) *Activities of Living Model of Nursing*. Edinburgh: Churchill Livingstone.

Roy, C. (1970) 'Adaptation: A conceptual framework for nursing', *Nursing Outlook*, 18(3): 43–5.

Wagner, D. and Whaite, B. (2010) 'An exploration of the nature of caring relationships in the writings of Florence Nightingale', *Journal of Holistic Nursing*, 28(4): 225–34.

World Health Organization (WHO) (1946) Preamble to the constitution of the World Health Organization as adopted by the International Health Conference, New York, 19–22 June 1946: signed on 22 June 1946 by the representatives of 612 states (Official Records of the World Health Organization No 2, p. 100) and entered into force on 7 April 1948. Geneva: WHO.

Yura, H. and Torres, G. (1975) 'Today's conceptual frameworks with the Baccalaureate nursing programs', *National League for Nursing Publication*, 15(1558): 17–75.

VALUE-BASED, PERSON- OR FAMILY-CENTRED CARE

CATHERINE DELVES-YATES

THIS CHAPTER COVERS

- What is value-based, person- or family-centred care?
- Compassion
- Caring
- Dignity

- Person-centred care
- Family-centred care
- Spirituality
- What to do if care is not value-based, person- or family-centred

> "
> The NHS belongs to the people ... It touches our lives at times of basic human need, when care and compassion are what matter most.
>
> **The NHS Constitution, DH (2013)**
>
> When I look back over my 94 years of life I have done many things – being part of the Fire Service during World War II; spending many years in Africa with my young family, who now have families of their own; welcoming both my mother and mother-in-law into my home to care for them when they couldn't care for themselves; and deciding at the age of 74 I was still young enough to be a blushing bride for the second time.
>
> Having moved from my own home to my son's when I came to be in need of extra help, and now relying on the care of others for many of my needs, what makes that care easier to accept is if it comes from those who don't just see me as an elderly lady but are able to appreciate me as a person. I am not just someone who needs help with a bath!
>
> **Joan Earley, patient**
> "

> "
> In my experience as a nurse, care, compassion and dignity are vital. These values help create a safe environment and reduce fear and anxiety at one of the most vulnerable times of a person's life.
>
> Delivering the nursing care I provide with compassion and dignity makes all the difference between working with humanity in partnership with patients and just completing a series of tasks.
>
> **Trish Mayes, adult nurse**
> "

Visit https://study.sagepub.com/essentialnursing2e to access a wealth of online resources for this chapter – watch out for the margin icons throughout the chapter. If you are using the interactive eBook, simply click on the margin icon to go straight to the resource.

INTRODUCTION

As identified by Joan, it is fundamentally important to deliver care with that special extra ingredient which makes it easily acceptable. That special extra ingredient is being compassionate and caring, delivering dignified care which is person- or family-centred and value-based. However, as we discuss in this chapter, it can be difficult to define exactly what we mean by these terms, and this is made even more complex by the fact that every patient you will nurse is an individual with unique needs and expectations regarding how they want those values to be expressed. It is very much easier to identify when compassion, care and dignity are missing, and it is to our professional shame that there have historically been many instances when we have failed those who depend on us.

Trish clearly highlights the importance of care, compassion and dignity in making patients feel safe at times at which they are most vulnerable. As she explains, the essence of nursing is not in completing a series of tasks, but in delivering care with humanity.

This chapter will discuss fundamentally important values in nursing practice. We will consider what compassion, caring, dignity, person- or family-centred care and value-based nursing practice are; how you can ensure your care upholds and promotes these values; and what to do if you observe care in which they are missing. We will also address the topic of spiritual care, deliberating its importance in holistic care and how you can deliver care designed to meet all of your patients' needs.

WHAT IS VALUE-BASED, PERSON- OR FAMILY-CENTRED CARE?

✓

ANSWER:
ACTIVITY 12.1

ACTIVITY 12.1: REFLECTIVE PRACTICE

If you were asked, 'What is value-based, person- or family-centred care and why is this important in nursing?' what would you say?

As you may have found in Activity 12.1, explaining value-based, person- or family-centred care is a monumental task. This is made more difficult because not only will nurses have differing views on what it is, but so will patients. It could be that we are setting ourselves an impossible task not only in trying to define this, but also in trying to deliver care based on these values. However, if we review our Code (NMC, 2015), the fundamental role which values hold in all aspects of nursing care becomes clearly evident.

So our quest, not only to define values, but also to find ways to ensure we deliver them as an everyday part of our nursing practice, continues.

The second part of Activity 12.1 – why is it important? – is actually much simpler. As Joan tells us at the very start of the chapter, a patient is not just someone who needs, for example, a bath; they have life histories and experiences that have made them unique individuals, which, in order to provide the care they find acceptable, we need to take into account. While pinning down exactly what the 'slippery' concepts of compassion, caring and dignity entail may be difficult, understanding their fundamental importance in every aspect of nursing care is not.

Just like the balls of wool used for knitting, the fundamental values of compassion, caring, dignity, person- or family-centred and value-based care are all strands of nursing care which need to be intertwined. However, as nurses, the end result we desire is not a jumper, but effective care that meets all of a patient's unique needs.

> Compassion, caring and dignity are the most important things in nursing because they help the patient to feel valued as a person. I always treat patients with compassion, care and dignity because I would expect that if I was ill and in hospital. I was doing the observations on placement and a lady asked me if it would be OK if she could have a shower before she went home. I said that it was fine and went to help her. She said that I treated her so well and she felt loved. This made me realise that it only takes a small amount of time to treat patients with compassion and respect and it makes all the difference to them.
>
> **Hannah Boyd, adult nursing student**

Just as we would all choose different colours of wool and different knitting patterns to suit not only a patient's needs but also our knitting ability, all of these values will be woven into the care that you deliver in a unique manner. As identified in the news headlines in Activity 12.2, it is often easier to realise what you *haven't* got – it is far more noticeable when a stitch is missing or a knitting pattern is incorrect than when all is perfect. However, as patients have the right to expect the care they receive to be of the highest standard, delivered by professionals (DH, 2013), our professional 'knitting' can only ever be perfect.

To enable us to understand what is meant by the terms compassion, caring, dignity, person- or family-centred care and value-based nursing practice, and how we can ensure they are promoted in our everyday nursing practice, we will now consider each term individually, starting with compassion.

ACTIVITY 12.2: REFLECTIVE PRACTICE

Undertake a search of the news headlines, either from your local area or from the national news. Find two news reports highlighting instances where patients were delivered nursing care that was not compassionate, caring, dignified, person- or family-centred or value-based:

- Read the reports and reflect on the details.
- What do you think was the cause of the fundamental lapse in care?
- What would you have done if you had seen this inadequate care being delivered?

COMPASSION

Compassion has been a value central to nursing since the profession was established, but it seems to be the one thing that the profession has been charged with losing, diluting and undervaluing as other priorities take its place.

As you will see discussed in many other chapters, the Francis Report (2013) and a number of other reports, such as that of Heslop et al. (2013), consider occasions when patients were not treated with the compassion they deserved, along with a number of other serious failings.

CASE STUDY 12.1: HECTOR

Hector is 9 years old, and while playing in the garden tripped and fell through a pane of glass in his grandfather's greenhouse. Luckily for Hector, he sustained only minor injuries, but he did need four sutures in a deep wound in his hand. When Hector was at his local hospital having the wound sutured, he was very scared and crying, because 'it hurt' and he 'didn't like seeing the blood'. The nurse suturing Hector's hand told him to 'stop being a baby' and as he was a 'big boy now he was not to cry', and said that 'the more he cried, the longer it would take, so the more it would hurt'.

Hector has arrived for an appointment to have his wound dressed at his GP's surgery, where you are on placement. The receptionist comes to find you and your practice educator to tell you that Hector, your next patient, has arrived, but he is hiding behind a chair in the waiting room, because he doesn't want to come and see 'the nasty nurses who hurt'.

ANSWER:
CASE STUDY 12.1

- What do you think might be the reason why Hector associates nurses with things that hurt?
- How are you and your practice educator going to deliver effective and compassionate care to Hector in order to help him realise that not all nurses are nasty and hurt?

Although the reports of Francis (2013) and Heslop et al. (2013) are the most recent examples of such failings, numerous other reports have repeatedly demonstrated similar inadequacies, ever since the poor conditions experienced by elderly patients in the 1960s were reported by Robb (1967). Learning from such appalling evidence is crucial. Promises that nothing like this will happen again are made repeatedly, but conscious effort is required to guarantee change. We must ensure this is the case.

Compassion, in a similar manner to caring, is directly derived from the ethical principle of beneficence. Beneficence is the ethical principle which requires that we seek to do or produce good for others. While the role of the nurse is diverse and multi-faceted, all nursing practice shares the same ultimate aim to improve the lives of those receiving care.

Let us consider a nursing activity – assisting a patient with a bath, for example, as Joan mentioned at the start of the chapter. The good done through this act is not just that of the direct effect of the patient being clean; it also depends on how the bath is given.

> In my ward placement I worked with patients that had had a stroke; some of these patients had temporarily lost the use of their voice and their ability to complete tasks of daily living. I had to try to understand what they needed and were trying to say as these patients were relying on me for their care. I could only try to understand how frustrating it must be to be unable to communicate their needs to me and others, and when they got irritated I accepted that and tried to make things better.
>
> **Sarah Parkes, LD nursing student**

Hector's experience with the nurse at the hospital is a clear demonstration that effective nursing involves far more than just carrying out tasks. The nurse sutured Hector's cut, so she successfully completed the task, but did so in a way that made a bad situation worse. She most certainly failed in her duty to make Hector's life better. Having a wound sutured in a compassionate or a non-compassionate manner can result in two very different experiences. Even if the amount of pain and discomfort for Hector had been the same, if the nurse had acted in a compassionate manner she would have done

Hector's 'inner being' far more good, showing him that nurses help when things are bad. She would also have gained Hector's trust, and so his experience of healthcare, including having his wound re-dressed by you and your practice educator, would have been far less stressful.

Having gained an understanding of the importance of compassion in nursing practice and ways to ensure you promote this value, we shall now consider caring.

WHAT'S THE EVIDENCE?

Reification and compassion in medicine: A tale of two systems

Smajdor, A. (2013) 'Reification and compassion in medicine: A tale of two systems', *Journal of Clinical Ethics*, 8(4): 111-18.

- The article by Smajdor (2013) asks if compassion has disappeared in healthcare, and, if so, what is emerging to fill its place.
- Reflect on your experiences of nursing: To what extent do you think you have witnessed nursing care being delivered compassionately?
- Now read the article and consider if the view expressed can be applied to your experience.

CARING

Caring is frequently described as being at the heart of nursing, but perceptions of what exactly that means appear to differ between nurses. Some nurses focus on attaining the skills which enable them to deliver care based on a range of specialist technical interventions, as they feel this is the most important aspect of care; others feel that caring means their ability to relate to their patients and 'be there for them'. Thus, there is disagreement between nurses as to which 'type' of caring is effective, which raises an interesting further question – who should be the judge of what is important about care? Patients, relatives and carers may have a very different perception. Baughan and Smith (2008: 53) highlight behaviours that are indicators of care, which can be integrated into your actions. These are:

- carrying out simple acts of kindness
- promoting dignity
- using and developing skills of empathy by 'tuning in' to the patient
- being able to move our gaze from the body (as an object of intervention) to the person (living a life)
- developing trust
- giving effective reassurance by giving the other person confidence in our ability to listen and to help them
- being proactive – asking patients what they need – not waiting to be asked
- recognising the limitations of one's own skills
- entering into a partnership with patients and their families to gain knowledge and share the 'power'
- engaging in anti-discriminatory practice by respecting another human being, irrespective of their age, gender, cultural origins, class, status or the condition from which they suffer.

As we have identified caring behaviours, we will now move on to consider dignity, the last of the three values, which must always be evident in the care you deliver.

ACTIVITY 12.3: REFLECTIVE PRACTICE

Reflect on an experience when you have been involved in delivering care:

- Can you identify any of the 'caring indicators' in the list above, in your experience?
- Which of the 'caring indicators' do you think you need to develop further?

> When people are in hospital, they are more vulnerable than when they are well at home due to being in an unfamiliar environment and being with unfamiliar people. It is therefore important that nurses show compassion to their patients to make them feel at ease and promote recovery. It is also vital to observe someone's dignity; nurses may require patients to unveil more of themselves than they would usually feel comfortable with, especially to a stranger. Nurses need to understand patients' preferences regarding personal hygiene so they know how best to respect people's privacy.
>
> **Michelle Hill, NQ LD**

DIGNITY

Dignity has been identified as important by patients in a wide range of settings, with patients who perceived their care as respectful and dignified reporting the highest levels of satisfaction. Further to this, healthcare professionals worldwide agree that promoting patient dignity is a fundamental element of their practice (Matiti, 2011). It is possible to conclude, therefore, that there is a shared view between not only nurses but also all healthcare professionals and their patients that dignity is important, with such a view enshrined in both legislation and professional guidance (see Table 12.1).

Table 12.1   Professional guidance and legislation identifying the importance of dignity

The Code: Professional Standards of Practice and Behaviour for Nurses and Midwives (NMC, 2015)
The International Council of Nurses' Code of Ethics for Nurses (2012)
Article 3 of the UK Human Rights Act (1998)
Article 1 of the United Nations International Bill of Rights (1996)
Amsterdam *Declaration on the Promotion of Patients' Rights* (WHO, 1994)
The European Regions of the World Confederation for Physical Therapy (2003)
General Medical Council guidance (GMC, 2013)
General Pharmaceutical Council Standards of Conduct, Ethics and Performance (2010)

Despite this agreement, however, the practicalities of promoting dignity within healthcare settings remain problematic, and it is not always achieved (Francis, 2013; Heslop et al., 2013). Potential reasons suggested for this are that the 'notion' of dignity is not clearly understood (Matiti and Baillie, 2011) and there is a need to aid healthcare professionals to identify practical ways of promoting patient dignity.

ACTIVITY 12.4: REFLECTIVE PRACTICE

- Look up dignity in three different dictionaries – either online or hard copy.
- Can you relate these definitions to the care you deliver to patients?

It is frequently stated that the word dignity comes from two Latin roots – *dignus* and *dignitas*. Both of these Latin roots have very similar meanings: *dignus* means 'worth' and *dignitas* means 'merit'. Hereby we meet our first problem. It is possible that when looking for definitions of dignity, the words you find need explanation themselves, and may not necessarily translate easily to the care you deliver to patients.

Matiti (2011: 21) helpfully outlines the meaning of dignity:

- Everyone has a unique and dynamic concept of dignity.
- Although there is no universal definition of dignity, there are commonly identified attributes of dignity through which it is maintained and promoted.
- Each individual perceives these attributes differently, depending on how they perceive the influencing factors.
- Perceptions of dignity are influenced by experiences in healthcare; the care environment procedures and healthcare workers' behaviour can all affect perceptions of dignity.

Matiti and Baillie show that not only can dignity often mean different things to different people, but it can vary depending on the context. Although this increases our understanding of the numerous aspects of practice where dignity is important, and of its subjectivity, we still do not have a concrete understanding of exactly what dignity is, or ways in which we can translate it to our care. If a concept – such as dignity – proves difficult to define, pointers to its meaning can be gained from considering the other theoretical concepts often used to describe its meaning (Ganter and Willie, 1998). In this way, it is possible for us to find the attributes (Chinn and Jacobs, 1983) of dignity (see Table 12.2), which we can then ensure feature in the care we deliver.

Table 12.2 The attributes of dignity

General attributes nurses must attain	Attributes felt by patients to be important
Respect	Self-respect and **self-esteem**
Effective communication	Independence
Autonomy	Personal standards are appreciated
Privacy	Control over surroundings and how others treat them
Worth	Able to make choices
Empowerment	Self-confidence and self-identity

So while we have to accept that it is difficult to define exactly what is meant by dignity, it is possible, by focusing on its attributes and turning these into practical actions, to understand the fundamental importance of dignity and ensure it is evident in our everyday nursing. In addition to focusing on the attributes, further assistance is offered by Matiti and Baillie (2011: 13), who develop the earlier work of

Haddock (1996) by producing a definition of dignity that can be applied to nursing practice: 'feeling and being treated as being important and valuable when in situations that are considered threatening.'

If we expand this definition to cover not only situations that are considered threatening, but also everyday activities, it is possible to demystify the concept of dignity and find a way to ensure it is always promoted in our care.

> I always try to involve patients in their own care, especially with elderly patients. I feel it can be quite undignified having someone making assumptions and doing everything for you – if that patient wants a shower rather then a wash by the bed, why not? And if they want to get dressed into their normal clothes rather then a hospital gown (circumstances permitting), surely that is a lot more dignified.
>
> Charlie Clisby, NQN

ACTIVITY 12.5: REFLECTIVE PRACTICE

Reflect on your most recent experience of patient care:

- How many of the attributes of dignity in Table 12.2 were present in the care you were involved in delivering?
- Would the patients whose care you were involved in say that they were 'feeling and being treated as being important and valuable when in situations that are considered threatening' and in everyday activities?

Effective nursing practice, although based on fundamental values, requires further structuring in order to ensure it can meet all of a patient's needs. To consider the structures within which we deliver care, we will now consider person-centred care, family-centred care and value-based nursing practice to identify the guiding features.

PERSON-CENTRED CARE

The 'person' is a frequently used foundation of many nursing theories and models. Person-centred care is an approach based on the work of Tom Kitwood (1937–1998), an English gerontologist, which respects and values the uniqueness of every individual and seeks to maintain their personhood. This is done by creating an environment in which personal worth, individuality, respect, independence and hope are all evident. The term 'person-centred care' is frequently used interchangeably with 'patient-centred care'; however, if this change in terminology is unaccompanied by an understanding of the foundations of person-centred care, there is a danger of misunderstanding its true importance. Person-centred care was devised as an approach that moved the provision of care away from a position in which personhood did not factor.

The features of person-centred care are:

- knowing the patient as a person
- enabling them to make decisions based on informed choices about what is available
- shared decision-making rather than exerting control over the patient

- providing information that meets the individual needs of patients
- supporting the person to express their choices
- ongoing evaluation to ensure that care remains appropriate for the individual.

FAMILY-CENTRED CARE

Family-centred care enables parents and other family members to be involved in the healthcare of their child, with care being planned around the whole family, not just the individual child. In this way, all of the family members are recognised as recipients of care.

This approach is beneficial! because it reduces anxiety and the negative effects of hospitalisation on both the child and the family, promotes the bond between parent and child and improves satisfaction with care. Family-centred care is delivered by children's nurses worldwide, recommended by children's nursing organisations and formally recognised in governmental policies in Ireland and England (DH, 2003; DHC, 2000).

Value-based practice

We all hold values and beliefs, which have been formed by our individual experiences throughout our lives so far. Our values and beliefs shape our attitudes, and so the ways that we think, feel and behave. As nurses, the values and beliefs we hold can have an impact on the care we deliver.

ACTIVITY 12.6: REFLECTIVE PRACTICE

- Reflect on what you have read so far in this chapter.
- What do you think is the relationship between the fundamental values of compassion, care and dignity and person- or family-centred care?

CASE STUDY 12.2: VALERY

Valery is 52 and has a long history of intravenous drug and alcohol dependency. She has 'lived' in a bus shelter for the past three weeks because she was asked to leave the hostel where she was staying after punching another resident and causing £1,584 of damage because she was in a 'rage'. Valery often has mood swings, one moment appearing to be calm and the next becoming angry, provocative and rude for no reason. She is frequently late or completely misses appointments. Today she walks into your clinic, shouting, three hours late.

When you see Valery, she is very dishevelled; her hygiene is poor and she smells overpoweringly of stale body odour and cigarettes. When she greets you, her speech is slurred, but you can just make out that she is saying: 'You! I have been waiting ages for you. There you are - wasting my time again. Just give me my drugs, you idiot, and get out of my way.'

(Continued)

- As you read the case story of Valery and imagined yourself as the nurse who she had come to see, what were your thoughts?
- Would your thoughts alter if you were to learn that Valery had been clean from drugs and alcohol for six months, and that the reason for this visit was to collect antibiotics for a recurrent chest infection and her slurred speech, forgetfulness, mood swings and poor hygiene were all due to pre-senile dementia?

There are no right or wrong answers in case study 12.2. The values you hold are your values and make you the person you are. However, you must remember that your values may not be the same as the patient's. Inflicting your values on a patient may be seen by them as judgemental and unprofessional (NMC, 2015), resulting in a negative effect on the care they receive from you.

As has been outlined so far in this chapter, the provision of healthcare is inseparable from values such as compassion, care and dignity. Considering the patient's or the family's values within this also plays a crucial role. At times, this can be challenging, as values can be complex and conflicting. This is particularly so when a patient's or family's values seem to be at odds with the evidence-based practice we wish to provide or the ethical principles most people uphold, or if a nurse's personal values have the potential to compromise the care delivered.

ACTIVITY 12.7: REFLECTIVE PRACTICE

- Watch the video case study on values and difficult personal choices, at https://study.sagepub.com/essentialnursing2e.
- Reflect on how this enables you to better understand how to support patients who need to make tough personal choices which may bring their values into question.

Value-based practice, a framework developed originally in mental healthcare, identifies the values we hold as being pervasive and powerful influences on the decisions made relating to care, and highlights that their impact is often underestimated (Petrova et al., 2006). Value-based practice suggests that some approaches to care enable us to ignore important displays of values because unless there is evidence of conflicting values, we presume they are shared. Value-based practice is an approach to supporting care that provides practical skills and tools for discovering an individual's values and negotiating ways in which these can be upheld in care delivery. It aims to introduce a wide range of views and enable the recognition of specific values that may be held by certain cultures, small groups, or those held only by certain individuals.

As we have previously discussed, in person-centred care, it is the values of the patient that dominate. However, one of the features of value-based practice is that the focus on the patient's values is supplemented by paying attention to a wider range of values, including those of the family, carers, healthcare professionals and society, as well as the values embedded in research, the organisation of services and policy documents. Awareness of such a range of values is important, as they all have the potential to hinder effective patient care. While we may like to think it is possible to 'hold back' our personal values, this is far from simple. Recognition of our own values is a necessary step in understanding the patient's. The more aware we are of our own values and personal beliefs, the more likely it becomes that the values that enhance effective relationships will be strengthened (Trenoweth et al., 2011).

Throughout the chapter so far, we have considered fundamental nursing values, how we can promote them in practice and the wider frameworks or structures of care that enable us to provide patients with effective nursing care. We will now move on to the topic of spirituality: an aspect of care that we need to deliver in order to work holistically with our patients, but one which is frequently overlooked.

SPIRITUALITY

Oldnall (1996) found that nurses are aware that patients have spiritual needs; however, they are unable to deliver spiritual care for two reasons: first, due to a lack of spiritual education within nursing education; second, due to the idea that spiritual care is an area dealt with by chaplains and other religious groups.

ACTIVITY 12.8: REFLECTIVE PRACTICE

Reflect on your most recent experience of caring for someone. Can you identify any care you delivered that could be described as spiritual?

It is possible that your reaction after reading Activity 12.8 could be 'Spiritual care? Is that really up to me?', or even 'Spiritual care – what exactly is that?'

First, let's answer the question as to whether spiritual care is a feature of nursing care. Throughout the whole of this book, a holistic approach has been emphasised and has been described as an important aspect of nursing care. In many chapters, it has been highlighted that:

- no matter where or with whom they practise, nurses always work in a holistic way
- when it is said that nurses deliver holistic care, this means that they consider the individual's physical, psychological, social, emotional, intellectual and spiritual needs.

From this we can see that spiritual care is an important aspect of a holistic approach, making this an area that, as a nursing student and then a registered nurse, you will need to incorporate within your care.

Second, we must actually answer the question of what spiritual care is – this is necessary before being able to consider the importance of spirituality in nursing care any further! If you ask many people what they understand by the word 'spirituality', they may well tell you that it 'relates to connecting with God', or is 'a search for the sacred' or 'religiousness'. But is this a contemporary understanding of the meaning?

ACTIVITY 12.9: REFLECTIVE PRACTICE

- Reflect on what the word 'spirituality' means to you. Do you see it as having a religious association or is your understanding more secular? Does spirituality have any links to other aspects of your everyday life?
- Make a note of your thoughts and compare them with the information presented in the rest of the chapter.

You may have found, in the thoughts you had when undertaking Activity 12.9, that the concept of spirituality is both broad and subjective, and maybe that you could write a very long piece explaining what spirituality means to you. This may be true for some people; others may have given it very little previous thought. Despite this, it is possible to identify common features of most individuals' answers when they are asked the same question, such as:

- hope
- meaning and purpose
- forgiveness
- beliefs and values
- spiritual care
- relationships
- belief in God or a deity
- morality
- creativity and self-expression. (McSherry, 2008)

When we consider these features, it becomes clear that spirituality can be seen to be associated with more than just religion. Spirituality can be viewed as an integral aspect of everyday life which can be relevant to all individuals – although we must take care to always remember that each individual will have their own unique view of spirituality, just as you noted down when you completed Activity 12.9. It also becomes evident that a formal association with religion may or may not be a feature in an individual's personal description of spirituality. An illness or crisis of any sort may be the catalyst that leads an individual to consider or re-evaluate their spirituality.

So, although we have to conclude that each individual's understanding of spirituality is complex, subjective and highly personal, we can view spirituality as relating to all activities that bring value and meaning to our everyday life and relationships. In addition to this, spirituality can be seen as a constant feature within our past, present and future. Thus, as nurses who care for patients while they experience a range of challenging situations, spirituality clearly becomes a fundamentally important aspect of the nursing care we provide.

How can I deliver spiritual care?

ACTIVITY 12.10: CRITICAL THINKING

Imagine the scene. You are at a wedding reception and have been seated at a table between two people you don't know. The conversation is becoming very stilted, so in an attempt to get everyone talking you say, 'Well, what shall we talk about – religion or politics?'

- What do you think their responses will be?
- Is your attempt to enliven the conversation likely to be successful?

ANSWER:
ACTIVITY 12.10

As we have already mentioned, spirituality is complex, subjective and highly personal. In the same way that you are unlikely to ask people about sensitive or intimate issues until you know them very well, if spirituality is mentioned – which many people often view as being linked to religion – it is possible that people will either stop talking or will feel they are being called to account for their personal views and become argumentative. So how can you manage to avoid reactions such as these and incorporate the spiritual dimension within the care you deliver?

If you study Figure 12.1, what do you see hidden in the middle of the word 'spirituality'?

Figure 12.1   Spirituality contains...

Source: McSherry (2008)

While it also has other meanings, ritual can be considered to relate to 'often repeated actions' which are concerned with the ordinary events and routines of everyday life. You may well have experienced some rituals during your experiences of caring for patients – nursing procedures that have been undertaken without consideration as to whether they are truly necessary, such as temperature, pulse and blood pressure being recorded at certain times of the day. Although the necessity of ritualistic nursing actions should be questioned, the structure and security provided by rituals can be positive. So, when considering the delivery of spiritual care, it can be very helpful to view it as an integral aspect of the rituals involved in the ordinary events and routines of everyday life.

If we take such an approach, it is not necessary to apply any specific additional models to enable us to deliver spiritual care. We can integrate it into the areas we already consider within the nursing process to assist us in delivering individualised, holistic, patient- or family-centred, evidence-based care.

Spiritual care is sometimes considered to be the same as psychological support. It is true that the two share many similarities, as psychological and spiritual wellbeing are intertwined – but spiritual care differs from counselling, for example. In fact, it is not possible for spiritual care to be described as any particular activity; it is far more complex, and actually is more about 'being' than doing.

In effect, it is about being caring, genuine and open in your communication with patients, offering them the opportunity to discuss any issues they feel are relevant and responding appropriately.

Rieg et al. (2006) suggest the very practical approach of asking questions of a patient:

- Ask open questions, focusing on how the patient is feeling. Good questions to get the conversation started are:
  - 'What do you find to be the most difficult part of your current situation?'
  - 'What hurts or angers you most at the moment?'
- Then find out what the patient believes would be helpful, by asking them:
  - 'What has helped you the most when you have felt like this before?'
  - 'Do your friends, family or faith help you?'

Such an approach will give an adult patient an opportunity to express a need for spiritual support. When caring for children or individuals with a learning disability, you may need to modify the language; possibly, with a child, you may need to ask the questions of their favourite teddy bear. In this way, it becomes clear that the questions you are asking relating to spiritual care are just the same as those you will ask relating to their physical or psychological comfort.

Thus, as seen earlier, asking a patient about their spirituality can be seen as an 'often repeated action' or ritual. Once you have discovered what the patient's needs are, just as with any other aspect of care, you can plan, implement and assess a range of actions to achieve the goal desired.

WHAT TO DO IF CARE IS NOT VALUE-BASED, PERSON- OR FAMILY-CENTRED

Throughout your nursing programme, you will see a wide range of care in a variety of settings. Your placements will ensure you gain the experience of being involved in delivering care in acute areas, such as general hospitals or specialist ones, and community environments, such as GP surgeries, patients' homes or residential care homes. The care you are involved in delivering will be emergency, long-term and short-term, and you will become an expert at assessing, planning, implementing and evaluating the care your patient needs. You will work with many nurses and be supported by a number of practice supervisors.

This experience is designed to ensure that when you become a registered nurse, you are capable of working without supervision to deliver competent care to the patients for whom you are responsible. While a nursing student, you will find some of the nurses and practice supervisors you work with to be inspirational. They will become your role models, whose standards and abilities you will aim to imitate throughout the rest of your career.

While you experience the delivery of care in this wide range of settings, you will observe nurses approaching the same tasks differently. Just because your current practice supervisor undertakes a nursing procedure in a different way from your previous practice supervisor, it doesn't necessarily make it wrong – it is just different. However, there may be times when you experience care that does not seem 'right' to you. As has been outlined throughout this chapter, and as you were asked to consider in Activity 12.2, not all care delivered to patients is good. Your role is to ensure that if at any time you feel the care you have seen is not 'right', not upholding the values of compassion, caring and dignity for example, you must:

- seek help and advice from a practice supervisor or lecturer when there is a need to protect people from harm
- seek help immediately from an appropriately qualified professional if someone for whom you are providing care has suffered harm for any reason
- seek help from your practice supervisor or lecturer if people indicate that they are unhappy about their care or treatment.

As nurses, we come into contact with vulnerable patients on a daily basis. Their protection is central to your role. Care which does not uphold the fundamental nursing values outlined in this chapter is never acceptable.

CONCLUSION

Compassion, care and dignity are fundamental nursing values which must be upheld in all aspects of our practice. Their exact meaning may be difficult to define, especially as they can be subjective, thus differing depending on the situation and the patient. However, it is possible to define certain features of nursing care which promote these values, and we must ensure they are evident in the care we deliver.

Person- or family-centred care and value-based nursing practice enable the nursing care we deliver to meet the unique needs of patients, while setting care within the wider values of contemporary society. In order to understand a patient's values, we need to be able to recognise our own.

Spirituality plays an important role in the delivery of holistic care; thus, we need to be able to discuss spiritual needs with patients and provide care to meet them. If we consider spirituality as an element of everyday ritual, it can provide structure and security, and we can address it in the same manner as any other aspect of care.

Throughout your nursing career, your primary role is, at all times, to protect those in your care. Any care that does not uphold the nursing values we consider to be fundamental can never be accepted.

CHAPTER SUMMARY

- Promoting compassion, care and dignity is fundamentally important in every aspect of nursing care.
- A number of serious failings of care can be identified within the history of nursing since the 1960s.
- Numerous nursing theories and models are based on person- or family-centred care, creating an environment where the uniqueness of each individual or family is recognised. While the terms 'person-centred care' and 'patient-centred care' are frequently used interchangeably, it should be remembered that person-centred care was devised as an approach that moved care provision away from a position in which personhood did not factor.
- We all hold values and beliefs which, because they shape the ways in which we think, feel and behave, can impact on the care we deliver.
- The more aware we are of our values and beliefs, the more likely it becomes that the values enhancing effective relationships with patients will be strengthened.
- Spirituality is both an integral aspect of daily life and a necessary consideration when delivering holistic nursing care. If it is considered as an everyday ritual, which provides security and structure, it can be incorporated into the areas of care that we already consider within the nursing process.
- As a nurse, your primary function is to protect those in your care. Care which does not uphold and promote fundamental nursing values is never acceptable.

CRITICAL REFLECTION

Holistic care

This chapter has highlighted the importance of compassion, caring, dignity, spirituality, a person- or family-centred approach and value-based practice when providing holistic care for a patient. Review the chapter and note down all the instances in which you think delivering compassionate, caring, dignified, spiritual, person- or family-centred and value-based nursing care will help meet the patient's physical, psychological, social, economic and spiritual needs. Think of a variety of different patients across the fields, not just those within your own field. You may find it helpful to make a list and refer back to it next time you are in practice, and then write your own reflection after your practice experience.

GO FURTHER

Books

Clarke, J. (2013) *Spiritual Care in Everyday Nursing Practice*. Basingstoke: Palgrave Macmillan. An interesting and informative text considering the spiritual needs of individuals in an everyday context.

Woodbridge, K. and Fulford, K.W.M. (2004) *Whose Values? A Workbook for Values Based Practice in Mental Healthcare*. London: The Sainsbury Centre for Mental Health. An excellent workbook which will help you to understand how diverse values relate, interact and impact on experiences, actions and relationships. While the workbook was designed specifically for mental healthcare, it is relevant to nursing care in all fields.

SAGE journal articles

FURTHER
READING:
JOURNAL
ARTICLES

Go to https://study.sagepub.com/essentialnursing2e for free online journal articles for this chapter. If you are using the interactive ebook, simply click on the book icon in the margin to go straight to the resource.

Gustafsson, L., Wigerblad, A. and Lindwall, L. (2014) 'Undignified care: Violation of patient dignity in involuntary psychiatric hospital care from a nurse's perspective', *Nursing Ethics*, 21: 176-86. An interesting article identifying seven themes which describe nurses' experiences of violation of patient dignity.

Other journal articles

Holloway, M. (2006) 'Death the great leveller? Towards a transcultural spirituality of dying and bereavement', *Journal of Clinical Nursing*, 15(7): 833-9. A very readable article which outlines four beliefs that overwhelmingly gave comfort to people who reported no religious affiliation at all.

Kantek, F., Kaya, A. and Gezer, N. (2017) 'The effects of nursing education on professional values: A longitudinal study', *Nurse Education Today*, 58: 43-6. An interesting article that aims to investigate the effects of nursing education on development of professional values.

Rieg, L.S., Mason, C.H. and Preston, K. (2006) 'Spiritual care: Practical guidelines for rehabilitation nurses', *Rehabilitation Nursing*, 31(6): 249-55. An informative article outlining practical guidelines for nurses when assisting patients to meet their spiritual needs.

Weblinks

FURTHER
READING:
WEBLINKS

Go to https://study.sagepub.com/essentialnursing2e for weblinks related to this chapter. If you are using the interactive ebook, simply click on the book icon in the margin to go straight to the resource.

www.thekairosforum.com – Kairos, a forum for people with intellectual or cognitive disabilities (KFICD), seeks to highlight and respond to the spiritual and religious needs of people with disabilities.

http://allnurses.com/nursing-and-spirituality/religion-culture-nursing-517282.html – a discussion board where views on spirituality and nursing are shared.

www.dignityincare.org.uk – website of the Dignity in Care network, which is led by the National Dignity Council. The website offers resources, support and a network of Dignity Champions: over 40,000 individuals and organisations who work to put dignity and respect at the heart of UK care services to enable a positive experience of care.

www.nursetogether.com – a website for nurses offering, amongst other things, interesting articles and stimulating discussion.

www.gov.uk/government/publications/the-nhs-constitution-for-england – the NHS Constitution, establishing the principles and values of the NHS in England.

www.show.scot.nhs.uk – NHS Scotland, highlighting the principles and values of the NHS in Scotland.

www.wales.nhs.uk – NHS Wales, highlighting the principles and values of the NHS in Wales.

http://online.hscni.net – the official gateway for Health and Social Care in Northern Ireland, highlighting its principles and values.

Video links

Have a break from the text and go to https://study.sagepub.com/essentialnursing2e for useful videos related to this chapter. If you are using the interactive ebook, simply click on the lightbulb icon in the margin to go straight to the resource.

VIDEO
LINKS

ACE YOUR ASSESSMENT

GREAT FOR
REVISION!

Review what you have learned by visiting the book's online resources at: https://study.sagepub.com/essential nursing2e If using your interactive ebook, just click on the icon in the margin to go straight there.

- Test yourself with multiple-choice and short-answer questions.
- Revise key terms with the interactive flash cards.

ONLINE
QUIZZES

REFERENCES

Baughan, J. and Smith, A. (2008) *Caring in Nursing Practice*. Dorchester: Pearson Education.

Chinn, P. and Jacobs, M. (1983) *Theory and Nursing*. St Louis, MO: Mosby.

Department of Health (DH) (2003) *Getting the Right Start: The National Service Framework for Children, Young People and Maternity Services – Standards for Hospital Services*. London: The Stationery Office.

Department of Health (2013) *The NHS Constitution*. London: DH.

Department of Health and Children (DHC) (2000) *The National Children's Strategy: Our Children – Their Lives*. Dublin: DHC.

The European Regions of the World Confederation for Physical Therapy (2003) Available at: http://www.erwcpt.eu/ (accessed 5 April 2018).

Francis, R. (2013) *Report of the Mid Staffordshire NHS Foundation Trust Public Inquiry*. London: The Stationery Office.

Ganter, B. and Willie, R. (1998) *Formal Concept Analysis: Mathematical Foundations* (trans. C. Franzke). Berlin: Springer-Verlag.

General Medical Council (2013) *Good Medical Practice*. London. General Medical Council.

General Pharmaceutical Council (2010) *Standards of Conduct, Ethics and Performance*. Available at: www.pharmacyregulation.org/ (accessed 5 April 2018).

Haddock, J. (1996) 'Towards a further clarification of the concept "dignity"', *Journal of Advanced Nursing*, 24(5): 924–31.

Heslop, P., Blair, P., Fleming, P., Hoghton, M., Marriott, A. and Russ, L. (2013) *Confidential Inquiry into Premature Deaths of People with Learning Disabilities (CIPOLD)*. Bristol: Nora Fry Research Centre. Available at: www.bris.ac.uk/cipold (accessed 18 February 2015).

International Council of Nurses (2012) *The ICN Code of Ethics for Nurses*. Available at: www.icn.ch/images/stories/documents/about/icncode_english.pdf (accessed 5 April 2018).

Matiti, M. (2011) 'The importance of dignity in healthcare', in M. Matiti and L. Baillie (eds), *Healthcare: Dignity in Healthcare*. London: Radcliffe Publishing. pp. 3–8.

Matiti, M.R. and Baillie, L. (2011) *Dignity in Healthcare*. London: Radcliffe Publishing.

McSherry, W. (2008) *Making Sense of Spirituality in Nursing and Health Care Practice*, 2nd edn. London: Jessica Kingsley Publishers.

Nursing and Midwifery Council (NMC) (2015) *The Code: Professional Standards of Practice and Behaviour for Nurses and Midwives*. London: NMC.

Oldnall, A. (1996) 'A critical analysis of nursing: Meeting the spiritual needs of patients', *Journal of Advanced Nursing*, 23(1): 138–44.

Petrova, M., Dale, J. and Fulford, B. (2006) 'Values-based practice in primary care: Easing the tensions between individual values, ethical principles and best evidence', *British Journal of General Practice*, 56(530): 703–9.

Rieg, L.S., Mason, C.H. and Preston, K. (2006) 'Spiritual care: Practical guidelines for rehabilitation nurses', *Rehabilitation Nursing*, 31(6): 249–55.

Robb, B. (1967) *Sans Everything: A Case to Answer.* London: Nelson.

Smajdor, A. (2013) 'Reification and compassion in medicine: A tale of two systems', *Journal of Clinical Ethics*, 8(4): 111–18.

Trenoweth, S., Docherty, T., Franks, J. and Pearce, R. (2011) *Nursing and Mental Health Care: An Introduction for All Fields of Practice.* Exeter: Learning Matters.

UK Human Rights Act 1998, Article 3. Available at: www.legislation.gov.uk/ukpga/1998/42/schedule/1/part/I/chapter/2 (accessed 5 April 2018).

United Nations International Bill of Rights (1996) Article 1. Available at: www.ohchr.org/Documents/Publications/FactSheet2Rev.1en.pdf (accessed 5 April 2018).

WHO (1994) *A Declaration on the Promotion of Patients Rights in Europe.* Amsterdam. World Health Organization.

PATIENT, SERVICE USER, FAMILY AND CARER PERSPECTIVES

KATRINA EMERSON AND RUTH NORTHWAY

--- THIS CHAPTER COVERS ---

- What it means to be a patient
- Types of carers

- How can healthcare professionals help?
- Planning care collaboratively

> My name is Frank and I am 59 years old. I moved to the UK in the 1960s with my parents, who came from the West Indies to find work and to give me a good education. I worked hard and got to university to study law and have worked as a barrister for my entire career. Recently, however, I have started to have difficulties with remembering things, which (in my job) is extremely problematic. My family also noticed that my moods were changing and instead of being even-tempered I had started to have outbursts of temper. In the end it was becoming such a problem at work that I went to the doctor. She referred me to a specialist and I was diagnosed as having the early stages of dementia. As you can imagine, this was devastating news – I knew that things would not get better and so I took early retirement from work so that I could leave with my head held high rather than making a big mistake. However, I feel as though I have been catapulted from being a person with a good job and a respected role to being a 'patient' who is going to get more and more dependent. I am worried about not being able to support my family and the demands my condition will make on them. The future looks very bleak and I am not sure where to go to get support.
>
> **Frank, patient**

> During my nursing course I have worked in a number of care settings and I have always thought that I had a pretty good understanding of what it was like to be a patient, a member of their family or a carer. Last month, however, my grandmother was admitted to one of the wards that I had worked on and I realised how different it feels to be on the receiving end of healthcare. The staff were very good and answered all my questions, as they knew me – nonetheless, I did wonder whether relatives who didn't know the questions to ask would have been able to get the information they need. Also, my grandmother was in a single room and, as a family, we noticed that staff didn't seem to come and check how she was on a regular basis. When we asked her she said that usually staff only come at meal times, to give her tablets and if she uses the call button. She added that she didn't like to use the buzzer as she knew the staff were busy. One day we arrived to find her quite distressed and feeling unwell, but she had not called the staff. I know how easy it can be to think someone else has given information to relatives and to not always check on side rooms. However, my experience in relation to my grandmother has made me determined to not take it for granted that someone else is taking responsibility for these aspects of care.
>
> **Sally, adult nursing student**

INTRODUCTION

Whichever field of nursing you are working in, one thing that is certain is that you will be in contact with 'patients' (as they are called within this book, but you will see later in this chapter that terminology can be challenging), their families and their carers. You are also likely to have personal experience of being either a patient or a family member of someone using the health service, and therefore have some insight into how this feels. However, people, their circumstances and the services they use are very different and, while our own experiences can help us to some extent, we need to understand a range of experiences in order to be effectively equipped to support others.

The student story at the beginning of this chapter highlights just how different it can be to be on the 'other side' of the care experience. Similarly, the patient story above reminds us how difficult it can be to have to take on the label of 'patient', and the impact it can have.

Working in partnership with people who use health and social care services, their families and carers is fundamental to nursing care. This means that we need to understand who they are and how we can best meet their needs. While this understanding will continue to develop throughout your nursing career, this chapter aims to help you start this process by considering the terminology we use, the needs of patients and their families and carers, and the implications for the planning and delivery of collaborative care.

ACTIVITY 13.1: CRITICAL THINKING

Take a few minutes to identify all the terms you have heard used to refer to those people who use the health service:

- Are there any you feel are better than others?
- Why is this?

ANSWER:
ACTIVITY 13.1

WHAT IT MEANS TO BE A PATIENT

You might think that it is fairly simple to identify a term that covers all those who use the health service and those people whom nurses may be involved in working with. However, even in writing this chapter it has been challenging to think of the most appropriate terms to use. Perhaps the most commonly used term is 'patient', particularly in hospital settings or when someone is receiving a particular treatment or intervention in the community (such as wound care). Indeed, we commonly refer to 'inpatients' and 'outpatients' in describing where people receive their care.

Most people would be happy to be referred to as a patient while they are within hospital; however, the appropriateness of using the term on a longer-term basis may not be so straightforward. For example, consider a woman who has a mastectomy, chemotherapy and radiotherapy because of breast cancer, who then receives oral hormonal treatment monitored at the hospital on a yearly basis for five years. She may still be taking medication, but is she a patient, as she goes about her day-to-day life in the way she did before her illness?

The term 'patient' seems more fitting where a particular illness or condition is having a significant impact on an individual's life and where ongoing intervention from a health professional is required. It may also be applied to a specific interaction with a health professional, such as in an outpatient setting. However, some people feel that 'patient' is a label that is inappropriately applied on a long-term basis, which then affects how they are treated by others. One area in which this has been particularly discussed is mental health settings: someone may experience acute phases of mental distress and require high levels of support during these periods, but once the acute phase subsides they may receive minimal support from mental health services. Indeed, they may hold down busy jobs and hold positions of considerable responsibility. To be viewed as a 'mental health patient' during such times may be experienced as stigmatising and as limiting the opportunities of the individuals concerned, since others view them as 'ill'. Other terms such as 'service user' and 'survivor' have therefore been used. These are not specific to mental health (for example, it is common to refer to cancer survivors), but this is one area where they have been widely used.

Even though these terms have very different connotations to that of 'patient', they too have given rise to some criticism. For example, McLaughlin (2009) argues that generally the term 'user' is linked to drug addiction, and therefore has its own negative connotations. He also notes that 'service users' is a term used to refer to a group of people who use a common service but who otherwise have little in common. Therefore, the diversity of need and experience within this group of people may be overlooked.

You may feel that the terminology used is not important as long as people receive a service. However, terminology has a number of important functions within the context of healthcare:

- Use of terminology can imply or lead to an imbalance of power in the relationship between those who are giving care and those who are receiving it. Traditionally, the doctor–patient relationship has been one where power and decision-making lay with the doctor, and this was reinforced by labelling the other party as 'the patient'. Doctors have been viewed as 'experts' and 'patients' have been expected (sometimes without question) to follow the doctor's advice. Moreover, if a 'patient' has stepped outside their designated role by questioning medical advice, they have run the risk of being viewed as difficult or non-compliant.
- It can give a message about how the people to whom the label is applied are viewed by others, which may influence how other people behave towards them. For example, until the early 1980s the qualification we now know as 'learning disability nursing' was referred to, in official nursing regulations, as 'mental sub-normality nursing'. Consider the image that portrayed of the people who were supported by such nurses.
- It might influence how the person to whom the term or label is applied sees themselves. For example, if someone in the early stages of dementia is admitted to a ward for investigations and constantly hears herself referred to as 'the dementia patient' by the ward staff, she may feel that the staff team see her as a condition rather than a person.

It is important that we consider these points when delivering care, as different people will prefer different terms. The 'What's the evidence?' box provides insight into how some recipients of mental health services feel about the use of terminology.

WHAT'S THE EVIDENCE?

Service user, patient, client, survivor or user: Describing recipients of mental health services

In this study, Simmons et al. (2010) surveyed people who used mental health services. A total of 350 questionnaires were returned from people using community and inpatient mental health services. Participants were asked whether they would like four different types of healthcare

(Continued)

professional (nurse, doctor, social worker or occupational therapist) to refer to them as a service user, patient, client, survivor or user. The possible responses were yes, no, unsure. They were then asked to rank the order of preference for the terms they would prefer a healthcare professional to regard them as.

In relation to how they would like each professional to refer to them, the term 'patient' emerged as a 'clear favourite', receiving the most positive endorsements and the least negative endorsements.

In relation to the four professional groups, 'patient' was the most frequently chosen option in relation to nurses and doctors and was slightly preferred to 'client' in relation to social workers and occupational therapists. The terms 'user' and 'survivor' received the least support in relation to the various professionals. A similar picture emerged from analysis of the ranking of preference.

It is concluded that despite the term 'service user' being used in most mental health policy documents, this term was not the most preferred in this study. It suggests that policy makers should recognise the evidence base for using the term 'patient'.

The findings of this research may surprise you, but it is worth bearing in mind that the people who completed the questionnaire in this study were currently receiving some form of active mental health intervention. Nonetheless, what this research does highlight is that people will have different views and expectations, and we need to be conscious of how we use language.

ACTIVITY 13.2: REFLECTION

Service user, patient, client, survivor or user?

- How do you refer to those you deliver care to?
- Why is this?
- Do you think the same findings would emerge if other groups of people who use health services were asked the same questions?
- What are your reasons for this conclusion?

ANSWER:
ACTIVITY 13.2

The need to respect different preferences draws our attention to the fact that patients are, first and foremost, people who have their own views, cultures, experiences, prejudices and expectations. In keeping with this, and in order to promote person-centred care, the new NMC *Standards for Pre-registration Nurse Education* (NMC, 2017) use 'person' to refer to those for whom nurses provide support and care.

To improve the quality of care provided and to enhance the experience of being a patient, recent approaches to care delivery have promoted a different approach to both nursing and wider healthcare. Kvåle and Bondevik (2008) argue that, while historically patients were viewed as passive recipients of healthcare, today the importance of acknowledging their values and perceptions in order to provide high-quality, evidence-based care is recognised. In their study, they sought to determine, from the views of patients themselves, what patient-centred care means. Three themes emerged: empowerment, shared decision-making and partnership in care.

Apply your knowledge of person-centred care by reading Jag's case study, at https://study.sagepub. com/essentialnursing2e.

CASE STUDY:
JAG

> As a child field student, I prefer to refer to them as 'young people/young person' – a 15- or 18-year-old may not like being called a child, as they are teenagers nearing adulthood. I feel the word 'patient' is very impersonal and makes everyone 'the same', and they are not – everyone is individual.
>
> **Siân Hunter, child nursing student**
>
> Wherever possible I try to refer to the people in my care by their name, as I think that is more personal and the person may not want others to know that they need staff to support and take care of them. If that is not possible, I look at the setting I am in and use 'patient' or 'service user'.
>
> **Sarah Parkes, LD nursing student**
>
> I do refer to individuals I care for as 'patients' but, with their permission, I do like to use their names – I feel this provides a much more personal and individual service, which patients react well to.
>
> **Charlie Clisby, NQN**

Kvåle and Bondevik (2008) use the term 'patient-centred care', but Manley et al. (2011) refer to 'person-centred care', and identify the following features of person-centred care:

- knowing the patient as a person
- enabling them to make decisions based on informed choices about what is available
- shared decision-making rather than exerting control over the patient
- providing information that meets the individual needs of the patient
- supporting the person to express their choices
- ongoing evaluation to ensure that care remains appropriate for the individual.

These elements of person-centred care are all evident in the new NMC Standards (NMC, 2017) and should therefore inform nursing practice.

CASE STUDY 13.1: MARK

I was diagnosed with HIV 20 years ago so I've experienced many changes, not just in the treatment options available but also the attitudes of healthcare workers towards people with HIV. I was given my diagnosis in a sexual health clinic and although everyone was very pleasant, I found attending the sexual health clinic reinforced my feelings of being 'dirty' or having 'done something wrong'. I was encouraged to join support meetings and attend service user groups but, from a purely personal perspective, I didn't really want to talk about my sexuality or meet other people with the same condition. I just wanted to be treated as an individual and get on with my life.

Maybe nurses need to question their assumptions about the type of support that people with HIV need and be aware that just because people share a diagnosis, they won't automatically have something in common. While some people with HIV want to focus on their condition, others try to ignore the virus and only think about it when a health check is due.

(Continued)

For me, it's important that when I have my hospital appointment it feels like an informal, friendly catch-up with a familiar face. Remembering my likes and dislikes, treating me as an equal and valuing my opinions about the care I would like to receive are important to me.

ANSWER: CASE STUDY 13.1

- Consider what Mark says about how he would like support to be provided. How can nurses support groups of patients while also addressing individual needs?

ACTIVITY 13.3: REFLECTION

Reflect on the care you have recently provided for one of your patients:

ANSWER: ACTIVITY 13.3

- How did it compare with the features of person-centred care identified by Manley et al. (2011)?
- What more could have been done to make the care and support more person-centred?
- What more could have been done to make the service more person-centred?

TYPES OF CARERS

Within the UK, we tend to use the term 'carer' to cover a wide range of people, including those who have a professional role (such as nurses), family members and friends, and people who are paid to provide care either in a range of care settings (such as day centres, residential homes and supported living) or in people's own homes.

The role of paid carers

Depending on the needs of the individual, paid carers may be involved in providing different aspects of care and support, such as:

- personal care – including meeting hygiene needs, providing assistance with dressing, attending medical appointments, supervising medication
- food preparation – assisting with shopping, preparation of meals, ensuring adequate diet and fluid intake
- socialising – assisting people to visit recreational facilities, supporting people to visit friends
- mobility – this might include assisting someone who is a wheelchair user and/or driving a car or assisting someone to use public transport
- employment – for example, assistance with administrative tasks or acting as a personal assistant to enable the individual to undertake a specific job
- emotional support – for example, providing encouragement to someone who has a phobia about going out or providing bereavement support.

Sometimes paid carers are referred to as 'unqualified', but many will have undertaken both on-the-job and other training. For example, a number will have completed NVQs in care or management, depending on their specific role. However, in contrast to nurses, they are not registered professionals.

Paid carers may spend considerable periods of time with the individuals they support, sometimes over a protracted time frame lasting even years. Although their role is not primarily one of providing healthcare, it can be seen from the list above that they can greatly influence the health of the people they support. For example, if someone with severe depression neglects their personal hygiene, refuses to take their medication and fails to eat an adequate diet, it is likely that their already impaired health will be further affected. A paid carer may be able to encourage the person and prompt them to eat, drink and attend to their hygiene. They may be able to identify when someone is beginning to develop health problems and alert the appropriate health professionals, thus having a key role in both helping to keep people healthy and prompting action if the health of the person they are caring for starts to deteriorate. This means that it is important for paid carers to have some basic health-related knowledge and understanding supported by educational initiatives, which are often provided by nurses working in related fields. Unfortunately, this does not always occur, and the recent *Confidential Inquiry into Premature Deaths of People with Learning Disabilities* (Heslop et al., 2013) identified gaps in knowledge and skills amongst some social care providers.

It is not always possible to prevent ill health, and in such instances it may be necessary for an individual to be admitted to hospital. A paid carer who knows the individual well can be an invaluable resource for hospital staff. Consider, for example, an elderly person with dementia who is admitted to hospital due to a respiratory infection. As well as feeling extremely unwell, they could be confused and unable to provide any information themselves. Or consider a person with a moderate learning disability, who may have little body awareness and complex communication needs. A paid carer may be able to inform the ward staff not only about the events leading up to the admission but also about the individual's likes and dislikes, their normal pattern of behaviour, how they express pain and many other important issues that are central to person-centred care. However, it is possible that the paid carer who is supporting the individual may not know them well; they may be a member of bank staff, for example, and it is essential to ask them rather than to assume. To assist the admission process, for people who have a learning disability, the acute hospital liaison nurse or a learning disabilities nurse from the local community team can help with the development of a hospital passport. These documents are ideally prepared in advance, in readiness for a potential admission. The care staff can keep them updated so, when the admission occurs, the essential information about the person is immediately available.

Paid carers can also be important in supporting people following their discharge from hospital. This may be for a temporary period if they are likely to recover their previous level of independence, or on an ongoing basis. In either situation, careful planning is important to ensure that an appropriate package of care is established before discharge and that good communication exists between agencies.

The role of informal carers

There are many people in our society who require care but who are not entitled to draw on the services of paid carers, choose not to do so or are unaware of such provision. Increasingly, there is also the issue of levels of paid care not being sufficient to meet needs. The escalating costs of providing care, limited resources and an ageing population have all resulted in an increasing number of people fulfilling the role of 'informal carer'. Historically, carers were drawn from the family of the patient, but changes within society over recent decades have impacted on families' ability to take this role. Issues such as employment, social mobility and divorce have all served to change the ways in which informal care is provided within a family. Today, carers are drawn from all sectors of society and include anyone of significance to the patient, such as family members, including children, partners and friends.

CASE STUDY 13.2: SARAH

We found out that Sarah had learning difficulties when she was 3 years old. As she was our first child, we hadn't realised she wasn't doing the things she should. We knew she wasn't doing as much as the babies of some of our friends, but everyone told us she was 'placid' or 'contented'. It took a long time for Sarah to be diagnosed with learning difficulties and even now we don't have a name for her disability; we just know that she needs a lot of help with things the rest of us take for granted. When Sarah was 4, she was admitted to hospital for tests (she has epilepsy). We were very anxious as she'd never been in hospital before and is easily upset.

Whenever we asked the nurses anything about her condition or the tests they were doing, we were told we needed to speak to a doctor. This was very frustrating as I wanted to be with my wife in case the news was bad, but I'm self-employed and didn't want to keep taking time off and losing money. The annoying thing was that when we saw the paediatrician, she said there wasn't anything new to tell us. Why couldn't the nurses have told us this? We knew if the news was bad the nurses couldn't tell us, but they might have given us a few words of reassurance or encouragement. There needs to be more transparency about what nurses can or can't tell you.

The other problem we have is that although we know what Sarah can, can't or won't do, whenever she goes into hospital her routine is changed. She will soon be a teenager; as she gets older it is more difficult for my wife and me to lift her, so it's really important to get her to do as much for herself as she can, but every time she comes home we have to start again. It feels like we are working against the hospital.

- How could the nurses work with the family to promote better communication?
- What could be done to maintain Sarah's routine as much as possible while she is in hospital?

ANSWER:
CASE STUDY 13.2

Each year, more than two million people become a carer for someone close to them (Carers UK, 2014). These informal carers provide a valuable service for which they are often untrained, unpaid and unsupported. Unlike healthcare workers, who choose to work in care, informal carers can find themselves doing so purely as a result of circumstances. Sometimes they may not even recognise themselves as carers, feeling instead that they are 'only' doing what any family member would do. There are a number of problems the informal carer may have to face:

- a lack of preparation or training
- a lack of recognition of the nature and extent of the role they play
- having to leave employed work in order to provide care, which can lead to financial difficulties, placing further strain on the carer
- an impact on family relationships – for example, there may be sibling rivalry or tensions between couples; being both a partner and a carer can be challenging if the role of carer results in the previous relationship with a partner being drastically altered
- the responsibilities of the role impacting on schoolwork and social development, where the carer is a child or younger person
- multiple caring responsibilities, such as caring for young children at the same time as caring for elderly, frail parents, which can give rise to difficult dilemmas regarding personal priorities
- isolation and loneliness due to limited opportunities for social engagement
- a neglect of their own health needs due to the demands of caring
- an imbalance of power between the carer and the cared-for due to increased dependency
- where the individual does not identify themselves as a carer, they may experience greater isolation, as they are unlikely to become part of a carer network or support group; they may feel a greater financial burden, as they may not be applying for the financial support available to carers. Commissioning groups and local services providers may not be aware of them as 'carers'; this may result in their needs not being assessed, which in turn influences local provision.

HOW CAN HEALTHCARE PROFESSIONALS HELP?

The priority in effectively supporting individuals and their carers is to recognise that their goals and requirements for care may differ from yours, and that the views of individuals and their carers can differ. The starting point must be to determine their wishes and expectations, to ensure all involved parties understand the professional support available and to negotiate care boundaries.

> Working with people with learning disabilities, their parents, families/carers are a valuable source of help. I have noticed that they can give you some tips on triggers that may upset the person you are caring for. I was once told that a young man was scared of public toilets as he had once got locked in one. Had I not known that when he needed the toilet while we were in the community, it could have caused some problems – we worked on trying to desensitise him to the problem.
>
> **Sarah Parkes, LD nursing student**

If a package of care is to be of any benefit, the first step is to establish that both parties are participating willingly and to be satisfied that there has been no coercion. It is a mistake to make assumptions about someone's willingness to care and about their acceptability as a carer for the patient. Caring for someone on a full-time basis can cause tensions and if either party is reluctant or unwilling to care, there is the potential for conflict and relationship breakdown – even abuse. It is important to remember, therefore, that legislation (such as The Care Act 2014 in England) makes provision for the needs of carers and their ability to continue providing care to be assessed, and places a duty on authorities to meet carers' needs for support.

Informal carers may find the skills and language used by healthcare professionals to be unfamiliar and confusing, but, alternatively, their caring role may have given them a level of knowledge and experience regarding their own situation that is greater than that of the professionals. This can lead to confusion and a blurring of roles; nonetheless, it is important to recognise each other's experience and expertise and, regardless of background, it is also important to keep messages clear and make meanings explicit. Preparing carers for the role and providing the right amount of support and guidance are essential. Consider the following points:

- There are a number of carers groups across the UK offering free courses for informal carers. Skills taught include nutrition, administering medication and minimal handling. These are also good ways of meeting other people with similar experiences.
- There are several registered charities offering support groups, days out and buddying services for young carers.
- Suitable respite care facilities may be available, although their availability does vary depending on the needs of the individual and local service provision. This might take the form of inpatient/residential respite care or identifying a home carer or volunteer for a couple of hours a week to allow the opportunity for personal time to meet friends, pursue hobbies or simply have time away.
- Make sure community services such as the GP have been notified and it has been recorded that the person has a caring responsibility. These professionals will take this into account when arranging visits and managing healthcare.
- Familiarise yourself with the range of local non-statutory support groups available. Many will happily provide help with a range of tasks, including shopping and transport. Remember that these services are usually free!
- Inform the carer of the availability of any benefits, grants or social work support, where appropriate. Point out organisations that can advise them, such as the Citizens Advice Bureau.

202 FUNDAMENTALS OF NURSING CARE

- Make sure that the carer is aware of their right to an assessment of their own needs.
- Remember to ask after the carer's health and wellbeing as well as that of the person they are providing care and support for.

PLANNING CARE COLLABORATIVELY

Developing a care plan which takes into consideration the needs of the patient and the role of both informal carers and healthcare professionals is essential. This is true whether a plan of care is being developed within a hospital or a community setting. A collaborative approach is required, along with clear acknowledgement of the roles and responsibilities of all parties. For example, there may be some aspects of care which the carer finds difficult to manage, in which case a suitable alternative needs to be in place. This will ensure that both the patient and their informal carer are central to the decision-making process and not inadvertently undermined or excluded. However, it is also important not to assume that carers will be able or willing to provide support, such as remaining with a patient in hospital in order to provide care. In this situation, it is essential that nursing staff gain a good understanding of the patient's normal routines, likes and dislikes in order to reduce disruption and so that needs do not go unmet. Acknowledging all the parties involved in a person's care and valuing their contribution and role will impact positively on all those involved. Be aware, however, that a paid carer accompanying someone into hospital may not have any healthcare training and may not always know the individual well – for example, they may be new in a post or working a bank shift.

CONCLUSION

You might think it is fairly simple to identify a term that covers all those who use the health service and those people with whom nurses may be working. However, it can be challenging to find the most appropriate terms to use. All of the individuals we deliver care to have differing circumstances, and the services they need vary. While our own experiences can help us to some extent, we also need to understand a range of experiences in order to be effectively equipped to support others. Taking on the label of 'patient' can be difficult and have a huge impact on your life.

Within the UK, we tend to use the term 'carer' to cover a wide range of people, who may be professional or informal carers. These informal carers provide a valuable service for which they are often untrained, unpaid and unsupported. Unlike professional healthcare workers who choose to work in care, informal carers can find themselves doing so purely as a result of circumstance.

As nurses, it is fundamentally important when planning and delivering care that we work in partnership with individual patients, their family and their carers to ensure that care is person-centred.

CHAPTER SUMMARY

- A range of terms is used to refer to people who use health and social care services.
- Some people have preferences regarding the terms that are used to refer to their relationship with the services.
- The support needs of individuals may be met by family/informal carers and people who are paid to provide care/support.
- Those who are paid to provide support may have an in-depth understanding of the needs of individuals, but they may not have healthcare training.

- Providing care can have an impact on family/informal carers and it is important that the needs of such carers are recognised and met.
- Such carers may not, however, view themselves as 'carers'.
- In planning and delivering nursing care, it is essential that we work in partnership with individual patients, their family and their carers to ensure that care is person-centred.

CRITICAL REFLECTION

Holistic care

Reflect on the healthcare that you have received or imagine you are receiving healthcare:

- Who would you want involved in your care planning and delivery to ensure it is both holistic and person-centred?
- Why?
- How will this reflection assist you to improve the care you deliver?

GO FURTHER

Books

Carter, B., Bray, L., Dickinson, A., Edwards, M. and Ford, K. (2014) *Child-centred Nursing: Promoting Critical Thinking*. London: SAGE. This book explores children and young people's experience of illness, consulting with children and young people about their care and approaches to nursing children, young people and their families.

Reed, A. (2011) *Nursing in Partnership with Patients and Carers*. London: SAGE. This book explores how the participation of patients and carers in nursing care can be promoted and how their experiences can be assessed.

SAGE journal articles

Go to https://study.sagepub.com/essentialnursing2e for free online journal articles for this chapter. If you are using the interactive ebook, simply click on the book icon in the margin to go straight to the resource.

FURTHER READING: JOURNAL ARTICLES

Coty, M.B. and Wishnia, G. (2013) 'Adjusting to recent onset of rheumatoid arthritis: A qualitative study', *Journal of Research in Nursing*, 18(6): 504-17. This article explores the experiences of people living with rheumatoid arthritis and identifies the key themes that emerge from their accounts.

Lambert, V., Glacken, M. and McCarron, M. (2013) 'Using a range of methods to access children's voices', *Journal of Research in Nursing*, 18(7): 601-16. This paper explores a range of approaches that can be used to support sick children to have a 'voice' within acute healthcare settings.

Moe, M., Hellzen, O. and Enmarker, I. (2013) 'The meaning of receiving home help from home nursing care', *Nursing Ethics*, 20(7): 737-47. This article explores the impacts on people of having to receive home nursing support, and the meanings they attach to this experience.

Weblinks

FURTHER READING: WEBLINKS

Go to https://study.sagepub.com/essentialnursing2e for weblinks related to this chapter. If you are using the interactive ebook, simply click on the book icon in the margin to go straight to the resource.

www.carersuk.org – Carers UK is a UK-wide organisation that represents and campaigns on behalf of carers.

www.ageuk.org.uk – Age UK is a third-sector organisation that provides a range of services for older people.

www.mencap.org.uk – the website of Mencap, an organisation that represents and campaigns on behalf of people with learning disabilities and their carers.

www.mind.org.uk – a mental health service-user group which provides a range of support and campaigns in relation to the rights of people with mental health problems.

www.discover4carers.eu – an online network connecting carers, DISCOVER aims to familiarise carers with digital technologies and embed them in their day-to-day lives.

www.easyhealth.org.uk – Easyhealth's aim is to ensure people know where to find 'accessible' health information.

Video links

VIDEO
LINKS

Have a break from the text and go to https://study.sagepub.com/essentialnursing2e for useful videos related to this chapter. If you are using the interactive ebook, simply click on the lightbulb icon in the margin to go straight to the resource.

ACE YOUR ASSESSMENT

ONLINE
QUIZZES

Review what you have learned by visiting the book's online resources at: https://study.sagepub.com/essential nursing2e If using your interactive ebook, just click on the icon in the margin to go straight there.

- Test yourself with multiple-choice and short-answer questions.
- Revise key terms with the interactive flash cards.

REFERENCES

Carers UK (2014) *Facts about Carers: Policy Brief.* Available at: www.carersuk.org/for-professionals/ policy/policy-library/facts-about-carers-2014 (accessed 31 October 2014).

Heslop, P., Blair, P., Fleming, P., Hoghton, M., Marriott, A. and Russ, L. (2013) *Confidential Inquiry into Premature Deaths of People with Learning Disabilities (CIPOLD).* Bristol: Norah Fry Research Centre.

Kvåle, K. and Bondevik, M. (2008) 'What is important for patient centred care? A qualitative study about the perceptions of patients with cancer', *Scandinavian Journal of Caring Science*, 22: 582–9.

McLaughlin, H. (2009) 'What's in a name? "Client", "patients", "customer", "consumer", "expert by experience", "service user" – what's next?', *British Journal of Social Work*, 39: 1101–17.

Manley, K., Hills, V. and Marriot, S. (2011) 'Person-centred care: Principle of Nursing Practice D', *Nursing Standard*, 25(31): 35–7.

Simmons, P., Hawley, C.J., Gale, T.M. and Sivakumaran, T. (2010) 'Service user, patient, client, user or survivor: Describing recipients of mental health services', *The Psychiatrist*, 34: 20–3.

ASSESSMENT, PLANNING, IMPLEMENTATION AND EVALUATION (APIE): THE PROCESS OF NURSING

REBEKAH HILL

THIS CHAPTER COVERS

- The role of APIE
- Assessment
- Planning

- Implementation
- Evaluation

> " [Y]ou get a doctor, they deal with the disease and the physical stuff ... but not the whole you, not the rest of the things that matter to you, like how you feel about things ... the nurse looks at all of you.
>
> **Monty, MH community patient** "

Visit https://study.sagepub.com/essentialnursing2e to access a wealth of online resources for this chapter – watch out for the margin icons throughout the chapter. If you are using the interactive eBook, simply click on the margin icon to go straight to the resource.

INTRODUCTION

While many healthcare professionals have a specific focus for their intervention, such as a physiotherapist concentrating on a patient's mobility or a pharmacist paying attention to drug administration, a nurse takes a holistic approach to patient involvement. Monty refers to this at the start of the chapter: he and other patients understand that nurses are distinctive in their perspective, in considering all aspects of a person. Nurses use a process by which they achieve effective patient care, the process consisting of assessing, planning, implementing and evaluating.

Assessment, planning, implementation and evaluation are skills fundamental to nursing; they enable person-centred, holistic care to be given, the provision of which is unique to nursing. It is a process that can be applied to individuals with diverse health needs within the differing fields of child, learning disability, mental health and adult nursing. This problem- or need-orientated approach to care is used in all nursing settings, whereby examination of a person takes place in order to identify any needs they might have, affording interventions to be provided to resolve the need identified. Assessment, planning, implementation and evaluation (APIE) is a framework, providing a structure to a nursing approach to care, to which we can attach a model.

Before reading this chapter, it might be helpful to read Chapter 12 for more information relating to the role of models in nursing.

THE ROLE OF APIE

Your approach to care is based on the needs of the person and the nursing context (DH, 2010, 2014). Each care setting might have a preference for identifying patients' needs using a different need-orientated assessment tool. Frameworks you might see for planning care include SOAP (subjective, objective, assessment, planning); SOAPIER (subjective, objective, assessment, planning, implementation, evaluation, response); DAPE (data, assessment, planning, evaluation) and PIRP (presenting, intervention, responses, plan) (Lloyd, 2010). Different fields of nursing use different frameworks. Throughout this chapter, we will use the APIE framework because it facilitates prompt identification of needs and is common to nursing practice in all fields.

Assessment, planning, implementation and evaluation are parts of a process known as the nursing process (Orlando, 1961). This is a problem- or need-solving framework enabling the provision of a systematic, individualised approach to care. Each stage of the nursing process is fundamental to the next; the cycle is continuous, as is each stage of it. Throughout the process, the nurse and patient work together, which is crucial to a person-centred approach to care. As a nurse, you continuously gather information about a patient; every look, every touch, every conversation is a data-collecting exercise from which you plan and give appropriate care, which is then evaluated. It is a cyclical process consisting of four stages – assessment, planning, implementation and evaluation – as shown in Figure 14.1. We will discuss this throughout the rest of the chapter.

ASSESSMENT

Making an accurate assessment is not an easy task, as you may find in doing Activity 14.1. Therefore, it is common to use a model to provide structure – an outline to help organise the data being gathered and logically order any questions asked. The use of a model encourages a systematic approach to assessment and also ensures that the physical, psychological, emotional and social aspects of activities are all considered. There are many different nursing models used, reflecting the differing fields of nursing, as the approach to care taken may vary according to the field.

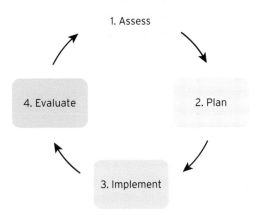

Figure 14.1   The nursing process

Approaches to care in learning disability tend to be based around person-centred planning, enabling the person to have as much control over their health as possible while accepting that there may well be multiple unmet health needs (DH, 2009). Similarly, mental health nursing adopts a person-centred approach to the care of people who have mental health problems, in which the emphasis lies on enabling people to cope with and find solutions to their problems (DH, 2011a, 2011b, 2012). The approach taken to the care of children recognises the importance of a partnership between health-care, the child and their family (DH, 2004). Adult nursing involves the nurse and the patient working in partnership to resolve healthcare problems, with the nurse empowering the patient to gain control over their needs (DH, 2012). Although the nursing models used within adult nursing vary, they are all tools which provide you with a means to perform a holistic and individualised assessment of a person (DH, 2012). For example, a frequently used tool, or nursing model, is Roper et al.'s (2008) Twelve Activities of Living, which provides 12 focal points upon which you can structure your assessment of the patient.

The model allows you to assess an individual and their performance of 12 activities which are considered important to living, considering levels of dependence and independence within each. Thus, the use of a nursing model provides you with a useful framework for your assessment.

Assessment is a process used to *appraise* a patient in order to identify their needs, both existing and potential. It involves gathering information about a person and using that information to make decisions about what nursing care interventions are required. Assessment is the foundation upon which all else is built and as such it is critical to the success of the nursing process. The assessment of a patient is a continuous process rather than a one-off event; it is ongoing. Furthermore, the type of assessment conducted will vary according to context. In an emergency following a traumatic injury, only an initial assessment of immediate physical need would be conducted on a child with a learning disability, but if the same child was being admitted to a care home for respite care they would require a full holistic assessment. Assessment types can vary and include the following:

- mini, when a quick physical assessment is required
- focused, when a specific problem is assessed
- comprehensive, an in-depth holistic appraisal of an individual
- ongoing assessment, which continuously monitors a patient's health. (Dougherty and Lister, 2015)

In a non-emergency situation, a thorough assessment is essential, encompassing every aspect of the person – physically, psychologically, emotionally and socially. An assessment should incorporate your examination of the patient's opinion and experiences, seeking their view to inform the care plan (DH, 2011a). Often, much of the information you gather in an assessment is verbal, such as a patient history and responses to questions. However, this is not always possible due to the nature of the person (e.g. an infant), their situation (e.g. unconscious) or the context (e.g. an emergency). An assessment should take into consideration the multiple aspects of a person as well as their individual responses to their problem or need. Features such as behaviour, emotions, psychological state and physical responses are all important in a holistic assessment.

> Assessing a patient holistically makes sure you are providing care for that individual as a whole, not just addressing one area of their life. This often has a much greater impact in improving health as different areas of an individual's life and health are often connected.
>
> **Charlie Clisby, NQN**

Using your senses

Assessment is actually a complex process, requiring the interplay and continuous appraisal of a number of your senses and skills. You will use your senses of speech, sight, smell, hearing and touch as well as your skills to question and explore, listen, observe, measure, examine, analyse and interpret. A good patient assessment gathers information from a variety of sources, rather like accumulating pieces of a jigsaw. A patient assessment is completed when all the pieces of the puzzle are drawn together to give a picture of the patient and their world.

CASE STUDY 14.1: JAINIL

Jainil is 4 years old and has become withdrawn and quiet, refusing to play or drink. He just wants to sit on his mother's lap and look at books, which is uncharacteristic for him as he is usually very active. When talking to his parents, it becomes apparent that Jainil has not had his bowels open for six days and that he has abdominal pain exacerbated by movement. Jainil's behaviour and his psychological and emotional responses have all been affected as a result of his physical pain.

- List the skills you need to perform an assessment on Jainil. Think about how you assessed the object in Activity 14.1 and relate these skills to performing an assessment of a patient.

ANSWER:
CASE STUDY 14.1

As is demonstrated in the case study of Andrew (14.2), the sources of information gathered for assessment might come directly from the patient or indirectly from a secondary source. Direct sources of information include a combination of observations, measurements and interview, while other people and current or previous records might contribute to secondary sources. The most important source of data regarding patient assessment is the individual themselves; however, there are circumstances in which other people will need to be consulted and other sources of information considered. When assessing a child or baby, a parent or guardian may provide most of the information you require. Similarly, in order to assess an adult who is unable to contribute to the process, you may need to obtain data from relatives, friends, ambulance staff or police. Confidentiality and informed consent must be maintained in all settings (NMC, 2015). Many patients admitted to hospital are accompanied by a letter from their GP, which provides valuable information. Previous medical notes, if available, can also be an important source of data. However, secondary sources of information should be used to supplement direct, primary sources from the patients themselves whenever possible.

CASE STUDY 14.2: ANDREW

Andrew is 24 years old and has been brought into an acute medical ward in an unconscious state. Staff Nurse Gray immediately looks at Andrew's face and chest, then puts her cheek down to Andrew's mouth and lays one hand on his forehead and another on his wrist.

- What information do you think the nurse was trying to ascertain by these actions?

Questioning and exploring

Effective communication skills are fundamental to a good assessment. There needs to be a therapeutic relationship between you and the patient, and the assessment must be ethical and respectful.

A comfortable interaction between you and the patient needs to be established; there has to be honesty, openness, trust and an understanding that you will not judge them (Lloyd, 2010). An assessment should appear to be a conversation. An experienced nurse will elicit information from what is apparently a chat, but is actually a crafted exchange aimed to draw essential assessment information.

Two types of questioning approaches are useful in a patient assessment: 'open questions' and 'closed questions'. Open questions invite a detailed response from the patient whereas closed questions can be answered 'yes' or 'no'. Initially, closed questions are useful to establish identity and baseline information; open questions then allow the patient to talk about their understanding. Once a need has been identified, it is then possible to use more probing open questions to elicit more information about that specific issue.

Open questioning enables the patient to elaborate and to provide their own account. Asking the patient to tell you why they have presented allows them to tell their story and provides you with important contextual understanding, such as an appreciation of what the patient knows about their admission to hospital or reason for consultation – a perspective which might be different from your own. Be mindful not to use medical terminology when assessing a patient, since it could be offputting for them. Similarly, ensure the questions you ask are appropriate – for example, a child's orientation to time, place and person could not be assessed by asking who the prime minister is; similarly, many adults might not know that either. There can be many further difficulties in assessing people, such as those who use non-verbal, sign or augmentative and alternative communication (AAC) or those who speak English as a further language; other difficulties may be encountered when assessing older people, people with learning disabilities or people with mental health needs, where there may be cognitive impairment or some other aspect which makes verbal communication difficult. It is necessary to ensure that the method of communication and the questions you ask take into account all of the possible difficulties encountered by the patient you are interviewing. This is more complicated than remembering to consider physical difficulties such as hearing or visual problems. It may be the case that an older person feels they should agree with the view of a professional, or that a patient with learning disabilities is unable to comprehend what you are asking.

If you do not consider these issues, the information you obtain will not truly reflect the patient's need.

Listening

It is fundamentally important that you are able to listen to what the patient has to say, giving them time to express themselves. Although it is sometimes time-consuming, by allowing the patient time to talk you will gain their unique perspective and an understanding of what is troubling them, which is often different from your presumption. Remember that people respond differently to things; working as a detective to solve a puzzle, you can look for clues and listen for them also. For example, paranoia might motivate one person to live in isolation, while the fear of transmitting a contagious disease may prompt another to live remotely from others. A person may cry in response to feeling happy, while another might cry in response to pain. If given the time, these responses can become apparent when you listen. So, it is important not only for you to allow time for the patient to express themselves, but also that you have time to listen and are attentive to what they say. You need to listen actively to patients rather than just hear what they say.

Observing

Observation of a patient provides vital sources of information, from assessment of general behaviour by observing non-verbal and verbal communication – such as noting facial expression indicative of pain or mood – to a more detailed assessment of perfusion by observing cyanosis within skin colour. Data obtained from observations might relate to any aspect of the person. It may vary from a general impression of a person's behaviour (if they are crying, for example) or appearance (torn and stained clothing) to a more precise observation (noting a bruising pattern on the skin).

Measuring

Measurement is a central aspect of assessment, providing important objective data. Measurement may take many forms, from using an assessment tool for depression, pain or distress to taking blood pressure and pulse to assess health. A number of assessment tools are often used within the assessment process, as part of an appraisal of risk. Such assessment tools are used to predict a person's level of risk of developing a specific problem or the possibility that their condition will deteriorate, so appropriate interventions can be deployed. Thus, you need to use tools that are appropriate both to the assessment and the patient being assessed.

The Paediatric Pain Profile (PPP) is a behaviour rating scale for assessing pain in children with severe physical and learning impairments.

Dis-DAT

Dis-DAT is a tool intended to help identify distress cues in people whose communication is severely limited because of cognitive impairment or physical illness. Assessment contains both objective and subjective data; both aspects are important and can complement each other when used together. Quantify your assessment where possible, such as using objective measurement to calculate a nutrition assessment, but qualify your assessment data also, by providing detailed factual descriptions of, for example, a patient's account of weight loss and the factors which surrounded it. Subjective accounts of a patient's behavioural response to a problem, or need, are important. The provision of both objective and subjective data is vital to making an accurate assessment.

Apply what you have learned in this chapter about using APIE in practice by reading John Smith's case study, at https://study.sagepub.com/essentialnursing2e.

CASE STUDY:
JOHN SMITH

Examining

A full patient examination provides important assessment information. Touch alone offers an assessment of circulation and temperature, while a full-body assessment of skin integrity is an important consideration for immobile patients. A 'top to toe' examination will provide a wealth of information which might complement or even conflict with verbal reports: something as subtle as loose-fitting dentures might indicate recent weight loss which a patient might well be oblivious to, while puncture marks might indicate denied drug use. Similarly, a patient may complain of feeling cold when touch reveals they are in fact pyrexial.

Analysing and interpreting

When analysing assessment data, remember to maintain a focus on the patient's viewpoint and remain as impartial as possible, meaning you need to be aware of your own biased interpretation of assessment data. Preserving the patient's perspective is vital; hear what the patient says rather than your own interpretation of what is said. For example, if a patient tells you they sleep for four hours a night, you, who sleeps for eight, may interpret this as poor; however, four hours' sleep may be normal and quite adequate for that patient.

Furthermore, awareness of your own influence on the assessment process is important, since it might affect what is divulged. An elderly male patient may find it uncomfortable to disclose his sexual dysfunction to a young female nurse, for example. Mindfulness of your body language, facial expressions and tone of voice is important, but paramount are your reaction, your attitude, your judgement and your preconceptions, all of which could influence your assessment of a patient.

While it is important that you carry out a fair and non-judgemental assessment, you must acknowledge that there may be factors that will impact on your ability to do this. These may include distractions, lack of time or resources, pain, confusion, anxiety, sensory impairment or severe learning disability, skills, knowledge or understanding, gender, language or culture (DH, 2011a). It is imperative that you, as a nurse, are respectful to a patient, regardless of their attitude towards you (NMC, 2015).

ACTIVITY 14.2: CRITICAL THINKING

The Twelve Activities of Living outlined in Roper et al.'s (2008) model are frequently used as a tool to assess a patient. They are:

- maintaining a safe environment
- communication
- breathing
- eating and drinking
- elimination
- washing and dressing
- controlling temperature
- mobilising
- working and playing
- expressing sexuality
- sleeping
- death and dying.

Within this assessment, when considering the activity of 'elimination', you may ask the patient when and how they use the toilet and listen to, analyse and interpret their response; you may measure and observe their urine, use your sense of smell to detect incontinence and examine their genitalia, if appropriate.

- How do you think you could assess a patient's ability to undertake the other 11 activities?
- How could you assess mental health, mood, behaviour, past medical and psychiatric history?
- How could you assess risk, or social issues?
- How could you include carers, family or other members of the healthcare team in an assessment?

As we have discussed so far, a thorough patient assessment requires you to use your senses and skills to question and explore, listen, observe, measure, analyse and interpret data. The information gathered in your assessment, and the gaps in it, will enable you to identify the patient's needs, from which a plan of how they might be resolved can be created.

CASE STUDY 14.3: GRAHAM

Graham is 34 and has moderate learning disabilities. He lives in a flat, supported by paid carers. Graham has physical disabilities and uses a wheelchair to get around. He has a history of urinary and faecal incontinence and his care staff assist him to manage his continence routine. He has recently lost weight.

- List all the possible ways you can collect data to enable a full assessment of Graham's needs to be produced.
- What tools would be useful to you in this assessment?

PLANNING

Planning is the approach a nurse takes to resolve a patient's needs. In planning, you need to translate the needs identified in the assessment into goals, the achievement of which can be measured in the implementation and evaluation stages of the process.

Through analysis of the patient assessment data, it is possible to identify the patient's needs. The needs identified will need to be prioritised and a plan devised in order for actions to help or resolve them to commence. The problem might be actual or anticipated, and the nurse will set a goal in relation to the problem identified. The goal that is set considers what can realistically be achieved to resolve the problem. When writing goals, SMART criteria can be used (Hamilton and Price, 2013), meaning the goal established ought to be:

Specific

Measured

Achievable

Realistic

Timed

Goal-setting must be specific to the problem, have the ability to be measurable and to be achieved, be realistic and be timed in order for it to be evaluated. The goal must be person-centred and stated in terms of the outcome for the patient if the goal is achieved. It is essential that the goals set are decided on in negotiation with the patient. Behavioural goal-setting involves identifying the person who will achieve the goal, the behaviour to be demonstrated, the conditions for the behaviour to occur, the conditions for how it will be evaluated and how often or by what time the behaviour has to be achieved (Lloyd, 2010).

Goal-setting can be short or long term, distinguishing between those goals which will be achieved immediately and those that will be achieved in the future. Having completed an assessment, planning of care and subsequent goal-setting involve you having to consider the level of need, the risk involved and the availability of resources.

Moving our focus away from planning for a moment in order to consider another, very important, issue that is raised by Graham's case study (14.3), it is known that when people with learning disabilities have a stay in hospital, they often leave dehydrated and malnourished. It is fundamentally important to assess a patient's level of independence and support needs as part of their original assessment. In extreme cases, failing to do this can result in their premature death (Heslop et al., 2013). While this is not the cause of Graham's problems in this case, unless you have assessed whether he needs support to eat and drink, it will be impossible to either effectively plan a goal for his nutritional needs or to provide him with effective care. It is always important to remember that patients can experience a whole spectrum of problems. Also, we need to remember that patients with learning disabilities and mental health needs can experience physical illness, and patients with physical illness can require support for their mental health.

Returning to the topic of planning, your priorities in your plan will depend on the nursing care setting and patient need. For example, in an emergency setting you would always act immediately and prioritise life-saving actions, but when there are no immediate threats to life it is important that prioritisation involves the patient.

CASE STUDY 14.4: GRAHAM REVISITED

Let's go back to Graham, whom you assessed earlier. It was identified that he had recently lost weight. Through a thorough assessment, it was recognised that he had lost 8 kg within the past three months and was malnourished and dehydrated.

Concerning Graham's dehydration, a specific, measurable, achievable, realistic and timed short-term goal could be that he will have an oral fluid intake of 2.5 litres every 24 hours for 72 hours. A long-term goal might be that he maintains hydration by achieving a daily oral intake of 2 litres of fluid.

ANSWER:
CASE STUDY 14.4

- Now write a SMART short-term goal for Graham's nutritional needs.

IMPLEMENTATION

Implementation is where the care prescribed to achieve the goal is put into action. Nurses put interventions into effect in order to resolve the problem identified by the assessment, just as we assess the weather in the morning and then decide what to wear for the day. We each have our own set of instructions which enable us to get dressed without ending up with our underwear on top of our clothes, for example (unless you are Superman). So you should follow the steps set in the implementation of care.

Implementation concerns the administration of the prescribed nursing interventions in order to accomplish the goal. The prescribed nursing interventions must be evidence-based, clear and specific.

The implementation plan relates to the plan of care the nurse needs to follow in order to achieve the goal. In doing this, nurses actually write a prescription; they prescribe the nursing actions which should be administered in order to accomplish the goal and meet the patient's needs. Upon evaluation, if the nursing actions have been ineffective in achieving the goal, they must be adjusted.

You may find it useful to use a framework when thinking about implementing care. REEPIG is an example of such a framework (see Table 14.1), which can be used in relation to the implementation of care (Hogston, 2011), to ensure that your prescribed interventions are Realistic, Explicit, Evidence-based, Prioritised, Involved and Goal-centred.

Table 14.1   REEPIG

Realistic	The plan of care must be realistic; any resources stated within the plan have to actually be available for use.
Explicit	The plan of care must be explicit – for example, in relation to a wound in need of dressing the plan must state the exact type of dressing to be used, the frequency of change and any specific technique to be incorporated so that each statement is qualified.
Evidence-based	The plan of care must be evidence-based, the research upon which the action is based and rationalised must be considered. Furthermore, the care interventions prescribed must reflect the best available evidence; for this you have to ensure you are up to date with contemporary research findings.
Prioritised	The most pressing need must be addressed first.
Involved	The patient and the members of the multi-disciplinary team should be involved since implementation could involve the coordination of a team of healthcare professionals in the delivery of care, such as when therapists are required in the rehabilitation of a patient; it could involve managing an environment, such as the provision of heating or cleanliness; it could involve organising resources, when a specific dressing is required for a wound, for example.
Goal-centred	You must ensure the plan of care meets the goals set.

Additionally, record-keeping is vital to the implementation of care; every care intervention must be recorded clearly, factually and accurately to reflect the professional standards for record-keeping (NMC, 2015).

CASE STUDY 14.5: GRAHAM'S WEIGHT

Remember Graham? He had lost weight and was found to be malnourished, and you set a SMART goal? Now you need to think about how you will achieve it. Let's say your goal stated that Graham gain a minimum of 0.5 kg per week and achieve a daily oral intake of 3,000 calories.

- Using the REEPIG criteria, write down what actions you will need to take in order to ensure this goal is achieved.

ANSWER:
CASE STUDY 14.5

EVALUATION

Evaluation is assessment of the response to the care implemented, to find out whether the goal has been achieved and the need resolved. It is an appraisal of the effectiveness of the interventions prescribed and implemented.

This monitoring of the response to the care implemented takes us right round the stages of the nursing process and back to assessment, since it involves a reassessment of the patient in order to evaluate a response. As with assessment, evaluation is continuous; also like assessment, there are many components to it, as it involves:

- patient assessment
- observation and monitoring
- using objective and subjective data
- appraisal of the goal and interventions
- patient involvement in assessing the effectiveness of care given from their perspective
- collaboration with the team involved in implementing the care
- effective record-keeping and documentation skills
- learning from the experience in order to improve future care.

The timing of evaluation could depend on the problem – or need – and the goal to be achieved. A potential problem might be evaluated differently from an actual problem, and similarly a short-term goal is likely to be evaluated more frequently than a long-term goal. Furthermore, just as goal-setting needs to be specific, measurable, achievable, realistic and timed in order for it to be evaluated, evaluation should be specific, measured, timed and stated in terms of whether the goal has been achieved.

It is important to quantify and qualify when evaluating. For example, it would not be meaningful to evaluate a mental health patient by stating that they seem happy; it needs to be quantified and expressed in terms of the person giving and maintaining eye contact and smiling appropriately in response to stimuli. When evaluating a child's newly diagnosed diabetes, it is necessary to qualify effectiveness by stating the range of blood glucose achieved following administration of the relevant drugs, which would then allow the care to be assessed for its effectiveness and achievement of the goal to be appraised.

If, following evaluation, the goal has not been achieved or the need resolved, reassessment is necessary to determine why. It could be that the need has changed, the goal was unrealistic or the intervention was ineffective. Whatever the reason, reassessment, resetting goals and reconsideration of the care to be implemented will be required. Evaluation enables a nurse to reflect on their actions to improve subsequent practice.

CASE STUDY 14.6: GRAHAM'S EVALUATION

Graham has been nursed by you for a week now, working in partnership with him (NMC, 2015), and you are evaluating his care plan:

ANSWER:
CASE STUDY 14.6

- What documents and data would you need in order to undertake this evaluation?
- How would you write your evaluation of Graham's care?

ACTIVITY 14.3: REFLECTION

Reflect on your experience of using APIE to care for Graham:

- How do you feel about using APIE?
- How did APIE enable you to care for Graham?
- Did you feel there were any limitations in using this approach?
- Did you consider the role of the carer during Graham's admission? Thinking about the need for Graham's care to continue when he goes home, might there be a need for his carers to receive further training?

CONCLUSION

The process of assessment, planning, implementation and evaluation (APIE) facilitates a person-centred and systematic delivery of patient care; such maintenance of a patient's best interest is fundamental to care (DH, 2011a). It ensures that patients receive appropriate and effective care aimed at resolving their needs by setting goals. This approach involves the most important people: the patients themselves. The cyclical nature of an APIE approach results in the implementation of effective care to meet needs.

CHAPTER SUMMARY

- Different fields of nursing adopt differing approaches to care to enable nurses to best meet the patient need.
- APIE is a generic process in all fields of nursing, regardless of the approach to care.
- The process of APIE is cyclical and ongoing.
- Assessment is fundamental to care; holistic assessment is essential for effective care to be delivered.
- Efficient planning of care is an important aspect of the process; SMART planning criteria allow patient needs to be translated into achievable goals.

- The implementation of evidence-based care is critical to resolve patient problems, and is a professional requirement of nursing.
- In evaluation, you assess responses to care, appraising whether goals have been met and problems resolved.

CRITICAL REFLECTION

Holistic care

APIE enables the provision of a holistic, person-centred approach to providing care. Reflect on the patient care you have been involved in and consider:

- how performing a thorough assessment enabled you to identify the patient's needs
- the importance of research in providing you with evidence-based care which could be implemented
- whether the patient's needs were met.

Now write a reflection focusing on this experience.

GO FURTHER

Books

Corkin, D., Clarke, S. and Liggett, L. (2011) *Care Planning in Children and Young People's Nursing*. London: Wiley-Blackwell. An excellent book focusing on care planning for children and young people.

Howatson-Jones, L., Standing, M. and Roberts, S. (2012) *Patient Assessment and Care Planning in Nursing*. London: SAGE. An excellent book which provides an overview of in-depth assessment considerations to be made when planning care.

SAGE journal articles

Go to https://study.sagepub.com/essentialnursing2e for free online journal articles for this chapter. If you are using the interactive ebook, simply click on the book icon in the margin to go straight to the resource.

FURTHER READING: JOURNAL ARTICLES

Cody, W. (2002) 'Critical thinking and nursing science: Judgement or vision?', *Nursing Science Quarterly*, 15(3): 184-9. This article considers the role of nursing theories and frameworks in enriching critical thinking in nursing practice.

Gilgun, J. (2004) 'Qualitative methods and the development of clinical assessment tools', *Qualitative Health Research*, 14(7): 1008-19. Two case studies are considered in order to highlight how assessment tools are incomplete if they do not include a qualitative component.

Turkel, M., Ray, M. and Kornblatt, L. (2012) 'Instead of reconceptualising the nursing process let's rename it', *Nursing Science Quarterly*, 25(2): 194-8. A discussion of the unique contribution nurses provide through their nursing language, theories and practice.

Weblinks

Go to https://study.sagepub.com/essentialnursing2e for weblinks related to this chapter. If you are using the interactive ebook, simply click on the book icon in the margin to go straight to the resource.

FURTHER READING: WEBLINKS

www.currentnursing.com - offering information and articles covering nursing research, models, theories and philosophy.

www.dh.gov.uk - the Department of Health website includes health directives and directions for care provision; it is an excellent source of information.

www.nice.org.uk – the NICE website contains much of the guidance upon which our care is based; it provides rich sources of evidence and reference to the studies from which some of the evidence is derived.

www.nmc.org.uk – the Nursing and Midwifery Council has an informative website which includes the standards which govern our nursing practice; it is an essential read.

www.rcn.org.uk – the Royal College of Nursing site offers access to a wide range of resources, including nursing models, theories and philosophy and their application to current practice.

www.communicationpassports.org.uk/About – provides information relating to personal communication passports.

Video links

VIDEO
LINKS

Have a break from the text and go to https://study.sagepub.com/essentialnursing2e for useful videos related to this chapter. If you are using the interactive ebook, simply click on the lightbulb icon in the margin to go straight to the resource.

ACE YOUR ASSESSMENT

ONLINE
QUIZZES

Review what you have learned by visiting the book's online resources at: https://study.sagepub.com/essential nursing2e If using your interactive ebook, just click on the icon in the margin to go straight there.

- Test yourself with multiple-choice and short-answer questions.
- Revise key terms with the interactive flash cards.

REFERENCES

Department of Health (DH) (2004) *Getting the Right Start: National Service Framework for Children.* London: HMSO.

Department of Health (2009) *Valuing People Now: A New Three Year Strategy for People with Learning Disabilities.* London: HMSO.

Department of Health (2010) *Equity and Excellence: Liberating the NHS.* London: HMSO.

Department of Health (2011a) *Essence of Care.* London: HMSO.

Department of Health (2011b) *The Mental Health Strategy for England.* London: HMSO.

Department of Health (2012) *Caring for our Future: Reforming Care and Support.* London: HMSO.

Department of Health (2014) *Five Year Forward View.* London: HMSO.

Dougherty, L. and Lister, S. (2015) *The Royal Marsden Hospital Manual of Clinical Nursing Procedures,* 9th edn. Oxford: Wiley-Blackwell.

Hamilton, P. and Price, T. (2013) 'The nursing process, holistic assessment and baseline observations', in C. Brooker and A. Waugh (eds), *Foundations of Nursing Practice: Fundamentals of Holistic Care.* London: Mosby.

Heslop, P., Blair, P., Fleming, P., Hoghton, M., Marriott, A. and Russ, L. (2013) *Confidential Inquiry into Premature Deaths of People with Learning Disabilities (CIPOLD).* Bristol: Norah Fry Research Centre.

Hogston, R. (2011) 'Managing nursing care', Chapter 1 in R. Hogston and B. Marjoram (eds), *Foundations of Nursing Practice: Themes, Concepts and Frameworks,* 4th edn. London: Palgrave Macmillan. pp. 1–21.

Lloyd, M. (2010) *Care Planning in Health and Social Care.* London: Open University Press/McGraw-Hill.

Nursing and Midwifery Council (NMC) (2015) *The Code: Professional Standards of Practice and Behaviour for Nurses and Midwives.* London: NMC.

Orlando, I.J. (1961) *The Dynamic Nurse–Patient Relationship.* New York: Putnam.

Roper, N., Logan, W. and Tierney, A. (2008) *The Roper-Logan-Tierney Model of Nursing Based on Activities of Daily Living.* Edinburgh: Churchill Livingstone.

CORE COMMUNICATION SKILLS

KAREN ELCOCK AND JEAN SHAPCOTT

THIS CHAPTER COVERS

- Why communication is so important
- Verbal and non-verbal communication
- Self-awareness

- Communicating with children
- Communicating with non-English speakers

> " A person can listen without caring but can't care without listening.
>
> **Anonymous** "

> " When I would tell particularly harsh or extreme things, she wouldn't show surprise or that she was appalled ... just kind of understanding and showing, just with her expression, that I was not so strange or different or bad ... making sure she had things clear. Like she would repeat back and say, 'Do I have that right?'
>
> **Mental health patients, in Shattell et al. (2006)** "

> " The importance of effective communication should never be under valued. It is intrinsic in every aspect of nursing, from reporting a deteriorating patient to a doctor (attention to detail is paramount) to having a chat with one of your patients (making them feel cared for and valued).
>
> **Charlie Clisby, NQN** "

Visit https://study.sagepub.com/essentialnursing2e to access a wealth of online resources for this chapter – watch out for the margin icons throughout the chapter. If you are using the interactive eBook, simply click on the margin icon to go straight to the resource.

INTRODUCTION

The voices above highlight the importance of good communication. Sadly, amongst the biggest criticisms by patients and carers is poor communication – not only in terms of how we communicate with them, but also in how we communicate important information to others who will be caring for them. This chapter introduces you to some of the core skills that are essential for effective communication to take place and ensure that you meet the expectations of the NMC Code on communicating clearly (NMC, 2015).

While most of us take our ability to communicate for granted, many of the patients with whom you will come into contact will have difficulties with communicating. These may be due to their age, language, physical disabilities which affect their ability to speak and/or hear, mental health problems that impact on the way they communicate with others, or developmental difficulties. Being aware of both verbal and non-verbal communication approaches and the importance of active listening will help you to develop the skills you will need to enable patients to feel heard and valued.

WHY COMMUNICATION IS SO IMPORTANT

Of all the skills a nurse must possess, the ability to communicate effectively is the most important. Failing to communicate effectively with patients, carers and other healthcare professionals can have serious consequences for all involved. Poor communication is in the top three most common complaints received from patients and their carers (Parliamentary and Health Service Ombudsman, 2015). As a nurse, the onus is on you to find effective ways of communicating with patients (NMC, 2015). You will therefore find that communication skills form a significant part of your nursing programme, and it is no surprise that they are one of the 6Cs of nursing identified by the Commissioning Board Chief Nursing Officer and DH Chief Nursing Adviser (2012: 13), who state:

> Communication is central to successful caring relationships and to effective team working. Listening is as important as what we say and do and essential for 'no decision about me without me'. Communication is the key to a good workplace with benefits for those in our care and staff alike.

Communication is an essential part of everyday life as well as a crucial element of good nursing care. In everyday life, communication helps to:

- establish relationships between healthcare professionals and patients, families and colleagues
- facilitate the gathering and sharing of information and ideas
- give meaning to the situation in which individuals find themselves. (Balzer-Riley, 2015)

Communication plays a fundamental role in patient safety and satisfaction, enables therapeutic relationships, allows nurses to collect important data regarding patients and facilitates nursing interventions and their evaluation.

What is communication?

Communication is a two-way process, which can be simultaneously simple and complex. In simple terms, the process consists of a 'sender' who wishes to transmit information (the 'message') to another (the 'receiver') (Bach and Grant, 2015). However, it is rarely as simple as that. Patients may be in severe pain, concerned about their health or being cared for in a busy inpatient area, all of which will impede communication. The aspects of any episode of communication that therefore need to be considered are not only the sender, message and receiver, as identified above, but also the 'channel' (or means) of communication, so-called 'noise' (which can be anything which interferes with effective communication) and 'feedback' (the response from the receiver to the message received) (Baughan and Smith, 2013).

> I would define communication as listening, responding to and interpreting people's actions, wants, needs, likes and dislikes, not only verbally but non-verbally – body language, facial expressions and tone of voice – also being able to communicate with others using tools such as pictures and eye pointing.
>
> **Siân Hunter, child nursing student**

In order to be an effective communicator, you need to have personal insight into your own way of behaving and communicating, demonstrate sensitivity to others and have knowledge of communication strategies appropriate to the different situations in which you will find yourself. These strategies generally fall into two categories – verbal and non-verbal.

VERBAL AND NON-VERBAL COMMUNICATION

Verbal communication relates to the use of the spoken word and is often extended to include the written word as well. What are important are not only the words used to communicate – which can reflect the age of the person, their culture and their level of development and education – but also how those words are spoken. Tone of voice, the pace at which someone is speaking, clarity of speech and volume are also relevant, particularly when considering the feelings of the individual. Non-verbal communication includes all aspects of body language – eye contact, posture, gestures, positioning, facial expressions, the way an individual presents themselves – with over two-thirds of what we communicate attributed to non-verbal cues (Leathers and Eaves, 2016). Individuals may be less aware of the messages they are transmitting in this manner than they are of those in their verbal communication. Non-verbal communication is particularly important for people with a learning disability and for people who have English as a second language or who use alternative and augmentative communication, both in getting messages across from you to them and in interpreting how they are feeling. Activity 15.1 will help you to understand this aspect of communication further.

ACTIVITY 15.1: REFLECTION

Which of the approaches identified could you use with patients for whom you have cared?

Active listening

There are a number of core skills you will need to develop in order to be an effective communicator. Of these, active listening is key and requires you to not only hear what has been said, but also to feed back what you hear to the speaker by way of re-stating or paraphrasing what you have heard in your own words. This will confirm what you have heard and that both you and the speaker have the same understanding.

There are three main skills involved in being an active listener – repeating, paraphrasing and reflecting. Repeating involves relaying the message back to the speaker using exactly the same words that they used. This can become somewhat irritating to the speaker, so an alternative is to paraphrase what the speaker said using similar words and phrases to those used by the speaker, or reflecting the content of the message back to them in your own words. 'Just listening' is important for all patients, but is especially valued by people who use mental health services (Morrissey and Callaghan, 2011).

If the meaning or context of the information being presented by the patient is unclear, the use of questions becomes important. There are two types of questions – open and closed. Open questions are used to elicit further information and enable a person to respond freely. Closed questions are direct, fact-finding questions and ask for specific information (Gault et al., 2017). Examples of open and closed questions are as follows:

- Open questions frequently start with words such as 'what', 'how' and 'why':

    o What are your strengths as a nursing student?
    o How do you think your next placement will develop your knowledge?
    o Why did you choose to study at your current university?

- Closed questions are those that can be answered with 'yes', 'no' or a one-word answer:

    o Are you a nursing student?
    o Where are you going for your next placement?
    o Do you like studying at your current university?

Communication skills contribute to a nurse's ability to demonstrate empathy, which is the ability to perceive the meaning and feelings of another and to communicate those feelings to the other person (Stein-Parbury, 2005). The ability to be empathetic can be influenced by a number of variables, including personality, gender, interpersonal style, culture, social confidence, environment and the level of communication skills that have been learned (Alligood and May, 2000). Empathy is essential for the development and maintenance of therapeutic relationships between nurses and their patients, whatever their age or health status, and is itself dependent on the skills to be explored in this chapter.

WHAT'S THE EVIDENCE?

Using a hospital passport tool to improve communication between people with a learning disability and hospital staff

WEBLINK: BELL (2012)

Bell, R. (2012) 'Does he have sugar in his tea? Communication between people with learning disabilities, their carers and hospital staff', *Tizard Learning Disability Review*, 17(2): 57-63.

Poor communication between different agencies, hospital staff and people with learning disabilities and their carers has been identified as playing a significant role in poor care and even loss of life for people with a learning disability. A hospital passport is a tool used widely in the UK to provide key information about a person with a learning disability who is being admitted to hospital. A document that uses pictures and symbols as well as text, it includes information about the individual's preferences and dislikes, routines, how to interpret their body language, fears and worries about their hospital admission, any reasonable adjustments they may require and key contacts.

Bell's (2012) qualitative study explored the impact of a hospital passport on the communication process through semi-structured interviews with 20 health and social care staff and carers and a focus group with adults with learning disabilities. The study found that the passport significantly improved communication between all the agencies involved in the care of people with a learning disability. Key recommendations were that the passport should be considered for other vulnerable groups such as older people and those with dementia; that there is a need for education and training in the different communication skills that can be used for people with a learning disability; and that passports should be used routinely in practice.

Now read the article and reflect on patients for whom you have cared who are unable to communicate easily:

- What strategies have you used to learn more about them as people or their individual preferences?
- How might the use of a passport be extended to include all patients?

SELF-AWARENESS

Self-awareness is an essential part of the repertoire of skills that a nurse requires in order to engage in a therapeutic relationship with patients. While there is no clear definition of self-awareness, there is general agreement that it is about an understanding of self in relation to feelings, attitudes and values (Eckroth-Bucher, 2010), and how these may impact on our behaviour with others. This is important in nursing, as without an understanding of how your feelings, values and attitudes may impact on others, it may be difficult to establish or maintain a therapeutic relationship (Mcabe et al., 2013; Thompson, 2015). There is strong support within the literature for the many benefits that awareness of self can bring (Eckroth-Bucher, 2010; Jack and Miller, 2008; Thompson, 2015), including:

- self-confidence, by understanding our strengths and our limitations and so developing appropriate coping mechanisms
- recognising how certain behaviours of others may impact on us and so how we might manage these (e.g. how we respond to people who are angry or aggressive)
- appreciating how others may perceive us (e.g. assertive, consistently apologetic) and so respond to us.

As a student learning disability nurse I was asked to produce a communication passport for a patient with learning disabilities who was to attend hospital to have an operation. The passport was shared in a best interests meeting and given to the hospital staff. With the information contained in the passport they could make reasonable adjustments for the patient and ensure a smooth transition into hospital. It enabled us, as a team, to understand her needs, communication and behaviours and ensure these were addressed with care and compassion. The passport worked well and her stay was a success. Communication passports are essential for all patients in our care as the more we understand and know about them the more we can adapt our care to their needs.

Julie Davis, LD nursing student

Strategies for developing self-awareness

There is a range of strategies and tools that can be used to develop self-awareness, and your choice will be down to individual preference, ease of use or availability.

Journals, diaries or logs (Thompson, 2015) can be a valuable record of activities, events, incidents that have taken place and our reactions to them, and can reveal a lot about you through what you choose to record and what you leave out. Repeated recording of specific types of incidents such as managing challenging situations may suggest that this is an area for development.

Reflective practice not only requires the skill of self-awareness, but will also further develop awareness of self as you reflect on experiences and your response to them, and others' responses to your actions or inactions.

Clinical supervision is defined as 'regular, protected time for facilitation [of] in-depth reflection on clinical practice' (Bond and Holland, 2010: 15) and is used widely in health and social care. It provides facilitated reflection with an experienced supervisor and can help nurses to develop self-awareness as they reflect on their clinical practice and the interpersonal relationships within it.

Experiential frameworks such as Johari windows or Jack and Miller's three-stage framework (Jack and Miller, 2008) are widely used to help explore what you know about yourself, what others may know about you and those aspects hidden from yourself and/or others.

Portfolios are recognised tools to hold a record and evidence of learning (Reed, 2015). They can be used to identify skills and competencies acquired, record feedback from lecturers, practice educators, patients and colleagues, and provide details of courses and study days attended and what was learned. You can use this information to review your progress in order to help you identify your areas of strength and areas for further development.

Case study 15.1 provides an example of how you can use the above strategies to develop self-awareness of your communication skills and to help you to identify areas for development.

CASE STUDY 15.1: JEN

Jen kept a reflective journal of her experiences in clinical practice. These included the following incidents:

- Feeling uncomfortable but saying nothing when she saw a member of staff simply tick things on a menu rather than asking the patient, because 'she was elderly and had dementia, so wouldn't remember what she'd ordered the next day'.
- Avoiding a patient in A&E who was shouting and talking to himself.
- Failing to speak up when staff laughed and joked during handover about a patient with a learning disability who had got really upset when his personal belongings had been rearranged on top of his locker.

When reviewing the reflections she kept in her portfolio, she found there was a constant theme, highlighting her difficulties in challenging the behaviour of staff she felt was unacceptable. She realised that she needed to develop her skills of challenging others and being assertive. Jen discussed this with her practice educator, who suggested that clinical supervision could be a strategy to use to help her explore the challenges she faced in being assertive and to help her better manage challenging situations.

- Review your reflections – can you find any common themes?
- What do these help you to learn about yourself?

Communication is an essential factor in the nursing role but miscommunication can happen; problems arise when we don't learn from miscommunication and continue to make the same mistakes. I feel that reflective practice is a really valuable tool in order to be able to develop my practice and my understanding of situations of care that I have been involved with. During my time as a student I cared for individuals whereby English was not their first language. I have found that it is important to find ways of communicating effectively and this may require the use of an interpreter or carers that can interpret where appropriate. I believe that this is important as it is giving them the opportunity to express themselves and be understood properly; very important elements of a person's main concerns can be missed as we can fill in what we don't understand with what we think they want to know based on our own values.

Samantha Vanes, NQ RNMH

COMMUNICATING WITH CHILDREN

A child's family or carer is a constant component of their life; therefore, any communication with a child is likely to be undertaken in the presence of an adult. One of the most important skills in ensuring effective communication in this situation is encouraging both child and parent(s) or carer to be actively involved in interactions. The resultant triadic interaction (Lambert, 2012) can become somewhat complex, since parents or carers can either be supportive of their child's participation in the conversation or try to prevent it.

Good communication is essential to children's ongoing development. Babies and very young children may be pre-verbal, and generally children use fewer words than adolescents or adults. They often struggle to express what they want to say and adults may find it hard to understand their language. Consequently, children's communicative styles are usually more demonstrative than verbal. When a child struggles to find the word they need to express themselves, they may instead demonstrate their thoughts through gestures, facial expressions, sounds and other forms of body language (Lefevre, 2010).

It is essential that nurses recognise these ways of communicating and adjust their own styles accordingly. Attention should be paid not only to the words that are used, but also to the ways in which they are used. Both the language and the approach of the nurse must be tailored to the age and developmental stage of the child to avoid confusing, frightening or patronising them (Naunton et al., 2017). A positive example of this can be seen when a nurse lowers themself to the level of the child to reduce the impact of the height difference and uses clear, simple and unemotional language.

It is also important that the nurse ensures the child understands what they have been told – and it is often not enough to simply ask the child, as they are likely to say 'yes' because that is what they think the nurse wants to hear. A child's understanding can be validated by asking them to repeat what was said to them, asking open questions to check understanding or asking an older child what they would tell a friend if they had to explain what has been said. Nurses should also recognise that an inability to gain full understanding does not justify a lack of discussion with a child who wants to know the situation (Hayes and Keogh, 2012).

Play is an important activity for all children and should not be underestimated as a means of communication (see Case study 15.2 as an example of how this can be used effectively). Engaging in play activities – for example, playing a game, drawing or storytelling – can facilitate a good relationship between a nurse and a child, even when their encounter is very brief (Coyne et al., 2009). If a child or a member of their family is to have an operation, the opportunity to use play to explore the situation can assist the child in becoming familiar with medical routines.

On my very first placement a young boy had been referred to PAU by his GP and had no grasp of English, and neither did his carer. I was very aware of how I approached him; I ensured my approach was slow and that my facial expression was kind and I smiled at him. As he smiled back I crouched down to his level as I am quite tall and I did not want to intimidate him, and ensured I was not too close as I did not want to invade his personal space. I considered my voice when I said hello, not loud and abrupt but soft, and gave him time to 'work me out' and respond. I asked him if he would like a book, and used my hands to try and demonstrate a book, which he appeared to understand and nodded. After this initial contact, it was the beginning of a therapeutic relationship. It was difficult, but all I had learnt in theory about communication enabled me to think on the spot and develop my knowledge on all the many aspects of communication, and then communicate effectively with what appeared to be a very frightened young boy who was in a lot of pain.

Siân Hunter, child nursing student

CASE STUDY 15.2: KIM AND KERRY

Zeb is a first-year nursing student who is accompanying his practice educator to visit a patient while on a community nursing placement. When they arrive at the house, the patient's 6-year-old twin daughters (Kim and Kerry) are clinging to their mum and seem rather tearful. Kim and Kerry refuse to leave their mother, which makes it difficult for Zeb's practice educator to provide the care she needs. Zeb positions himself where Kim and Kerry can see what he is doing and starts to draw a picture in his notebook. When he has finished, Zeb asks the twins what he has drawn. Although reluctant to engage at first, they become very excited when they realise he has drawn a picture of them.

Kim then asks Zeb to draw a picture of their older brother, Jake. She says he is very tall and has long legs and arms, and Kerry adds that he has lots of black curly hair. Zeb asks what Jake's favourite clothes are and Kim says emphatically: 'Jeans that don't fit him and his red baseball cap, back to front of course.' Next, Zeb asks what Jake likes to eat and, in chorus, Kim and Kerry say 'pizza!'

Then Zeb shows them his picture – Jake has very long arms and legs, but hardly any body, and Kim and Kerry can't see his face because of his black curly hair. He is sitting inside a big pair of jeans that clearly don't fit him, with a back-to-front baseball cap on his head. In front of him is the most enormous pizza! 'Does this look like Jake?' Zeb asks, and Kim and Kerry start to laugh and tell him about their brother.

Zeb's practice educator has now finished talking to Kim and Kerry's mother, who tells them that the nurses have to leave, but that the practice educator will come again soon. On hearing this, Kim and Kerry turn to the practice educator and say 'You can only come back if Zeb comes with you!' As they leave, Zeb takes the two pictures out of his notebook and gives one each to Kim and Kerry.

This scenario demonstrates the importance of what some might consider 'non-conventional' communication skills.

ANSWER:
CASE STUDY 15.2

- When communicating with children in healthcare settings, how might play benefit the therapeutic relationship between the nurse and the child?
- What non-conventional communication approaches might be used in other fields of practice?

When considering communication with children, it is important not to forget adolescents, who are in the final years of childhood. Nurses need to strike a balance between stereotypical views of young people and the reality that many of these individuals have a problem-free adolescence, are just 'normal' people and are good communicators (Coleman and Hagell, 2007). Effective communication can be hindered by negative attitudes or by focusing on the parent rather than on the young person's day-to-day life, education and emotional wellbeing (Fallon, 2012). Robinson (2010) identified a range of communication skills that young people expect nurses to display, which included being available, accepting, informed and informative, empathic and able to ensure privacy and dignity. Although in this case these were applied to communication with young people, they are indeed the skills required by any nurse when communicating with children of any age.

COMMUNICATING WITH NON-ENGLISH SPEAKERS

The UK is becoming an increasingly multicultural country (McClimens et al., 2014) and therefore it is highly likely that you will meet patients for whom the national language, English, is a second language, or who have only a limited grasp of it (Activity 15.2 will help you identify the key nationalities and languages spoken in your area). This can pose a number of challenges for you, not only in communicating at the simplest level, but also in understanding the different cultural beliefs and values that can influence the individual's understanding of our healthcare system and further impact on effective communication (Lakhani, 2008). Different cultures will have different beliefs about the causes of illness and disease – for example, in some cultures, people with mental health problems are believed to be possessed. It can be helpful therefore to learn about the culture of your patient so that you are aware of culturally sensitive issues, such as the use of eye contact and touch.

ACTIVITY 15.2: REFLECTION

Go online and search for neighbourhood statistics. This will enable you to search for data on people in your local area, including country of birth, ethnic group and main language spoken, and give you an overview of the potential for meeting patients who may be less familiar with our healthcare system due to being born in another country.

- How familiar are you with the different cultural beliefs of the range of ethnic groups in your area?
- How might this influence your ability to give culturally sensitive care?

> I would ensure I used a translator if I had to communicate complicated or detailed information. However on a 1:1 basis I have used facial expressions, body language, gestures and pointing. I have also used photos to enable the patient to communicate their needs to me. I have also learnt simple body part names in their language when I have built up a relationship with them, to enhance communication.
>
> **Julie Davis, LD nursing student**

It is important to remember that just because an individual can speak the national language, this does not mean that they are literate in it – no matter which culture they come from – and so they may not be able to understand written information (Szczepura et al., 2005). To assist those who do not speak the national language, most healthcare organisations now provide information leaflets in a range of languages, as well as interpreting services.

Use of interpreters

Interpreters should always be professionals, who have been trained for interpreting within healthcare settings; although there may be staff in the healthcare setting who can speak the same language as the patient, they should only be asked to interpret in an emergency. An approved professional interpreter should always be used over a family member where important information is being asked for or given, in order to be sure of accurate interpretation; additionally, if the information being asked for is sensitive and a family member is interpreting, the patient may not feel able to express themselves fully. Children should never be used to act as interpreters.

Thinking outside the box helps with this situation. It's important where possible not to rely on relatives to interpret for the patient. Red Cross emergency translation handbooks can help identify people's languages and help with basic questions. Telephone interpreters are the best method for interpretation. However gestures and Google Translate have also been used in situations I have witnessed.

Laura Grimley, adult nurse

Situations in which an approved interpreter should be used are admission assessment, consent for treatment, explanation of diagnosis, treatment or medications and discharge information. Interpretation can be provided over the phone or face to face, depending on the circumstances: for example, when breaking bad news, face-to-face interpretation would always be required.

Key points to remember when using an interpreter are:

1. Discuss expectations with the interpreter.
2. Look at the patient when you speak.
3. Speak clearly at a normal pace. Do not shout!
4. Address them by name or say 'you', not 'he' or 'she'.
5. Check that the interpreter is managing your speed of communication.
6. Avoid medical jargon.
7. Check for understanding.

Unfortunately, an interpreter cannot be present 24 hours a day, and therefore you will need to use other strategies to ensure that effective communication takes place when delivering routine care or social interaction, such as:

- sign language
- communication passport
- hospital communication book

- asking an interpreter (preferably) or family member to write down basic questions in English and their own language so that you and the patient can point to the relevant one, e.g. 'Do you have pain?'
- picture boards
- learning a couple of key words in the patient's own language
- remembering that smiling is a universal form of communication.

Finally, regardless of who you are communicating with, there is a key lesson for all of us that came from Dr Kate Granger, who whilst in hospital as a patient found that many staff failed to introduce themselves before delivering care, an essential first step in any therapeutic relationship. Kate started a campaign – #hellomynameis (see Activity 15.3) – which has had over 1.6 billion impressions since the campaign started and has been picked up across the world.

ACTIVITY 15.3: REFLECTION

Take a look at the website http://hellomynameis.org.uk:

- Do you always introduce yourself before starting a care activity?
- How could you ensure this becomes an intrinsic part of your communications with the people you care for?

HELLO MY
NAME IS

CONCLUSION

This chapter has introduced the primary importance of communicating effectively when caring for patients. The fundamental skills required for effective communication and strategies for communicating with particular patient groups have been outlined, with the need for self-awareness highlighted. Within your role as a nurse, the onus is on you to communicate effectively with the patients in your care. In Chapter 16, you will find these skills are explored in more depth and applied to challenging situations that you may encounter as a nurse.

CHAPTER SUMMARY

- The ability to communicate effectively is the most important skill a nurse can possess.
- Communication plays a role in patient safety and satisfaction, facilitates therapeutic relationships, enables nurses to collect important data regarding patients and facilitates nursing interventions and their evaluation.
- Observing non-verbal cues is important, especially with children and patients who are unable to communicate verbally or may not have the vocabulary to accurately communicate their thoughts and feelings.
- The use of journals, reflection on practice and clinical supervision are valuable strategies for developing insight into your values and beliefs, as well as your strengths and areas for development.
- The UK is becoming increasingly multicultural; this requires nurses to not only develop strategies for communicating with those who do not speak the national language, but also to understand how different cultural beliefs can impact on a person's understanding of healthcare and treatment.

CRITICAL REFLECTION

Holistic care

This chapter has highlighted the importance of communication in holistic patient care. Reflect on a situation in which:

- reading non-verbal cues was particularly important. How can you sensitise yourself to observing and interpreting these?
- you had difficulty in communicating with a patient. What were the problems and how might you have managed them more effectively?

GO FURTHER

Books

Bach, S. and Grant, A. (2015) *Communication and Interpersonal Skills in Nursing*, 3rd edn. London: SAGE/ Learning Matters. This book covers key topics in communication and interpersonal skills linked to the NMC's *Standards for Pre-registration Nursing Education*, with useful case studies and activities to help apply theory to practice.

Gault, I., Shapcott, J., Luthi, A. and Reid, G. (2017) *Communication in Nursing and Healthcare*. London: SAGE. An excellent book which explores communication in relation to a wide range of situations and client groups that will be valuable throughout your degree.

Moss, B. (2017) *Communication Skills in Health and Social Care*, 4th edn. London: SAGE. A practical guide which is presented in a unique and easy to use dictionary format.

Goldbart, J. and Caton, S. (2010) *Communication and People with the Most Complex Needs: What Works and Why this is Essential*. London: Mencap. A report based on the views of carers, researchers and service providers which presents a range of strategies for communicating with people with profound intellectual impairments, severe autism and challenging behaviour, including the use of passports, intensive interaction, the use of switches and the picture exchange system.

SAGE journal articles

FURTHER
READING:
JOURNAL
ARTICLES

Go to https://study.sagepub.com/essentialnursing2e for free online journal articles for this chapter. If you are using the interactive ebook, simply click on the book icon in the margin to go straight to the resource.

Rodriguez, C.S. Spring, H.J. and Rowe, M. (2014) 'Nurses' experiences of communicating with hospitalized, suddenly speechless patients', *Qualitative Health Research* 25(2): 168-178. A research study into the challenges nurses have had in communicating with people who have suddenly lost the power of speech.

MacDonald, L.M. (2016) 'Expertise in everyday nurse-patient conversations: The importance of small talk', *Global Qualitative Nursing Research*, 3: 1-9. An interesting research article on the way nurses use small talk and its importance.

Other journal articles

Lambert, V., Glacken, M. and McCarron, M. (2011) 'Communication between children and health professionals in a child hospital setting: A child transitional communication model', *Journal of Advanced Nursing*, 67(3): 569-82. An ethnographic study of the nature of communication between children and health professionals in a child hospital setting which challenges views on how active children want to be in the communication process.

Padfield, B. (2013) 'Assessing communication on a mental health unit', *Nursing Times*, 7 May. Available at: www.nursingtimes.net/nursing-practice/clinical-zones/mental-health/assessing-communication-on-a-mental-health-unit/5058256.article. Describes how the *Essence of Care* benchmarking toolkit was used to enhance communication interventions on an acute adult mental health ward.

Weblinks

Go to https://study.sagepub.com/essentialnursing2e for weblinks related to this chapter. If you are using the interactive ebook, simply click on the book icon in the margin to go straight to the resource.

www.mefirst.org.uk – Me First is a really useful website to help healthcare professionals improve their communication with children and young people.

www.businessballs.com/johariwindowmodel.htm – this is a useful overview of the Johari window, a simple tool for understanding and developing self-awareness.

www.nhs.uk/CarersDirect/guide/communication/Pages/Communicating.aspx – the NHS Choices website has useful guidance on communication problems due to illness or physical disabilities, as well as information on interpreting services.

www.mencap.org.uk/ – this web page provides a range of useful resources on how to communicate with people who have a learning disability, and the use of communication resources.

Royal College of Speech and Language Therapists (2013) *Five Good Communication Standards*. London: RCSLT. Available at: www.rcslt.org/news/docs/good_comm_standards. This document outlines the reasonable adjustments to communication that patients with a learning disability and/or autism should expect to receive in both hospital and residential settings.

FURTHER
READING:
WEBLINKS

Video links

Have a break from the text and go to https://study.sagepub.com/essentialnursing2e for useful videos related to this chapter. If you are using the interactive ebook, simply click on the lightbulb icon in the margin to go straight to the resource.

VIDEO
LINKS

ACE YOUR ASSESSMENT

Review what you have learned by visiting the book's online resources at: https://study.sagepub.com/essential nursing2e If using your interactive ebook, just click on the icon in the margin to go straight there.

ONLINE
QUIZZES

- Test yourself with multiple-choice and short-answer questions.
- Revise key terms with the interactive flash cards.

REFERENCES

Alligood, M. and May, B. (2000) 'A nursing theory of personal system empathy: Interpreting a conceptualization of empathy in King's interacting systems', *Nursing Science Quarterly*, 13: 243–7.

Bach, S. and Grant, A. (2015) *Communication and Interpersonal Skills in Nursing*, 3rd edn. London: Learning Matters.

Balzer-Riley, J. (2015) *Communication in Nursing*, 8th edn. New York: Elsevier Mosby.

Baughan, J. and Smith, A. (2013) *Compassion, Caring and Communication: Skills for Nursing Practice*. Harlow: Pearson.

Bell, R. (2012) 'Does he have sugar in his tea? Communication between people with learning disabilities, their carers and hospital staff', *Tizard Learning Disability Review*, 17(2): 57–63.

Bond, M. and Holland, S. (2010) *Skills of Clinical Supervision for Nurses: A Practical Guide for Supervisees, Clinical Supervisors and Managers*, 2nd edn. Maidenhead: Open University Press.

Coleman, J. and Hagell, A. (2007) 'The nature of risk and resilience in adolescence', in J. Coleman and A. Hagell (eds), *Adolescence, Risk and Resilience: Against the Odds*. Chichester: Wiley. pp. 1–16.

Commissioning Board Chief Nursing Officer and DH Chief Nursing Adviser (2012) Compassion in Practice: Nursing, Midwifery and Care Staff: Our Vision and Strategy. Available at: www.england. nhs.uk/wp-content/uploads/2012/12/compassion-in-practice.pdf (accessed 23 February 2015).

Coyne, I., Hayes, E. and Gallagher, P. (2009) 'Research with hospitalised children: Ethical, methodological and organisational challenges', *Childhood*, 16: 413–28.

Eckroth-Bucher, M. (2010) 'Self-awareness: A review and analysis of a basic nursing concept', *Advances in Nursing Science*, 33(4): 297–309.

Fallon, D. (2012) 'Communicating with young people', in V. Lambert, T. Long and D. Kelleher (eds), *Communication Skills for Children's Nurses*. Maidenhead: McGraw-Hill. pp. 34–48.

Gault, I., Shapcott, J., Luthi, A. and Reid, G. (2017) *Communication in Nursing and Healthcare*. London: SAGE.

Hayes, V. and Keogh, P. (2012) 'Communicating with children in early and middle childhood', in V. Lambert, T. Long and D. Kelleher (eds), *Communication Skills for Children's Nurses*. Maidenhead: McGraw-Hill. pp. 19–33.

Jack, K. and Miller, E. (2008) 'Exploring self-awareness in mental health practice', *Mental Health Practice*, 12(3): 31–5.

Lakhani, M. (2008) *No Patient Left Behind: How Can We Ensure World Class Primary Care for Black and Minority Ethnic People?* London: DH.

Lambert, V. (2012) 'Theoretical foundations of communication', in V. Lambert, T. Long and D. Kelleher (eds), *Communication Skills for Children's Nurses*. Maidenhead: McGraw-Hill. pp. 1–18.

Leathers, D. and Eaves, M. (2016) *Successful Nonverbal Communication*, 4th edn. Abingdon: Routledge.

Lefevre, M. (2010) *Communicating with Children and Young People: Making a Difference*. Bristol: Policy Press.

Mcabe, C., Timmins, F. and Campling, J. (2013) *Communication Skills for Nursing Practice*, 2nd edn. London: Palgrave Macmillan.

McClimens, A., Brewster, J. and Lewis, R. (2014) 'Recognising and respecting patients' cultural diversity', *Nursing Standard*, 28(28): 45–52.

Morrissey, J. and Callaghan, P. (2011) *Communication Skills for Mental Health Nurses*. Maidenhead: Open University Press.

Naunton, P., Martin, K. and Reid, J. (2017) 'Me first: promoting children and young people centred communication in health and social care using innovative educational resources', *Archives of Diseases in Childhood*, 102(S3): A4.

Nursing and Midwifery Council (NMC) (2015) *The Code: Professional Standards of Practice and Behaviour for Nurses and Midwives*. London: NMC.

Parliamentary and Health Service Ombudsman (2015) *Complaints about Acute Trusts 2014–15*. London: The Stationery Office.

Reed, S. (2015) *Successful Professional Portfolios for Nursing Students*. London: SAGE.

Robinson, S. (2010) 'Children's and young people's views of health professionals in England', *Journal of Child Health*, 144: 310–26.

Shattell, M., McAllister, S., Hogan, B. and Thomas, S. (2006) '"She took the time to make sure she understood": Mental health patients' experiences of being understood', *Archives of Psychiatric Nursing*, 20(5): 234–41.

Stein-Parbury, J. (2005) *Patient and Person: Developing Interpersonal Skills in Nursing*, 3rd edn. Sydney: Elsevier.

Szczepura, A., Johnson, M., Gumber, A., Jones, K., Clay, D. and Shaw, A. (2005) *An Overview of the Research Evidence on Ethnicity and Communication in Healthcare: Final Report*. UK Centre for Evidence in Ethnicity, Health and Diversity (CEEHD), Warwick University.

Thompson, N. (2015) *People Skills*, 4th edn. London: Palgrave Macmillan.

COMMUNICATION AND INTERPERSONAL SKILLS IN CHALLENGING CIRCUMSTANCES 16

STEVE TRENOWETH AND WASIIM ALLYMAMOD

--- **THIS CHAPTER COVERS** ---

- Challenging situations in nursing
- Healthcare environments and communication challenges

- Handling challenging situations

> One of the biggest challenges I face as a nurse is trying to understand what my patients are trying to tell me. As a child nurse, I have found that children tend to communicate emotionally when they are not well – they may cry or scream when in pain, or sometimes they go very quiet. This makes trying to find out what is wrong really difficult at times. I know it is vitally important to speak to the parents here – they can provide so much information that can help you to understand what the child may be experiencing. However, they are, understandably, often very anxious and stressed when their child is not well, and I find myself having to use all my nursing skills to calm and support them before they can chat to me. And all the time I'm aware that their child is not well and that calming the parents down can delay the treatment of their child – vital minutes may be ticking away. But of course we have to be very careful not to communicate anxiety. This I find one of the most challenging aspects about my job – how to communicate with people at highly stressful times, while trying to keep a professional and calm outward appearance. I have become very aware of how I present to others since I became a child nurse – and I have thought long and hard about what I say and how I say it.
>
> Heidi, nurse

Visit https://study.sagepub.com/essentialnursing2e to access a wealth of online resources for this chapter – watch out for the margin icons throughout the chapter. If you are using the interactive eBook, simply click on the margin icon to go straight to the resource.

INTRODUCTION

As we saw from the previous chapter, communication is a core skill of nurses and we must remember that communication occurs whether we intend it or not! That is, as nurses we must be mindful of unintended communication (which may undermine the messages we wish to send) and mindful of how we can use our skills to communicate effectively with our patients (which may promote the messages). We must also be receptive to the communication which our patients are sending to us, and sensitive to how their symptoms and wider healthcare experiences might undermine the messages they intend to send. On occasions, as a result of these healthcare experiences and other factors, adults, children and adolescents may present in ways which we may interpret as 'challenging'. In this chapter, we explore these challenging situations in nursing and how we can ensure that our verbal and non-verbal communication and behaviour demonstrate our professionalism as nurses, and that such challenges reinforce our primary goal in nursing – to care for all people, adults, children and adolescents alike, who experience health difficulties and distress.

CHALLENGING SITUATIONS IN NURSING

ANSWER:
ACTIVITY 16.1

ACTIVITY 16.1: REFLECTIVE PRACTICE

Make a list of situations that you find challenging in nursing. Why do these situations feel challenging? How many of these situations involve communication with other people?

There are many challenging situations in nursing and everyone is likely to feel a range of emotions. Often, the most challenging situations for us as nurses involve communication issues – not being able to understand what is being said to us or not being understood (or being misunderstood) in return. There are many potential barriers to communication (or 'filters' as Hindle (2003) calls them) and difficulties may arise from many sources.

ANSWER:
ACTIVITY 16.2

ACTIVITY 16.2: REFLECTIVE PRACTICE

What barriers are there in our communication with each other? Consider circumstances when you feel you have been misunderstood or when you have misunderstood someone. Why did this happen?

Language

The first and most obvious communication barrier is not being able to understand another person because they speak (and perhaps can only speak) a different language. This can seriously impact on the patient's ability to engage actively with nurses in their care and treatment, and can lead to confusion and frustration, and even anxiety and fear.

ACTIVITY 16.3: REFLECTIVE PRACTICE

How might you overcome linguistic barriers in communicating with others?

ANSWER:
ACTIVITY 16.3

It is important to ensure that information is readily available to all patients and service users. Key written information should be available in all common languages and interpreters should be accessible to explain healthcare interventions. Family members may be useful here to help form a bridge between the patient and healthcare staff. However, the words that we use – that is, our verbal language – are in fact only one part of how we communicate with other people. There is a considerable amount of information which we convey to others in our gestures, facial expressions, eye contact, and so forth. There are, of course, further challenges here as non-verbal communication and behaviour are often culturally imbued and this is, of course, open to misunderstanding and misinterpretation. That is, what may be considered acceptable and appropriate in one culture may be considered offensive in another.

Culture

The benefit of using language is, of course, the ability to directly clarify the messages that we transmit so as to reduce misunderstandings. However, different cultures are likely to have different expectations about social interaction and conduct. There is a danger here that such misunderstandings may lead to prejudicial assumptions which can dramatically undermine the nurse–patient relationship (McCabe and Timmins, 2013). Nurses who work in multicultural countries such as the UK need to be *culturally competent*. Papadopoulos et al. (1998) describe such cultural competence as stemming from cultural awareness, cultural knowledge and cultural sensitivity.

Cultural awareness

Cultural awareness stems from an examination of how culture (including our own) helps to structure beliefs, attitudes and behaviours. This helps us to understand that there are many equally valid interpretations of the world and that our own culture is one amongst many.

Cultural knowledge

Cultural knowledge stems from an understanding of the beliefs, traditions and behaviours of different communities, including their healthcare beliefs and practices. Cultures also differ in terms of what is considered socially acceptable around personal space and contact, gender roles, attitudes towards ageing and older people, eye contact, gestures, volume/rate of speech, and so on.

Cultural sensitivity

When we are being culturally sensitive, we have an acceptance and empathic understanding of another person; we seek to build a trusting relationship, based on respect; and we are able to use our interpersonal and communication skills in a way which does not cause offence.

The nurse who is culturally competent actively challenges discriminatory practice and is sensitive, aware and has a fundamental cultural knowledge which underpins their nursing skills, including their assessment, care and treatment. The nurse here may find the input of family members invaluable in helping them to understand the cultural frame of reference of their patients.

Consciousness

Clearly, people who have fluctuating levels of consciousness, or who are unresponsive, pose considerable communication challenges for the nurse. There are a number of points of good practice here. Always assume that the person can hear and understand what is going on around them. Some people who have regained consciousness have recalled conversations that took place around them whilst they were unconscious (Leigh, 2001). In providing direct patient care, you must ensure that you continue to interact with the person and explain to the person what you will be doing, even if they are unconscious and apparently unresponsive, and encourage family members to do the same (Leigh, 2001).

As in any nursing intervention, the person must be centre of attention. Never refer to the person in their presence as 'he' or 'she' – that is, in the third person. Imagine for a moment how you would feel if someone were referring to you in this way. It is likely that you would feel ignored and not valued. The person must be the centre of your attention when attending to their needs.

Sensory impairments

Nurses must possess the ability to communicate with a wide range of people, including those who have sensory impairments, such as people who are deaf, blind or cannot speak. If a person uses some form of aid (for example, glasses, a hearing aid) to facilitate communication, then it is vital that these are fitted and that they are working properly. This must form a part of a comprehensive nursing assessment and family members and carers may also be consulted for advice. Of course, people with sensory impairments may manage to live their lives and communicate with others perfectly adequately. The challenge is really for us in ensuring that we can be understood and that we can receive the messages that our patients/service users are sending. This is compounded by possible healthcare issues and symptoms that the person is currently facing.

It is important to ensure that the environment is conducive to communication and here clear signage, appropriate lighting and so on may be helpful. If you are communicating with a person with a sensory impairment, then it is vital to ensure that the person can actually understand what you are saying – for example, speaking clearly with appropriate volume or ensuring that you face a person who lip reads. A note pad and pen may be helpful to the person who finds verbal expression difficult. Augmented or alternative methods of communication (AAC) may be helpful for people with disabilities, such as photographs or images; and using sign language, even with a simple 'hello', can be very reassuring to a person who signs.

CASE STUDY 16.1: PROFESSOR STEPHEN HAWKING

For many years, Professor Stephen Hawking suffered from **Amyotrophic Lateral Sclerosis (ALS)** (one of the most common types of motor neurone disease), the symptoms of which include an atrophying of muscles and difficulty with swallowing, breathing and speaking (dysarthria). Professor

Hawking used his cheek muscles to control a device which allowed him to communicate one word per minute. However, this did not prevent him from writing books (such as *The Grand Design* (with Mlodinow, 2010)) and contributing to/presenting television programmes. His ability to receive and understand messages from other people and his environment was not impaired.

- What challenges do you foresee that nurses may have in communicating with a person diagnosed with motor neurone disease?

ANSWER:
CASE STUDY 16.1

Mental health problems

Sometimes, a person may be impaired in their communication with us (and we may also be unable to communicate effectively with them) as they may be experiencing mental health problems. It is important to recognise that people who experience mental distress may not necessarily have a formal psychiatric diagnosis. That is, not everyone who is mentally distressed has a diagnosable mental health problem and, of course, vice versa. As nurses, we should not be guided by whether or not a person has received such a diagnosis, and be more concerned with the person's immediate presenting needs.

The nurse needs to understand that their patient's mental ill health can pose significant communication challenges for both parties. As an example, let's consider how we communicate with a person who is low in mood – that is, experiencing a *depressive episode*. An understanding of the features of a depressive episode will be essential for the nurse in order for them to appreciate the patient's internal world, and how they may subsequently adjust their communication strategy. The *International Statistical Classification of Diseases* (ICD-10) (World Health Organization (WHO), 2004) describes different forms of depressive episodes of varying severity – from 'mild' to 'severe' episodes (which in the latter case may be accompanied by, for example, 'psychosis', strange beliefs and bizarre behaviour). It is a common mental health problem and symptoms of a depressive episode can include:

- feelings of sadness and despair
- a loss of sense of hope for the future
- appetite disturbances, often with weight loss
- sleep disturbances
- social withdrawal
- loss of interest or pleasure in activities that are normally pleasurable
- decreased libido
- decreased energy
- an inability to concentrate
- feelings of guilt
- suicidal thoughts.

However, it is important to distinguish between feeling 'down' and being depressed. A diagnosis of depression can only be made if many of the above symptoms persist for a period of time (typically at least two weeks); are abnormal for the individual; present for most of the day (and almost every day); and are largely uninfluenced by environmental circumstances (WHO, 2004).

People who experience a depressive episode typically appear very sad. They do not tend to engage voluntarily in communicating with others and may even actively avoid social interactions. There is always a danger that in busy healthcare environments, the needs of such people may be overlooked. The nurse must ensure that the person who is low in mood is not neglected and must make every effort to engage with the person. Neurocognitively, people who are low in mood tend to have a problem with processing information, that is, it often takes a longer period of time than normal for the person to understand what has been said to them, and likewise to think of a response. It is thought that this is due to either a depletion of certain chemicals (known as neurotransmitters) which facilitate the flow of information in the brain or the inability of neurons to fully utilise neurotransmitters which again reduces the brain's ability to function effectively. (In fact, this is how anti-depressants are thought to work – they work at a neuronal level to increase levels of transmitters in synapses and subsequently the brain's ability to send and receive messages.)

This can lead to conversations seeming rather stilted and slow. It is important for the nurse to realise that conversing with the person who is low in mood may take a longer period of time than for non-depressed patients, and they must take this into account in their communication strategy. There is a tendency when we are busy or pressured to seek to obtain quick answers, particularly in very acute settings, but with the person who is low in mood this is not usually possible. We would advise you not to rush the process, as this will not be helpful, and it is most likely that the person who is low in mood will still be processing the first question whilst you are asking the second. So, when talking to a person who is low in mood, it is important to consider how many questions you ask and how frequently you ask them. This is known as *pacing*.

First of all, we should be aware that sometimes when people are unwell (physically, mentally or both) their ability to comprehend what is happening to them may be diminished and they may seem less tolerant to frustration. There may be symptomatic experiences (such as pain, breathlessness or fatigue) or confusion or fear surrounding a diagnosis, or worry and concern about a health problem which they or a loved one may be facing. They may be frustrated by the inability of healthcare staff to give reassurance or answers to their questions regarding the cause of their illness or the trajectory or prognosis of a disease. In short, the person may be experiencing considerable stress or distress. The social conventions of interpersonal communication may be challenged at such times and the nurse needs to have empathy with, and an understanding of, the emotional experience of their patients. It is important to be able to recognise and anticipate that people may have such experiences, and that we consider how to communicate with people who may be on edge and therefore more prone to emotional outbursts.

HEALTHCARE ENVIRONMENTS AND COMMUNICATION CHALLENGES

CASE STUDY:
HARRY
(STUDENT)

In healthcare practice, we get accustomed to how things work. As we develop increasing expertise, we develop a sophisticated understanding of health and illness. We use increasingly complex healthcare terminology and acronyms with confidence and ease. We take for granted the healthcare environment, and systems and departments and their functions. And we sometimes forget that our patients do not have the same understanding of themselves! What may seem obvious or 'common sense' to us is not necessarily seen the same way by our patients. Without care, we may communicate in 'jargon', leading to further confusion and anxiety. Healthcare systems, including the role and function of specialist departments, can also be confusing in the extreme to people who are not 'in the know'.

ANSWER:
ACTIVITY 16.4

ACTIVITY 16.4: REFLECTIVE PRACTICE

Consider, for example, the difference between 'aural' and 'oral' care. How might this lead to confusion?

Healthcare services and departments may also be very specialised and, as a consequence, referrals may be made by one department to another department which may delay diagnosis or treatment, increasing levels of anxiety. So, not only must we consider the emotional experiences of our patients, we must also be aware of situations in healthcare which may lead to increased levels of frustration, confusion, anxiety or even fear.

HANDLING CHALLENGING SITUATIONS

The first step in handling challenging situations is being able to find out why such situations are challenging for the person and what is concerning the person. This may seem obvious but it may be missed when the person's behaviour is being focused on. Often, situations which involve conflict in healthcare involve misunderstandings of some sort. The person may feel they lack information, or may feel excluded from decision-making. There may have been a mistake or an error or omission. Here, an apology, coupled with explanations and information, swiftly and sincerely given, can resolve many issues. However, there are times when finding solutions to problems can be more complex. For example, a person may feel aggrieved or may feel that they have not received the treatment or intervention that they wanted and here a resolution may not be within the role of the nurse who should, supportively, informatively and with clarity, direct the person to the complaints procedures of the hospital, Trust or service. This should not be perceived negatively and the nurse should respect the wishes of the person and their desire to resolve their problems at a higher level.

WHAT'S THE EVIDENCE?

WEBLINK: NMC

NMC Children's Nursing: Field Specific Competencies. Available at: www.nmc-uk.org/global assets/sitedocuments/registration/overseas/childrens-nursing-field---specific-competencies.pdf (accessed 5 June 2017).

The NMC has provided important advice when working with children, young people and their parents. For the NMC, the care of children, young people and their parents must be our first concern, treating them as individuals and respecting their dignity. Developing relationships built on trust and respect is an important part of this process, and being able to effectively communicate with children and young people is a fundamental part of managing challenging situations. For example, in communicating with young people, the NMC advises:

- treating people as individuals and collaborating with them, maintaining clear professional boundaries
- being open, honest and consistent in your interactions with children, young people and their parents, and with colleagues
- making time to get to know the child/young person and their parents, communicating directly with them, working in partnership, listening and responding appropriately to what they say themselves, assisting them in talking openly to others and sharing their own information
- being friendly, professional and compassionate
- recognising and acknowledging the beliefs of children, young people and their parents; if there are choices, helping children and young people to make them using play and other appropriate means of communication

(Continued)

- asking the child/young person how they want you to communicate sensitive information
- recognising the knowledge and skill held by parents (and by the child/young person) in relation to their child and their illness, disability or treatments
- taking steps to identify and overcome any barriers to understanding, whether this is the result of language, disability or stage of development
- empowering children and young people and their parents through providing information and giving them time for making decisions; giving information as early as possible; being prepared to repeat this and to discuss any concerns – consent must be voluntary and without coercion; checking that the child/young person and their parent/carer understands the information they have been given; and being prepared to explain complex concepts which are not understood and document the discussions
- documenting discussions, any disagreements and the action you have taken to resolve such issues and the outcome
- working effectively as part of a team, communicating with colleagues in the care setting and with the child/young person and their parents about your plan of care, safeguarding and promoting the welfare of children and young people at all times
- ensuring that the physical environment and environmental safety are appropriate for children, young people and their families, and highlighting safety concerns where you are not able to take immediate action to remove, reduce or manage risk
- providing a high standard of evidence-based practice and holistic care, acting openly, honestly and with integrity at all times.

There are a number of general principles which are important to be aware of when attempting to handle challenging situations. As we can see from the above advice from the NMC (2013), they involve being able to manage one's self; building relationships; communicating effectively, both verbally and non-verbally, in managing angry and/or aggressive behaviour; and maintaining good professional boundaries. Let's start by exploring how we may manage ourselves in challenging situations.

Managing one's self

In nursing, we often talk about 'managing' challenging situations or circumstances. However, one of the key elements is being able to manage one's self. Here, we need to think about our own responses in the face of challenging behaviour. We can, at particularly stressful and challenging times, 'leak' information. By this we mean that, if we are not mindful, we can unconsciously send messages (both negative and positive) to another person, and this is particularly true of our emotions, which are mostly communicated non-verbally. This can both inflame and calm a situation and there may be implications for how we are seen by another if there is a disparity between what we say and how we act. We may be perceived by another person as being 'deceitful' (or 'inauthentic'). This has clear implications for building a caring and therapeutic relationship with patients/service users as the person may not trust us.

As a rule of thumb, in any challenging situation the nurse needs to try to remain as calm as possible and to be mindful of their own communication (both verbal and non-verbal), as well as of what is being communicated by the other person. The nurse needs to ensure that, even under very trying circumstances, they remain focused on demonstrating professionalism, care and compassion, whilst maintaining the person's dignity and acting in a way which is in keeping with what is in the best interest of their patient (NMC, 2015). This is by no means easy, requires considerable expertise and is one of the many reasons why nursing is such a skilled and valuable profession – we respond not only to the physical needs of our patients, but also to their psychological and emotional needs as well.

Building relationships

In handling challenging situations, it is important to convey a clear message that you are a trustworthy person, and to instil confidence that you are able to help. Similarly, it is important to try to establish a psychologically safe and calm environment within which a relationship can develop. Establishing trust, building relationships and developing rapport must be seen as a core role for nurses, and this is particularly important with people who may be seen as 'challenging' or reluctant to accept treatment. The use of therapeutic touch can be very positive in nursing in building relationships. However, in challenging situations, such as when a person is angry, this is not advisable and should be avoided as touch in these circumstances may be seen as a threatening gesture.

Communicating effectively

Early intervention is the best way of handling any challenging situation. By this we mean 'nipping things in the bud' and trying to intervene before a situation escalates from a concern to an angry out-burst. However, before we can effectively communicate with another person, we need to hear what they are saying. As Kirby and Cross (2002: 195) put it:

> All our patients have a tale to tell. They are tales of survival – survival from the most over-whelming mental and physical conditions … It is through the re-telling of these narratives and focusing on problems, that we can help to find an alternative and more meaningful way to live. We simply need to learn to listen.

Listening helps us to develop an understanding of the person's point of view. It helps us to develop empathy and ensure that we respond in a compassionate and helpful way.

Once we have listened and understood, establishing and commencing dialogue is an important next step. Most people will simply want to have their concerns aired and do not want to be angry or aggressive. Ensure that you adopt a respectful tone and that the dignity of the person is not compromised. It is vital to remember the emotional state of the person and that they may be motivated by fear, frustration or confusion. When faced with such challenging situations, it is a good idea to start by asking the permission of the patient to talk (Nelson-Jones, 2015). A number of 'door-openers' to a conversation are dependent on whether you are wanting to take a formal or an informal approach. Consider how the person likes to be addressed and use the person's title (Mr/Mrs, etc.) if you are unsure. It is a good idea to reflect back to the person how they are presenting, but this must not be done in a way which is accusatory, critical or condemnatory; simply state, for example, that the person is shouting, or that they seem angry. Reassure the person that you wish to try to resolve their concern and listen to their problem. Telling the person to 'calm down' tends to have the opposite effect! Often, when you do not know a person very well, you will tend to be more formal in your approach – for example:

> Mr Jones, I can see that you are really quite angry at the moment. Would you like to tell me what the problem is, please? I would like to understand what it is that is troubling you. There is no need to shout – I'm here to listen. Perhaps if we had a chat, I may be able to help you.

Of course, if you already know a person, you may already have established a rapport and relationship which you can build on in a challenging situation – for example:

> Fred, is there something on your mind? You seem quite angry today. I'd really like to talk to you to see what we can do to help. Would that be OK?

Listen very carefully to the person's responses. This is known as *active listening* – demonstrating that you are listening to the person and hearing what they have to say. You may find that this is best conducted in a quiet, comfortable room – this maintains confidentiality and helps to reduce the overall levels of stimulation in the environment which may maintain or inflame the situation. Of course, there are often other people in the vicinity who may be receiving care and treatment, who may be distressed by angry outbursts. Here, some thought is needed about a suitable venue and you must be mindful of your own personal safety. If you are going to use a quiet room, make sure that the rest of the team know where you have gone. A room which has an alarm and ideally two exits would be best (if this is not possible, then you must make sure that you sit closest to the door in case you need to make a hasty exit, if the person appears to be getting angrier and you are concerned for your own safety).

Nelson-Jones (2015) recommends that you pay attention to your body language when encouraging the person to talk. He suggests:

- adopting a relaxed and open body posture
- leaning slightly forward
- using an appropriate gaze and eye contact (try not to stare)
- conveying appropriate facial expressions (smiling, for example)
- trying to limit gestures such as waving your hands about (they may be perceived as aggressive)
- being sensitive to personal space (remember, angry people need more personal space).

Here, the focus should be on trying to establish what is concerning the person. There are some techniques which can help the person to talk. For example, you could use *reflective statements* which reflect back what the person has said, and are an important skill in active listening (Miller and Rollnick, 2002; Nelson-Jones, 2015). Reflective statements can help to check assumptions about what the patient has said, help to clarify meaning and also allow the client to hear 'again' what they have said. *Repeating* is simply repeating what the client has said. For example:

> Patient: I'm so angry at being in hospital. Nobody ever listens to me.
>
> Nurse: You are angry that nobody ever listens to you.

This, of course, can be irritating if used often! There are other reflective statements which could also be used, such as *rephrasing* (where a remark is reflected back to the patient in a slightly different way using synonyms, for example):

> Patient: I'm so angry at being in hospital. Nobody ever listens to me.
>
> Nurse: It upsets you that no one seems to hear what you are saying.

Another core reflective statement is that of *paraphrasing*. Here, the meaning of the client's remark is inferred and reflected back, and a good paraphrase can reflect back to the person underlying meanings and emotions (Nelson-Jones, 2015). For example:

> Patient: I'm so angry at being in hospital. Nobody ever listens to me.
>
> Nurse: You feel that you would like to be able to make more decisions about your life.

Clearly, this is quite a skill which requires practice and training, but can be very powerful in getting to what may be the heart of the problem. But a note of caution here: the less you understand about the patient and their situation, the more cautious you need to be in reflecting back the meaning within their remarks – if you do not accurately reflect what people are saying, they may feel you are not listening or do not understand.

There are of course other techniques which may be helpful in trying to understand what is troubling the patient. Questioning is a useful skill, but you should always place an emphasis on encouraging the patient to express themselves and allow them to do most of the talking. 'Open-ended' questions are very helpful in this regard as they are seen to be 'door-openers' and encourage a narrative answer, for example:

- What concerns do you have at the moment?
- What's on your mind?
- What can we do for you?
- How can we help?

Closed questions, by contrast, invite brief or yes/no answers which tend to halt the flow of the conversation and tend not to encourage talk if they are over-used. They should be used sparingly and only when you would like a direct answer to a specific question. Examples include:

- Do you have any concerns at the moment?
- Do you feel angry?
- Are you in pain?

Other techniques include using *affirming statements*, which are a way of demonstrating an empathic understanding, recognition and acknowledgement of the difficulties the patient is experiencing or has experienced. They are a means of providing direct, *genuine* support and encouragement. For example:

- Things must be very difficult for you at the moment.
- I think if I were in your position, I would also find that very difficult.
- You certainly have had a lot to cope with – more than most people perhaps.

Of course, there will be a need to close the conversation and here it is a good idea to *summarise* what has been said and to acknowledge the concerns of the patient. Summarising is the process of drawing together material that has been discussed and it shows that you have been listening actively. You should always check that your summary is an accurate representation of the patient's views. For example:

> I'd like to pull together some of the things that you have said. Let me know if I have mis-interpreted something or if I have missed something out. So, you feel that … is that a fair summary? Have I left anything out?

There are times, however, when the person does not want to sit down and discuss what is on their mind. Here, a different set of skills is required to defuse and de-escalate the situation, and to resolve conflicts. It is important to consider not only what you say but also how you say it. You must adopt a non-critical and non-threatening approach tone. Approach the person cautiously, making sure that you do not startle the person. It is vital not to be seen as confrontational or provocative, either in words or behaviour – this will only inflame the situation further. Be aware of personal space. People who are angry need more personal space and the situation may escalate if you stand too close.

WHAT'S THE EVIDENCE?

The National Institute for Health and Care Excellence (NICE) has offered the following good practice advice for de-escalating potentially aggressive situations (NICE, 2005: 9): one staff member should assume control of a potentially disturbed/violent situation. This staff member should:

- consider which de-escalation techniques are appropriate for the situation
- manage others in the environment (for example, removing other service users from the area, getting colleagues to help and creating space) and move towards a safe place
- explain to the service user and others nearby what they intend to do, giving clear, brief, assertive instructions
- ask for facts about the problem and encourage reasoning (attempt to establish a rapport)
- offer and negotiate realistic options
- avoid threats
- ask open questions and ask about the reason for the service user's anger
- show concern and attentiveness through non-verbal and verbal responses
- listen carefully
- not patronise and not minimise the service user's concerns
- ensure that their own non-verbal communication is non-threatening and not provocative.

Maintaining professional boundaries

It is during times of challenge that your professionalism as nurses is most tested. From a nursing point of view, we need to consider our professionalism in handling challenging situations and that our respect for our patients is undiminished by their behaviour. That is, we need to ensure that we maintain good professional boundaries.

Assertion is a very important nursing skill which can be a very useful technique in managing challenging situations. It is very important to be able to distinguish between *assertiveness* and *aggressiveness*. Assertiveness is an interpersonal behaviour that 'attends to and informs others of one's own needs and feelings, and sends the message to the other in such a way that neither person is belittled, put down or blamed' (Porritt, 1990: 98).

There are some very important ideas here – assertiveness is an honest and positive means of expressing your own viewpoint clearly whilst listening to other people and respecting their views. When we are being assertive, we may agree to disagree. This, of course, does not rule out the possibility of negotiation and compromise.

It is very important to ensure one's own professional and ethical behaviour and professional boundaries when being assertive and when attempting to manage challenging situations, and to ensure that one works at all times within the spirit and letter of The Code (NMC, 2015).

Support

Attempting to resolve challenging situations and conflict can be emotionally and psychologically draining (McLaughlin et al., 2013) and can lead to a loss of self-esteem, reduced confidence and 'burnout'. It is vital that if you have been involved in such situations you are offered and receive support. Of course, everyone has their own mechanisms for coping, but it is vital for the psychological health of the nurse that they are able to discuss any issues that may impact on their ability to function as a nurse.

The first step in obtaining support is to first acknowledge that you need support. There is sometimes a feeling that nurses should be able to cope with anything and that any stress and distress they experience is 'part of the job'. This is simply not the case and there is always a possibility that nurses who do not receive support (both practical and emotional) at times of stress are at an increased risk of burnout. If you feel your exposure to challenging situations has led you to feel distressed, it is important that this is brought to the attention of your manager or, if you are a student, to your practice educator and/or personal tutor. Support is readily available to help you to discuss your feelings and you should not feel shame or embarrassment in accessing this if you feel it is appropriate.

CONCLUSION

In this chapter, we have explored a number of challenging situations in nursing. We have looked at the barriers to communication (such as language, mental health problems, unconsciousness, sensory impairments, culture, and so forth) and how we may overcome such barriers. We have discussed how we can ensure that our verbal and non-verbal communication and behaviour demonstrate our professionalism as nurses. We have also explored a number of techniques which could be used in attempting to resolve challenging situations, such as the nurse's ability to manage themselves, being able to build relationships, effective communication and maintaining professional boundaries. Finally, we stressed the importance of the nurse being able to access and receive emotional support.

———————————— CHAPTER SUMMARY ————————————

- There are many barriers to communication in nursing which nurses need to identify and learn how to overcome.
- There are professional and personal skills, knowledge and attitudes needed to handle challenging situations, including communication and interpersonal skills and the skills needed to de-escalate potentially aggressive situations.
- Being able to maintain professionalism during times of conflict is a reflection of the professional role of the nurse.
- Nurses need to have good professional boundaries during challenging situations.

———————————— CRITICAL REFLECTION ————————————

- Consider reasons why people's experiences of healthcare services can sometimes lead to frustration, confusion and anger. Think about nursing services you may have worked in from the viewpoint of patient/clients/service users and their carers and/or relatives. What could be done, do you think, to reduce the possibility of conflict between patients and healthcare staff?
- What level of support should nurses receive following their involvement in challenging situations?

GOING FURTHER

Books

A background understanding of how to utilise and develop effective communication skills is essential in nursing. The following books are particularly helpful in this regard:

McCabe, C. and Timmins, F. (2013) *Communication Skills for Nursing Practice*, 2nd edn. Basingstoke: Palgrave Macmillan. An excellent book which takes the reader through various aspects of communication in nursing practice. It is very easy to read and informative, and the section on conflict is very useful.

Nelson-Jones, R. (2015) *Basic Counselling Skills: A Helpers Manual*, 4th edn. London: SAGE. Nelson-Jones' approach is clear, practical and informative. The book is packed with useful examples and exercises to help you develop the fundamental skills of counselling which can be used in a wide variety of nursing situations.

SAGE journal articles

FURTHER
READING:
JOURNAL
ARTICLES

Go to https://study.sagepub.com/essentialnursing2e for free online journal articles for this chapter. If you are using the interactive ebook, simply click on the book icon in the margin to go straight to the resource.

Schmidt Bunkers, S. (2010) 'The power and possibility in listening', *Nursing Science Quarterly*, 23(1): 22–27.

Other journal articles

Bonner, G. and McLaughlin, S. (2007) 'The psychological impact of aggression on nursing staff', *British Journal of Nursing*, 16(13): 810–14. This excellent article looks at the impact of aggression and suggests ways in which nurses and organisations can support people who have been involved in challenging situations.

Duxbury, J. and Whittington, R. (2005) 'Causes and management of patient aggression and violence: Staff and patient perspectives', *Journal of Advanced Nursing*, 50(5): 469–78. This article looks at the various reasons why conflict may occur in hospital settings and how patients and staff may perceive the events (and their causation) differently.

Lowe, T., Wellman, N. and Taylor, R. (2003) 'Limit-setting and decision-making in the management of aggression', *Journal of Advanced Nursing*, 41(2): 154–61. This study explores nursing staff's perceptions of, and preference for, various interventions in the management of aggressive behaviour.

Weblinks

FURTHER
READING:
WEBLINKS

Go to https://study.sagepub.com/essentialnursing2e for weblinks related to this chapter. If you are using the interactive ebook, simply click on the book icon in the margin to go straight to the resource.

National Institute for Health and Care Excellence (NICE) (2005) *Violence: The Short-Term Management of Disturbed/Violent Behaviour in In-patient Psychiatric Settings and Emergency Departments*. Available at: www.nice.org.uk/CG25. While this resource tends to focus on reducing violent behaviour, there is much here which will be helpful in understanding best-practice responses to angry and aggressive behaviour.

Other useful weblinks include:

www.asrn.org/journal-nursing-today/356-dealing-with-the-difficult-patient.html – this link presents a number of strategies and points to consider when communication between nurse and patient becomes difficult.

www.ausmed.com.au/blog/entry/every-nurses-nightmare-dealing-with-difficult-patients – within this link very useful tips are given upon how to manage challenging behaviour.

www.nursingcenter.com/lnc/journalarticle?Article_ID=1090605 – it is not only the patient who you need to communicate effectively with, relatives can become stressed and may be challenging. This link offers advice and strategies that you will find helpful in managing challenging situations with a patients relative.

ACE YOUR ASSESSMENT

Review what you have learned by visiting the book's online resources at: https://study.sagepub.com/essential nursing2e If using your interactive ebook, just click on the icon in the margin to go straight there.

ONLINE
QUIZZES

- Test yourself with multiple-choice and short-answer questions.
- Revise key terms with the interactive flash cards.

REFERENCES

Hawking, S. and Mlodinow, L. (2010) *The Grand Design*. New York: Bantam Books.

Hindle, S. (2003) 'Psychological factors affecting communication', in R. Ellis, B. Gates and N. Kenworthy (eds) *Interpersonal Communication in Nursing Theory*, 2nd edn. London: Churchill Livingstone.

Kirby, S.D. and Cross, D. (2002) 'Socially constructed narrative interventions: A foundation for therapeutic alliances', in A.M. Kettles, P. Woods and M. Collins (eds) *Therapeutic Interventions for Forensic Mental Health*. London: Jessica Kingsley Publishers. pp. 187–205.

Leigh, K. (2001) 'Communicating with unconscious patients', *Nursing Times*, 97(48): 35–6.

McCabe, C. and Timmins, F. (2013) *Communication Skills for Nursing Practice*, 2nd edn. Basingstoke: Palgrave Macmillan.

McLaughlin, S., Pearce, R. and Trenoweth, S. (2013) 'Reducing conflict on wards by improving team communication', *Mental Health Practice*, 16(50): 27–9.

Miller, W.R. and Rollnick, S. (2002) *Motivational Interviewing: Preparing People for Change*, 2nd edn. New York: Guilford Press.

National Institute for Health and Care Excellence (NICE) (2005) *Violence: The Short-Term Management of Disturbed/Violent Behaviour in In-patient Psychiatric Settings and Emergency Departments*. Available at: www.nice.org.uk/CG25 (accessed 1 August 2017).

Nelson-Jones, R. (2015) *Basic Counselling Skills: A Helpers Manual*, 4th edn. London: SAGE.

Nursing and Midwifery Council (NMC) (2013) *Working with Young People*. Available at: www.nmc-uk. org/Nurses-and-midwives/Regulation-in-practice/Regulation-in-Practice-Topics/Advice-for-nurses-and-midwives-working-with-young-people (accessed 1 August 2017).

Nursing and Midwifery Council (NMC) (2015) *The Code: Professional Standards of Practice and Behaviour for Nurses and Midwives*. Available at: www.nmc.org.uk/standards/code (accessed 1 August 2017).

Papadopoulos, I., Tilki, M. and Taylor, G. (1998) *Transcultural Care: A Guide for Health Care Professionals*. Dinton, Wilts: Quay Books.

Porritt, L. (1990) *Interaction Strategies: An Introduction for Health Professionals*, 2nd edn. Melbourne: Churchill Livingstone.

World Health Organization (WHO) (2004) *ICD-10: International Statistical Classification of Diseases and Related Health Problems – Tenth Revision*. Vol. 2, 2nd edn. Available at: www.who.int/classifications/icd/ICD-10_2nd_ed_volume2.pdf (accessed 1 August 2017).

ENSURING QUALITY AND EFFECTIVE MANAGEMENT OF RISK

17

MELANIE FISHER, MARGARET SCOTT AND KAREN ELCOCK

THIS CHAPTER COVERS

- What is quality?
- Quality in health and social care settings
- Why quality monitoring is important
- The concept of risk assessment
- What is risk assessment?

- Risk assessment: the skills required
- Managing risk
- Risk management in practice
- The contribution of incident reporting to the risk-management process

> " Assessing risk is very important in mental health nursing, individuals that are in need of specialist care from mental health services may be at a point where they are of a high risk to themselves or others. It is part of my role to be able to assess for risk factors and changes in how a person is presenting and deliver care according to their needs. If a person is feeling very low in mood and has a history of self harm I would need to consider if this person needs to have extra support at that time, whether they are at an increased risk of harming themselves and what care needs to be considered to help them through this. Assessing risk can be a complex process and I feel that it is important to discuss risk as a multidisciplinary team in order to effectively deliver care.
>
> **Samantha Vanes, NQ RNMH** "

> " It was the Francis Report that finally opened my eyes to the importance of monitoring quality in healthcare. Until then I'd seen it as a real nuisance that took me away from my patients. Now I appreciate not only why it is important to monitor quality but more importantly why it is important to act upon the results.
>
> **Nikolas, charge nurse, medical ward** "

Visit https://study.sagepub.com/essentialnursing2e to access a wealth of online resources for this chapter – watch out for the margin icons throughout the chapter. If you are using the interactive eBook, simply click on the margin icon to go straight to the resource.

INTRODUCTION

The purpose of this chapter is to examine quality and safety in healthcare delivery. As a registered nurse, you will play a key role in meeting people's needs for high-quality, safe care. Our aim is to introduce the concept of quality in nursing and also to examine the importance of effective risk assessment and management of risk.

Patient safety and effective risk assessment are key to the assurance of quality in healthcare delivery. Risk assessment and the management of risk cannot be viewed in isolation – both concepts have specific definitions and functions but each concept is multi-faceted and it would be unlikely to have one without the other. You will learn that within healthcare risks do exist and that no matter how hard we try to eliminate risk, having no risk at all is just not achievable. There is little doubt that the Francis Report on the failings at the Mid Staffordshire NHS Foundation Trust (Francis, 2010, 2013) has again raised the importance of not only how organisations monitor the quality of the care they deliver, but also how they respond to issues of concern, as well as where accountability lies – at all levels of healthcare organisations – when problems arise. In particular, there is a call for promotion of a culture in healthcare delivery which is candid, transparent and open. Francis (2015) reminds everyone engaged in healthcare delivery that we have a responsibility to 'speak up' and raise concerns if we witness sub-optimal care, and this includes student nurses.

WHAT IS QUALITY?

The concept of quality within healthcare is challenging to define, as it is something that will have different meanings to different people: the government, finance teams, healthcare professionals, patients and carers, to name but a few.

ACTIVITY 17.1: REFLECTIVE PRACTICE

- Reflect on your own experience as a user of healthcare.
- What are your views on what constitutes a quality service?

The World Health Organization (WHO, 2006) uses a definition of healthcare quality developed by the Institute of Medicine (IOM) in the USA in 2001 (IOM, 2001) that identifies six dimensions for healthcare quality: to be effective, efficient, accessible, patient-centred, equitable and safe. Did your answer to Activity 17.1 include any of these areas? Each country in the UK has different organisations responsible for the monitoring of quality in healthcare organisations but common to all is a framework of clinical governance.

QUALITY IN HEALTH AND SOCIAL CARE SETTINGS

A focus on quality in health and social care settings is, rather surprisingly, relatively new, arising in the late 1990s as a direct response by the Labour government of the time to a number of serious failings within healthcare, such as those found in the Bristol Inquiry and the Shipman Inquiry and at Liverpool Children's Hospital. These failings led to investigations that identified not only variations in the quality of service provision between different organisations, but also a lack of accountability within them. The investigations led to the Labour government publishing its white paper, *The New NHS: Modern, Dependable* (DH, 1997), which, for the first time, put quality at the centre of the NHS, and following this up by setting out its plans to realise that vision in *A First Class Service: Quality in the New NHS* (DH, 1998). This was soon followed by an enquiry into how risk is managed in the NHS and the publication of the report *Organisation with a Memory* (DH, 2000).

The framework set out by the government in these publications centred on a system of clinical governance, with chief executives – on behalf of their board – made accountable for the clinical quality of their organisation in addition to its financial performance (which had previously been their main responsibility and focus (Dixon et al., 2012)).

WHY QUALITY MONITORING IS IMPORTANT

The argument for the importance of the ongoing monitoring of quality in health and social care is put very simply by Sir Bruce Keogh in his foreword to the draft report by the National Quality Board (NQB), *Quality in the New Health System: Maintaining and Improving Quality from April 2013*, in which he says:

> A relentless focus on quality means a relentless focus on how we can positively transform the lives of the people who use and rely on our services. In contrast, a failure to focus on quality and to make it our primary concern can result in lasting emotional and physical damage to patients and even death. The appalling failures at Mid Staffordshire NHS foundation trust and at the independent hospital, Winterbourne View, provide stark reminders that when we fall short on our responsibilities in respect of quality, the consequences for patients, service users and their families can be catastrophic. (NQB, 2013: 4)

At both Mid Staffordshire and Winterbourne View, there was failure at all levels to monitor quality outcomes and key risk indicators, with senior management focusing on the organisations' financial matters rather than on quality through clinical governance (DH, 2012; Francis, 2013). Clinical governance is therefore seen as key to quality monitoring, but there are a number of different approaches to monitoring quality, some of which will involve you, both as a student and as a registered nurse.

How is quality monitored?

The quality of healthcare is monitored at two levels: independent bodies at a national level which monitor an organisation as a whole, and each healthcare organisation's own internal systems and processes of monitoring through a framework of clinical governance.

While the central aim of clinical governance is to improve quality and safety in healthcare, the most important element is to make clear the accountability of everyone involved in the delivery of healthcare, from practitioners (including students) to managers at the topmost level (Pridmore and Gammon, 2007). Despite this, there remains a lack of clarity about the responsibility that staff at different levels in healthcare organisations have in implementing clinical governance. In the UK, this is compounded by the fact that England, Scotland, Wales and Northern Ireland have developed different clinical governance frameworks and processes for implementation and monitoring, and use slightly different terms, driven by country-specific policies (Pridmore and Gammon, 2007). For students, this can be problematic, as much of the literature tends to be based on the approach used in England. In addition, much of the literature focusing on clinical governance as a topic in its own right is now relatively old, as the focus has moved to publications on discrete elements of clinical governance and each change in government has led to changes in the bodies with responsibility for or charged with providing guidance on clinical governance. It is therefore important for you not only to be aware of the current underpinning policies and approaches used within your own country, but also to understand the different components of clinical governance and utilise these terms when undertaking literature searches, to ensure that your understanding is both contemporary and relevant to the country in which you are practising. The key components of clinical governance are patient and public involvement, risk management, clinical standards, staffing, education, accurate information and clinical audit. Clinical audits are widely used in practice and you may have come across these whilst on placements.

ACTIVITY 17.2: REFLECTION

Discuss with your practice educator and the staff at your placement what nursing audits are undertaken in their area, and ask if you can participate in one. Reflect on the findings and the implications of the results on care in that area.

ACTIVITY 17.3: CRITICAL THINKING

Explore the website of an organisation where you have recently had a placement. You will find that they publish key reports on patient and staff surveys, on their quality outcomes and from quality inspections:

- Have any areas of risk been identified that the organisation needs to take action on?
- How do these relate to your own experience there?

The ability to recognise where an individual or group of patients may be at risk is essential to ensure that the patients you care for do not come to harm, and therefore it is important that you know how to both assess for risk and manage it.

THE CONCEPT OF RISK ASSESSMENT

There are many activities and actions that can be used to minimise and reduce risks, and by appropriately assessing and managing risk we can significantly improve patient satisfaction and outcome. Risk assessment tools are one element of risk assessment; other core nursing skills which contribute equally to a robust and accurate risk assessment will be discussed. Evidence-based research, policy drivers and legislation are explored in relation to risk assessment and this is applied to clinical practice through the use of activities.

Consideration is given to the ways in which risk is managed, drawing on case studies and activities to help readers think about what risk and risk management mean to them, relating general principles to their own practical experience. We acknowledge that, as humans, errors and mistakes are made. It is believed that, through reporting mistakes, valuable learning can take place to prevent the same mistakes from occurring again. We will take into account the contribution of 'incident' reporting to the risk-management process, and that, through reporting, patient satisfaction and care can improve dramatically.

Assessment of and managing risk play a large part in nursing and patient safety. We take risks every day – whether crossing the road, driving a car or using other modes of transport. People will generally take risks if they feel that there is an advantage or benefit, so how does this apply to nursing and healthcare in general?

Risk is the chance that any activity or action could happen and harm you. When patients consider having a procedure, intervention or screening, they need to know not only the benefits but also the risks involved, so that they can make an informed decision. If a patient decides to undergo a procedure, their informed decision-making forms the basis of their decision to give informed consent. It could appear that many patients will have a large degree of control over this situation, as they will have already given due consideration to the benefit of a procedure and whether or not these outweigh the risk. However, we must not forget that many of those we care for are vulnerable patients. They may not be able to give informed consent because of mental health needs or a learning disability, for example, or will simply give their consent to anything because they think that is what is expected of them. Many patients, including those who when you meet them do not seem vulnerable, would not feel able to question or challenge a nurse or other healthcare provider.

It is important to remember that we, as nurses, along with all healthcare professionals, have a responsibility to warn patients of the known risks of any procedure, care or treatment. This responsibility isn't altered by the risk being very small. If you fail to do this, you may be liable to an accusation of negligence (Fisher and Scott, 2013).

There are also aspects of healthcare delivery where patients have little or no control over risk, for example contracting an infection during a hospital stay, or a piece of equipment malfunctioning and injuring them. So, when caring for patients, although it is impossible to eliminate all risks, we have a duty to protect patients as far as is 'reasonably practicable'. This means that when caring for patients you must always avoid any unnecessary risk.

Zero risk does not exist

As we have found, there is no such thing as zero risk, so we need to recognise that all care and treatment carry some risk that cannot be avoided or escaped. However, it is best to focus on the risks that really matter – those with the potential to cause harm. When we consider risk, we need to do so in partnership with benefit. This then aids us to work out whether the risk is acceptable.

To calculate what an acceptable risk is, we need to find the balance between the possible adverse effects or degree of harm with the expected benefits. If the possible adverse effect or degree of harm seems a risk worth taking in order to achieve the expected benefits, the risk becomes acceptable (see Figure 17.1).

There is, however, a personal element in this, as some individuals are more accepting of others. For example, in June 2012 Nik Wallendar felt that the risk of walking across Niagara Falls (Canada) on a tightrope was an acceptable one. His gamble paid off and he became the first person to walk right over the Falls. Such acceptance of huge risk has no place in nursing, so, to assist us to provide safe care by applying an evidence-based approach, when caring for patients we undertake a risk assessment.

Figure 17.1   An acceptable risk

Image © Robin Lupton

WHAT IS RISK ASSESSMENT?

Statistics tell us that patients do come to harm due to exposure to risk, some of which is unforeseen but some of which is foreseeable. There are 24,000 serious incidents of healthcare harm in the NHS each year (DH, 2017). When harm is foreseeable, there are steps we must take to minimise it. To do this, there are a number of risk assessments that enable us to manage risk, thus improving the quality and safety of patient care.

ACTIVITY 17.4: CRITICAL THINKING – RISK

ANSWER:
ACTIVITY 17.4

- Think about your experience during your last placement.
- What types of risks were the patients you were involved in caring for exposed to?

Whilst advances and innovations in healthcare increase our ability to successfully treat patients with more complex illnesses, they also bring the potential for greater risk and harm. In its simplest form, risk can be described as the potential for an unwanted outcome. An example of this is if you decided to cross the road 10 metres away from a pedestrian crossing and got knocked over by an oncoming car. You have taken a risk, because you ignored the increased safety offered by the pedestrian crossing. The unwanted outcome for you is that you got knocked over, with the potential of causing irreversible harm.

Everyday nursing practice can present similar risks. For example, whilst you are escorting a patient who requires assistance to walk to the bathroom, you notice that another patient has spilled their drink on the floor. The potential for someone to slip on the wet floor is evident but there is no one else around to wipe up the spillage. However, once again, in the same way as when you crossed the road without using the pedestrian crossing, you take a risk. You continue to escort the patent safely to the bathroom.

In choosing to do this rather than wipe up the drink, you have allowed there to be a potential for another patient or member of staff to slip on the wet floor, again an unwanted outcome.

The risk in this case is foreseeable and, as we have discussed, you should always undertake the actions necessary to minimise any potential harm to others. The action you should have taken was to ensure that the patient you were escorting to the bathroom remained safe, by, for example, seating them comfortably on a chair, then wiping up the spilt drink. By recognising the opportunity to act proactively and prevent problems by applying an evidence-based approach, the risk of harm can be reduced. You had the opportunity to cross the road using an evidence-based approach that would reduce the risk of harm (the pedestrian crossing), and then to be proactive and prevent problems (by wiping up the spill). Whilst neither of these actions was in itself anything out of the ordinary, they both had the potential to deliver a far more positive outcome than your choices brought you.

Oh dear, you really are not having a good day!

In daily nursing practice, not all risks are as easy to identify as a slippery floor, so to help us assess and manage risks for those in our care we use a wide range of risk assessment and management tools.

Examples of tools used to assess and manage risk are:

- malnutrition screening – MUST
- early warning scores
- falls risk assessment
- pain assessment
- pressure ulcer assessment
- suicide behaviours questionnaire
- swallowing assessment.

This is not an exhaustive list. You are likely to be familiar with some of the above; other risk identification tools or methods might be less obvious, for example risk assessments for clients at risk, or with a risk of violence. We also refer to other useful sources of data to help us identify risk:

- incident reports
- audit reports
- patient complaints and feedback
- policies and procedures.

ACTIVITY 17.5: DECISION-MAKING

Gregor is 85 years old and has Alzheimer's disease. Until recently, he has been cared for at the home of his daughter who is 63. However, she has found it increasingly difficult to manage Gregor as he has become increasingly confused, aggressive at times, and refuses to eat and take his medication. He has suffered weight loss, clearly looks emaciated and his mobility is poor.

You have been asked to admit Gregor to the nursing home you are on placement at and complete his nursing assessment:

- What potential risks do you think Gregor may be exposed to?
- What assessment tools would you use for his risk assessment?

ANSWER:
ACTIVITY 17.5

RISK ASSESSMENT: THE SKILLS REQUIRED

Whilst, as we have seen, there are a number of risk assessment tools available to assist nurses in identifying risk factors in groups of patients, these are only part of our risk assessment tool kit. It is important to recognise that assessment tools are only effective if they are used in conjunction with your own clinical decision-making and professional judgement, and in collaboration with the patient and others involved in providing care. The ability to perform a robust and accurate assessment is a core nursing skill and significant data must not be missed.

CASE STUDY 17.1: CATHERINE

Catherine is a 50-year-old teacher who has been admitted to the surgical investigation unit for an exploratory endoscopy following a number of visits to her GP with gastric problems. She recently moved 200 miles away from her home town, where she had lived since she was born, because her husband had changed his job. She has just started a new job herself but is finding it hard to adjust to so many changes.

Catherine attended the **pre-assessment clinic** a week ago where she was assessed by a registered nurse and a healthcare assistant (HA) to ensure she was fit to undergo an exploratory endoscopy. They asked her a number of questions regarding her general health, and her blood pressure, pulse and temperature were taken and recorded.

When Catherine returns on the morning of her procedure, she is greeted by Jane, a different registered nurse, and asked to put on a hospital gown and wait by a bed. After looking through Catherine's notes from her pre-assessment, Jane notes that her pulse is a bit higher than she would have expected – 105 beats per minute, so she decides to take it again. This time Catherine's pulse is 110 and the beats are irregular. When Jane speaks to the registered nurse and HA who performed the pre-assessment observations, it becomes apparent that the HA had used an automated machine to measure Catherine's pulse, which would not have detected that it was irregular.

Jane alerts the doctor and a decision is made to postpone the procedure until further investigations are performed. Catherine is very upset that her endoscopy has been cancelled.

- What are the risk issues arising from this case study?
- What skills did Jane use to assess and manage the risks associated with Catherine's care?

As a nurse, in order to accurately assess risk, we need to possess a number of fundamental skills:

- observational skills
- clinical decision-making and professional judgement
- effective communication skills
- a contemporary evidence-based knowledge which includes an understanding of relevant policy, procedure and legislation.

Observational skills

As Florence Nightingale (1859/1946) points out, 'The most important practical lesson that can be given to nurses is to teach them what to observe – how to observe'. Being able to make accurate observations as a nurse is one of the most important and frequently used skills. These observations will relate to every aspect of a patient, not just those identifying their physiological status, such as temperature, blood pressure and pulse.

When assessing risk, we need to observe a patient's general appearance, psychological status, nutritional status and habits, to name just a few. All of the risk assessment tools we use require us to accurately observe an aspect of a patient's functioning. If we are unable to do this, no matter how good the tools are, they will not assist us to deliver safe and effective care.

Clinical decision-making and professional judgement

Nursing involves planned as well as unplanned decisions, so clinical decision-making and professional judgement are key components of nursing care. Clinical decision-making involves reviewing the potential consequences (risks and benefits) of possible alternative actions before committing oneself one way or another. Professional judgement is used to review options before a decision is made (Standing, 2017). This includes recognising your own limitations and lack of experience.

CASE STUDY:
WILL

Professional judgement is particularly important when delegating care. In order to delegate the appropriate task to the appropriate person, nurses must be aware of their own accountability and the role of others. When delegating an activity of care to another person, you must be certain that they are competent and have received adequate and appropriate training to perform the activity. We saw this not to be so in the care given to Catherine at her pre-admission clinic visit. The registered nurses judged it was safe to delegate taking Catherine's pulse to the healthcare assistant. However, due to a lack of knowledge the healthcare assistant used an automated machine, which did not detect that Catherine's pulse was irregular. This could indicate that there was a problem with her heart. So, if Catherine had undergone the procedure as planned, she might have been harmed due to the registered nurses' error in judgement.

Effective communication skills

As is outlined in Chapters 15 and 16, out of all the skills a nurse must possess, the ability to communicate effectively is the most important. Failure to communicate effectively with patients, carers and other healthcare professionals can have serious consequences for all involved. Within your role as a nurse, the onus is on you to communicate effectively with the patients in your care. We must ensure that our verbal and non-verbal communication reinforces our primary nursing goal – to deliver safe care for all patients at all times. Thus, accurate risk assessment has to be built on effective communication.

A contemporary evidence-based knowledge which includes an understanding of relevant policy, procedure and legislation

The decisions we make about care must be based on the latest evidence and best practice. Using the latest evidence and best practice available in all aspects of your nursing practice promotes care delivery that is both safe and effective.

This, in a similar manner to observation, communication and clinical decision-making and professional judgement, is fundamental to accurate risk assessment. If your knowledge base is not contemporary or you have no understanding of relevant policy, procedure and legislation, no matter what tools you apply in your risk assessment you will not be able to deliver safe care.

So, it becomes very clear that risk assessment cannot be viewed in isolation. Further to this, if we are aiming to provide the best possible care for patients, then we must also consider the most appropriate way to manage those risks that have been identified.

MANAGING RISK

Although it may now seem surprising, the essentials of risk management, which linked processes for identifying, analysing and controlling risk, were not evident in the NHS until the mid-1990s.

In 1995, the NHS Litigation Authority (NHSLA) was established in order to manage the Clinical Negligence Scheme for Trusts (CNST). The CNST handles clinical negligence claims against all NHS Trusts. The NHSLA has two main responsibilities which are:

- working towards improving risk management practices in the NHS
- handling negligence claims made against NHS organisations.

Consider the news headlines below in relation to your own practice experiences.

News headlines

During 2012–13, it was found that 16,006 relatives of patients had lodged claims against the NHS, up from 13,517 a year earlier.

The chief executive of the Patients Associated states that 'most people only pursue legal action when every other avenue has failed … people who contact us say that all they wanted was an explanation of what went wrong, and changes made so that nobody else would suffer'. (Donnelly, 2013)

These facts and figures might not come as a surprise, but there is a significant yearly increase in the number of claims lodged against the NHS. Initially, risk management was designed to control the cost of litigation, but now, more importantly, the aims have been extended to reducing incidents of harm and improving the quality of care delivered.

The current approach of the NHSLA is to assess Trusts against a set of standards that aim to improve processes and risk management systems. However, it is worth noting that limitations within the existing standards and assessment process have been recognised and the fact has been acknowledged that even if a risk management system exists which complies with the existing NHSLA standards, it does not in itself mean that the Trust is safe.

Several high-profile system failures, in which major lapses in the quality of care have resulted in serious injuries to patients, have done much to raise public and professional awareness about the risks of healthcare and the need to actively explore ways of making healthcare safer for both patients and staff.

ACTIVITY 17.6: CRITICAL THINKING – SYSTEM FAILURES

ANSWER:
ACTIVITY 17.6

What high-profile system failures can you think of that have highlighted the risks associated with healthcare?

There has been a great deal learned from these high-profile system failures, part of which has resulted in the recognition that there are numerous important factors when considering safety, and although effective risk management processes are important, they are only one of many things that should be considered when assessing whether practices are safe.

RISK MANAGEMENT IN PRACTICE

Once a potential for harm has been identified and to some degree measured through risk assessment, a plan is designed and implemented to avoid risks and reduce the likelihood of damage and loss. Although risk management does not have a secret recipe, it involves acting on those areas that have been identified as potentially 'risky' or harmful by changing a set of circumstances, the environment or behaviour to reduce the potential for and amount of risk. The result of appropriately managing risk is improved patient satisfaction and outcomes.

We know that healthcare is inherently risky and we have established that there is no such thing as zero risk, but there are many activities and actions that can be taken to minimise and reduce those opportunities for errors to occur.

EXTRA
CASE STUDY!

CASE STUDY:
JENNA

ACTIVITY 17.7: CRITICAL THINKING – DEFINING RISK MANAGEMENT IN YOUR PRACTICE

There are many variations when defining risk management in practice:

- How would you define the term 'risk management' in relation to the care you were involved in providing on your last placement?

ANSWER:
ACTIVITY 17.7

Three common themes present in nearly all definitions of risk management, which are the

- identification
- evaluation and
- correction

of potential risks. Risk management can be both *proactive*, which is the avoidance and prevention of risk, and *reactive*, which relates to loss or subsequent damage following an event that has caused harm or an undesirable outcome.

CASE STUDY 17.2: EMILY

Emily is 29 years old and has physical and intellectual disabilities due to **Down's syndrome**. She has severely impacted wisdom teeth and has been admitted to hospital to have them removed. Emily has significant cardiac problems due to the Down's syndrome and takes a range of medication to support

(Continued)

her heart. Therefore, the decision has been made to first attempt to remove her wisdom teeth in the operating theatre under local anaesthetic, as this will put less strain on her heart. Only if this is not possible will a general anaesthetic be administered.

The theatre team prepare for Emily's arrival and in doing so they prepare the necessary equipment and drugs for both a local anaesthetic and a general anaesthetic, should this be required.

To ensure that there is no possibility of Emily contracting an infection, it is routine for an antibiotic to be administered, regardless of whether her teeth are removed under local or general anaesthetic. The antibiotic and the induction agent – a drug given at the start of a general anaesthetic to make a patient unconscious – are drawn up into two separate 20 ml syringes. The colour of each drug is identical and the only way to distinguish between the two syringes is by using different-coloured labels – antibiotic (white label) and induction agent (yellow label).

Emily arrives in theatre and all goes well, with her teeth removed under local anaesthetic. The anaesthetist then administers the routine antibiotic. Thirty seconds later, Emily becomes unconscious.

The induction agent had been given in error. Even though the drugs had been clearly and appropriately labelled, a momentary 'lapse in concentration' occurred and Emily was given the wrong drug. The incident occurred due to an error in human performance.

- Could this situation have been avoided?

Case study 17.2 illustrates an example of *reactive* risk management. Fortunately, Emily did not come to any harm despite her cardiac problems, but an undesirable outcome occurred following an event. The anaesthetic team would need to support Emily's airways and monitor her cardiac function until the drug had worn off and she was able to breath unaided.

To avoid situations, such as those described in Emily's case, healthcare organisations use a variety of methods to manage risks. The success of any risk management programme depends on:

- creating and maintaining safe systems of care
- improved human performance
- designing systems where adverse events or situations that can cause harm are reduced.

As we outlined at the start of the chapter, just as when you choose not to wipe up a spilled drink and allow another nurse to slip, we are all responsible for taking the correct action when we see a potentially unsafe situation or environment. It is important that we report such incidents so that the correct steps can be taken to avoid similar incidents in the future. We know from 'News headlines' that the majority of people who pursue legal action would have preferred some sort of acknowledgement that 'changes would be made so that nobody else would suffer', rather than the emotional and lengthy process of litigation.

It is important to move away from a culture of blaming individuals to one where we learn from mistakes and complaints. Acknowledging the fact that errors and mistakes do happen because we are *human* is an opportunity to improve the quality of care and to implement improvements.

Effective risk management involves everyone within a healthcare system, so we all need to understand risk management and the objectives of strategies to reduce risk.

ACTIVITY 17.8: CRITICAL THINKING – EMILY

Re-read case study 17.2 and consider Emily's story in relation to the three common themes present in most definitions of risk management:

- identification
- evaluation
- correction.

How do you think the risks present could have been identified – are there any *assessment tools* that you could use?

- Now consider the *evaluation* component of the incident. What do you think this actually means?
- What factors could have influenced the undesirable outcome for Emily?
- Think about *correction*. What recommendations could you suggest to reduce the likelihood of a similar situation occurring again?

THE CONTRIBUTION OF INCIDENT REPORTING TO THE RISK-MANAGEMENT PROCESS

As we saw from the incident involving Emily, human error is inevitable. Reducing the likelihood of harm occurring and minimising the consequences of any harm that does occur are best achieved by learning from errors, rather than attributing blame. By collecting information from incidents, errors and near misses (it almost happened, but didn't) and feeding that information into management systems, it is possible to drastically reduce the chances of future incidents, or at least minimise the impact of any errors or incidents that do occur.

ACTIVITY 17.9: CRITICAL THINKING – YOUR PLACEMENT

Think about your last placement:

- What systems were in place to report incidents?
- Would you feel confident in reporting an incident which directly involved you?
- What, if any, are the barriers to reporting incidents?

We are only human

Studying human error can be a very powerful tool for preventing disaster or harm. 'Human factors' is a strategy that is being implemented to improve patient safety and it is gaining great momentum in the UK. Human factors is essentially an umbrella term which encompasses all those factors that influence people and their behaviour, such as the environment, organisational and job factors, design and individual characteristics which influence behaviour at work (Patient Safety First, 2009).

Focusing on human factors can lead to improvements in day-to-day clinical operations through an appreciation of the effects of teamwork on human behaviour and the application of this to the healthcare setting (Clinical Human Factors Group, 2017). Putting it simply, human factors can be thought of as a concept of designing things to make it easy for people to use and do the right thing. The design of the workplace, equipment and ways in which we work should be based on human characteristics and abilities – how we process information, communicate, make decisions and remember things, rather than expecting people to adapt to the poorly designed world around them (Norris, 2009).

What if you witness practice that is sub-optimal or compromises patient safety?

As a student nurse, you are required to act in the patient's best interest in the same way you will be required to as a registrant. In order to register, you are required to demonstrate that you are able to understand and act in line with local and national frameworks, legislation and regulations for assessing, managing and reporting risks, ensuring that appropriate action is taken. The NMC *Standards of Proficiency for Registered Nurses* (2018) require that you:

6.8 Demonstrate an understanding of how to identify, report and critically reflect on near misses, critical incidents, major incidents and serious adverse events in order to learn from and influence future practice.

6.10 Apply an understanding of the differences between effective risk management and risk aversion to avoid compromising quality of care and health outcomes.

6.11 Acknowledge the need to accept and manage uncertainty, and demonstrate awareness of strategies that develop resilience in themselves and others.

It is expected that you will speak up on behalf of people in your care as an everyday part of your role. Failure to report concerns may bring your fitness to practise into question. However, it is generally acknowledged that nurses and students in particular find raising concerns challenging for a variety of reasons. Raising concerns is often referred to as 'whistleblowing' and this can often have negative connotations. Nonetheless, Francis (2015) advocates that students are ideally placed to recognise substandard practice because they bring 'fresh eyes' to the practice placement.

In order to support students and registrants to raise a concern, the NMC (2015a) issued guidance to nurses which should be read in conjunction with the Code (NMC, 2015b). In addition, healthcare organisations have policies in place on whistleblowing. Providers of education in nursing raise awareness of this in their curricula. It is important that you are aware of policies and procedures in relation to raising concerns and you should also be aware of who to report your concerns to.

CASE STUDY 17.3: MR SENGUPTA

You have been allocated to a busy colorectal ward for an eight-week placement. Tuesdays are particularly busy, with an all-day operating list, and your practice educator has asked you to work alongside the health care assistant (HCA) to ensure that all post-surgical patients have vital observations taken regularly. At first glance, the HCA appears to be very competent and efficient, completing several sets of observations while you have only managed to complete one full set. You become concerned as you know that you are spending time to complete the observations accurately, which prompts you to double-check the HCA's documentation of vital observations. It is apparent that the HCA has been directly copying previous observations, without actually undertaking the observations herself. While you are double-checking Mr Sengupta's post-surgical vital observation, it very quickly becomes apparent that he is deteriorating, his blood pressure has dropped, and his pulse rate has increased, as has his respiratory rate. The HCA recorded only two minutes earlier that all observations were within normal limits, identical to the observations recorded 30 minutes earlier. You check Mr Sengupta's surgical dressing and drains, noticing that there is almost one litre of fresh blood in one of the drains. It is obvious that Mr Sengupta is bleeding internally and needs to return to theatre as soon as possible. You alert your practice educator to the situation. Mr Sengupta returns to theatre and the bleeding is arrested. You are commended on your vigilance and management of the situation.

ACTIVITY 17.10: CRITICAL THINKING – MR SENGUPTA

Read case study 17.3 and consider the following:

- Has the HCA done anything wrong?
- Do you know how to access your university policy and trust policy on raising concerns?
- If you witness substandard practice, would you know who to report it to?
- Which section of the NMC *Standards of Proficiency for Registered Nurses* (2018) applies to this particular case study?

CONCLUSION

This chapter has introduced you to the concept of quality care and risk assessment. The quality of care delivered to patients and how concerns are responded to, are of fundamental importance. As technology advances and life expectancy increases, so too has the need to carefully consider levels of risk been heightened. Risk assessment and risk management are so closely intertwined that they cannot be viewed as two separate entities. Put simply, they are two sides of the same coin, which can work together to provide safe care, patient satisfaction and positive outcomes.

Risk assessment and risk management are both multifaceted and complex and the success of a safer NHS depends on many factors. Learning valuable lessons in relation to risk can only serve to benefit healthcare organisations and the patients and staff that work within them.

CHAPTER SUMMARY

- To deliver quality care, we must remain risk-aware and develop skills to enable us to carry out effective risk assessment and manage risk appropriately.
- As nurses, we will work with a variety of patients, some of whom are more vulnerable than others, and therefore we must develop skills of assessing and managing risk.

- Sound decision-making and professional judgement are very important in managing risk.
- Students must be aware of relevant legislation and policy drivers in relation to risk management.
- Students must understand the relationship between risk assessment and risk management.
- Students must acknowledge the value of reporting and learning from incidents that occur in everyday clinical practice.
- It is imperative that students value and recognise the importance of contemporary evidence-based knowledge, policy, procedure and legislation.

CRITICAL REFLECTION

If you are asked to carry out a specific risk assessment on a patient, for example malnutrition screening (MUST) or using the Suicide Behaviours Questionnaire (SBQ-R), how would this influence the overall care of the patient?

GO FURTHER

Books

Fisher, M. and Scott, M. (2013) *Patient Safety and Managing Risk in Nursing*. Exeter: Learning Matters.
Gottwald, M. and Lansdown, G.E. (2014) *Clinical Governance: Improving the Quality of Healthcare for Patients and Service Users*. Maidenhead: Open University Press.
Hart, C. (2014) *A Pocket Guide to Risk Assessment and Management in Mental Health*. Abingdon: Routledge.

Report

Francis, R. (2013) *The Mid Staffordshire NHS Foundation Trust Public Inquiry*. London: The Stationery Office. Available at: www.gov.uk/government/publications/report-of-the-mid-staffordshire-nhs-foundation-trust-public-inquiry. A pivotal report focusing on the events at Mid Staffordshire Hospital. Within the report are a number of recommendations which all nurses need to be aware of.

SAGE journal articles

FURTHER READING: JOURNAL ARTICLES

Go to https://study.sagepub.com/essentialnursing2e for free online journal articles for this chapter. If you are using the interactive ebook, simply click on the book icon in the margin to go straight to the resource.

Ramsden, S. (2012) 'The NHS reform agenda and patient safety', *Clinical Risk*, 18(2): 43–5. This article explores the relationship between the traditional governance-based approach to managing safety and the more proactive transformational approaches that utilise improvement science.
Schwendimann, R., Milne, J., Frush, K., Ausserhofer, D., Frankel, A. and Sexton, J.B. (2013) 'A closer look at associations between hospital leadership walkrounds, and patient safety climate and risk reduction: A cross sectional study', *American Journal of Medical Quality*, 28(5): 414–21. A study of the relationship between leadership walkrounds and patient safety. The leadership walkround is a concept practised in the USA which is gaining wider recognition and implementation in the UK.

Other journal articles

McSherry, R., McSherry, W. and Pearce, P. (2013) 'Can clinical governance act as a cultural barometer?', *Nursing Times*, 109(19): 12–15. Discusses the importance of learning from the Francis report and how clinical governance can be used to measure the culture of healthcare environments.

Weblinks

Go to https://study.sagepub.com/essentialnursing2e for weblinks related to this chapter. If you are using the interactive ebook, simply click on the book icon in the margin to go straight to the resource.

FURTHER
READING:
WEBLINKS

www.rcn.org.uk/clinical-topics/clinical-governance – the Royal College of Nursing's clinical governance site offers a range of valuable resources and details country-specific strategies, standards and agencies.

www.nmc.org.uk/standards/safeguarding/introduction-to-safeguarding-for-adults – this web page provides guidance on safeguarding resources and best practice in each of the four countries of the UK.

www.patients-association.org.uk – the Patient Association works in partnership with the NHS to improve the care that is delivered. It supports people in raising concerns through the NHS complaints system. The website offers booklets, publications and research reports, as well as patient stories.

www.nrls.npsa.nhs.uk/resources/?entryid45=59840 – this website has useful information in relation to foresight training, offering comprehensive paper- and video-based scenarios; it provides pre-and post-registration nurses with the opportunity to develop and practise the skills to identify 'risk-prone' situations.

www.nrls.npsa.nhs.uk/resources/?EntryId45=59825 – here you will find an easy-to-use healthcare risk assessment tool which aims to promote awareness in identifying risk and the ways in which risk can be minimised. Suggestions and guidance are offered as to how greater consistency can be achieved in the way risk assessment is applied across all sectors of the NHS.

www.CHFG.org – a useful website with links to other resources related to human factors in healthcare.

Video links

Have a break from the text and go to https://study.sagepub.com/essentialnursing2e for useful videos related to this chapter. If you are using the interactive ebook, simply click on the lightbulb icon in the margin to go straight to the resource.

VIDEO
LINKS

ACE YOUR ASSESSMENT

Review what you have learned by visiting the book's online resources at: https://study.sagepub.com/essential nursing2e If using your interactive ebook, just click on the icon in the margin to go straight there.

ONLINE
QUIZZES

- Test yourself with multiple-choice and short-answer questions.
- Revise key terms with the interactive flash cards.

REFERENCES

Clinical Human Factors Group (2017) What is Human Factors? Available at: http://chfg.org/about-us/what-is-human-factors (accessed 17 September 2017).

Department of Health (DH) (1997) *The New NHS: Modern, Dependable*. London: HMSO.

Department of Health (1998) *A First Class Service: Quality in the New NHS*. London: HMSO.

Department of Health (2000) *Organisation with a Memory*. London: The Stationery Office.

Department of Health (2012) *Transforming Care: A National Response to Winterbourne View Hospital – Department of Health Review Final Report*. London: HMSO.

Department of Health (2017) *Draft Health Service Safety Investigations Bill*. Available at: www.gov.uk/government/publications/health-service-safety-investigations-bill (accessed 17 September 2017).

Dixon, A., Foot, C. and Harrison, T. (2012) *Preparing for the Francis Report: How to Assure Quality in the NHS*. The King's Fund. Available at: www.kingsfund.org.uk/sites/files/kf/field/field_publication_ file/preparing-for-the-francis-report-jul2012.pdf (accessed 17 September 2017).

Donnelly, L. (2013) NHS negligence claims rise by 20 per cent in just one year. *The Telegraph*. 2 June.

Fisher, M. and Scott, M. (2013) *Patient Safety and Managing Risk in Nursing*. Exeter: SAGE/Learning Matters.

Francis, R. (2010) *Independent Inquiry into Care Provided by Mid Staffordshire NHS Foundation Trust*. January 2005–March 2009, Volume I. London: The Stationery Office.

Francis, R. (2013) *Report of the Mid Staffordshire NHS Foundation Trust Public Inquiry*. London: The Stationery Office.

Francis, R. (2015) *Freedom to Speak Up: An Independent Review into Creating an Open and Honest Reporting Culture in the NHS*. London: The Stationery Office.

Institute of Medicine (IOM) (2001) *Crossing the Quality Chasm: A New Health System for the 21st Century*. Washington, DC: National Academies Press.

National Quality Board (NQB) (2013) *Quality in the New Health System: Maintaining and Improving Quality from April 2013*. Available at: www.gov.uk/government/publications/quality-in-the-new-health-system-maintaining-and-improving-quality-from-april-2013 (accessed 17 September 2017).

Nightingale, F. (1859/1946) *Notes on Nursing: What Nursing is, What Nursing is Not*. Philadelphia, PA: Lippincott.

Norris, B. (2009) 'Human Factors and safe patient care', *Journal of Nursing Management*, 17(2): 203–11.

Nursing and Midwifery Council (NMC) (2015a) *Raising Concerns: Guidance for Nurses and Midwives*. London: NMC.

Nursing and Midwifery Council (2015b) *The Code: Professional Standards of Practice and Behaviour for Nurses and Midwives*. London: NMC.

Nursing and Midwifery Council (2018) *Standards of Proficiency for Registered Nurses*. London: NMC.

Patient Safety First (2009) *The 'How to Guide' for Implementing Human Factors in Healthcare*. London: The Health Foundation.

Pridmore, J. and Gammon, J. (2007) 'A comparative review of clinical governance arrangements in the UK', *British Journal of Nursing*, 16(12): 720–3.

Standing, M. (2017) *Clinical Judgement and Decision Making in Nursing*. London: SAGE/Learning Matters.

World Health Organization (WHO) (2006) *Quality of Care: A Process for Making Strategic Choices in Health Systems*. Geneva: WHO.

RECORD-KEEPING AND DOCUMENTATION

18

JILL BARNES AND ROBERT JENKINS

THIS CHAPTER COVERS

- What is record-keeping?
- What is accurate record-keeping?
- Legal and professional issues related to record-keeping

- Ensuring you keep satisfactory records
- Consequences of poor record-keeping
- The role of the nursing student in record-keeping

> Do you think I have time to sit down and write pages and pages of what I did all day? No thank you, I would rather spend precious time with the children and their families.
>
> **Martin, children's nurse**

> I came into nursing to care for people, not write about it; besides, nothing much changes when caring for older people, so what is there to write?
>
> **Zara, mental health nurse**

> Nobody reads it anyway and if they did they wouldn't understand some medical terms. I think patients may get upset if they read the full extent of their condition – best if they don't have access to their records and are left well alone.
>
> **Michael, adult nurse**

> I think it is difficult to write person-centred records which are both comprehensive nursing records but can also be understood by the person they are written about.
>
> **Edie, learning disability nurse**

> I like to add notes about each patient's care on my handover sheet and update notes using this every 3–4 hours. It's a good idea to write 'between the hours of 8 and 12 the patient received the following care', as this saves you having to put individual times on every aspect. It can also be handy to break your documentation down into bullet points, 1 being nutrition, 2 continence, etc.
>
> **Charlie Clisby, NQN**

Visit https://study.sagepub.com/essentialnursing2e to access a wealth of online resources for this chapter – watch out for the margin icons throughout the chapter. If you are using the interactive eBook, simply click on the margin icon to go straight to the resource.

INTRODUCTION

Some of the above nurse voices illustrate that nurses across all fields of practice may not fully appreciate the importance and relevance of record-keeping in nursing practice. Record-keeping – or, rather, poor record-keeping – is the third highest reason why registered nurses are removed from the professional register. Nurses often cite pressure of work or other more important activities as reasons for not making accurate recordings of various aspects of nursing care. In order to maintain your registration when you qualify, you will need to be competent in record-keeping. However, it is not just a case of you potentially losing your registration; poor record-keeping can lead to negative outcomes for the patient and in some instances may lead to premature death.

This chapter aims to develop your knowledge and skills in relation to how to keep accurate and 'good' records, and to help you understand the professional and legal requirements associated with record-keeping.

WHAT IS RECORD-KEEPING?

Accurate record-keeping helps to promote high standards and improves continuity of care. The records should tell us what problems the patient has, what care and treatment they need, what progress they are making and what their plan of care is. Effective records promote better communication of information between members of the multi-disciplinary healthcare team. Records must provide an accurate account of treatment, planning and care delivery, particularly in areas such as patients' wishes, capacity and consent. They should enhance the ability to detect problems, such as changes in the patient's condition at an early stage (for example, observation charts). Overall, they must provide a contemporaneous account of the patient's journey.

ACTIVITY 18.1: CRITICAL THINKING

- Discuss with your fellow students why you think it is important to keep good records about patients.
- How does this form part of caring for a patient?

The Nursing and Midwifery Council (NMC) revised *The Code: Professional Standards of Practice and Behaviours for Nurses and Midwives* in 2015 and highlighted in point 10 that nurses and midwives must keep clear and accurate records relevant to their practice. Record-keeping is an integral part of nursing practice and is essential to the provision of safe and effective care. It is not an optional extra to be fitted in if circumstances allow. Record-keeping is a fundamental aspect of a nurse's role and, as such, is part of their professional duty of care owed to the patient (Dimond, 2015). Stevenson et al. (2010) identify that documentation has always been an essential part of the profession of caring, and highlight that as far back as the 1800s doctors kept records in ward notebooks; in the 1850s, during the Crimean War, Florence Nightingale kept the first patient-orientated health records. The importance of accurate record-keeping was highlighted within the NMC guidelines for records and record-keeping (2009: 12) (see Table 18.1). These identify that accurate record-keeping has many important functions. These guidelines have subsequently been replaced by point 10 of the

NMC (2015) Code, which states that nurses and midwives must 'keep clear and accurate records relevant to your practice. This includes but is not limited to patient records. It includes all records that are relevant to your scope of practice.

To achieve this, you must:

10.1 Complete all records at the time or as soon as possible after an event, recording if the notes are written some time after the event.

10.2 Identify any risks or problems that have arisen and the steps taken to deal with them, so that colleagues who use the records have all the information they need.

10.3 Complete all records accurately and without any falsification, taking immediate and appropriate action if you become aware that someone has not kept to these requirements.

10.4 Attribute any entries you make in any paper or electronic records to yourself, making sure they are clearly written, dated and timed, and do not include unnecessary abbreviations, jargon or speculation.

10.5 Take all steps to make sure that all records are kept securely.

10.6 Collect, treat and store all data and research findings appropriately.'

ACTIVITY 18.2: CRITICAL THINKING

- What types of records are used in relation to patients?
- Make a list of the various types of records you have seen or are aware of in clinical practice.

ANSWER:
ACTIVITY 18.2

Table 18.1 NMC guidelines for records and record-keeping

- Helping to improve accountability
- Showing how decisions related to patient care were made
- Supporting the delivery of services
- Supporting effective clinical judgements and decisions
- Supporting patient care and communications
- Making continuity of care easier
- Providing documentary evidence of services delivered
- Promoting better communication and sharing of information between members of the multi-professional healthcare team
- Helping to identify risks and enabling early detection of complications
- Supporting clinical audit, research, allocation of resources and performance planning
- Helping to address complaints or legal processes

Source: NMC (2009: 12)

Note: Although these guidelines have been replaced by the 2015 Code, the general principles of how records support care remain the same.

What is a record?

Basically, any information you record about a patient is a record. The Data Protection Act 1998 defines a health record as 'consisting of information about the physical or mental health or condition of an identifiable individual made by or on behalf of a health professional in connection with the care of that individual'.

There is now a move towards electronic patient records and documentation. The transition to electronic records has not taken place as quickly as planned, however, and in many areas paper records are still the main form of communication. You will read more about the use of electronic records later in this chapter.

WHAT IS ACCURATE RECORD-KEEPING?

ANSWER:
ACTIVITY 18.3

ACTIVITY 18.3: CRITICAL THINKING

What do you feel are the main principles of accurate record-keeping? Consider areas such as safety, practicalities, key information, storage, language and legal and ethical considerations.

In relation to each of the four fields of nursing, what additional considerations would you need to make? For example, consider children or people with learning disabilities, dementia or mental health needs.

The NMC previously provided guidance in relation to record-keeping. Table 18.2 summarises the main principles identified by the NMC (2009: 4) for accurate record-keeping. These principles have been integrated within the revised Code (NMC, 2015), and although the 2009 guidance for record keeping is no longer available, the points in Table 18.2 should be used as a guide to assist you as a student to maintain accurate records.

Table 18.2   Principles of accurate record-keeping

Ensure your handwriting is legible	Ensure your records enable you to communicate fully and effectively with your colleagues to ensure they have all the information they need about the people in your care
Sign all entries to records and ensure your name and job title are printed alongside the first entry	Do not alter or destroy any records without being authorised to do so
Put the date and time on all records. This should be in real time and chronological order, and be as close to the actual time as possible	In the unlikely event that you need to alter your own or another healthcare professional's records, you must give your name and job title, and sign and date the original documentation. You should make sure that the alterations you make, and the original record, are clear and auditable
Your records should be accurate and recorded in such a way that the meaning is clear	Where appropriate, the person in your care, or their carer, should be involved in the record-keeping process
Records should be factual and not include unnecessary abbreviations, jargon, meaningless phrases or irrelevant speculation	The language you use should be easily understood by the people in your care. This is a very important consideration when caring for children and young people and vulnerable adults, such as patients with dementia or a learning disability, as the language used within the records must facilitate the patient's and carer's involvement and not alienate them from active participation in care

You should use your professional judgement to decide what is relevant and what should be recorded

Records should be readable when photocopied or scanned

You should record details of any assessments and reviews undertaken, and provide clear evidence of the arrangements you have made for future and ongoing care. This should also include details of information given about care and treatment

You should not use coded expressions of sarcasm or humorous abbreviations to describe the people in your care

Records should identify any risks or problems that have arisen and show the action taken to deal with them

You should not falsify records

When you consider the points in Table 18.2, they are not difficult to interpret and not difficult to adhere to; disappointingly, though, many nurses fail to maintain a satisfactory standard of record-keeping. NMC professional conduct hearings often quote poor record-keeping as a contributing factor in other misconduct issues. So, what are the legal and professional requirements in relation to record-keeping?

> Always date and sign everything, always have a black ballpoint pen in your pocket. Write clearly, be succinct and accurate, do not use abbreviations and do not write down irrelevant information.
>
> **Siân Hunter, child nursing student**

> I like to add notes about each patient's care on my handover sheet and update notes using this every 3–4 hours.
>
> **Charlie Clisby, NQN**

LEGAL AND PROFESSIONAL ISSUES RELATED TO RECORD-KEEPING

The first principle to remember is: 'if it is not recorded, it has not been done'. Some nurses often believe that if care is routine, it does not need to be recorded. This can be quite a problem in areas where the same person is cared for over a long period of time. All fields of nursing (learning disabilities, mental health, children and adult) have such environments. It may become standard practice not to record activities of daily living as you may be recording the same information day after day. Interestingly, that may well indicate that the type of service you provide needs reviewing. The courts take the view that if it is not documented it did not happen, so a daily bath did not occur unless, every day, the records identify that the patient had a bath.

ACTIVITY 18.4: CRITICAL THINKING

When you are next in practice, look at a patient's record of care and then answer the following questions:

- If you did not know the patient, would the record accurately inform you of what they were like, what treatments they had received and how they responded?
- If possible, look at different patient groups – children, older people, people with learning disabilities, etc. – and repeat this exercise.

A claim for negligence resulting in personal injury can be made up to three years from the knowledge of the harm (the Limitation Act), and in the case of a child, up to three years after a child reaches 18. Records are usually kept for a minimum of eight years, and in the case of a child, until they have at least reached their 21st birthday. So if you were involved in caring for a child when they were aged 4, you could be called to give evidence in an inquiry when the child is 20. The question is – would you be able to remember what care you gave and the outcome of the care 16 years after the event? That would be extremely doubtful, hence the need for comprehensive and accurate records to be maintained. The records you keep may assist or hinder your defence against a claim of negligence in areas such as coroner's inquests, criminal proceedings, NMC fitness-to-practise committee hearings, health board or trust investigations, disciplinary investigations, Protection of Vulnerable Adult (POVA) inquiries, and so on.

There are three main legal aspects underpinning record-keeping: data protection, confidentiality and freedom of information. The recently introduced General Data Protection Regulations (GDPR) (2018) states that all staff have responsibility for ensuring that data are kept securely and not disclosed unlawfully, and that also means you as a nursing student. The GDPR has a number of key principles which states that personal (patient) data that must be:

- processed fairly and lawfully in a transparent manner
- collected and processed only for a specified purposes
- adequate, relevant and limited to what is necessary in relation to why it is being processed
- accurate and kept up date. Inaccurate data should be deleted or rectified as soon as possible
- not kept longer than necessary
- protected by appropriate security

For a fuller explantion of the principles and regulations see Information Commissioners Office link on this live document at https://ico.org.uk/for-organisations/guide-to-the-general-data-protection-regulation-gdpr/.

Further to protecting patient data is the need to ensure you maintain confidentiality. All staff, including you as a student, have a duty to protect the confidentiality of patient records and are governed by the Caldicott principles (HSCIC, 1997), which can be found in Figure 18.1.

It is very important that you maintain confidentiality in relation to patient records and do not leave them in public places for unauthorised persons to view. This also includes any notes you make about patients. Sometimes during handover or 'report', staff and students will be allowed to make notes about the patients; you may write down their name, diagnosis, maybe some results or tests they are due to have, or what you need to do for the patient that shift. What do you then do with that paper at the end of the shift – what if you left it lying on another patient's locker or on the bus on the way home? You would clearly be breaching confidentiality. Such pieces of paper are best avoided, but if you need to make notes about patients, encode their identity and make sure the paper goes into confidential waste when you have finished with it and is not taken home with you.

Justify the purpose of using patient information
Only use patient information when absolutely necessary

Use the minimum information required
Access to patient information should be on a strict 'need to know' basis

All staff handling patient information should understand their responsibilities
All staff handling patient information should understand and comply with the
law relating to patient information

Figure 18.1   The Caldicott principles

Source: HSCIC (1997)

> If I have taken notes about a patient during the day I make sure that I put them in the shredder at the end of the day to protect the patient and me. This also helps to protect me because I am not leaving with patient information.
>
> **Hannah Boyd, adult nursing student**

> All the personal notes that are kept for service users are done electronically in the trust where I have had my placements and now where I currently work. All the computers and the patient records can only be accessed by a personal password which has to be changed regularly. I do not discuss my password with anybody or allow anybody to access service user notes through my log-in details and I always make sure the computer screen is locked when I am not at the computer. I also ensure that I document clearly discussions and events in service user notes that are accurate.
>
> **Samantha Vanes, NQ RNMH**

ACTIVITY 18.5: REFLECTION

Considering the patients you have been involved in caring for, think about the advantages and disadvantages of them holding their own records. For the purpose of this activity, think of paper records only.

The third legal aspect relating to record-keeping is the Freedom of Information Act (FOIA) 2000. This act changed the way the nursing and medical profession handled information. In the past, patients had been told very little about their condition or diagnosis and treatment, with the idea that 'ignorance is bliss'. Care plans and case notes were hidden away and, if a patient attempted to even cast a gaze on the observation chart at the end of the bed, it was removed from them. It was almost a secret society, with the recipient of care on one side and those delivering care on the other. However, the introduction of the FOIA changed this culture of secrecy and gave patients in the UK the right to know about their care. Patients had the right to confidentiality, the right to public administration, the right to be told if a piece of information exists and the right to receive the information.

Thus, the emphasis in providing patients with information has changed considerably, and now patients are active and equal participants and decision-makers in their care, not just passive and silent recipients of care. There is now a greater emphasis on patients holding their own records – this practice has been operating in midwifery for some time. People with a learning disability will have hand-held, person-centred records. These usually include a person-centred plan, comprising their one-page profile, health action plan and hospital passport. These records are often kept in addition to the 'patient record' system in your workplace. Remember to complete these person-held records in such a way that the person and their carers can understand what is written without the need for further clarification.

In addition to ensuring you adhere to the legal requirements for record-keeping, both as a nursing student and when you become a registered nurse, you have a professional duty to maintain accurate and legible records at all times. Dimond (2015) states that failing to maintain reasonable standards of record-keeping can be construed as professional misconduct and can result in being summoned to appear in front of a professional conduct committee. Unfortunately, this is not an uncommon occurrence: in one year alone (2010 to 2011), the NMC fitness-to-practise panel removed 28 nurses from the professional register for poor record-keeping.

CASE STUDY 18.1: CLAIRE AND IAN

Consider each of the situations below:

- What decision did the professional conduct committee reach and what sanction do you think was applied?

The stories of Claire and Ian are based on true cases, and the actual outcome is online, so don't look at this until you have judged for yourself!

Claire

Claire has been a health visitor for 20 years and was an adult nurse prior to that. She has worked in many inner-city locations within the UK and has a great deal of experience in caring for families in deprived areas.

She was reported to the professional conduct committee because it was alleged that:

- She removed patients' records and kept them in her car and at home.
- Her records lacked detail and were partially or wholly illegible.
- Records were unsigned.
- Records contained no evidence of the action taken by her; for example, she failed to record when a child had been made subject to a child protection plan.

This was the second time Claire had been reported to the professional conduct committee. She had been subjected to a supervision of practice order following her previous offence.

Ian

Ian has been a mental health nurse for two years. He has worked since he completed his nursing programme within a small community team in a rural location. He was reported to the professional conduct committee because he was alleged to have:

- incorrectly made an entry relating to patient B in patient A's notes, then removed the page, photocopied the page and replaced the page in patient B's notes
- then destroyed the original entry.

Now that you have judged the cases, go online and find out the outcomes for Claire and Ian.

CHECK YOUR ANSWERS!

ANSWER:
CASE STUDY 18.1

ENSURING YOU KEEP SATISFACTORY RECORDS

So, how can you ensure your records are of satisfactory standard? After all, you would not wish to be removed from a professional register that you have worked so hard to get on. Therefore, it is important to develop accurate record-keeping skills, as follows:

1. Your handwriting must be legible; it is of little use if no one other than you can read the entry. If your writing is difficult to read, print rather than use joined-up writing.
2. You must use black pen, not pencil, as it could be erased. There may be occasions when the area in which you are working requires you to use a red pen for specific entries – make sure you are aware of when this would be.
3. You must sign the entry and print your name and designation; as a nursing student, you must have each entry counter-signed by a registered nurse until you are deemed competent in record-keeping.
4. You must put the time and date (the time should be in the 24-hour clock); the records should be in chronological order.
5. Your records must be clear, factual and accurate, with sufficient detail to enable you in ten years' time to understand exactly what had happened to the patient during the time you were caring for them and how they responded.
6. The record should be written up as soon as possible after the episode of care and any temporary note-taking, for example in an emergency situation, should be formalised within 24 hours.
7. You should avoid unnecessary abbreviations, jargon, meaningless phrases or irrelevant speculation. You should also avoid using text language or slang.
8. You must not erase or alter records with correction fluid or remove pages from records.

To help remember how to make accurate records, Glasper (2011) suggests the use of the mnemonic CIA (see Figure 18.2). Glasper (2011) also suggests that you follow the **No ELBOW** rule when making notes (see Figure 18.3).

How often should an entry be made?

The frequency of entries is governed by local policies, changes in the patient's condition and professional judgement. The latter may be difficult for you as a student until you develop competence

Figure 18.2   CIA

Figure 18.3   No ELBOW

in determining what information to record and when. More frequent entries will be required for patients who:

- present with complex problems
- show a deviation from the norm
- are vulnerable or at risk of harm or abuse
- require more intensive care than normal
- are confused and disorientated or generally give cause for concern.

When working with patients who are subject to mental health legislation, records must be maintained in accordance with the Mental Health Act Commission for England and Wales, the Mental Welfare Commission for Scotland and the Mental Health Commission for Northern Ireland.

CONSEQUENCES OF POOR RECORD-KEEPING

Dimond (2015) identified a number of common problems related to record-keeping, such as absence of clarity, complaints, missing information, spelling mistakes, inaccurate information, use of jargon, not recording details of phone calls and failing to record patients' special needs. Poor record-keeping or information-sharing may lead to fatal outcomes: for example, not recording allergies to certain drugs or products may lead to the sudden death of a patient. In many child protection inquiries, a failure to record and share information has been noted as a contributory factor in failing to prevent the child's death (Department of Health and Home Office, 2003).

Apply your knowledge of what is good and bad record-keeping by reading the case study on Mary Davis, at https://study.sagepub.com/essentialnursing2e.

CASE STUDY: MRS MARY DAVIES

Poor record-keeping has also been a factor in many adult abuse inquiries, such as the Francis Report (2013) and *The Confidential Inquiry into Premature Deaths of People with Learning Disabilities* (Heslop et al., 2013). The Care Quality Commission's (2013) Mental Health Act annual report highlighted that some patients were not involved in care planning and had no idea what was in their care plan. In other instances, some detained patients were not made aware of the grounds for their detention or received no information on discharge from hospital.

ACTIVITY 18.6: REFLECTION

Some records use statements that are difficult to determine the exact meaning of.

Spend a couple of minutes with some of your fellow students thinking about what each of the following mean; note down what they mean to you and then compare the answers with those of your colleagues:

- poor dietary intake
- diarrhoea
- satisfactory fluid intake
- slept well.

It is very likely that you will have found that your answers differ: 'satisfactory fluid intake' will mean one thing to one nurse and something different to another. However, if the entry states that the patient has had a total of 2,800 ml oral intake in the past 24 hours, everyone is clear about the patient's fluid intake.

THE ROLE OF THE NURSING STUDENT IN RECORD-KEEPING

As a nursing student, you must take personal accountability for accurate record-keeping. You must be supervised in this activity and all of your entries must be counter-signed by a registered nurse until such time as your practice educator deems you competent. Further clarity in relation to this can be found on the Royal College of Nursing website.

However, this may vary, depending where you are on a practice placement, with some areas' local policies requiring a registered nurse to counter-sign your entries throughout your time as a student. You must ensure you adhere to the professional and legal requirements for record-keeping. The rule of thumb is: if you are unsure or do not feel competent, then seek advice from your practice educator or another qualified practitioner.

The acceptable and unacceptable use of nursing and medical terminology

If at all possible, jargon, abbreviations and nursing and medical terminology should be avoided, especially as we want to encourage patients to be active participants and decision-makers in their care. The use of this type of terminology puts up barriers to effectively enabling this, particularly when caring for vulnerable groups of people such as those with learning disabilities, those with dementia, or children. Indeed, some abbreviations can be dangerous or have more than one meaning.

I have become more familiar with confusing terminology and abbreviations but not memorised them all yet, there are so many!! I think the important thing is not to be afraid to ask what they are, you need to be sure what they mean, and technically they should not be used. On placement I asked all the time, I always said first what I thought it may be, but always sought confirmation as a misunderstanding could be quite dangerous for a patient.

Siân Hunter, child nursing student

For example, CNS could stand for central nervous system or clinical nurse specialist. More worrying is DNR, which may be district nurse referral or do not resuscitate – you would not want to interpret that one incorrectly.

STEVENSON
ET AL
(2010)

WHAT'S THE EVIDENCE?

Use of electronic patient records

Stevenson, J.E., Nilsson, G.C., Petersson, G.I. and Johansson, P.E. (2010) 'Nurses' experience of using electronic patient records in everyday practice in acute/inpatient ward settings: A literature review', *Health Informatics Journal*, 16(1): 63-72. Available at: http://jhi.sagepub.com/content/16/1/63.refs.html (accessed 23 February 2015).

Stevenson et al. (2010) is a very interesting literature review relating to the nurse's experience of using electronic patient records. It summarises the findings of five main studies and found that generally nurses were critical of using electronic records as they felt they were not user-friendly, were too remote from the patient's bedside and often used systems which were out of sync with the way nurses think and work.

However, on the positive side, some of the findings identified that electronic record-keeping had led to a decreased workload and improved the quality of documentation, and that this had the potential to lead to improved safety and patient care.

- Read the 'Discussion' section of the article (pp. 68-70) for particularly useful information which will increase your understanding of the advantages and disadvantages of using electronic records.

Some terminology, however, is acceptable, as long as the patient understands it. For example, you can use accurate terminology for diagnosis – such as hypertension, meningitis – and for observations – such as TPR, BP. You must only use the terminology and abbreviations if they make sense to all who will access the records and it is permitted within local policy. Remember, it is no longer a secret language. Patients have a right to be fully informed of all aspects of their care and to see all of their records, whether they are in paper or electronic form.

Finally, this chapter will consider the move to electronic record-keeping and the current research in relation to this.

When thinking of student nurses in particular, Baillie et al. (2012) carried out a study exploring nursing students' experiences of electronic record-keeping. The study used focus groups and was conducted specifically with midwifery, adult and mental health field nursing students. The study found that positive experiences of using electronic records during their pre-registration education programme were more likely to have a positive impact on their implementation post-qualifying.

ACTIVITY 18.7: REFLECTION

Access this article: Baillie, L. Chadwick, S., Mann, R. and Brook-Read, M. (2012) 'Students' experiences of electronic health records in practice', *British Journal of Nursing*, 21(21): 1262-9:

- Reflect on the students' experiences in the study and your own experiences of electronic records to date.

CONCLUSION

Accurate and legible record-keeping is an integral part of nursing practice and essential to the provision of safe and effective care. There are important legal and professional issues relating to accurate and legible record-keeping and the NMC (2015) outlines key principles that you must, at all times, apply to the records you keep. Poor record-keeping or information-sharing can lead to fatal outcomes for patients and serious charges of professional misconduct for nurses.

Patients have a right to be fully informed of all aspects of their care and to see all of their records, whether they are in paper or electronic form. If at all possible, jargon, abbreviations and nursing and medical terminology should be avoided. As a nursing student, you must take personal accountability for accurate record-keeping. A good rule of thumb to remember is: if you are unsure or do not feel competent, then seek advice from your practice educator or another qualified practitioner.

CHAPTER SUMMARY

- It is important to maintain accurate patient records which provide a contemporaneous account of a patient's journey in order to improve and monitor care.
- The Nursing and Midwifery Council (NMC) states that record-keeping is an integral part of nursing practice and is essential to the provision of safe and effective care.
- Nurses have to complete a number of different records, depending on the nature of the patient and the service provided.
- The principle is that if the care given is not recorded, it is presumed not to have occurred.
- All parties involved in providing care should be involved in record-keeping – patients, carers, nurses and other health professionals.
- Patient records must be kept safe and stored appropriately to maintain confidentiality.
- Poor record-keeping can result in you being held accountable to your professional body, particularly if harm comes to a patient.
- Within healthcare settings, there is now a move towards electronic record-keeping.

CRITICAL REFLECTION
Holistic care

- Reflect on your most recent placement experience.

Although this chapter has considered how to ensure accurate record-keeping:

- What factors can you identify that may work against this in clinical practice?
- What impact does poor record-keeping have on the provision of holistic patient care?

GO FURTHER
Books

Dimond, B. (2015) 'Record keeping, statements and evidence in court', Chapter 9 in *Legal Aspects of Nursing*, 7th edn. London: Pearson. pp. 219–36. An interesting textbook with an excellent chapter on the importance of accurate record-keeping.

Griffith, R. and Tengnah, C. (2013) 'Record keeping', Chapter 11 in *Law and Professional Issues in Nursing*, 3rd edn. Exeter: Learning Matters. pp. 206–22. An excellent chapter outlining the legal and professional issues relating to record-keeping.

Journal articles

St. Aubyn, B. and Andrews, A. (2017) 'Advanced care planning in palliative care coordination: The NMC code and record keeping', Review article, *Nursing and Palliative Care* 2 (6): 1–3. Available at: www.oatext.com/pdf/NPC-2-172.pdf. This short review article provides a good discussion on how nurses working in palliative care can adhere to the NMC code with regards to record keeping. It specifically focuses on three advance practice areas - care planning, patients who refuse treatment and patients not for active resuscitation.

Beach, J. and Oates, J. (2014) 'Maintaining best practice in record-keeping and documentation', *Nursing Standard*, 28 (36): 45–50. This CPD article explores a range of important issues in regards to best practice in nurse record keeping in areas such as collaborative approaches to planning and evaluating care, patient ownership of records, implications of increased use of electronic records, digital storage and recent developments in information governance.

The two articles listed below identify the most common mistakes encountered with record-keeping and suggest ways in which nurses can develop accurate record-keeping skills:

Glasper, A. (2011) 'Improving record keeping: Important lessons for nurses', *British Journal of Nursing*, 20(14): 886–7.

Prideaux, A. (2011) 'Issues in nursing documentation and record keeping practice', *British Journal of Nursing*, 20(22): 1450–4.

Weblinks

Go to https://study.sagepub.com/essentialnursing2e for weblinks related to this chapter. If you are using the interactive ebook, simply click on the book icon in the margin to go straight to the resource.

FURTHER
READING:
WEBLINKS

Heslop, P., Blair, P., Fleming, P., Houghton, M., Marriott, A. and Russ, L. (2013) *The Report of the Confidential Inquiry into Premature Deaths of People with Learning Disabilities (CIPOLD)*. Bristol: Norah Fry Research Centre/University of Bristol. Available at: www.bris.ac.uk/cipold. Poor record-keeping has also been a factor in many recent adult abuse inquiries; this report identifies many lapses in accurate record-keeping.

www.rcn.org.uk/development/health_care_support_workers/professional_issues/accountability_and_delegation_film - as a nursing student, you must take personal accountability for accurate record-keeping. You must be supervised in this activity and all of your entries must be counter-signed by a registered nurse until such time as your practice educator deems you competent. Further clarity in relation to this can be found at the web link above.

Care Quality Commission (2013) *Mental Health Act Annual Report*. Available at: www.cqc.org.uk. The Care Quality Commission's recent Mental Health Act Annual Report highlighted that some patients were not involved in care planning and had no idea what was in their care plan.

ACE YOUR ASSESSMENT

Review what you have learned by visiting the book's online resources at: https://study.sagepub.com/essential nursing2e If using your interactive ebook, just click on the icon in the margin to go straight there.

ONLINE
QUIZZES

- Test yourself with multiple-choice and short-answer questions.
- Revise key terms with the interactive flash cards.

REFERENCES

Baillie, L., Chadwick, S., Mann, R. and Brook-Read, M. (2012) 'Students' experiences of electronic health records in practice', *British Journal of Nursing*, 21(21): 1262–9.

Care Quality Commission (CQC) (2013) Mental Health Act Annual Report. Available at: www.cqc. org.uk (accessed 23 February 2015).

Department of Health and Home Office (2003) *The Victoria Climbie Inquiry: Report of an Inquiry by Lord Laming*. London: The Stationery Office.

Dimond, B. (2015) *Legal Aspects of Nursing*, 7th edn. London: Pearson.

Francis, R. (2013) *Report of the Mid Staffordshire NHS Foundation Trust Public Inquiry*. London: The Stationery Office. Available at: www.midstaffspublicinquiry.com (accessed 23 February 2015).

Glasper, A. (2011) 'Improving record keeping: Important lessons for nurses', *British Journal of Nursing*, 20(14): 886–7.

Health and Social Care Information Center (HSCIC) (1997) Resources for Caldicott Guardians. Available at: http://systems.hscic.gov.uk/infogov/caldicott/caldresources (accessed 23 February 2015).

Heslop, P., Blair, P., Fleming, P., Houghton, M., Marriott, A. and Russ, L. (2013) *The Confidential Inquiry into Premature Deaths of People with Learning Disabilities (CIPOLD)*. Bristol: Norah Fry Research Centre/University of Bristol. Available at: www.bris.ac.uk/cipold (accessed 23 February 2015).

Nursing and Midwifery Council (NMC) (2009) *Record Keeping: Guidance for Nurses and Midwives*. London: NMC.

Nursing and Midwifery Council (2015) *The Code: Professional Standards of Practice and Behaviour for Nurses and Midwives*. London: NMC. Available at: www.nmc.org.uk/standards/code (accessed 10 May 2018).

Stevenson, J.E., Nilsson, G.C., Petersson, G.I. and Johansson, P.E. (2010) 'Nurses' experience of using electronic patient records in everyday practice in acute/inpatient ward settings: A literature review', *Health Informatics Journal*, 16(1): 63–72. Available at: http://jhi.sagepub.com/content/16/1/63.refs.html (accessed 23 February 2015).

CLINICAL DECISION-MAKING

GEMMA HURLEY

--- **THIS CHAPTER COVERS** ---

- Clinical decision-making
- Types of decisions
- How nurses make sound decisions

- The decision-making process
- The role of patients

> "
> My name is Mrs Davidson, I am 88 years old and live with my cat Lexy in a ground-floor maisonette. I have had four hospital admissions in the past six months due to problems with my breathing. I have a condition called chronic obstructive pulmonary disease (COPD) and also heart failure. Recently, the community matron and my doctor admitted me onto a 'virtual ward' as they said it would be a better way of looking after me at home and prevent unnecessary hospital admissions. The nurses visit me often and they give me the ongoing care and support I need so I feel safe and well looked after. They do the same things as if I was on the hospital ward, such as weigh me regularly, check my breathing and manage my medications, so that I am able to feel well enough to potter around my home with Lexy.
>
> **Mrs Davidson, patient**
> "

> "
> My name is Shristi and I am a first-year nursing student, nearing the end of my first community practice placement. My previous practice placement was in a surgical ward based within an acute healthcare trust.
>
> At the beginning of the community placement I felt quite anxious as this setting was unfamiliar to me. I felt privileged to be working with patients in their homes, but I also found it unsettling – and making decisions took me so much longer than the registered nurses. I was always seeking affirmation from the nursing team and I was starting to lose the confidence I had gained from my previous placements.
>
> I was really worried that others would think I lacked interest and commitment and I kept checking the protocols and health assessment tools before making any decisions. My practice educator was instrumental in making me feel welcome and reassured me that it was normal to feel like this in a new setting. He also explained to me that my limited experience in this placement meant that I was not able to make rapid decisions based on pattern recognition, which expert nurses use in the decision-making process. However, as time progressed and I was continuously supported by the nursing team I became more satisfied with my ability to make the correct decisions. I also realised how the skills and experience I had acquired in my previous placement, such as measuring vital signs, could help me to make more in-depth decisions, as I did have the knowledge to interpret and make sense of relevant findings.
>
> **Shristi, first-year nursing student**
> "

Visit https://study.sagepub.com/essentialnursing2e to access a wealth of online resources for this chapter – watch out for the margin icons throughout the chapter. If you are using the interactive eBook, simply click on the margin icon to go straight to the resource.

INTRODUCTION

Are you able to identify with Shristi's feelings of anxiety? Do you find that on entering a new placement you worry about making right and timely decisions about patients' care? Starting a new placement can be daunting and challenging for any health professional, but making decisions relating to patient care is an acquired and transferable skill. Mrs Davidson's story above shows that many of the decisions that are made are based on skills that can be used anywhere, regardless of the healthcare setting.

The type of decisions we make as nurses may be unique to a particular placement and require field-specific knowledge, but the process by which we form our decision-making strategies is based on common elements utilised by all nurses. Furthermore, the depth and the way in which we develop our decision-making are influenced by our level of expertise. In nursing, professional growth and skill acquisition progress through five distinct stages: novice, advanced beginner, competent, proficient and expert (Benner, 2001). The novice nurse is new to nursing, as in the case of Shristi, and uses a set of rules to form a decision that takes a long time, whereas the expert nurse, such as her practice educator, uses his experience and knowledge to intuitively grasp the situation and make rapid decisions.

This chapter will discuss what we mean by clinical decision-making and some types of decisions that nurses make. It highlights key drivers that influence our role in decision-making and demonstrates nurses' responsiveness to the changing landscape of the National Health Service. Throughout the chapter, case studies and activities will help you to link theoretical ideas with patient care, in order to enable you to make sense of how to make decisions safely and effectively.

CLINICAL DECISION-MAKING

Nurses are responsible for making a large number of decisions in their daily duties and this often involves them understanding:

- their level of competency
- their attitudes and behaviour
- the evidence
- the patient's wishes and beliefs
- the environment, which includes the available resources and expertise.

Furthermore, the types of decisions nurses are required to make have expanded over the past decade and are influenced by public expectation, increasingly complex patient needs, healthcare policy, staff shortages, employer demands and the nature of the nurse's role. For example, some nurses have expanded their role in non-medical prescribing and are working in settings such as urgent care treatment centres, which means they are required to make decisions on prescribing medications following diagnostic reasoning. Other nurses working in public health settings, such as health visitors, may be involved in making decisions promoting the health and wellbeing of children and their families.

Clinical decision-making involves the processes of critical thinking, problem-solving and reflective practice, thus utilising several 'ways of knowing', which have been described by Carper (1978) as:

- personal
- intuitive
- experiential
- empirical
- ethical
- aesthetic.

For the nurse, decision-making has an integral role in ensuring patient-focused care and requires the ability to sift, synthesise and organise the information gathered.

What decisions will you make?

Pre-registration nursing courses are designed to foster critical thinking and analytical reflection as part of the unique learning partnership that exists between healthcare providers and universities. The dynamic and active learning in which you will participate during your nursing course prepares you to engage in decision-making that is responsive to the changing landscape of healthcare provision, at an embryonic stage in your career.

The nature of the decisions made by a nursing student would depend on their stage of the course, the care environment, the practice educator/student relationship and expectations. For example, a first-year nursing student on their first ward placement may be alerted to the identification of patients who need assistance with eating and drinking through the red tray system. At meal times, they will be expected not only to assist those individuals with their meals but also to adapt decisions in accordance with the patient's preferences and abilities. The patient may express preferences about drinking through a straw instead of a beaker, for example, and so care decisions would be adapted to accommodate the patient's preferences. A third-year nursing student may recognise malnutrition in this patient through application of screening tools such as the Malnutrition Universal Screening Tool (MUST) (BAPEN MAG, 2003), and would alert qualified staff to the need to refer the patient to specialist services such as a dietician.

As your nursing education and experience progress, the patient care-related decisions you will be involved in making will become more refined and intricate. Furthermore, to ensure decision-making is effective there needs to be a balance between experience, self-awareness, knowledge, evidence-based practice and application of appropriate assessment tools, on the one hand, and collaborative inter-disciplinary team working on the other. For example, when using the MUST tool that screens for malnutrition, the qualified nurse will integrate current relevant evidence, utilise fundamental ways of knowing that are unique to nursing and combine this with their knowledge of themselves when working with others, such as a dietician, to formulate decisions that are holistic and patient-focused.

A substantial part of the nurse's role in decision-making revolves around direct and holistic patient care, as is demonstrated in Figure 19.1.

I attended a best interest meeting at a hospital for a service user with cancer. We discussed her long-term prognosis and the need for a hip operation with the family, ward staff and surgeon. We contributed our opinions and what was in her best interests. This led to the operation and the smooth transition for her from home to hospital. This meeting taught me that it is important to think about the ethical issues and quality of life for people with terminal illnesses.

Julie Davis, LD nursing student

ACTIVITY 19.1: REFLECTION

Reflect on the decision-making skills you have engaged during your experience of patient care so far:

* Can you identify an aspect of a decision-making skill gained in one setting that you have been able to apply in a different setting?

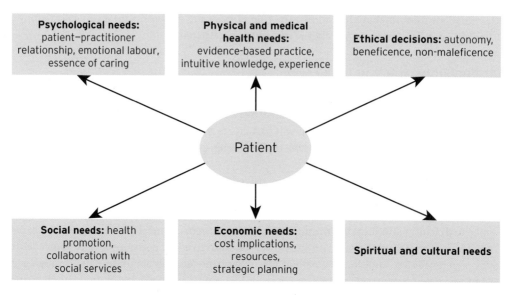

Figure 19.1 The nurse's role in decision-making

CASE STUDY 19.1: BIANCA

Bianca is a 14-year-old girl who has attended a sexual health clinic. She is accompanied by her friend Abby, who is of the same age. Bianca admits to having unprotected sexual intercourse (UPSI) two days ago and is requesting the emergency contraceptive pill. Her boyfriend is of a similar age (15) and she admits that they were both under the influence of alcohol at the time of UPSI, so condoms were not used.

Bianca is adamant that her parents must not be informed as, due to their religious beliefs, they do not agree with sex before marriage. This was her first sexual encounter and she says she bitterly regrets it. She says: 'I know I have let my parents down – I feel so bad'. She also says that since the episode of UPSI, she has been getting a stinging sensation when she passes urine.

Sharon, the nurse, asks a series of open-ended questions which allow Bianca to explore her feelings so her emotional needs can be assessed. This also enables Sharon to appreciate the patient's spiritual and cultural health beliefs, so these can be considered when making decisions about her care.

Bianca's physical needs are assessed by asking relevant questions and taking specimens for clinical tests. These indicate that Bianca has a urinary tract infection and that, as her last menstrual bleed was two weeks ago, she is mid-cycle and so at high risk of pregnancy.

In assessing Bianca, Sharon decides that she is **Fraser-competent**. Bianca has stated that she did not feel coerced and that both partners consented to sexual activity, although she now regrets it.

Sharon encourages Bianca to consider talking to her parents or a responsible adult whom she feels safe to confide in.

The emergency contraceptive pill is prescribed for Bianca, with follow-up advice on sexual health screening. Sharon is also aware of the high incidence of teenage pregnancies in the UK and their financial and emotional impacts, and so she talks to Bianca about awareness of the use of long-term reversible contraception. Furthermore, she invites Bianca and her friend to attend the youth clinic that she runs alongside voluntary and public health organisations.

ANSWER:
CASE STUDY 19.1

- Using Figure 19.1, can you identify the core aspects of the holistic care provided to Bianca?

TYPES OF DECISIONS

Nurses are continuously making decisions with and for patients at all levels of the NHS. Their role demands active participation as decision-makers at both strategic and grassroots levels. For example, in case study 19.1, it can be seen that Sharon, the nurse, was involved in making direct decisions that were centred on Bianca, but she was also involved at a strategic level in developing access services for young people.

ACTIVITY 19.2: REFLECTION

Can you identify a situation in which you have been involved where a holistic approach to decision-making has been applied?

The nature of the decisions made by nurses and the frequency with which they are involved in being decision-makers depend on their work environment, their perception of their role and organisational autonomy. For example, a night nurse site manager may perceive part of their role as being able to make decisions on diagnosis and the management of exacerbation of certain conditions, and they may be given organisational support in making decisions that involve requesting and interpreting diagnostic tests.

Thompson and Stapley (2011) suggest that the types of decisions nurses make can be categorised as described in Table 19.1.

CASE STUDY 19.2: TONY

Tony is a 19-year-old male, newly diagnosed with type 1 diabetes who has been admitted to the ward due to a third episode of ketoacidosis. Initially, Tony was given intravenous fluids and put on a sliding scale insulin infusion pump so that his blood glucose and dehydration could be corrected.

Once ketoacidosis was corrected, it was hoped that Tony would be willing to take control of his health and actively take part in the decision-making process for his care.

However, Tony seemed withdrawn and distant. He did not make eye contact when the nurse delivered his care and refused to take part in checking his blood glucose or self-injecting his insulin. Tony says he 'doesn't see the point in any of it' as having diabetes has 'stunted his dreams and ambitions'.

The nurse decided that Tony would benefit from seeing a counsellor to explore his feelings and come to terms with his diagnosis. A referral was made to a counsellor, with Tony's consent.

- What decision types has the nurse used in caring for Tony? (Use Table 19.1 for reference.)
- What factors do you think influenced the nurse's decision to refer Tony to a counsellor?

ANSWER:
CASE STUDY 19.2

Table 19.1   Types of decisions nurses make

Decision type	Examples of decisions of this type that you may need to make as a nursing student	Factors influencing the decision
Intervention/Effectiveness	The non-pharmacological interventions that should be implemented in helping patients with diabetes maintain the required blood glucose levels	Evidence-based practice, resources, patient choice, ethics
Targeting	Identifying which patients are at risk of developing diabetes	Policy drivers, protocols, evidence-based practice, specialist/expert advice, equipment, patient involvement
Prevention	Exploring health-promotion techniques, for example to prevent a further cardiovascular event, such as smoking cessation	Guidelines, patient choice/motivation, resources, skills and training, incentives/targets to be achieved
Timing	Knowing when is the best time to, for example, weigh patients, such as in the early morning before breakfast	Patient participation and preference, evidence-based practice
Referral	Deciding which professional team to refer to with a specific diagnosis – for example, a patient with chronic, uncontrolled psoriasis may require a dermatology referral	Resources, evidence-based practice, accessibility, protocols, patient choice
Communication	Communicate with patients and their families on, for example, the discharge planning process, including deciding the best ways of communicating information to all persons involved, such as the patient, family, GPs, district nurses, social services	Patient and family involvement, multi-agency working, team meetings
Service organisation and delivery process		Policy, protocol
Assessment	How to accurately and objectively assess, for example, the level and nature of pain	Pain assessment tools, communicating with patients
Diagnosis	Taking a relevant history of signs and symptoms that are related to a specific condition	Intuitive knowledge, pattern recognition, practice knowledge, evidence base
Information-seeking	Seeking further information before a decision is made	Resources, patient's choice, evidence, aesthetics and ethics, local guidelines
Experience, understanding, or critical exploration – the interpretation of cues in the process of care	Exploring ways of effectively managing the risk of suicide in a patient with depression, for example	Evidence, resources, knowledge and recognising red flags

Source: Adapted from Thompson and Stapley (2011)

HOW NURSES MAKE SOUND DECISIONS

It is argued that, for the experienced nurse, decision-making is often done without conscious awareness. However, on reflection, this complex process of decision-making can be unravelled and can show how patient care-related decisions are influenced by a number of factors. According to Benner and Tanner (1987), amongst these are:

- knowledge
- evidence-based practice
- experience
- intuition
- ethics
- the nurse–patient relationship
- the professional role
- organisational rules and culture.

Each of these will now be discussed in turn, identifying how it affects the decisions nurses make.

Knowledge: This is formed of both objective technical knowledge and tacit knowledge that is embedded in practice. It is unique to the profession and often difficult to define, as much of it is hidden in our daily activities. The way in which nurses acquire this knowledge is complex and is gained from a wide range of sources: biological and social sciences; personal and life experience; intuition; scientific enquiry; nursing experience; and formal education.

Evidence-based practice: The nurse applies scientific knowledge through analysis and synthesis of research-based findings in the decision-making process. However, it is appreciated that evidence-based practice includes both objective scientific enquiry and interpretative theories that enable the nurse to link research to patient care. For example, the nurse may be influenced by quantitative studies that examine the statistics suggesting a connection between abnormal blood glucose and blood pressure measurement in the development of vascular disease in patients with diabetes. In addition, the nurse may be influenced by qualitative studies that seek to understand the patient's behaviour and experiences that contribute to poor control of their blood sugar levels. The knowledge gained from both the quantitative and qualitative research paradigms informs the nurse when making decisions, which will help a patient to control their blood glucose and blood pressure.

Nursing knowledge and skill acquisition come from both formal education and practice-based learning, but often implementing decisions is a challenge that involves many factors. For example, some studies suggest that sometimes nurses feel constrained when making decisions due to hierarchical influences and economic pressures (Traynor et al., 2010). Furthermore, the constantly changing landscape of healthcare demands that nurses adapt and expand their roles, which requires a balance between scientific knowledge and practice-based learning. Pre-registration nurse education recognises this and, as a result, nursing students spend equal time in the classroom and practice settings. Knowledge gained in this way enables the nursing student to apply scientific data learned in the classroom to the practice setting, with the support of experienced practice educators, as seen in the case of Shristi. The use of guidelines, protocols, computer decision support systems and care pathways means that evidence-based practice is a fundamental aspect of the decision-making process.

Experience: Experiential knowledge allows nurses to make rapid decisions, offering wider treatment choices and in-depth care plans. This rich bank of knowledge is usually gained over time. Through reflection, mentorship and clinical supervision, the nurse is able to integrate this acquired knowledge into the decision-making process. This type of knowledge is normally passed on from experienced nurses and can be gained from observation, role models, handovers, mentorship and team meetings.

Intuition: Expert nurses also use intuition to inform the decision-making process. This relies on the nurse's perception of the situation, unconscious thought processing and pattern recognition, and is often expressed as 'a gut feeling', 'a sixth sense' or 'I just know but can't explain how' (Nyatanga and Vocht, 2008). The use of intuitive knowledge has been challenged and defined as being somewhat mystical, because it does not use the analytic processing seen in scientific knowledge. Further to this, it is unique to the individual and involves personal feelings that often do not have a rationale. For example, in case study 19.2, in addition to the nurse having a good understanding of the scientific knowledge, she may, through unconscious thought, have been picking up on subtle cues that informed her decision to refer Tony for counselling.

> When with the respiratory nurse the nurse stopped and helped a patient who was short of breath. The patient was a COPD patient and very often out of breath. However the specialist nurse intuitively knew that the patient was having a panic attack and was able to talk to them and reduce their breathing problems.
>
> **Laura Grimley, adult nursing student**

Ethics: There are core principles of medical ethics that should be applied in the decision-making process: *beneficence* – an obligation to do good; *non-maleficence* – an obligation to do no harm; *respect for autonomy* – respecting decisions made by individuals who are mentally competent; and *justice* – ensuring equality and moral obligation. Obtaining informed consent that is free from coercion, maintaining confidentiality and respecting the values and wishes of the patient are integral components of ethical decision-making. There is an ethical dimension within the decision-making process, as it is necessary to act in the patient's best interest by being their advocate, representing the patient's beliefs and wishes in situations where they are unable to voice their opinions for themselves. Nurses' responsibility of advocacy is outlined in the Code (NMC, 2015), which states the importance of nurses always acting as advocates for those they are caring for, assisting them to access relevant care, support and information.

Nurse–patient relationship: This is a dynamic and complex relationship in which trust, respect and professional boundaries must be maintained in order for effective care to be delivered. It is a therapeutic relationship that puts the needs of the patient at the forefront and involves being professionally intimate with a patient when helping them with personal care, being empathetic by offering them understanding and always being able to provide competent, high-quality care. Although a power imbalance may exist in this unique relationship, where the nurse may have specialised knowledge and information on the healthcare resources available, it is crucial that active patient participation and collaboration are embraced in the decision-making process (NMC, 2015).

Professional role: Role recognition is fundamental in ensuring nurses are aware of their level of competence and their limitations in making and implementing decisions. It must always be remembered that nurses are accountable for their actions and omissions at professional and organisational levels (NMC, 2015).

The novice nurse utilises a more scientific approach in forming their decisions, especially when there is a high level of uncertainty – as can be seen in the case of Shristi – when compared with an experienced nurse who is able to integrate intuitive knowledge, thus making rapid decisions without conscious thought. Shristi's practice educator recognised that nursing students often feel anxious due to unfamiliar healthcare settings and their lack of experience. These contribute to the lengthier time spent making decisions. However, when nursing students are offered ongoing support and facilitation they are able to develop their means of knowing, as described above, and can integrate these into their decision-making processes. Shristi's practice educator may have served as a role model and through coaching and providing opportunities to reflect, may help her confidence to develop.

Organisational rules and culture: Creating a culture that is receptive and responsive to shared decision-making has been recognised to increase patient satisfaction due to partnership working and greater transparency (AQA, 2013). There are instances, however, when – due to traditional norms and beliefs – a patient may assume a passive role in their care. Furthermore, there can be occasions, due to a lack of time and staff shortages, when nurses rely heavily on one aspect of knowledge, such as protocols, in making decisions, instead of integrating their mastery into the clinical reasoning process. The nursing student needs to recognise organisational challenges while optimising their use of the resources put in place to help develop their decision-making strategies, such as IT decision support systems, preceptorship and clinical supervision.

THE DECISION-MAKING PROCESS

The decision-making process can be grouped into two key areas, the intuitive and the analytical paradigms, as outlined in Table 19.2.

WHAT'S THE EVIDENCE?

FURTHER READING: DECISION-MAKING PROCESS

How do nurses make decisions and how does this decision-making process change during the different stages of nursing development?

Jewel, A. (2013) 'Supporting the novice nurse to fly: A literature review', *Nurse Education in Practice*, 13: 323-7 explored the existing literature relating to the support offered to novice nurses, what they find difficult and how they can be assisted to apply their knowledge to patient situations, make decisions and respond with appropriate actions.

Ellis, N. (2017) 'Decision making in practice: Influences, management and reflection', *British Journal of Nursing*, 26(2): 109-12.

- Reflect on the support you have been offered, what you have found difficult and how you were helped to apply your knowledge to patient situations, make decisions and respond with appropriate actions.
- What do you think is needed to help novice nurses develop their clinical decision-making skills?
- Now read the Ellis article and consider whether your thoughts echo those it highlights.

The analytical framework uses a structured process in the gathering and processing of information, with hypotheses generated and tested in the process of reaching the decision.

Table 19.2   The two key areas of the decision-making process

Analytical	Intuitive
Rules or guidelines are applied to the situation	Pattern recognition, experiential, gut feelings
Conscious data gathering and organisation	Emotional intellect, making connections
Thought process follows a logical sequence	
Information processing and **metacognition**	Rapid, unconscious processing of cues
Hypothesis generation and testing	
Use of decision trees, **algorithms**	
Diagnosis	

Carroll and Johnson (1990) suggest that there are significant stages in the decision-making process (Figure 19.2) and, within the analytical framework, decision-making often begins with identifying that a problem exists.

The ways in which the decision-making stages are applied to the situation being considered will be dependent on the nurse's knowledge and experience and may be informed by both the analytical and intuitive reasoning processes.

It must be noted that this framework is not a sequential process, but can start at any point and can be repeated or backtracked depending on the situation. The problem is broken down into segments, making it easier to understand; the way in which this is done is influenced by the nurse's qualities, such as experience and intuition.

In the analytical clinical reasoning paradigm, the novice nurse may consciously use scientific information, such as a protocol or guidelines, in order to enable them to recognise a patient's signs and symptoms and to formulate an explanation. This is described as hypothetico-deductive reasoning. This form of clinical reasoning follows sequential steps: cue recognition, hypothesis generation, cue interpretation and hypothesis evaluation (Tanner et al., 1987). A novice nurse will collect all of the information before making a decision and planning patient care: a process which is known as backward reasoning. An expert nurse, however, will work from a hypothesis and then collect information to either confirm or refute this.

The hypothetico-deductive approach does not include the action and feedback stages defined by Carroll and Johnson (1990) (Figure 19.2). Carroll and Johnson's model also allows the nurse to make pre-decisions about the situation, to consider if a problem exists at all and, if it does, to explore various solutions to that problem.

The intuitive framework is often used by experienced nurses, where 'immediately knowing' occurs without conscious thought. Benner and Tanner (1987) argue that it is this intuitive thinking that differentiates the expert nurse from the novice, as they are able to make sense of the situation without relying on processing analytical principles. Cognitive theorists have suggested that intuitive decision-making is dependent on the cognitive continuum, which has three dimensions: complexity of the task; ambiguity of the task; and form of the presenting task (Hamm, 1988). It essentially means that how we make decisions is largely influenced by the nature of the task and the time available. Therefore, if the task is familiar to the nurse, lots of information is available and there are time pressures, the nurse is more likely to use intuition in making decisions.

Apply your understanding of intuitive skills in action by reading Tina's case study, at https://study. sagepub.com/essentialnursing2e.

CASE STUDY: TINA

The graphical diagram in Figure 19.3 provides a visual explanation of the two poles of decision-making. It is suggested that decisions are often based on a combination of intuitive and analytical thinking, which offers a 'middle ground' or 'quasirationality' in formulating nursing decisions.

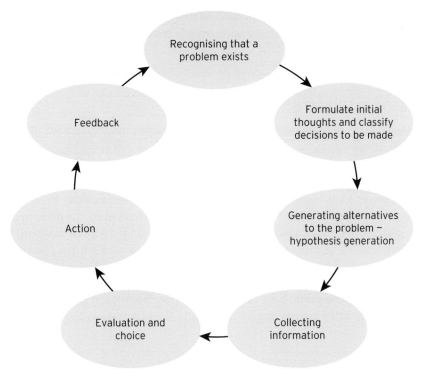

Figure 19.2   Descriptive model of decision-making

Source: Adapted from Carroll and Johnson (1990)

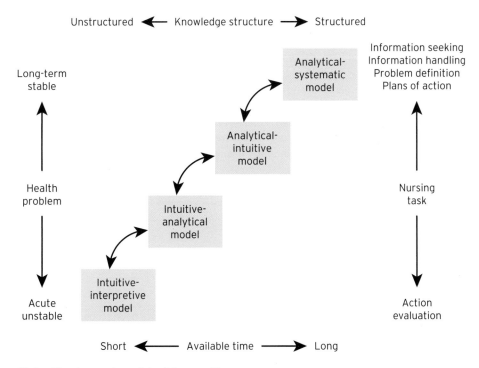

Figure 19.3   The two poles of decision-making

Source: Hamm (1988)

This theoretical perspective on patient care-related decision-making suggests that if lots of information cues are required to make a decision and the task is poorly structured, with limited time available, it is more likely that intuitive decision-making will be applied.

THE ROLE OF PATIENTS

Patient involvement within healthcare is a statutory responsibility in some parts of the UK, with governmental health policies outlining the need for services to be geared around the patient, promoting their active participation (DH, 2000).

A study by Thompson (2007) suggests that the extent of patient involvement in care-related decision-making may vary between five distinctive levels, with varying degrees of patient–practitioner power existing in each. This ranges from no involvement by the patient, at the lowest level, to the practitioner giving the patient the necessary information to make informed decisions about their care, at the highest level. Furthermore, the extent of patient involvement in the decision-making process may be dependent on the individuals' level of education and literacy skills. Patients with a higher level of education often consider themselves to have joint active responsibility in making decisions about their care, whereas those of lower educational attainment can see their level of involvement as merely consenting to options provided by the doctor (Smith et al., 2009).

CASE STUDY 19.3: STEVEN

Steven is a 19-year-old man recently diagnosed with schizophrenia. His condition was diagnosed during his first year of university, which Steven's parents found devastating. Ruomei, the mental health nurse in charge of his care, spent a lot of time with Steven and his parents, offering them timely information and support that helped them to understand the condition and provided them with continuous reassurance. Ruomei worked collaboratively with Steven and his family, the university and the mental health team in organising and coordinating his care, following informed consent.

Nine months later, with a good support network, Steven was able to resume his studies. Ruomei continues to have regular reviews with Steven, and his parents now feel confident that he will be able to lead a full and happy life. Steven and his parents agree that because Ruomei had specialist knowledge about schizophrenia and continuously involved them in Steven's care, they felt reassured at a time when they felt most vulnerable.

- Reflect on a situation in which you actively involved a patient's family in the patient's care.
- Did this alter the way you made decisions when planning the patient's care?

Empowerment

To enable successful patient involvement in decision-making, patients need to be empowered, which involves providing:

- the information necessary to make informed choices about health
- the opportunity to voice opinions on how services can be shaped.

A demonstration of this is the Expert Patient programme, through which people with long-term conditions gain the confidence, knowledge and skills to actively work in partnership with health professionals in managing their health condition. Joint decision-making has significant benefits at both an organisational and an individual level. For example, discharge planning that involves the patient and their families at the outset enables their needs to be prioritised, resources to be cost-effectively sourced and potential problems identified early on, with systems put in place to prevent unnecessary re-admission, which has a direct impact on reducing organisational costs.

CONCLUSION

Nurses make a large number of patient care-related decisions, using a range of strategies specific to the particular situation. Throughout your nursing course, your ability to make decisions will develop, based on your increasing knowledge and practice-based learning.

The types of decisions made by nurses may be unique to a particular placement and require field-specific knowledge, but within the process by which decision-making strategies are formed, common elements utilised by all nurses can be identified.

Patient care-related decisions are based on a combination of analytical and intuitive thinking; alongside critical reflection, this enables constant development so that eventually it is possible to progress to become an expert, as described by Benner (2001).

Patients and their family or carer may need to be empowered to be able to be involved in decision-making. Thus, it is an important aspect of the nurse's role to provide both the information necessary for those involved to make informed choices about health and the opportunity for them to voice opinions on how services can be shaped.

CHAPTER SUMMARY

- Effective decision-making is an important aspect of the provision of high-quality nursing care.
- Nurses in all fields and all settings make a large number of decisions.
- Decision-making involves the integration of theory and practice.
- A number of strategies can be applied to assist in developing the core skills required to make decisions that are holistic and patient-focused.
- Engagement of the patient and their family in the decision-making process is essential.

CRITICAL REFLECTION

Holistic care

- This chapter has highlighted the importance of effective decision-making in providing holistic care for your patient.
- Review the chapter and note down all the instances in which you think making effective patient care-related decisions will help you to meet the patient's physical, psychological, social, economic and spiritual needs.
- Think of a variety of different patients across fields, not just within your own field. You may find it helpful to make a list and refer back to it next time you are in practice, and then write your own reflection after your practice experience.

GO FURTHER

Books

Benner, P. (1984) *From Novice to Expert: Excellence and Power in Clinical Nursing Practice*. Menlo Park, CA: Addison-Wesley. This book provides sound insights into how the nurse progresses through skill acquisition to develop distinctive levels of proficiency. It is useful to assist you to understand and appreciate your journey in developing professionally and gives examples of how nursing judgement and decision-making grow through skill acquisition.

Eraut, M. (1994) *Developing Professional Knowledge and Competence*. London: Falmer Press.

Mezirow, J. (1990) *Fostering Critical Reflection in Adulthood: A Guide to Transformative and Emancipatory Learning. 'How Critical Reflection Triggers Transformative Learning'*. San Francisco, CA: Jossey-Bass.

Sharples, K. and Elcock, K. (2011) 'Decision-making', Chapter 15 in *Preceptorship for Newly Registered Nurses*. Exeter: Learning Matters. pp.137–48. This chapter is useful in demonstrating the different approaches used in the decision-making process and shows how nursing judgement guides the decisions made. It gives examples of how shared decision-making can be enhanced through the use of patient decision aids.

Thompson, C. and Dowding, D. (2009) *Clinical Decision-Making and Judgement in Nursing*. London: Churchill Livingstone/Elsevier. This book offers nurses further details of the knowledge and skills required to develop their decision-making strategies.

SAGE journal articles

FURTHER
READING:
JOURNAL
ARTICLES

Go to https://study.sagepub.com/essentialnursing2e for free online journal articles for this chapter. If you are using the interactive ebook, simply click on the book icon in the margin to go straight to the resource.

Dowding, D., Gurbutt, R., Murphy, M., Lascelles, M., Pearson, A. and Summers, B. (2012) 'Conceptualising decision-making in nurse education', *Journal of Research in Nursing*, 17(4): 348–60. This article shows how critical thinking underpins clinical decision-making and conveys how this can be developed through innovative teaching methods. It is useful for nursing students as it provides an insight into how, through varying teaching strategies such as simulation and problem-based learning, decision-making skills can be enhanced.

Other journal articles

Banning, M (2008) 'A review of clinical decision making: Models and current research', *Journal of Clinical Nursing*, 17(2): 187-195.

Carper, B. (1978) 'Fundamental patterns of knowing in nursing', *Advances in Nursing Sciences*, 1(1): 13-23.

Griffith, R. (2015) 'Accountability in district nursing practice: Key concepts', *British Journal of Community Nursing*, 20(3): 146-149.

Gillespie, M. (2010) 'Using the situated clinical decision-making framework to guide analysis of nurses' clinical decision-making', *Nurse Education in Practice*, 10(6): 333–40. This framework is useful as it provides you with another way in which you could combine key elements – contextual factors, foundational knowledge, decision-making and thinking processes – in developing your decision-making skills.

Standing, M. (2007) 'Clinical judgement and decision-making in nursing: Nine modes of practice in a revised cognitive continuum', *Journal of Advanced Nursing*, 62(1): 124-34. An interesting article discussing how to combine nursing judgement with the decision-making process. It provides examples of nursing decisions and is useful in helping you to link theoretical knowledge to patient care.

Weblinks

Go to https://study.sagepub.com/essentialnursing2e for weblinks related to this chapter. If you are using the interactive ebook, simply click on the book icon in the margin to go straight to the resource.

FURTHER READING: WEBLINKS

http://personcentredcare.health.org.uk – this website facilitates ways by which shared decision-making may be enhanced and helps health professions to build a person-centred approach to decision-making.

www.rcn.org.uk – this website provides nurses with a learning zone that uses web-based resources to help develop evidence-based practice and critical thinking.

www.thecochranelibrary.com – this website is useful as it provides a wide range of critically appraised evidence that can be applied to decision-making.

www.nmc-uk.org – the professional nursing organisation's site is useful in providing guidance and ensures that professional standards are maintained in the decision-making process.

——————— ACE YOUR ASSESSMENT ———————

Review what you have learned by visiting the book's online resources at: https://study.sagepub.com/essential nursing2e If using your interactive ebook, just click on the icon in the margin to go straight there.

ONLINE QUIZZES

- Test yourself with multiple-choice and short-answer questions.
- Revise key terms with the interactive flash cards.

REFERENCES

Advancing Quality Alliance (AQA) (2013) Shared Decision-Making. Available at: www.advancing qualityalliance.nhs.uk/sdm/about-shared-decision-making (accessed 7 December 2013).

Benner, P. (2001) *From Novice to Expert: Excellence and Power in Clinical Nursing Practice*. Upper Saddle River, NJ: Prentice Hall Health.

Benner, P. and Tanner, C. (1987) 'Clinical judgment: How expert nurses use intuition', *American Journal of Nursing*, 87(1): 23–31. Available at: www.effectivepractitioner.nes.scot.nhs.uk/home.aspx (accessed 24 June 2013).

British Association for Parenteral and Enteral Nutrition Malnutrition Advisory Group (BAPEN MAG) (2003) *Nutritional Screening of Adults: A Multidisciplinary Responsibility*. Worcester: BAPEN.

Carper, B. (1978) 'Fundamental patterns of knowing in nursing', *Advances in Nursing Science*, 1(1): 13–23.

Carroll, J. and Johnson, E. (1990) *Decision Research: A Field Guide*. Thousand Oaks, CA: SAGE.

Department of Health (DH) (2000) *The NHS Plan: A Plan for Investment, A Plan for Reform*. London: The Stationery Office.

Ellis, N. (2017) 'Decision making in practice: Influences, management and reflection', *British Journal of Nursing*, 26(2): 109–12.

Hamm, R.M. (1988) 'Clinical intuition and clinical analysis: Expertise and the cognitive continuum', in J. Dowie and A. Elstein (eds), *Professional Judgement: A Reader in Clinical Decision-Making* (pp. 78–105). Cambridge: Cambridge University Press.

Jewel, A. (2013) 'Supporting the novice nurse to fly: A literature review', *Nurse Education in Practice*, 13: 323–7.

Nursing and Midwifery Council (NMC) (2015) *The Code: Professional Standards in Practice and Behaviour for Nurses and Midwives*. London: NMC.

Nyatanga, B. and Vocht, H.D. (2008) 'Intuition in clinical decision-making: A psychological penumbra', *International Journal of Palliative Nursing*, 14(10): 492–6.

Smith, S.K., Dixon, A., Trevena, L., Nutbeam, D. and McCaffery, J. (2009) 'Exploring patient involvement in healthcare decision-making across different education and functional health literacy groups', *Social Science & Medicine*, 69(12): 1805–12.

Tanner, C.A., Padrick, K.P., Westfall, V.E. and Putzier, D.J. (1987) 'Diagnostic reasoning strategies of nurses and nursing students', *Nursing Research*, 36(6): 358–63.

Thompson, A.G.H. (2007) 'The meaning of patient involvement and participation in health care consultations: A taxonomy', *Social Science and Medicine*, 64(6): 1297–1310.

Thompson, C. and Stapley, S. (2011) 'Do educational interventions improve nurses' clinical decision-making and judgement? A systematic review', *International Journal of Nursing Studies*, 48(7): 881–93.

Traynor, M., Boland, M. and Buus, N. (2010) 'Professional autonomy in 21st century healthcare: Nurses' accounts of clinical decision-making', *Social Science and Medicine*, 71: 1506–12.

SAFEGUARDING

ROBERT JENKINS AND JILL BARNES

20

THIS CHAPTER COVERS

- What do we mean by the term 'safeguarding'?
- Safeguarding adults
- Safeguarding children

- The legal framework
- Abuse
- The safeguarding role of nurses

> " The system as a whole failed in its most essential duty – to protect patients from unacceptable risks of harm and from unacceptable, and in some cases inhumane, treatment that should never be tolerated in any hospital.
>
> **Robert Francis QC (DH, 2013a)** "

> " This Public Inquiry [Francis] not only repeats earlier findings but also shows wider systemic failings so I would like to go further as Prime Minister and apologise to the families of all those who have suffered for the way that the system allowed such horrific abuse to go unchecked and unchallenged for so long. On behalf of the government – and indeed our country – I am truly sorry.
>
> **Rt Hon David Cameron MP (DH, 2013a)** "

Both voices from the initial government response to the report of the Mid Staffordshire NHS Foundation Trust Public Inquiry (DH, 2013a: 5)

> " Vulnerability comes in many forms and it is a nurse's duty to safeguard individuals who may come to harm, be at risk or not have their care needs met. Nurses are in a position that allows vulnerabilities to be recognised and the need for safeguarding to be identified; we have a responsibility to our patients to report any concerns.
>
> **Charlie Clisby, NQN** "

Visit https://study.sagepub.com/essentialnursing2e to access a wealth of online resources for this chapter – watch out for the margin icons throughout the chapter. If you are using the interactive eBook, simply click on the margin icon to go straight to the resource.

INTRODUCTION

Safeguarding in nursing has been given top priority due to a number of recent negative press reports highlighting both poor and abusive practices in a number of healthcare settings. As is outlined by the voices from the Department of Health inquiry (2013a) at the start of the chapter, there have been huge failings in care and patients have not been kept safe. There is the potential for this to happen to any person receiving care, but it is a particular danger for those classed as vulnerable, such as children, those with a learning disability, those with mental health needs or older people. Indeed, some individuals may need safeguarding across their lifespan, from cradle to grave.

When it comes to safeguarding in the United Kingdom, there are two important things to keep in mind. The first is that the legal and policy context may be different in the four countries (England, Scotland, Wales and Northern Ireland) that make up the UK. Second, there are also key differences between child and adult protection approaches, particularly with regard to policy and procedures. In spite of the differences, however, all areas adopt a multi-agency approach to safeguarding. This chapter will therefore explore the safeguarding role of nurses in caring for and supporting a range of vulnerable persons.

WHAT DO WE MEAN BY THE TERM 'SAFEGUARDING'?

ACTIVITY 20.1: CRITICAL THINKING

Safeguarding is ...

- What do you understand by the term 'safeguarding'?
- What are the main differences between child and adult safeguarding?

The Care Act 2014 defines safeguarding as upholding an adult's right to live in safety, free from abuse and neglect. The NMC (2016) describes safeguarding as: 'a range of activity aimed at upholding a person's fundamental right to be safe. It means protecting patients and their families from all forms of harm, abuse and neglect, including poor practice'.

This statement seems to adhere to the notion that the patient is viewed as somewhat passive, with the nurse protecting or guarding them from harm. However, this reactive stance is far from the case: the Department of Health (2011) views the safeguarding role of health professionals as involving more than just protecting people from harm, and advocates six key principles (see Figure 20.1). Safeguarding is viewed as more of a proactive approach in which nurses work in partnership with patients through an empowering relationship in order for them to be more than just mere passive recipients of care practices and interventions. This strategy may be further enhanced by a person- or patient-centred approach to care in which positive risk-taking through proportionality is promoted.

Safeguarding adults is different from safeguarding children, in that adults are presumed to have mental capacity, whereas children are generally regarded as lacking capacity and therefore being in need of protection (Baeza, 2011).

SAFEGUARDING ADULTS

All adults are deemed to have capacity until determined otherwise, and are therefore entitled to make their own decisions and choices even if other people consider them unwise. Adults are considered capable of safeguarding themselves from potential harm. However, adults who are vulnerable and lack the capacity to make decisions independently are provided with additional protection under the Mental Capacity Act (MCA) 2005. The legislation applies to everyone involved in the care, treatment and support of people aged 16 and over living in England and Wales (excludes Scotland and Northern Ireland) who are unable to make all or some decisions for themselves, and is designed to protect and restore power to those vulnerable people who lack the capacity to make decisions. All professionals have a duty to comply with the Code of Practice.

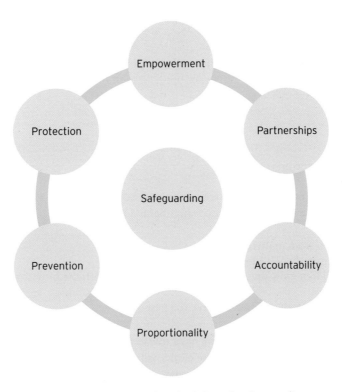

Figure 20.1   Department of Health's (2011) six principles of safeguarding

CASE STUDY 20.1: PEESHE

Peeshe is a 75-year-old man who lives at home with his wife. He has three sons, two daughters, seven grandchildren and three great grandchildren. Peeshe has recently been diagnosed with dementia. His wife, many friends and neighbours had suspected for some time that there was something not 'quite right' with Peeshe at times, as he had become very forgetful and confused and had difficulty with his verbal communication. At other times, he is still the life and soul of the party and keeps his family entertained with his passion for music and singing. He has always been a very healthy and active person. Peeshe and his wife have visited their family doctor for a medication review, and the doctor is concerned Peeshe may not have the capacity to consent to the new medication regime.

(Continued)

- Referring to the Mental Capacity Act 2005, what would you do if you were concerned Peeshe lacked the capacity to reach a decision about his care or treatment?
- Consider the impact of Peeshe's dementia on each of the following people:

  o   wife
  o   children
  o   grandchildren and great-grandchildren
  o   friends and neighbours.

- Do you think they would all feel the same about Peeshe? In regard to safeguarding, who is likely to be in the best position to safeguard Peeshe and why?

ANSWER:
CASE STUDY 20.1

A lack of mental capacity may, for example, be due to a stroke or brain injury; dementia; a learning disability; a mental health problem; confusion, drowsiness or unconsciousness because of an illness or treatment of it; or substance misuse.

SAFEGUARDING CHILDREN

In terms of safeguarding children, HM Government (2013a) issued guidance in order to promote children's welfare and protect them from harm. It highlighted four key areas:

- *protecting* children from maltreatment
- *preventing* impairment of children's health or development
- *ensuring* that children grow up in circumstances consistent with the provision of safe and effective care
- *taking action* to enable all children to have the best outcome.

The government further stated that everyone has a role to play if they come into contact with children and their families. This is actually the same for adults, with the NMC (2016) stating that safeguarding is everyone's business. However, there are fundamental differences between adult and child safeguarding in areas such as legislation, policies and procedures, terminology and definitions used.

THE LEGAL FRAMEWORK

In England, Wales and Northern Ireland, the legal structures for safeguarding adults are rather disjointed, with no single overriding piece of legislation. Instead, a framework of policies has been introduced to safeguard vulnerable adults and protect them from abuse.

In Scotland, the situation is different and legislation (the Adult Support and Protection [Scotland] Act 2007) has been introduced which seeks to safeguard adults who are at risk and unable to safeguard their own interests. This places a duty on local authorities to make enquiries where someone is thought to be at risk, including giving them power to enter premises to check on the safeguarding needs of vulnerable adults. The legislation also includes assessment, removal and banning orders. The Welsh Government's Social Services and Well-being (Wales) Act 2014 and the English equivalent The Care Act 2014 both created local authority duties to make inquiries and decide if action needs to be taken to protect an 'adult at risk'. The Welsh Act goes a stage further by also creating an adult protection and support order.

Vulnerability or adults at risk?

The Department of Health (2011) states that vulnerability is affected by three key elements:

- personal circumstances, e.g. disability or ill health
- environmental risks, e.g. level of social contact, quality of care, adaptations and service received
- resilience factors, e.g. support networks, personal strengths and coping mechanisms.

Nurses should not assume that, just because a person has an illness or a disability, they are automatically vulnerable. Many individuals are able to demonstrate that they are capable of safeguarding their own interests. However, a significant number of people have additional 'vulnerability factors' which mean that they probably need to be safeguarded by professionals. For example, an older adult may live independently with minimal support, but may become more vulnerable when they develop an infection. If additional vulnerability factors exist, such as the individual living in poverty or having no close family, their vulnerability will be further heightened. It is important to emphasise that, as these factors will fluctuate over time, so will a person's level of vulnerability (Jenkins and Davies, 2011). Currently, there is a move away from the term 'vulnerability' towards one of 'adults at risk'. This is because it is felt that the term 'vulnerability' has become almost meaningless, due to different interpretations in areas such as mental capacity, environment and social situations. The focus of safeguarding should be more on risk factors which make the individual open to abuse.

ACTIVITY 20.2: CRITICAL THINKING

In view of the discussion relating to vulnerability or adults at risk, what reasons can you think of why people with learning disabilities, older people, children and people with mental health needs may be more at risk of being vulnerable to abuse?

It is possible that individuals are more vulnerable due to the stigma of their diagnosis or label. This may make others feel that such groups are inferior, too needy, or to be feared. Many such individuals may have poor communication skills and are often reliant on others for daily living needs. On occasion, this may create huge amounts of pressure, leading to intolerable levels of stress and burnout, which, in turn, may lead carers to abuse those they care for. Apply what you have learned about working with vulnerable adults by reading Rosie's case study, at https://study.sagepub.com/essentialnursing2e.

CASE STUDY: ROSIE

Perceived 'differences' or behaviours may also act as triggers for others to abuse vulnerable people. One research study, undertaken by people with learning disabilities (Northway et al., 2013), provides insight into the daily abuses that some vulnerable groups of people face, and what we can do to help.

WHAT'S THE EVIDENCE?

Keeping safe and providing support

Northway, R., Jenkins, R., Jones, V., Howarth, J. and Hodges, Z. (2013) 'Researching policy and practice to safeguard people with intellectual disabilities from abuse: Some methodological challenges', *Journal of Policy and Practice in Intellectual Disabilities*, 10(3): 188–95.

FURTHER READING: KEEPING SAFE

(Continued)

The research in Northway et al. (2013), undertaken in 2010-13 by people with learning disabilities, highlights three key messages:

- **LISTEN** to us. Do not ignore us!
- **BELIEVE** us. Believe what we say!
- **DO** something. Help change things!
- Watch the video or read the article and reflect on how you can implement the three key messages highlighted.

ABUSE

Most nurses would have an idea of what abuse means, in that it is an unwelcome act or activity. However, it can be difficult to define precisely. The most widely used definition of adult abuse in the past was provided by the Department of Health (2000) document *No Secrets* and the National Assembly for Wales (NAfW, 2000) document *In Safe Hands*, both of which stated: 'Abuse is a violation of an individual's human and civil rights by another person or persons.'

This definition was felt to be too wide-ranging and led to too much uncertainty on what type of abuse had taken place (DH, 2009; Magill et al., 2010). Specifically in terms of healthcare settings, despite a number of high-profile abuse scandals (see, for example, the Francis Report, 2013), there has been little research in the UK exploring this issue, although in Sweden Brüggemann et al. (2011: 130) have undertaken work in this area and state:

> Abuse in health care is defined from patients' subjective experiences of encounters with the healthcare system, characterised by events that lack care, where patients suffer and feel they lose their value as human beings. The events are most often unintentional and nurtured and legitimised by the structural and cultural contexts in which the encounter takes place. The outcomes of abuse in health care are negative for patients and presumably for staff and the health care system as well.

This definition provides a patient's perspective, in that abuse somehow makes the individual on the receiving end feel less than human. This is often the result of nurses not treating patients with dignity and respect, as well as ignoring their needs. It may well be the case that abuse in healthcare is not normally intentional – although if you are on the receiving end, this may make very little difference to you. Sadly, it is also possible that there may be indifference to abuse being carried out on the part of both professionals and organisations, as was seen in the Francis Report (2013).

While it remains difficult to find a universal definition for abuse, there are a number of established categories or types which provide a focus in most new multiagency safeguarding policies:

Physical abuse: Examples include hitting, slapping, pushing or kicking, excessive force, overuse of medication, inappropriate use of physical restraint.

Sexual abuse: Examples include rape or non-consensual sexual assault, buggery, incest, touching of sensitive areas of the body and coercing or encouraging vulnerable people to participate in or watch pornographic material.

Psychological abuse: Examples include insults, humiliation, harassment, bullying, threats of harm, isolation, deprivation of contact, persecution, controlling, intimidation, withdrawal from services or supportive networks, coercion and active denial of rights.

Financial/material abuse: Examples include theft or fraud as well as exploitation, inappropriate use or misappropriation of a person's financial resources, property, inheritance, pension, allowances or insurance.

Neglect and acts of omission: Examples include the intentional or unintentional act of withholding basic forms of care and necessities of life, resulting in malnutrition, dehydration, poor hygiene, isolation, sleep deprivation and/or pressure sores. This can include a failure by professionals to access appropriate healthcare on behalf of patients.

Discriminatory abuse: Examples include discriminatory attitudes in areas such as gender, race, sexual orientation, disability, religion and culture.

Institutional abuse: Examples include rigid and inflexible routines, treating adults like children, lack of choice, lack of dignity and respect; and the rights of patients becoming secondary to the organisation's priorities. Essentially, this involves the development of a culture of care which allows poor practice and abuse to flourish.

Physical, sexual, psychological, financial, discriminatory and institutional abuse, plus neglect or acts of omission, are mentioned in most multi-agency policies on safeguarding those at risk from abuse. Some policies also include reference to spiritual abuse, female genital mutilation (FGM), forced marriage, human trafficking and slavery. There are also two other forms of abuse which are usually situated outside adult protection and safeguarding work but which may impact on safeguarding activities. These are hate crime and domestic violence.

Hate crime

Hate crime is where abuse of the person is motivated by prejudice or hostility towards an identifiable group of people. Currently, this relates to areas such as disability, race, religion and belief, sexual orientation and transgender identity.

ACTIVITY 20.3: CRITICAL THINKING

The Francis Report (2013), a public inquiry into the Mid Staffordshire NHS Foundation Trust, and Winterbourne View (DH, 2013b), a review of the standards of care provided to residents in a home for people with learning disabilities, highlighted a large number of disturbing features in the care provided. These included a tolerance of poor standards, greater concern about business priorities than the quality of patient care, poor communication, a lack of accountability, an inward-looking and neglectful culture, poor monitoring of standards, defensiveness and a general lack of candour when dealing with concerns or complaints. Many recommendations for improvement were made: some were more general, while others were specific recommendations for nursing.

- Read the recommendations from the Francis Report presented in Table 20.1.
- What type of abuse do you think was evident in the care the Mid Staffordshire NHS Foundation Trust delivered to some patients?

ANSWER:
ACTIVITY 20.3

Table 20.1 Some key recommendations made in the Francis Report (2013)

General recommendations	Recommendations for nursing
Foster a common culture shared by all in the service of putting the patient first	Increased focus on a culture of compassion and caring in nurse recruitment, training and education through the establishment of national standards
Ensure openness, transparency and candour throughout the system relating to matters of concern	Training and continuing professional development for nurses should apply at all levels (from student to director)
Ensure that the relentless focus of the healthcare regulator is on policing compliance with accepted standards	The professional voice and leadership in nursing need to be strengthened, for example by ensuring that ward nurse managers work in a supervisory capacity and are not office-bound, so they have a greater awareness of patient needs
Make all those who provide care for patients - individuals and organisations - properly accountable for what they do and to ensure that the public is protected from those not fit to provide such a service	Consideration should be given to the introduction of a new professional qualification related to care of the older person

Domestic violence

Domestic violence can be a complex area of safeguarding practice (McGarry et al., 2011) and may involve both adults and children. It is often a hidden problem and tends to occur behind closed doors in the family home. It has been defined by HM Government (2013b) as:

> Any incident or pattern of incidents of controlling, coercive or threatening behaviour, violence or abuse between those aged 16 or over who are or have been intimate partners or family members regardless of gender or sexuality. This can encompass, but is not limited to, the following types of abuse: psychological, physical, sexual, financial [and] emotional.

The government wanted to address current concerns in this new definition by including young persons (aged up to 16 years old) and coercive behaviour. This very much reflects the multicultural nature of domestic violence in areas such as 'honour'-based violence, female genital mutilation (FGM) and forced marriage. It must be remembered, however, that victims are not confined to one gender or ethnic group. (Access the following link for more information: www.gov.uk/guidance/domestic-violence-and-abuse#domestic-violence-and-abuse-new-definition.)

THE SAFEGUARDING ROLE OF NURSES

ACTIVITY 20.4: CRITICAL THINKING

- Read the Nursing and Midwifery Council's (NMC) (2015) *The Code: Professional Standards of Practice and Behaviour for Nurses and Midwives*. London: NMC.
- What are nurses' safeguarding responsibilities contained in this guidance?

As nurses, we are all responsible and accountable for our practice, and for ensuring that we are fit to practise.

Our nurses' Code (NMC, 2015) identifies a number of areas that are related to our safeguarding responsibilities, such as:

- 17 Raise concerns immediately if you believe a person is vulnerable or at risk and needs extra support and protection.
- 2.3 Encourage and empower people to share decisions about their treatment and care.
- 2.5 Respect, support and document a person's right to accept or refuse care and treatment.
- 4.1 Balance the need to act in the best interests of people at all times with the requirement to respect a person's right to accept or refuse treatment.
- 14.1 Act immediately to put right the situation if someone has suffered actual harm for any reason or an incident has happened which had the potential for harm.
- You work within the limits of your competence, exercising your professional 'duty of candour' and raising concerns immediately whenever you come across situations that put patients or public safety at risk. You take necessary action to deal with any concerns where appropriate. (p. 11)
- 16.3 Tell someone in authority at the first reasonable opportunity if you experience problems that may prevent you working within the Code or other national standards, taking prompt action to tackle the causes of concern if you can.
- 14 Be open and candid with all service users about all aspects of care and treatment, including when any mistakes or harm have taken place. (NMC, 2015a)

I feel sad because the majority of the time the care that patients receive is good and it is just a few nurses that don't do things correctly. When I see these things it makes me more determined to care for patients the best I possibly can.

Hannah Boyd, adult nursing student

I used to feel really deflated when I saw such negative coverage, and still find it sad when I hear stories about poor care, however, now I always keep in mind the 6Cs: Competence, Commitment, Communication, Care, Compassion and Courage, and that we're a new generation of nurses that can and will make a difference.

Siân Hunter, child nursing student

One of the most unacceptable aspects of the failings at the Mid Staffordshire NHS Foundation Trust (Francis Report, 2013) and Winterbourne View (DH, 2013b) is that nurses were perpetrators of abuse as well as witnessing poor and abusive practice.

Raising and escalating concerns

As a nurse, you will be constantly exposed to a whole range of human experiences, some of which may cause you to question the actions of yourself and others. In an ideal environment, you will be encouraged to ask questions and raise legitimate concerns. You should be able to do so without fear of censure, reprisal or ridicule. Healthcare settings and environments should foster feelings of dignity, respect and compassion in care. Everyone, including student nurses, should be able to question clinical practice and receive a timely response. The NMC (2017) highlights the important role that clinical leaders play in promoting an open work environment in which staff are both accountable and encouraged to raise concerns about the safety of people in their care. Student nurses who have concerns should always seek help and advice from a practice educator or tutor when there is a need to protect people from harm, or if you are unhappy about any aspects in the care and treatment of patients while on placement.

Figure 20.2 illustrates the five main stages which the NMC suggest you should follow if major issues such as safeguarding need to be raised in practice.

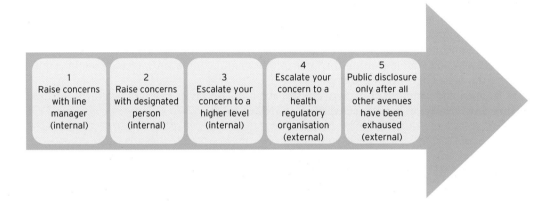

Figure 20.2   Five stages for raising and escalating concerns

Source: NMC (2017)

CASE STUDY 20.2: JAKE, KEVIN AND GERTRUDE AND YOU

Consider each of the stories carefully and then answer the questions at the end of the box.

Jake

While on placement in a children's nursery, you notice Jake, a 4-year-old boy, playing on his own for long periods of the time, or just staring out of the window. He is never taken out on trips and instead the nursery staff leave him with very young children (aged 1–3 years).

When you ask a nursery nurse why they do this, she states that he has autism and 'such children are all like that'. She then laughs and says that you should know this and they don't teach you much at university.

Kevin and Gertrude

While on placement with a community mental health nurse, you visit Kevin, a 54-year old man with schizophrenia living in his family home. He lives with Gertrude, his 70-year-old mother. You notice that Gertrude looks pale, smells strongly of urine and has bruising on her face and leg. You speak to the community nurse and he tells you he just deals with the mental health side of things with Kevin, and that Gertrude is always falling over the clutter in the house.

You

This is your last day of placement on a busy ward in a large general hospital. Today, there has been insufficient time to provide adequate care to all of the patients, due to a cardiac arrest and two patients falling. Most of the older patients you are helping your practice educator care for require full continence care. You have noticed that three patients appear wet or soiled, but it has not been possible to have the assistance you need to change them for over four hours. The ward team is also behind in assisting people with their meals and bathing and there are two patients still in the corridor waiting to be admitted to the ward.

Your practice educator tells you that you will have to work late to help out and, although it is your final day, she will not have time to complete your assessment today, so you will have to come back at a later date.

Questions to consider for Jake, Kevin and Gertrude and you

- Do you have any concerns regarding poor or abusive practice in any of the cases? If so, what forms of abuse have occurred?
- If you did have concerns, what actions would you take?
- What potential barriers may prevent you from raising a concern?
- How would you overcome such barriers?

In each of the cases of Jake, Kevin and Gertrude and you, there is enough information to ask questions or raise concerns about people at risk of being harmed. It is important to remember that when you are asking questions or raising concerns, which is all you are doing. You are not acting as a kind of judge and jury, deciding who is guilty or not. As a nursing student, you should be encouraged to question practice, and as a registered nurse you should be able to justify all of your actions. Good practice is often evident in environments or cultures which foster openness and honesty in a constant endeavour to enhance the quality of care. Effective leadership is also a key feature in such areas (Northway and Jenkins, 2017). Nurses should always prioritise time to reflect on their own practice and learn from their experiences.

In terms of what constitutes good, poor or abusive practice, or simply 'the good, the bad and the ugly' (Northway and Jenkins, 2017), there are different perspectives. In the case studies of Jake, Kevin and Gertrude and you, it is possible to see potentially poor or abusive actions, and you may wonder if there is any good practice here. The good practice comes from you raising concerns, reflecting and ensuring patients are protected from harm. It is never easy to question the practice of those who are more senior, experienced or assertive. Doing nothing has never been an option and you must overcome your fears or your lack of action may call your fitness to practise into question (NMC, 2015).

To assist you in this, remember that you will have a wide range of support systems available while you are on placement, including your personal advisor. There is also specific legislation in place to protect potential whistleblowers if you have concerns which have not been dealt with sufficiently.

> As a newly qualified nurse I came across an elderly woman who suffered from MS; she had severely decreased mobility, which inhibited her ability to care for herself. She came into hospital for a routine procedure and I was going through her admission paperwork with her. I noticed that she was very unkempt; she smelled of urine and had lots of visible cuts and bruises. I asked her who looked after her and she told me she lives at home with her husband, who is her main carer. I decided to refer her to the adult safeguarding team within the hospital. At first I must admit I thought this patient was suffering abuse at the hands of her husband and even felt angry that she had been mistreated, but it turned out that he also had a disability and was not coping with being her main carer. They had never asked for help as they thought they would be split up and put into care homes. In the end home care was organised to assist with the wife's care needs and they were able to stay in their home. This taught me to approach situations like this professionally and non-judgementally.
>
> Charlie Clisby, NQN

CONCLUSION

Nurses play an important role in safeguarding and supporting a range of vulnerable persons. Safeguarding adults can be more problematic for the practitioner in that there are limited powers to intervene if the adult has mental capacity. On the other hand, children and vulnerable adults who are deemed to lack capacity are afforded greater protection. However, no matter whether you come into most contact with adults or children, safeguarding is everyone's business.

Just because a person has an illness or a disability, we should not assume that they are automatically vulnerable or that they lack capacity; many of the individuals for whom we care are able to demonstrate that they are capable of safeguarding their own interests.

The serious case review into the abusive conduct of the care and nursing staff working at Winterbourne View (DH, 2013b) and the Francis Report (2013), a public inquiry into the Mid Staffordshire NHS Foundation Trust, highlighted a large number of disturbing features in the care provided. One of the most unacceptable aspects of these reports was that many nurses must have witnessed poor and abusive practice, but remained silent and chose not to raise concerns.

As a nurse, you will be constantly exposed to a whole range of human experiences, some of which may cause you to question the actions of yourself and others. Healthcare settings and environments should foster feelings of dignity, respect and compassion, enabling everyone to feel able to question clinical practice without fear of negative consequences.

CHAPTER SUMMARY

- Effective safeguarding requires a proactive approach to nursing practice, which is more than just simply protecting vulnerable people from harm.
- The six key principles of safeguarding are empowerment, partnership, protection, prevention, proportionality and accountability.
- There are both similarities and differences in children's and adults' safeguarding. Essentially, adults are presumed to have mental capacity while most children are not.
- It is important that you understand the safeguarding policy and legislation that apply in the country in which you are practising.
- We are all potentially vulnerable depending on personal circumstances, environmental risks and our own resilience.

- Research by vulnerable adults informs us that we must listen to them, believe what they say and ultimately do something about their concerns.
- The Winterbourne View serious case review (DH, 2013b) and the Francis Report (2013), a public inquiry into the failings of the Mid Staffordshire NHS Foundation Trust, highlighted widespread institutional abuse of patients.
- Questioning and reflective practice should always be encouraged.
- Seek help immediately if someone for whom you are providing care has suffered harm for any reason.

CRITICAL REFLECTION

Holistic care

- Much of this chapter has concerned poor or abusive practice, but what exactly constitutes good, holistic practice?
- Some people may be more at risk of harm due to being viewed as 'vulnerable'. Do you think, as a student nurse, that you too may be vulnerable to harm? If so, how?

GO FURTHER

Books

MacIntyre, G., Stewart, A. and McCusker, P. (eds) (2018) *Safeguarding Adults: Key Themes and Issues*. London: Palgrave Macmillan. This text explores some of the emerging approaches to adult safeguarding in a number of multi professional practice areas such as mental health, older people and people with learning disabilities.

Northway, R. and Jenkins, R. (2017) *Safeguarding Adults in Nursing Practice*, 2nd edn. London: SAGE/ Learning Matters. This textbook has been specifically developed for student nurses and all chapters have been updated with this second edition and are linked to the NMC competencies and Essential Skill clusters related to safeguarding issues.

Wate, R. and Boulton, N. (2015) *Multi-agency Safeguarding in a Public Protection World: A Handbook for Protecting Children and Vulnerable Adults*. Hove: Pavilion. This textbook provides an overview of interagency working in both areas of child and adult safeguarding.

Report

Department of Health (2011) Safeguarding Adults: The Role of Health Service Practitioners. Available at: www.gov.uk/government/uploads/system/uploads/attachment_data/file/215714/dh_125233.pdf. This document sets out the key principles of safeguarding for healthcare professionals.

Journal articles

Brüggemann, A.J., Wijma, B. and Swahnberg, K. (2011) 'Abuse in health care: A concept analysis', *Scandinavian Journal of Caring Sciences*, 26(1): 123-32. An interesting Scandinavian perspective on the concept of abuse related to healthcare.

Hood, R., Price, J., Sartori, D., Maisey, D., Johnston, J., and Clark, Z. (2017) 'Collaborating across the threshold: The development of interprofessional expertise in child safeguarding', *Journal of Interprofessional Care*, 31 (6): 705-713.

This interesting research study explored how teachers, nurses and social workers work together in order to safeguarding children. A number of important findings were identified in areas such as decision making, risk taking, responsibility, assessment, relationships, conflict and uncertainty.

Ion, R., Smith, K., Moir, J. and Nimmon, S. (2016) 'Accounting for actions and omissions: A discourse analysis of student nurse accounts of responding to instances of poor care', *Journal of Advanced Nursing*, 72(5): 1054–64. This account discusses the issues and decision-making process of student nurses on how and whether they should raise concerns about poor care.

Weblinks

Go to https://study.sagepub.com/essentialnursing2e for weblinks related to this chapter. If you are using the interactive ebook, simply click on the book icon in the margin to go straight to the resource.

The two weblinks below are to organisations who wish to improve the dignity and respect shown to those who are cared for by professionals, particularly in residential or hospital care:

www.dignityincare.org.uk/about
http://myhomelife.org.uk
The following links are to websites of organisations which support victims of abuse or are concerned with improving safeguarding:

www.victimsupport.org.uk – Victim Support is an independent charity which offers information and support to victims of crime and traumatic events.
www.nationaldomesticviolencehelpline.org.uk – a 24-hour national service helpline for women experiencing domestic violence, run in partnership between Women's Aid and Refuge.
www.nmc.org.uk/standards/guidance/safeguarding – this NMC web page provides helpful guidance on safeguarding issues.
www.scie.org.uk/adults/safeguarding – the Social Care Institute of Excellence web page has some very helpful resources and information on adult safeguarding.
www.nspcc.org.uk – the NSPCC website has some very helpful resources and information on child safeguarding.
www.elderabuse.org.uk – Action on Elder Abuse is a national charity devoted to fighting the abuse of older people.
www.cqc.org.uk/contact-us – CQC provides full whistleblowing guidance for people who work for providers registered with CQC.
www.pcaw.org.uk – Public Concern at Work is the leading independent UK authority on whistleblowing. It provides confidential advice to individuals who witness wrongdoing at work and are unsure about whether or how to raise a concern.
www.mencap.org.uk/campaigns – Mencap fights for equal rights for all people with a learning disability. Campaigns have included 'Out of Sight', seeking to help stop the abuse and neglect of people with a learning disability in institutions like Winterbourne View; the 'R-word campaign' to stop verbal abuse using offensive names; health; and the 'Stand by me' campaign to tackle disability hate crime.

Video links

VIDEO
LINKS

Have a break from the text and go to https://study.sagepub.com/essentialnursing2e for useful videos related to this chapter. If you are using the interactive ebook, simply click on the lightbulb icon in the margin to go straight to the resource.

ACE YOUR ASSESSMENT

Review what you have learned by visiting the book's online resources at: https://study.sagepub.com/essential nursing2e If using your interactive ebook, just click on the icon in the margin to go straight there.

ONLINE
QUIZZES

- Test yourself with multiple-choice and short-answer questions.
- Revise key terms with the interactive flash cards.

REFERENCES

Baeza, S. (2011) 'Learning from safeguarding children', in A. Mantell and T. Scragg (eds), *Safeguarding Adults in Social Work*, 2nd edn. Exeter: Learning Matters. pp. 81–93.

Brüggemann, A.J., Wijma, B. and Swahnberg, K. (2011) 'Abuse in health care: A concept analysis', *Scandinavian Journal of Caring Sciences*, 26(1): 123–32.

Department of Health (DH) (2000) *No Secrets: Guidance on Developing and Implementing Multi-agency Policies and Procedures to Protect Vulnerable Adults from Abuse*. London: The Stationery Office.

Department of Health (DH) (2009) *Safeguarding Adults: Report on the Consultation on the Review of 'No Secrets'*. London: DH.

Department of Health (DH) (2011) *Safeguarding Adults: The Role of Health Service Practitioners*. London: DH.

Department of Health (DH) (2013a) *Patients First and Foremost: The Initial Government Response to the Report of the Mid Staffordshire NHS Foundation Trust Public Inquiry*. London: DH.

Department of Health (DH) (2013b) *Winterbourne View Hospital: Department of Health Review and Response*. London: TSO. Available at: www.gov.uk/government/publications/winterbourne-view-hospital-department-of-health-review-and-response (accessed 2 May 2017).

Francis, R. (2013) *Report of the Mid Staffordshire NHS Foundation Trust Public Inquiry*. London: TSO. Available at: www.midstaffspublicinquiry.com/sites/default/files/report/Executive%20summary.pdf (accessed 2 May 2017).

HM Government (2013a) Working Together to Safeguard Children: A Guide to Inter-agency Working to Safeguard and Promote the Welfare of Children. Available at: http://media.education.gov.uk/assets/files/pdf/w/working%20together.pdf (accessed 20 April 2017).

HM Government (2013b) *Guidance: Domestic Violence and Abuse*. Available at: www.gov.uk/guidance/domestic-violence-and-abuse#domestic-violence-and-abuse-new-definition (accessed 20 April 2017).

Jenkins, R. and Davies, R. (2011) 'Safeguarding people with learning disabilities', *Learning Disability Practice*, 14(1): 32–9.

Magill, J., Yeates, B. and Longley, M. (2010) *Review of In Safe Hands: A Review of the Welsh Assembly Government's Guidance on the Protection of Vulnerable Adults in Wales*. Pontypridd: University of Glamorgan.

McGarry, J., Simpson, C. and Hinchliff-Smith, K. (2011) 'The impact of domestic abuse for older women: A review of the literature', *Health and Social Care in the Community*, 19(1): 3–14.

National Assembly for Wales (NAfW) (2000) *In Safe Hands: Protection of Vulnerable Adults in Wales*. Cardiff: NAfW.

Northway, R. and Jenkins, R. (2017) *Safeguarding Adults in Nursing Practice*, 2nd edn. London: SAGE/ Learning Matters.

Northway, R., Jenkins, R., Jones, V., Howarth, J. and Hodges, Z. (2013) 'Researching policy and practice to safeguard people with intellectual disabilities from abuse: Some methodological challenges', *Journal of Policy and Practice in Intellectual Disabilities*, 10(3): 188–95.

Nursing and Midwifery Council (NMC) (2015) *The Code: Professional Standards of Practice and Behaviour for Nurses and Midwives*. London: NMC.

Nursing and Midwifery Council (NMC) (2016) Safeguarding Fact Sheet. Available at: www.nmc.org. uk/globalassets/sitedocuments/safeguarding/toolkit/safeguarding-fact-sheet.pdf (accessed 19 April 2017).

Nursing and Midwifery Council (NMC) (2017) *Raising and Escalating Concerns: Guidance for Nurses and Midwives*. London: NMC.

PROMOTING HEALTH

CHARLENE LOBO, DARYL EVANS AND HELEN WALKER

THIS CHAPTER COVERS

- Nurse's role in health promotion
- Defining health promotion
- Health-promotion theory applied to nursing
- Promoting health at an individual level

- Promoting health at community level
- Promoting health at population level
- Nurses as role models

> I'm really annoyed, and confused about the lack of a clear message concerning alcohol consumption. I don't think I drink too much, just socially. I'll maybe have a few glasses of red wine of an evening and a couple of gin and tonics at the weekend. What's wrong with that? The trouble is, every time I read one of those women's magazines or newspapers about drinking I get worried. Am I drinking too much?
>
> We keep being told that red wine is good for you, but how much? When I asked the practice nurse she looked it up for me on the internet and told me two small glasses a day, and not every day. That's a bit mean, you can't go out for a meal and just have two small glasses.
>
> **Emer, patient**

> The more patients I care for the more I realise how important it is to be able to explain symptoms to patients in a way they comprehend, because then they can begin to help themselves recover. We can do so much to help but we need to encourage the patients' understanding to promote independence.
>
> **James, first-year mental health nursing student**

INTRODUCTION

Over the last few decades, since the inception of the National Health Service (NHS), there has been a shift in the health of the nation. In the early part of the twentieth century, infectious diseases were a major cause of death and health outcomes were greatly influenced by biomedical advances in vaccinations and antibiotics, the formation of the NHS, the expansion (and professional education) of health professions, and advances in treatments and medical technologies. The early 1960s saw the emergence of conditions associated with lifestyle – today, the main causes of premature death come from lifestyle diseases and illnesses such as hypertension, type 2 diabetes, chronic obstructive pulmonary disease (COPD) and HIV. It stands to reason therefore that there is a requirement for a greater impetus to focus on promoting health, avoiding ill health and minimising the complications of existing conditions, which is reflected in the nursing proficiencies (NMC, 2017).

Within this chapter, the importance of health promotion as part of the nurse's role is explored, and how nurses can use theoretical principles of health promotion to empower patients to become more aware of and adopt healthier behaviours. Throughout the chapter, the focus is on raising awareness of health risks and improving the health of individuals, families, communities and populations, in both acute and community settings.

NURSES' ROLE IN HEALTH PROMOTION

ACTIVITY 21.1: REFLECTION

Before reading this chapter any further, reflect on your experiences of healthcare, either as a patient or as a provider of healthcare:

- Can you identify any care you have either received or provided as being health promotion?
- How effective has this been?

Nurses have an obligation and accountability to promote health for patients, families and the wider community, encouraging health and influencing positive outcomes at individual, community and population levels in a variety of care settings:

> Registered nurses make an important contribution to the promotion of health and the prevention of ill health by empowering people to exercise choice, take control of their own health decisions and behaviours and manage their own care where possible. (NMC, 2017: 10)

Nurses also work from a broader perspective, understanding the wider determinants of health and health inequalities. They work with patients and recognise that they are the experts on their illnesses, as well as with other professionals and organisations and recognise that nurses can't improve health on their own, both in hospital and community settings.

DEFINING HEALTH PROMOTION

Health promotion has been defined by the WHO (1986: 1) as 'a process of enabling people to increase control over, and to improve, their health'. This puts the emphasis on the principle of enabling people, rather than telling them what to do or controlling what they can and cannot do, although it is argued that an element of controlling activity actually helps people to make healthier choices. For example, the ban on smoking in enclosed public areas and workplaces enabled smokers to begin to quit, as well as preventing passive smoking to an extent. Controls on advertising cigarettes, alcohol and snack foods (in the latter case to children) have an impact on people's choices.

It is interesting to consider whether nurses prefer to see themselves as enabling or controlling. It would certainly have an impact if patients did as they were told in terms of health behaviour: if they gave up smoking, looked out for early signs of cancer, ate less salt, fat and sugar and lost weight appropriately. In reality, it is just not as simple as this. Behaviour change is hard to achieve in the face of long-term habits, poor living circumstances and a lack of support. Some might argue that in the relatively short time frame within which the majority of nursing care is delivered, especially in acute settings, nurses can't actually have that much of an influence. At a very baseline health-promotion level, nurses should ensure that they raise all patients' awareness of risk and assist them to begin the process of moving to a healthier lifestyle.

The definition of health promotion has been further defined by the World Health Organization (WHO, 2005: 1) as 'the process of enabling people to increase control over their health *and its determinants*, and thereby improve their health'. This incorporates the more recent acknowledgement of the impact of inequalities in health and the wider (social) determinants of health. Nurses who can aid this process are equally powerful political movers and shakers, even if only in small ways. Enabling a patient to see that getting retrained and preparing to find a job will improve their ability to eat more healthily, undertake physical activity and gain social support, is a real breakthrough. Similarly, helping a parent to understand that their living environment limits their choice of food, activity and the safety of their child, could be beginning a development of community action to improve the geographical area and thus improve health. These kinds of health-promotion activities, that work with communities and on a population level, are often considered in the context of public health practice (other areas include disease control and surveillance, research and management of systems).

When working with the community team we worked with a client who was smoking heavily every day. We discussed how he was feeling in himself both physically and mentally. We noted his responses and asked him what interests he had and what he enjoyed doing. We then supported him to read and listen to music instead of going outside to smoke. We came back to him after a couple of weeks and discussed how he felt physically again. He had noticed he was coughing less and did not become as breathless when doing things as he had previously, he had also saved money! He decided to continue to cut down his cigarettes as he did feel better. We also gave him tools to help deal with stressful situations. Health promotion is extremely important as it gives our patients control over their own wellbeing and health, leading to a better quality of life and less health complications as they get older.

Julie Davis, LD nursing student

Health promotion in the UK

In the UK, central government at Westminster decides what happens in England in relation to the health strategy. Wales, Scotland and Northern Ireland have their own parliamentary systems which produce strategic plans for their own countries, while still acknowledging central government policy and guidance. The World Health Organization (WHO) has played a significant role in setting the direction and leading the way internationally for governments to set their health strategies. A list of WHO health promotion conferences and an outline of the outcomes from the

CASE STUDY:
MR PATEL

most influential conferences that have influenced health promotion strategies worldwide and in particular in the UK is available at www.who.int/healthpromotion/conferences/en.

In England, Public Health England (PHE) has the responsibility for giving direction and setting out the government's policy on health in their strategic plan (Public Health England, 2016). One of the key aims of the current policy is to work with healthcare professionals to develop their roles in illness prevention through the All Our Health and Make Every Contact Count campaigns.

FURTHER
READING:
WHO/PHE

ACTIVITY 21.2: CRITICAL THINKING

Look at the WHO website on past global conferences at: www.who.int/healthpromotion/conferences/en and make a list of the key outcomes of each conference.

Look at the PHE website and read the strategic plan for the UK at: www.gov.uk/government/uploads/system/uploads/attachment_data/file/516985/PHE_Strategic_plan_2016.pdf.

- What actions in the strategic plan reflect the outcomes from the WHO conferences?
- What actions have the UK government outlined for the NHS?
- What interventions are in place in your last placement that reflect the government's strategic plan?

Defining health

When we discuss health promotion, it is important to consider in the first instance what exactly we mean by 'health'. The WHO (1948: 1) once defined health as 'a state of complete physical, mental and social wellbeing and not merely the absence of disease or infirmity'. This definition has been seen as idealistic and limited in the sense of being an impossible state, as many would argue that perfect or total health is not attainable. The important point to consider here is the move away from a medical model of health, where health is viewed as the absence of illness or disease, to recognising that people can have an illness but still consider themselves to be healthy. For example, a patient with well-controlled diabetes, asthma or **bipolar disorder** who manages to live well may see themselves as being perfectly healthy.

The WHO changed its definition in 1986 to a more realistic one which relates more effectively to people's lives, stating that health is 'a resource for everyday life, not the objective of living, making it a positive concept, emphasizing social and personal resources, as well as physical capabilities' (p. 1). This later definition suits the goals of nursing more closely, as nurses can see themselves enabling the attainment of health in terms of a resource to help people live as well as they can more readily than they can enable completeness of health and the absence of disease. This also identifies that people living with long-term altered health states, such as diabetes, asthma or bipolar disorder, can be healthy.

FURTHER
READING:
HEALTH
PROMOTION

ACTIVITY 21.3: CRITICAL THINKING

- Using your personal view of what health entails, write a definition.
- Now read R. Labonte's (1993) seminal work on health promotion and empowerment at: www.researchgate.net/publication/246362374_Health_Promotion_and_Empowerment_Practice_Frameworks (more specifically Chapter 2). Consider your answer in relation to his writing: would you change anything about your original definition?

HEALTH-PROMOTION THEORY APPLIED TO NURSING

Whether planning action for one patient, a group of patients who share a common experience – such as heart disease – or a community of people, theory is essential for quality practice. Health-promotion practice, as in all nursing practice, should be theoretically based to ensure that a sound ethical and systematic approach is applied to practice. There are a vast number of theories, models and frameworks that can be used in promoting health, incorporating psychological, social and educational theory in their construction, and it can be very confusing to decide which theory to use in practice. The theory that might be selected to underpin practice could be based on the client group or the objective of the intervention, and influenced by one's own values and beliefs. Hubley and Copeman (2008) present a useful overview of health-promotion theory, categorising it in relation to client group (Table 21.1).

Table 21.1 Overview of health-promotion theory

Client group	Theory/model
Individual	Biological models Motivation theory Cognitive dissonance Health belief model Stages of change/behaviour change model
Family/friends	Social learning theory Theory of reasoned action Social network theory
Community	Social capital theory Communication of innovations
Nation/society	Normative models Culture-based models Economic/legal models

Katz et al. (2000) categorise theory in a different way, based on the approaches that might be used in the delivery of the intervention (Table 21.2).

Table 21.2 Categorisations of theory

Approach	Theory/model
Descriptive models	Ewles and Simnett (2003) Tannahil (2009) Tones and Tilford (1994)
Educational/ behaviour change models	Prochaska and DiClimente (1982) Health belief model (Becker, 1974) Theory of reasoned action (Ajzen and Fishbein, 1980) Health action model (Tones, 1995)
Analytical models	Caplan and Holland (1990) Beattie (1991)

PROMOTING HEALTH AT AN INDIVIDUAL LEVEL

CASE STUDY:
BUGS

At an individual level, there are three main ways in which nurses promote health:

1. They help people make informed choices through understanding their illness and its impact.
2. Through proactively raising awareness of health risks and promoting healthier choices and opportunities.
3. Helping people engage in behaviour change to adhere to therapeutic interventions, self-manage their illness or engage in a healthier lifestyle.

Helping people make informed choices

Before we can help people make choices, we need, first, to understand what 'health' means to them and, second, to get an understanding of their capacity and capability. We cannot assume that all people have the same level of understanding, thus the first step is always to assess the situation fully and establish which information and approach would be useful to the patient. We need to consider things like: the patient's age (children learn differently from adults); their capacity to learn (the person may have a condition that impairs capacity, such as a learning disability, dementia, substance use, a head injury); and the stage in the patient's journey (for instance, they recently discovered they have an illness and it is something they know little about, or it is a long-standing chronic condition about which they are knowledgeable). The extent to which people have the capacity to obtain, process and understand the basic health information and services needed to make appropriate health decisions is known as health literacy.

CASE STUDY 21.1: TIM

Tim is a 49-year-old salesman from the south of Scotland who is outgoing and gregarious, often described as the 'life and soul of the party'. He lives with his wife and two sons in a rural village and travels extensively to his work territory in the North of England. He started to lose weight rapidly and then appeared to catch a bug which caused him to be violently sick and bedridden within a few days. Tim had extreme difficulty breathing and could barely walk to the toilet. His GP sent him to hospital, where he arrived in a confused state and literally collapsed onto a bed. After a very brief consultation with nursing staff, they tentatively suggested he was suffering from type 1 diabetes; this was later confirmed by the consultant.

Tim spent the next four days in hospital in the high dependency unit. Prior to discharge, he and his wife met with the clinical nurse specialist who explained the basics of managing diabetes. Since Tim's job meant he had to drive many miles, he was required to contact the DVLA and advise them of his condition. The first month at home was relatively uneventful, and then Tim began to experience violent spasms in his feet and lower legs. He was unable to sleep or work and subsequently became extremely depressed.

*   Should the nurses have suggested a diagnosis prior to the consultant's assessment?
*   What information would you provide Tim's family with to assist them in supporting him?

Health literacy is an important concept in promoting health because, as Berry (2016) says, 'Put simply, how can we expect someone with type 2 diabetes to confidently self-manage their condition when

FURTHER
READING:
JONATHAN
BERRY BLOG

they are unaware there is a link between it and the food they are eating?' (see his full blog at www.england.nhs.uk/blog/jonathan-berry).

Health literacy can be defined as 'the personal characteristics and social resources needed for individuals and communities to access, understand, appraise and use information and services to make decisions about health' (WHO, 2016). So, for people to understand their health, they need to know where to find the information, the information needs to be in a format they can understand, they need to understand the range of choices, the impact of these choices and then they need to be able to work out if the information or services match their needs and preferences. The Royal College of General Practitioners (2014) produced a report which highlighted that 43% of adults (those aged 16–65 years) cannot fully understand and use written health information, increasing to 61% when numeracy is included. The report claims there is a mismatch between expectations of patients' behaviour and communicating in a way that enables patients to understand those expectations.

ACTIVITY 21.4: IMPROVING SKILLS IN HEALTH LITERACY

To improve your skills in health literacy, go to https://learn.nes.nhs.scot/1449/elearning-digital/health-literacy-tools-and-techniques and complete the e-learning module.

WEBLINK:
HEALTH
LITERACY
TOOLS

Raising awareness of health risks and promoting healthier choices

Raising awareness of health risks and promoting healthier choices has always been part of nursing practice, sometimes known as health education and sometimes as health promotion. These two terms have been used interchangeably in the nursing literature and in practice, despite there being an important difference between them. According to Whitehead (2004), health education tends to have a stronger bio-medical focus and a predominant mode of practice, especially in the acute setting, whereas health promotion recognises the wider socio-political and economic determinants that influence health. It is also argued that health education leans toward a power imbalance in favour of the educator and health promotion is a more egalitarian model of learning that puts the patient at the centre of the interaction. Current practice supports the notion of 'health coaching' as a way of promoting health in an empowered way. Coaching is a form of development that encourages a person to maximise their performance; it is more a way of helping people to learn rather than teaching them to learn. Traditionally, health education has been more focused on passing on information from 'expert' to patient; it has been about advising and telling people what they should/need to do. Coaching is about supporting people to work out for themselves what they should/need to do and facilitating the achievement of their own goals.

As identified earlier, health coaching as a concept is gaining increasing importance in healthcare delivery – it encourages professionals to use evidence-based skills (such as motivational interviewing, behaviour change theory and communication strategies) to underpin conversations between a healthcare practitioner and a patient. Nurses are constantly interacting with people and therefore have a huge number of opportunities to engage in positive coaching conversations.

WEBLINK: BETTER
CONVERSATION

ACTIVITY 21.5: REFLECTION

- Listen to what patients and professionals say about effective conversations at www.better conversation.co.uk.
- Think of two interactions you have had with a patient in your last placement. How could you have changed the focus to make it a 'better conversation'?

Health Education England has introduced a campaign called 'Make Every Contact Count', suggesting that professionals should use every opportunity to undertake 'opportunistic chats' to deliver healthy lifestyle messages and encourage people to take positive steps towards making a lifestyle change and/or signposting them to services that can support them. The focus of this approach is to engage in a conversation that has an empowering effect.

> Educating patients can empower them to manage their health and saves time because they can help themselves stay fit and healthy and therefore spend less time seeing their doctors because they have prevented ill health. This would then reduce the waiting lists and prevent further demand on the services in later years.
>
> **Julie Davis, LD nursing student**

WEBLINK: MAKING
EVERY CONTACT
COUNT

WEBLINK:
E-LEARNING
RESOURCE

ACTIVITY 21.6: MAKING EVERY CONTACT COUNT

- Read the fact sheet www.makingeverycontactcount.co.uk/media/1129/mecc-factsheet.pdf and listen to what patients and professionals say about effective conversations at www.better conversation.co.uk.
- Improve your skills by accessing the elearning resource www.e-lfh.org.uk/programmes/making-every-contact-count.

A model of behaviour change: Prochaska and DiClemente (1982)

Prochaska and DiClemente (1982) developed their Transtheoretical Stages of Change model to explain how people go through distinct stages in the process to change to healthier behaviours (see Figure 21.1).

The model suggests that, at first, a person does not wish to change or cannot see the reason to do so (pre-contemplation). Something may then make them reconsider and think about perhaps changing (contemplation). This stage could last a while before the person begins to plan to change and looks for ways to do it (preparation). Before too much looking around happens, hopefully the person will make the difficult decision to try some method of change (making a change). If that trial is successful, showing some results, or at least being not objectionable, the person may keep it up (maintaining a change). At any time in this process, a problem may occur, causing the person to give up (relapse) and revert to one of the previous stages.

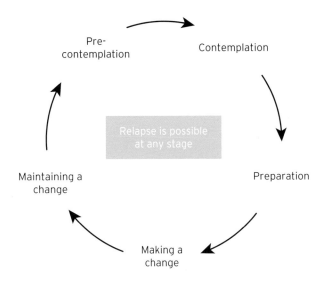

Relapse is possible at any stage

Figure 21.1   Prochaska and DiClemente's (1982) Transtheoretical Stages of Change model

This is a very important model to understand and use as it is very patient-centred and much of the government guidance on promoting health is based on this model. The model can also be used in group situations; it is popular in smoking-cessation programmes, which is what the authors developed the model for. The aim of this model is for the nurse to be able to judge which stage a person has reached and to deliver an intervention suitable to that stage, enabling the person to move on to the next stage or return from relapse. Application of the model is demonstrated in Table 21.3. It identifies the stage of the model, how you might recognise the person is at this stage from what you might see in their behaviour and what you might hear them say. It identifies what the aim of the intervention at this stage is and what you could say and do to motivate the person to move on to the next stage.

Table 21.3   Applying Prochaska and DiClemente's (1982) model

Stage 1: Pre-contemplation – not interested in change

What you might see:

- Clients may feel attacked and react by being defensive and angry
- They may not see that the health risks or the benefits of stopping have anything to do with them personally
- They may feel it is harder and harder to find a place where they can smoke in peace

Your aim:

Encourage them to consider the possibility of stopping

What you could say:

- In what way do you think this behaviour affects your health?
- What risks are you running by continuing to act in this way?

What you might hear:

- I don't want to
- I'm not ready to stop
- I'm not really interested
- I tried it once and didn't like it
- It doesn't work
- You've got to die of something

(Continued)

Can you imagine yourself in … years from now?

What do think will be the price to pay for continuing to be this way?

How do you feel when people nag you about this?

<u>Brief message</u>

Stopping smoking/losing weight is the single best thing you can do to improve your health. If you decide to stop in the future, we will help you all we can

<u>Actions</u>

Engage in a critical awareness exercise

Stage 2: Contemplation – thinking about change

What you might see:

Clients may have been thinking about changing behaviour for a long time, possibly years

They may be afraid and wonder how they would cope

They may have many doubts, asking themselves questions such as:

Can I do it?
What if I fail?
Will I feel I'm missing something?

What you might hear:

I've been thinking about it for some time

I'm not sure I could do it

I'll probably do it sometime

I would like to do it some day

Your aim:

Encourage them towards taking action in the near future

What you could say:

What good things do you think you will find if you stop?

What do you enjoy about smoking/eating?

What are the things you don't like about it?

What worries or concerns you about smoking/being overweight?

What are the things you feel you might lose?

<u>Brief message</u>

I am glad that you want to change some day. I would like you to think about trying to change soon

<u>Actions</u>

Urge changes, i.e. delay smoking for 30 mins

Offer carbon monoxide test

Provide leaflets and record and ask at next visit

Stage 3/4: Preparation – preparing to and making change

What you might see:

Clients will begin to see that the benefits of giving up are greater than the costs

They will begin to believe that changing behaviour is worthwhile and that they can do it, but they may still have some fears that they won't succeed

What you might hear:

I'd like to try the patches

I'm planning to…

I'm trying to find…

I had my last cigarette on…

I've just stopped smoking/started a diet

Your aim:

Help them to make decisions about when and how to change and to look for alternatives to smoking/eating. Encourage them to plan effectively and to reinforce determination and motivation

What you could say in preparation:

Have you tried changing behaviour before?

> How long did it last?
>
> How did you feel during that time?
>
> What benefits did you notice when you weren't smoking/lost weight?
>
> Why did you start again?
>
> What did/didn't work?
>
> Are you changing your behaviour for yourself or somebody else?

What you could say in planning:

- When will you have your last cigarette/start your diet/start exercising?
- Do you need people around you to support you? If so, how?
- What things might trip you up?
- How will you cope with these?
- How can you keep going?
- Devise a plan
- Treatment options

Brief message

Well done, we can do this together, let's see what works for you

Actions

Clear plan with small achievable goals

Stage 5: Maintaining change

What you might see:

- Maybe continuing to make changes
- For some this remains a struggle for some time, and others may relapse into their old behaviour patterns again

What you might hear:

- I'm doing OK
- I've stopped for a while now
- I'm getting there, but it's not easy
- I still really miss it
- I think I'll manage to keep going
- I haven't smoked in the last...

Your aim:

Reinforce the motivation to remain changed, and boost confidence in what has been achieved so far

What you could consider:

- Remind about the temptation to have just one...
- Look at the positive signs of success
- Go back over the reasons for changing in the first place
- Encourage rewards for what has been accomplished
- Invite the smoker to do a CO test to provide encouragement
- Invite the dieter to measure and compare weight circumference
- Look for ways of getting extra help and support

Brief message

Keep going, I am really interested and want to see you regularly

Actions

Offer regular support

(Continued)

Relapse

What you might see:

Clients may have an all-or-nothing approach and be back to square one

They may have had a small relapse, smoking one or two cigarettes, or had one large meal

What you might hear:

I was OK until...

It doesn't work ... I can't do it

I tried but it was too hard

I was doing fine until...

Your aim:

Encourage them to see relapse as a normal part of the change process and to learn from the experience so that the chances of success are greater next time

What you could consider:

Revisit why they stopped

Help them to see that a temporary lapse or slip is not the same as a permanent setback

Remind them that the more times they try, the more likely they are to win through in the end

If they have slipped back to the thinking or preparing to change stages, help them to start moving forwards again

<u>Brief message</u>

Don't give up giving up!

<u>Actions</u>

Reassure and look to start back into any stage of the cycle

WHAT'S THE EVIDENCE?

Helping people to change health behaviour

WEBLINK:
NICE

National Institute for Health and Care Excellence (NICE) (2014) Behaviour Change: Individual Approaches. Available at: www.nice.org.uk/guidance/PH6 (accessed 12 November 2017).

NICE (2014) outlines that professionals providing behaviour change programmes should ensure interventions meet individual needs by:

- giving patients clear information on behaviour change interventions and services available, and how to use them – if necessary, people should be helped to access the services
- ensuring services are acceptable and meet patients' needs – this includes any needs in relation to a disability or another 'protected characteristic' in relation to equity
- recognising times at which people may be more open to change, for instance at a life-changing moment (such as becoming a parent) or when hearing a medical diagnosis (such as heart disease or diabetes)
- ensuring that those leading behaviour change programmes keep in touch with patients to help them maintain the changes they have made and support them if they are struggling – they need to be ready to help people who are having difficulties with fresh ideas and advice.

Reflect on the health-promotion programmes you have experienced, either as a nursing student or before starting your course:

- How effectively did these programmes achieve the points identified in the NICE guidance?
- Now read the NICE guidance in full and consider how you can implement the points identified in your practice.

PROMOTING HEALTH AT COMMUNITY LEVEL

Promoting health at community level often means working with the wider family and groups of people to achieve positive health outcomes. Tones and Tilford's (1994) empowerment model offers a good framework to do this.

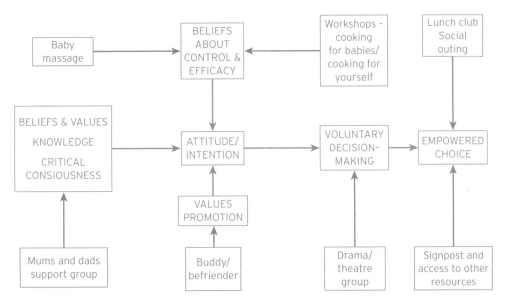

Figure 21.2   Adaptation of Tones and Tilford's (1994) education process of empowerment

The model proposes that people's knowledge, beliefs and values influence their attitudes, which in turn influence their decisions on the choices they make, therefore health promoters can engage in a range of activities that influence values, beliefs and knowledge to change people's attitudes and influence them to make positive choices. This model is considered an empowerment model in the way it uses educational interventions to develop social and cognitive skills and competencies, which in turn increases people's self-worth and enhances their sense of power and self-determination. Table 21.4 is an explanation of the above model using a range of activities to empower a group of vulnerable mothers to enhance their parenting capacity.

CASE STUDY 21.2: DAN

You are currently visiting Dan weekly with your practice educator, a district nurse, to check the healing of a varicose ulcer and to ensure he is taking his anti-depressants. Dan is 46 years old, has a long history of depression and is estranged from his family. He is employed on a casual basis only (minimum wage) in the building trade. Dan lives in a big city, in hostel accommodation, which means he has no permanent home. The area he lives in is a deprived one. Most of the shops and facilities are closed and boarded up. The only food shops are small general stores at variable, but not discount, prices – in fact, some are more expensive because the businesses are struggling.

(Continued)

CHECK YOUR
ANSWERS!

ANSWER:
CASE STUDY 21.2

Dan says he generally eats sausage rolls and pies bought from a local convenience store. There are only limited communal cooking facilities at the hostel and he shares a room with another man.

- How could you help Dan to eat more healthily?
- In your plan, make sure you consider:
  o Dan's reasons for not eating healthily
  o Dan's motivation to change
  o the environmental and structural barriers to improving Dan's diet.

Table 21.4 Activities to empower mothers

Activity		Aim	
Support groups	Opportunities for facilitated discussion	Raise critical consciousness	Influence change in knowledge, values and beliefs
Counselling	Opportunities to have individual counselling or a referral for counselling	Raises critical consciousness and self-esteem	Influences change in knowledge, values and beliefs
Buddy/befriender	Individual support and opportunities to demonstrate positive reinforcing behaviours	Provides modelling	Promotes values, self-worth and self-esteem
Baby massage	Baby massage classes	Provides modelling	Enhances beliefs about control and efficacy
Workshops	A range of workshops on cooking, reading, health literacy, etc.	Provide health and life skills teaching	Enhance beliefs about control and efficacy
Social outings/ lunch clubs	Opportunities to develop social relationships	Build social and self-regulatory skills and competence	Enhance self-esteem and self-worth
Signposting other resources			Enhances environmental and social support

Source: Adapted from Tones and Tilford (1994)

ACTIVITY 21.7: REFLECTION

Think about a patient you have cared for and consider how you could apply this model.

PROMOTING HEALTH AT POPULATION LEVEL

Promoting health at population level is also considered public health practice.

Tannahill (2009): A health-promotion model

Tannahill's (2009) model of health promotion (see Figure 21.3) emerged from the mid-1980s vision of promoting health as a united set of principles. Not far removed from the ideas in the Ottawa Charter,

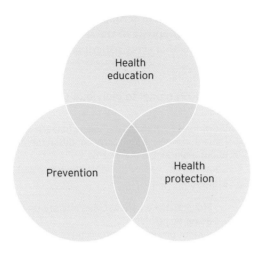

Figure 21.3 Tannahill's (2009) model

Tannahill suggested that existing health education and prevention services needed to be enhanced by setting public policy to protect health.

The three overlapping spheres of Tannahill's model can be used to identify important health-promotion actions when nursing individuals, patient groups or communities (see Table 21.5).

The model could also be used to form a structure for the entirety of a health-promotion project. It is often used as a framework to set a strategy, incorporating several interventions to achieve an overall aim. A community-based project focusing on, for example, osteoporosis in women could be constructed as follows:

- *Health education sphere*: a campaign of posters and leaflets, with talks being given to all women's groups in the local area.
- *Prevention sphere*: promoting good nutrition and physical activity for girls in school; encouraging women to recognise their risks and request screening; supporting women to take up weight-bearing exercise.
- *Health protection sphere*: developing policy to provide low-cost exercise facilities for women, lobbying for the strategic planning of a comprehensive screening programme.

Tannahill's (2009) model can also be used to assist in the planning required for an organisation to become a 'healthy organisation'. This is a settings-based approach to health promotion. The WHO began this approach with its Healthy Cities programme in the 1980s, taking a whole-systems view of promoting health where people live, work, travel, study, etc. A setting may be a school, a hospital, a prison or a neighbourhood. As a nurse, it would be possible to apply this idea to the setting of just one ward, clinic, practice, nursing home or hospice. With a settings-based approach, the focus is on health topics relevant to the people in the setting. Those people include patients, their families and, of course, staff. Some ideas could include:

- *Health education sphere*: displaying health information in an easily accessible way, such as through leaflets, posters, showing DVDs, having discussions. To keep things fresh, the calendar of events would be based on, for example, Men's Health Week or National Smile Week.
- *Prevention sphere*: this would mean health-promotion practices such as providing healthy food, enabling physical activity, limiting alcohol, banning smoking, creating access to health screening.

- *Health protection sphere*: this would involve setting standards based on national strategic plans and policies and creating policies appropriate to the setting – for example, providing staff access to low-cost gym sessions or ensuring that every patient receives education about their condition.

Table 21.5   Applying Tannahill's (2009) model to individuals, patient groups or communities

Health education sphere (teaching people about healthy lifestyles and preventing disease)	• Individuals – a parent who needs to learn about healthy eating for children • Patient groups – a long-term condition mental health patient group learning about maintaining oral health • Communities – an education campaign about using condoms for safe sex

Prevention sphere (providing primary services such as immunisation, secondary services such as screening and tertiary services such as support for people living well with a diagnosis)	• Primary prevention:
	  ○ Individuals – a patient being advised on the correct sun protection before going on holiday
	  ○ Patient groups – the provision of low-fat, -salt and -sugar food in a supported living home for people with learning disabilities
	  ○ Communities – nurse-led laughter and happiness project for the elderly in the local library
	
	• Secondary prevention:
	  ○ Individuals – advising a woman to attend cervical screening
	  ○ Patient groups – patients attending a stroke club being screened for depression
	  ○ Communities – promoting smoking cessation
	
	• Tertiary prevention:
	  ○ Individuals – patient education about their condition and its management
	  ○ Patient groups – supporting informal carers' groups in order to prevent any problems for them and the people in their care
	  ○ Communities – an exercise and eating project devised for obese children

Health protection sphere (creating policies, strategies and best practice guidelines for different preventable health issues)	• Individuals – talking with a parent about school policy on sex education and provision of the 'morning after pill' • Patient groups – working with drug users on an outreach programme about infection control in local hostels • Communities – raising awareness in a low-income area about availability of low-cost and free physical activity provision

ACTIVITY 21.8: REFLECTION

Reflect on your most recent placement area, the patients you were involved in caring for, their families and the staff:

- Using the three overlapping spheres of Tannahill's (2009) model, how could you turn this placement into a healthy organisation?

NURSES AS ROLE MODELS

Whether nurses should be role models is a potentially controversial and often debated issue, which needs to be dealt with sensitively as it can cause conflict and hurt. We can all recognise, without people adopting a blaming or accusatory stance, that it would be good if all nurses were 'in a state of complete' health. But, as has already been discussed in this chapter, such a state is not achievable. Health is best considered as a 'resource for living' as effectively as we can. The debate about whether nurses should be role models and follow the health behaviours they promote to others raises a number of questions, many of which are complex.

Starting with the simpler questions, for example: do nurses have to be 'free from disease'? It is possible to answer no, as there are many nurses working with various conditions and disabilities, and they could be considered excellent role models in their ability to effectively undertake a demanding professional role at the same time as managing their condition or disability. A similar question is whether nurses always have to remain healthy. Once again, it is possible to answer no, since we all get colds and have accidents occasionally.

Having answered these questions, we move on to consider what lies at the core of this controversial issue – whether fat nurses, smoking nurses, nurses who enjoy a drink and nurses who are couch potatoes are able to promote health to others. Interestingly, most of the blame seems to be attached to those nurses with visible or obvious poor health behaviours. How often is it considered that nurses who are constipated, nurses who do not practise safe sex or nurses who do not attend screening opportunities cannot promote the health of others?

So, it is necessary to take a sensible approach to this debate – otherwise we could end up saying that a nurse who has not had a baby or reared a child could be viewed as unable to act as a role model to a parent. A parent could say to such a nurse, 'You don't understand what I'm going through', but even if the nurse had children, the parent could say: 'Your experience was not like mine, you don't understand'. There are huge dangers in such an approach: not only would it be impossible to try to match any patient's experience, but one of the important aspects a nurse can bring to any patient's situation is their objective view.

Let us return to the issue of nurses who have visible signs of poor health: a nurse who is fat, for example. Can a fat nurse help a fat patient to lose weight? Let's imagine the scene – a patient says to a fat nurse, 'You obviously can't help because you can't do it for yourself'. However, if the fat nurse is sufficiently secure in themselves, they can use their own experience to show empathy and share experiences – 'Did you ever try the X diet? Wasn't it awful, and it didn't work anyway'. Now imagine the scene again, but with a slim nurse. They may not be able to use their experience in the same fashion to demonstrate that they understand what the patient is going through, and in this situation the patient may say, similarly to the parent in the previous discussion, 'What do you know about it?', or may feel intimidated and less able to openly discuss their unhealthy eating behaviours. Even if this slim nurse was once fat and has lost weight, they may not fare any better, as the patient could feel they were being shown up for failing.

This demonstrates how easy it becomes for this debate to be sidetracked and removed from the important issue of encouraging patients to strive to attain the best health possible. Possibly the best way forward is for nurses to focus on becoming role models for self-esteem, motivation, trying hard and active learning, rather than role models for perfect health.

CONCLUSION

Health promotion is something all health professionals and their assistants and students must become involved in. Health promotion is as much a goal of nursing and part of providing holistic care as is the provision of quality care related to the patient's condition. Improving the health of people while they are in your care improves patients' quality of life and makes best use of health service resources. Nurses need to understand the principles, theory and evidence of health promotion in order to deliver optimal care in the same way they would provide any other evidence-based care.

CHAPTER SUMMARY

- Health promotion involves enabling people to gain the best health they can, regardless of illness or inequalities, and is an essential part of the nurse's role.
- Health is an attainable condition but is never complete.
- International policies are used to design health-promotion projects and interventions.
- A range of theoretical models can be used to help structure health-promotion interventions.
- Health promotion is an aspect of public health.
- Behaviour change is an important goal in promoting health.
- Health promotion is applicable in all settings and in all fields of nursing.

CRITICAL REFLECTION

Holistic care

This chapter has highlighted the importance of health promotion in providing holistic care for patients:

- Think of a patient for whom you have cared recently. For each aspect of care you gave, note which health-promotion opportunities arose. For example, when washing the patient, did you take the opportunity to teach them about hand hygiene?
- How would your care need to be adapted for a patient from another field of nursing – learning disability, adult, child or mental health?
- Now write a reflection on how you integrated health promotion into your nursing care.

GO FURTHER

Books

Evans, D., Coutsaftiki, D. and Fathers, C.P. (2014) *Health Promotion and Public Health for Nursing Students*, 2nd edn. Exeter: Learning Matters. A readable and concise book covering all aspects of health promotion in nursing practice.

Hubley, J. and Copeman, J. (2008) *Practical Health Promotion*. Cambridge: Polity Press. A very good overview covering practical application of health promotion. This book considers in detail the concept of communicating for health.

Report

HEALTH
LITERACY
REPORT

The Royal College of General Practitioners (2014) Health Literacy Report. Available at: www.rcgp.org.uk/clinical-and-research/resources/a-to-z-clinical-resources/health-literacy-report.aspx.

Journal article

Rush, K.L., Kee, C.C. and Rice, M. (2005) 'Nurses as imperfect role models for health promotion', *Western Journal of Nursing Research*, 27(2): 166–83. Research into the idea of nurses as healthy role models.

Whitehead, D. (2004) 'Health promotion and health education: Advancing the concepts', *Journal of Advanced Nursing*, 47(3): 311–20. Good analysis on the difference between the concepts of health education and health promotion and aids understanding of why the notion of empowerment in practice is so important.

Weblinks

Go to https://study.sagepub.com/essentialnursing2e for weblinks related to this chapter. If you are using the interactive ebook, simply click on the book icon in the margin to go straight to the resource.

FURTHER
READING:
WEBLINKS

The four websites of the overall public health and health promotion organisations throughout the nations of the UK are listed below, followed by other useful web pages:

www.gov.uk/phe – Public Health England
www.publichealthwales.wales.nhs.uk – Wales
www.healthscotland.com – Scotland
www.publichealth.hscni.net – Northern Ireland
www.gov.uk/government/uploads/system/uploads/attachment_data/file/516985/PHE_Strategic_plan_2016.
    pdf – the latest news from the Department of Health, which is relevant to the whole of the UK.
www.nice.org.uk – the National Institute for Health and Care Excellence is the organisation which
    produces guidance for the UK government on public health (including health promotion) practice.
www.nhs.uk/Pages/HomePage.aspx – NHS Choices is a very good website for both you and patients to
    find out about both lifestyle issues and diseases.

ACE YOUR ASSESSMENT

Review what you have learned by visiting the book's online resources at: https://study.sagepub.com/essential
nursing2e If using your interactive ebook, just click on the icon in the margin to go straight there.

ONLINE
QUIZZES

- Test yourself with multiple-choice and short-answer questions.
- Revise key terms with the interactive flash cards.

REFERENCES

Ajzen I. and Fishbein M. (1980) *Understanding Attitudes and Predicting Social Behaviour.* Englewood Cliffs, NJ: Prentice-Hall.

Beattie, A. (1991) 'Knowledge and control in health promotion: A test case for social policy and social theory', in J. Gabe, M. Calnan and M. Bury (eds), *The Sociology of the Health Service.* London: Routledge.

Becker, M.H. (1974) 'The health belief model and sick role behavior', *Health Education and Behavior*, 2: 409–19.

Berry, J. (2016) Does Health Literacy Matter? Blog, 19 October. Available at: www.england.nhs.uk/ blog/jonathan-berry (accessed 29 November 2017).

Caplan, R. and Holland, R. (1990) 'Rethinking health education theory', *Health Education Journal*, 49(1): 10–12.

Ewles, L. and Simnett, I. (2003) *Promoting Health: A Practical Guide*, 5th edn. London: Balliere Tindall.

Hubley, J. and Copeman, J. (2008) *Practical Health Promotion.* Cambridge: Polity Press.

Katz, J., Peberdy, A. and Douglas, J. (2000) *Promoting Health, Knowledge and Practice*, 2nd edn. London: OU in association with Palgrave.

National Institute for Health and Care Excellence (NICE) (2014) Behaviour Change: Individual Approaches. Available at: www.nice.org.uk/guidance/PH6 (accessed 12 November 2017).

Nursing and Midwifery Council (NMC) (2017) *Draft Standards of Proficiency for Registered Nurses*. London: NMC.

Prochaska, J.O. and DiClemente, C. (1982) 'Transtheoretical therapy: Toward a more integrative model of change', *Psychotherapy: Theory, Research and Practice*, 20: 161–73.

Public Health England (2016) *Strategic Plan for the Next Four Years: Better Outcomes by 2020*. London: Public Health England.

Royal College of General Practitioners (2014) *Health Literacy*. London: Royal College of Health Practitioners.

Tannahill, A. (2009) 'The Tannahill model revisited', *Public Health*, 123(5): 396–9.

Tones, B. (1995) 'Making a change for the better: the health action model', *Healthlines*, 27: 17–19.

Tones, K. and Tilford, S. (1994) *Health Education: Effectiveness, Efficiency and Equity*, 3rd edn. Cheltenham: Nelson Thornes.

Whitehead, D. (2004) 'Health promotion and health education: advancing the concepts', *Journal of Advanced Nursing*, 47(3): 311–20.

World Health Organization (WHO) (1948) *Constitution*. Geneva: WHO.

World Health Organization (1986) *Ottawa Charter*. Geneva: WHO.

World Health Organization (2005) *Bangkok Charter for Health Promotion in a Globalized World*. Geneva: WHO.

World Health Organization (2016) *Promoting Health in the SDGs*. Geneva: WHO.

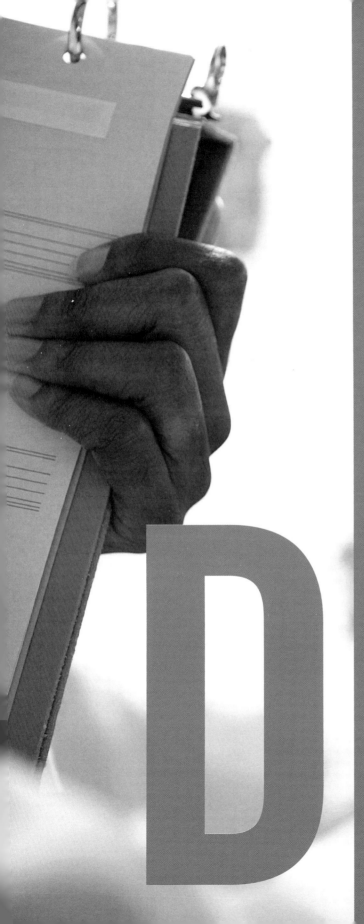

SKILLS FOR NURSING CARE

D

The aim of this part of the book is to introduce you to a range of practical skills and procedures that you will use, many on a daily basis, throughout your nursing course and during the rest of your nursing career.

In nursing, practical skills and procedures are a sound foundation for all of the care we deliver. However, it is fundamentally important that we supplement these skills with a range of other aspects of nursing, such as acting in a caring and compassionate manner, being professional, providing holistic care while listening to what patients tell us and always treating each patient as an individual.

This part of the book covers the core skills nurses use every day as part of their toolkit to deliver effective patient care. These are a diverse set of procedures, ranging from preventing and controlling infection, managing pain, taking clinical measurements and applying the principles of moving patients safely to assisting with the most intimate daily care needs of hygiene and elimination.

As Jo, Caroline and Joseph all remind us, in nursing the emphasis is not only on the ability to carry out a practical skill correctly, but also on being able to carry out a practical skill in a caring, compassionate and person-centred way. This is the true essence of nursing, which ensures patients always receive the best care possible. The voices below highlight the importance of these issues – read them and keep them in mind as you read through the chapters in this part of the book.

INFECTION PREVENTION AND CONTROL (IPC)

ROSE GALLAGHER

THIS CHAPTER COVERS

- IPC and standard precautions
- Hand hygiene
- Standard precautions and gloves

- Your responsibilities as a waste producer
- Management of used linen

REQUIRED KNOWLEDGE

Before reading this chapter, it will be helpful to:

- read key policies relating to infection prevention and control in your placement and any relevant information relating to hygiene, glove use, dermatitis or latex allergy
- spend a couple of hours with a local specialist IPC nurse to discuss hand hygiene and

glove use and accompany them if audits of practice are being undertaken
- find out who your local hospital waste manager is and arrange to spend time with them to discuss the waste hierarchy and how this is being met.

My name is Liam. I am 16 years old and have chronic kidney disease. I have dialysis four times a week and know how vulnerable I am to infection.

I joined a patient group and used the internet to get information about patient safety in dialysis units. We have hand-washing drummed into us by the staff all the time! Everyone wears gloves and uses those alcohol gels. I showed my nurse a website on my iPad after finding some patient information on gloves and how they can be dirtier than hands. I was worried about this, but she was really good and explained why gloves were worn and how staff should use them. Now I am much happier! I can see that everyone does the same thing and that everyone is treated the same as everybody else.

Liam, patient

Infection prevention and control is the responsibility of every healthcare professional – it is very important that germs with the potential to cause infections are not passed on to patients. Knowing and adhering to your hospital's policies on IPC is a must; we need to protect our patients from dangers seen and unseen.

Charlie Clisby, NQN

INTRODUCTION

The prevention of infection is central to patient safety and underpins the safe provision of care in every nursing field and care setting. This chapter covers several practical clinical skills that are fundamental to nursing care and which you will need to incorporate into your everyday practice. IPC is a huge field, so it is not possible to cover all of the relevant issues within this chapter, but we can ensure that you understand the essential principles.

IPC can succinctly be described as the practical application of microbiology in clinical practice. Humans have always lived alongside micro-organisms, a relationship which can, at times, be beneficial and, at times, harmful to the host (us humans) – and possibly, and occasionally, you, as a nurse caring for a patient. Bacteria, viruses and fungi (commonly referred to as germs) deserve the greatest respect at all times. Our challenge as nurses is to manage their presence in the context of care settings wherever these may be, all of which offer opportunities for risks to patients and, on occasion, ourselves. It is important to remember that we can only ever reduce, not eradicate, the presence of germs which can lead to infection.

This chapter will assist you in thinking about the care you deliver to each patient in terms of IPC risks. Whatever care setting you are in – acute or community – and no matter what your field of nursing, the fundamental principles apply.

IPC AND STANDARD PRECAUTIONS

Several essential and commonly performed clinical practices are central to what is known as 'standard precautions'. This term is generic and describes practices that, when used consistently and routinely for all patients, regardless of known or unknown infection status, are effective at interrupting the transmission of micro-organisms. **Note: this is not the same as assuming all patients are infectious!** When used properly, these precautions prevent the transfer of germs between patients and staff, and, of course, vice versa. This principle of interrupting the development of infection is central to the 'chain of infection'.

Standard precautions commonly include but are not limited to:

- hand hygiene
- appropriate use of personal protective clothing (PPE) such as gloves, disposable aprons, respiratory masks and visors/goggles (as required for individual patients only based on the situation and risk presented)
- safe handling and disposal of sharps
- waste disposal
- management of linen.

We will start with hand hygiene, as this is a core element of standard precautions.

HAND HYGIENE

Hand hygiene is the most frequently talked about and contentious of IPC practices. As a student, you will witness both good and poor hand hygiene practice, so it is important that you have a sound understanding of the theoretical and practical aspects of hand hygiene and are confident both in your own practice and in recognising when others may be putting patients at risk. Think of your hands as tools that are used for work – they need to be clean, safe and cared for to maintain their use.

For the purposes of this chapter, we will define hand hygiene as a process for reducing or destroying the number of micro-organisms present on the hands through hand-washing or the use of hand sanitisers such as alcohol gel.

Hand hygiene on its own as an intervention to prevent infection will not be successful. It is one of a number of core practices that need to be undertaken together as a 'package' to protect both patients and staff. In practice, hand hygiene is frequently combined with other practices, such as the use of gloves, aprons and masks and aseptic technique. Glove use in particular is integral to hand hygiene, as gloves also have direct contact with patients and can become contaminated through care activities. Think gloves – think hands!

The importance of hand hygiene

Hand hygiene is important both within healthcare and in wider non-healthcare settings as a public health intervention to reduce the spread of communicable diseases (e.g. influenza) and infections caused via the faecal–oral route, such as norovirus.

The patient environment (be it their own home or another care setting) is important as a factor in the spread of infection. Contamination of the environment by the bacterial flora (for example, from the skin, bowel or respiratory tract) of patients or staff occurs easily due to their presence and the care activities undertaken. As staff move from one patient to another, or have contact with a patient's immediate care environment (the area immediately surrounding the patient's cot/bed/chair), hands 'pick up' micro-organisms which, if not removed though hand hygiene, can be passed to the next patient or deposited elsewhere. One of the most challenging aspects of hand hygiene is that the impact of not undertaking it may not become apparent for some time after the event – even if it can ever be conclusively attributed to a lack of hand hygiene. This absence of immediate visible consequences for patients, together with a lack of visible contamination of hands by micro-organisms, provides challenges to improving hand hygiene compliance.

> Frequent hand-washing is vital for the protection and safety of all patients. If infection is spread it can be life-threatening, especially to the most vulnerable of patients. As nurses who follow the Code we are there to do no harm, and I believe excellent hand hygiene skills are an element of upholding it.
>
> **Alice Rowe, NQ RNMH**

Gloves are a central element of standard precautions and are classified as personal protective equipment (PPE) when used for the protection of staff, but not when used to protect the patient. You will see gloves being used in nearly every care setting and speciality. Concerns exist, however, that gloves are used inappropriately in nursing practice, with their use and overuse putting both patients and staff at risk.

Serious risks exist when multiple care tasks are undertaken with the same patient, which involve moving from one part of the patient's body to another. An excellent example of this is the provision of wound care following urinary catheter care. If hand hygiene is not performed following the urinary catheter care, any bacteria present on the hands (or gloves) of staff will be directly transferred to the wound area, which may result in infection with bacteria from the patient's groin/perineal area.

Understanding why hand hygiene helps reduce the risk of infection

Our hands always have germs present on them. It is impossible to physically remove or destroy all of them, although we can significantly reduce their numbers. Germs present on hands are predominantly bacteria, but occasionally may include spores (from fungi or bacteria) or viruses (e.g. the common cold) if hands are in contact with a contaminated surface, body area or fluid. The bacteria on our hands can be divided into two categories: resident and transient bacteria. Resident bacteria are those that live on our hands permanently. The resident bacterial flora (also known as microbiota) play a protective role by helping to prevent non-resident bacteria from establishing permanently on the skin.

Transient bacteria are those most frequently associated with the spread of infection in healthcare and also the home or social environments. These transient bacteria become loosely attached to the outer skin layers of the hands following physical contact with people, equipment or environmental surfaces and, if not removed or destroyed, they will easily be transferred from one place or person to another, as highlighted in Table 22.1.

WHAT'S THE EVIDENCE?

WEBLINK:
KLEBSIELL
SPECIES

Casewell, M.W. and Phillips, I. (1977) 'Hands as a route of transmission for *Klebsiella* species', *British Medical Journal*, 2: 1315-17.

   In this seminal paper, Casewell and Phillips (1977) demonstrated a link between nursing care activities, the contamination of hands and the colonisation or infection of patients. The study focused on obtaining evidence of how one specific bacteria (**Klebsiella spp**) was being transmitted between patients and staff.

Table 22.1 Contamination of nurses' hands by different *Klebsiella spp* following care procedures

Patient	Care activity	*Klebsiella* types colonising patients	*Klebsiella* types recovered from nurses' hands
A	Lifting patient	21, 47, 10	47, 10
B	Taking blood pressure and pulse	21	21
	Physiotherapy	21	21, 28
	Washing patient	21	24, 28
	Taking oral temperature	21	21
	General nursing	21	21
C	Radial pulse	21	21
	Touching shoulder	21	21
	Touching groin	21	21
D	Washing patient	21, 45, 9	21, 45
E	General nursing	15	15
	Extubation	15	15
	Touching groin	15	15, 19
F	Touching hand	55, 47	55

Source: Adapted from Casewell and Phillips (1977)

The results showed that *Klebsiella spp* were recovered from the hands of nurses and body sites of patients. As is shown in Table 22.1, specific nursing procedures were identified that resulted in the contamination of nurses' hands following contact with patients.

The introduction of routine hand-washing with chlorhexidine by staff resulted in sustained reductions over time of colonisation of patients with *Klebsiella spp*.

- Reflect on the essential care activities that you undertake, such as those illustrated in Table 22.1. Do you ever think about how contaminated your hands might be, even when there are no visible signs of dirt?
- When you are next on placement, for a four-hour period keep a record of how often you wash your hands and the reasons for doing so. Reflect on the results: do you think you washed your hands too infrequently, too often, or was your practice in line with local policies?
- Now read the rest of the chapter and see if you are correct!

How and when to perform hand hygiene

In this chapter, we are considering what is known as 'social hand-washing' with non-medicated soap. There is another form, which is known as surgical hand-washing (or scrubbing). This has not been included because social hand-washing is suitable for nurses in most situations, apart from the preparation of hands for invasive procedures undertaken with strict asepsic techniques, such as in operating theatres.

The aim of hand-washing is to remove transient germs (bacteria, viruses, fungi and spores) from the surface of the hands using mechanical friction as a result of the application, rubbing and removal of soap and water during the process of washing. Hand drying using paper towels also physically removes germs from the hands. This contrasts with the application of hand sanitisers, which chemically destroy or inactivate bacteria present on the surface of the hands. Currently, the use of hand sanitisers is not promoted for patients suspected or known to have viral gastroenteritis (e.g. norovirus) or an infection due to *Clostridium difficile*. Hand-washing with soap and water is recommended in these circumstances.

Hand-washing

A technique adapted from research evidence provides a framework for hand-washing. This technique (see Figure 22.1) enables good coverage of the hands with soap or hand sanitiser and a systematic technique to support effective hand hygiene.

As a further aid to effective hand-washing, Taylor (1978) identified areas of the hands which were most frequently missed during hand-washing. Her findings are still used today to help teach and improve hand-washing techniques (see Figure 22.2).

Guidelines

There are various guidelines and expectations relating to practice that you must be aware of when cleaning your hands. These include:

- infection control policies
- local programmes such as hand hygiene campaigns/strap lines.

1. Wash palm to palm

2. Rub back of both hands

3. Rub back of fingers interlaced

4. Wash both thumbs

5. Rub palms with fingertips

6. Wash wrists

Figure 22.1   Ayliffe's six-step hand hygiene technique

Source: Adapted from Ayliffe et al. (1978)

To ensure you always wash your hands effectively, follow the steps outlined in Clinical Skill 22.1.

Sometimes missed   Frequently missed

Figure 22.2   Areas of the hands most frequently missed during hand-washing

ACTIVITY 22.1: REFLECTION

Reflect on the effectiveness of the technique you use to wash your hands:

- Do you follow the six steps outlined by Ayliffe et al. (1978) (Figure 22.1)?
- Do you miss the areas identified by Taylor (1978) (Figure 22.2)?

Use of hand sanitisers

The use of alcohol-based hand rubs and foams has increased dramatically over the past ten years. They are far more effective than soap and water in reducing the numbers of transient bacteria on hands. The application and distribution of hand sanitiser can follow a similar technique as for the application of soap and water (Figure 22.1); however, hand sanitisers must be left to dry naturally on the hands and not washed off, because the action of evaporation is important.

Hand sanitiser gel is a convenient and highly effective method for the decontamination of hands, as you are able to apply it, rub it into your hands and move to the next patient or physical location without stopping to do hand-washing. This was a key factor in the promotion and adoption of hand sanitisers in healthcare facilities in the UK, in addition to the fact that they also offer a convenient portable alternative in environments where soap and water may not be readily available, such as in remote locations or ambulances.

It is important to remember that hand sanitisers are not suitable to use in all circumstances and that the physical contamination of hands by dirt or body fluids must be managed by first removing this by hand-washing (or use of hand wipes in community settings). This is most important as organic material is known to inactivate alcohol. Hand sanitisers can be applied once the hands are clean to ensure they are safe for the next patient. To ensure you always do this effectively, follow the steps outlined in Clinical Skill 22.2.

When to perform hand hygiene

When to perform hand hygiene remains a matter of much debate. Central to this are the risks that touching different potential sources of contaminants, either patient or environmental, bring. Long lists of indications about when to wash your hands have been replaced with an emphasis on assessing the potential risk. The concept of 'reference points' for hand hygiene linked to space/time (Sax et al., 2007) led to the development of the World Health Organization (WHO, 2009) framework of the '5 moments for hand hygiene', which has been widely but not exclusively adopted as a contemporary standard to apply:

1. Before touching a patient
2. Before clean/aseptic procedure
3. After body fluid exposure
4. After touching a patient
5. After touching patient surroundings.

One of the advantages of the '5 moments' is that it takes a patient-centred approach. It can also be adapted to situations outside of hospitals where the focus remains on the patient, be it a patient sitting in a chair or ambulance, or a baby in a cot.

STEP-BY-STEP CLINICAL SKILL 22.1: HAND-WASHING

☑ Before you start

Consider, is it beneficial to inform the patient that you intend to wash your hands? The patient and their relatives or carers may be reassured that you are taking steps to protect them from the transmission of infection via hands.

☑ Essential equipment

Running tepid water, soap, hand towels (preferably disposable, but patients may offer you a clean hand towel in community settings).

☑ Field-specific considerations

Washing your hands is an essential skill within the care of patients from all fields. The principles outlined in this skill will not vary depending on the field.

☑ Care-setting considerations

Facilities for hand-washing will vary considerably between care settings and patients' homes.

Always be prepared for a lack of running water, soap and clean hand towels.

In community settings, carry your own supply of hand towels or hand wipes to support hand-washing. Always carry hand sanitiser for situations when this is appropriate.

Keep hand sanitisers out of the reach of children or those with impaired mental capacity. Refer to Clinical Skill 22.2, below.

☑ What to watch out for and action to take

Do not apply soap directly to dry hands as this can result in sore hands and poor coverage of soap.

Staff with broken skin should cover it with a plaster. Staff unable to perform hand hygiene (because of sore hands) should not be working in clinical environments due to the risks to patients and themselves. Staff suffering from dermatitis and/or sore hands should seek advice from their local occupational health department.

Always use the foot pedal of the bin (if available) - never dispose of hand towels by lifting the lid using your fingers because this will result in recontamination of your hands.

STEPS AND THE REASONS FOR THEM IN HAND-WASHING

Identify the need for hand hygiene to be performed
Undertake an assessment to ascertain whether there is a need for hand-washing to take place

Turn on taps and select a comfortable temperature
Water that is too hot or too cold can impact on compliance with the hand-washing technique

Wet hands
Prepare hands to receive soap and facilitate an even covering of soap for the next stage

Apply soap
Apply one dose of liquid soap to cupped hands.
   If bar soap is the only option available, then this may be used, depending on its quality. Community staff may carry small amounts of soap with them in containers

Rub hands together and evenly distribute soap coverage following steps set out in Figure 22.1
Rubbing hands together produces mechanical friction. This results in all areas of the hands coming into contact with soap and transient micro-organisms being lifted from the outer layers of the skin into the soap solution on the hands

Rinse hands
To remove the transient micro-organisms present in the soap solution from the hands

Dry hands
Dry the skin of the hands and remove any remaining transient organisms as a result of mechanical friction. Ensure all areas of the hands are dry

Dispose of hand towels
Dispose of used materials correctly without re-contaminating your hands

Source: Loveday et al. (2013); NICE (2012)

It should be noted, however, that even though this approach offers a theoretical improvement, its application in practice for complex interactions, such as the delivery of a baby, remains controversial, and 100 per cent compliance is doubtful and unachievable in all situations.

Monitoring hand hygiene compliance

As a nursing student, it is almost certain that you will have your hand hygiene compliance monitored at some point, most likely in an inpatient setting. Hand hygiene is a priority area for the improvement and monitoring of infection prevention as it is thought to reflect overall standards of infection prevention.

Audits of hand hygiene vary in their methodology, but direct observation remains the current standard. This method, however, is not practical in settings where staff work alone – for example in GP surgeries, practice nurse or midwife clinics, or community settings such as patients' own homes. Direct observation is also fraught with practical difficulties and bias, particularly if staff are aware they are being observed.

Healthcare organisations frequently report high compliance scores for hand hygiene, but audits undertaken by infection prevention teams often show much lower results.

STEP-BY-STEP CLINICAL SKILL 22.2
USING HAND SANITISER

☑ Before you start

Consider whether it is appropriate to inform the patient that you are going to use sanitiser on your hands so the patient and their relatives or carers are reassured that you are taking steps to protect them from the transmission of infection via hands.

☑ Essential equipment

Hand sanitiser (this may be carried personally, available at the point of care or wall-mounted).

☑ Field-specific considerations

Ensuring your hands are free from transient micro-organisms is an essential skill within the care of patients from all fields. The steps outlined in this skill will not vary depending on the field.

☑ Care-setting considerations

Facilities for hand hygiene will vary considerably between care settings and patients' homes.

Always be prepared for a lack of running water, soap and clean hand towels. In community settings, carry your own supply of hand towels or hand wipes to support hand hygiene. Always carry hand sanitiser for situations in which this is appropriate.

Keep hand sanitisers out of the reach of children or those with impaired mental capacity. The ingestion of alcohol hand sanitisers that has resulted in the death of patients has been recorded (HM Coroner, 2017).

☑ What to watch out for and action to take

Any cuts, open wounds or dry skin on hands will sting following the application of hand sanitiser. Staff with broken skin should cover it with a plaster. Staff unable to perform hand hygiene (because of sore hands) should not be working in clinical environments due to the risks to patients and themselves. Staff suffering from dermatitis and/or sore hands should seek advice from their local occupational health department.

STEPS AND THE REASONS FOR THEM IN HAND HYGIENE

 Identify the requirement for hand hygiene to be performed
Assess whether hand hygiene needs to take place.
    The decision to use sanitiser will depend on being:

- confident that the hand sanitiser will be effective to decontaminate hands. Remember, if a patient has diarrhoea or a gastrointestinal infection such as *C. difficile*, hand sanitiser may not be effective. Wash hands first, if possible, then apply hand sanitiser if needed. Visibly soiled hands should be cleaned with soap and water, if available, or a hand wipe prior to application of sanitiser
- able to access hand sanitiser at the point and time of need

 Apply the hand sanitiser to all surfaces of the hands and rub hands together to support evaporation following steps set out in Figure 22.1
All surfaces of the hands come into contact with the hand sanitiser to ensure transient micro-organisms are destroyed. This six-step technique is more effective than other less standardised techniques (Reilly et al., 2016)

 Allow the hand sanitiser sufficient time to dry (evaporate) prior to next patient contact
The hand sanitiser needs adequate time to be effective and destroy micro-organisms on hands

Source: Loveday et al. (2013); NICE (2012)

Improving hand hygiene

A number of barriers to hand hygiene have been recognised, which include:

- a perception that other patient needs take priority
- time pressures
- the impact of hand hygiene products on staff skin
- poor role models promoting hand hygiene
- inadequate staffing
- scepticism about the benefits of hand hygiene
- inappropriate glove use.

ACTIVITY 22.2: REFLECTION

- How would you feel if you observed another member of staff not complying with hand hygiene or appropriate use of gloves?
- Do you have a responsibility to raise this issue on every occasion or just those that you feel are particularly important?
- How would your actions impact on the risk to patients?

Patient and public knowledge

Patient empowerment and knowledge of hand hygiene have increased tremendously over the past ten years, as Liam's voice at the start of the chapter showed us. This has arisen due to greater public awareness of infection prevention, media messages and education relating to hand hygiene. For patients, the focus should be both on supporting them to clean their hands so as to prevent endogenous infection, for instance wound infections caused by removing or picking at dressings, and on encouraging good hygiene practices such as hand-washing before meals and after using the toilet. Within both hospital and home or community settings, practical obstacles exist in encouraging good patient hand hygiene.

> I lead by example by regularly washing my hands; I give them advice and use gentle persuasion.
>
> **Julie Davis, LD nursing student**

CASE STUDY 22.1: GRAZIELLA

Being admitted to hospital can be a very frightening time for both patients and their families. We put our trust and faith in the staff caring for us. Therefore, it is important to make patients feel safe and secure and feel that everything possible is being done.

Of course, no one wants to be in hospital; patients are there to be treated for a variety of conditions and in most cases the outcome will be fine. However, this is not always the case – complications may occur, prolonging an admission, which can make patients more susceptible to a whole host of problems. Infections are the major problem. I know this only too well because someone very dear to me sadly lost her life due to one of these infections.

My grandmother went into hospital to be treated for a urine infection, something that should have been easy enough to treat; however, antibiotics, a less than clean environment and staff who were not adhering to IPC measures were to blame for my grandmother contracting **C. difficile** infection. Within a period of ten weeks, my grandmother fought hard to overcome many problems but she could not fight *C. difficile*. She died as a result of the infection.

Watching her suffer in the way she did is something I will never forget. Of course, we all have to die, and at the age of 93 my grandmother had lived her life, but no one should have to suffer in the way she did.

Could my grandmother's infection have been avoided? I think so. Thirty patients became infected with *C. difficile* during the period in which my grandmother was in hospital. Staff did not know how to control it but something as simple as washing their hands could have prevented so many patients becoming infected.

Hand hygiene is one of the most basic ways of helping to keep patients safe. Something that only takes a couple of minutes of your time can be the key in ensuring that your patient is being protected from infection. That is the least any patient can expect from staff looking after them.

- Next time you are busy caring for patients, time exactly how long it takes you to perform hand hygiene.
- Performing effective hand hygiene has the potential to save a patient's life. Are you really so busy that this is a risk worth taking?

STANDARD PRECAUTIONS AND GLOVES

As mentioned previously, gloves are a core element of what is currently known as 'standard precautions'. Gloves provide a physical barrier between the user (you) and the substance originating from the patient (e.g. excreta, bodily fluids or chemicals used in care practices that they may come into contact with). The potential harm from biological risks relates to micro-organisms that may be present (e.g. blood-borne viruses or bacteria) which, when transmitted, are capable of causing infection in either other patients or staff.

We will differentiate between the two main glove types by using the term 'examination gloves' to describe disposable single-use gloves used for routine clinical practice, and 'protective gloves' to refer to single-use gloves that are used to protect the wearer from exposure to harmful chemicals or drugs. The latter are required to meet additional testing standards to those of standard 'examination' gloves, to prevent the risk of permeation of chemicals. A common example is 'nitrile' gloves. We will not be discussing the use of sterile gloves for surgical procedures.

It is important to understand the different types of gloves available and the differences between them. On your placements, you will come across many different nursing activities, and gloves may vary considerably between settings and patient groups.

Ideally, different glove types should be provided, to enable nurses to choose which to use based on a risk assessment of the requirements of the activity being undertaken. Within healthcare organisations, different staff groups will have different needs – for example, porters will need heavy-duty protective gloves when collecting or transporting waste; theatre staff require surgical gloves; nurses administering chemotherapy agents may require 'protective' gloves because of their exposure to hazardous drugs. In some settings, such as mental health, gloves may be very infrequently worn and contact with chemicals will be limited. In other nursing fields, the use of gloves may be more common.

Being clear on employer and employee responsibilities

Health and safety legislation requires both employers and employees to undertake risk assessments of potential risks in the workplace, and to eliminate these where possible. In the case of healthcare, it is not possible to remove these risks, such as caring for a patient and the micro-organisms they may be carrying, or a patient's need for chemotherapy drugs. Where risks cannot be eliminated or managed by engineering controls (e.g. safety needles), measures should be put in place to reduce the impact of those risks that remain. Gloves are, therefore, when used correctly, one example of a control measure used to protect both staff and patients from risk.

Glove types and sensitivity to their components

Single-use disposable gloves may be manufactured using different components – natural rubber latex, vinyl or synthetic rubbers such as nitrile and neoprene are all frequently used. Gloves may also be powdered or unpowdered and sterile or unsterile.

Sensitivity and reactions to glove components are important issues for those working in healthcare, particularly nurses. The most well-known example is natural rubber latex, but many people do not realise that sensitivity can also develop to other, non-latex gloves. Sensitivity to chemicals used in the manufacturing process of gloves is another example. Natural rubber latex proteins are considered hazardous to health (HSE, 2012) and therefore need to be managed under the Control of Substances Hazardous to Health Regulations (COSHH) guidelines (2002, updated 2013). Currently, the use of latex gloves is not banned but many organisations have moved away from, or are in the process of moving away from, latex.

When to use gloves

As with hands, gloves can act as a vehicle for the transmission of micro-organisms and therefore it is important to change gloves if moving from one patient to another, or when undertaking multiple care tasks on the same patients. Gloves are not a substitute for hand hygiene!

The use of gloves has increased tremendously over the past 30 years and indiscriminate use is now recognised as a significant risk to both patients and nurses (Loveday et al., 2013) which undermines hand hygiene (Fuller et al., 2011).

Indications for glove use are:

- when anticipating contact with blood or body fluids
- when anticipating contact with non-intact skin or mucous membranes
- when a risk of contact with hazardous chemicals or drugs exists.

Reasons for the unprecedented rise in glove use are not really known; however, in discussion with students and registered nurses, it appears that some nurses feel they must wear gloves with all patients regardless of any established risk. This means that nurses are often observed wearing gloves for routine bed-making, feeding patients or even bathing them – when no contact with specific risks, as highlighted previously, exists. It seems that a perception of a 'dirty task' overrides the rationale and evidence base that hand hygiene is sufficient for all other 'non-identified risk' situations.

> While it is our duty to ensure that our practice is up to date, at times you will experience working with practice educators who have been trained differently to us and as such may well use gloves in different circumstances to us or will not wear gloves. If this occurs and you are unsure what to do read the local policies to guide your practice or simply ask your practice educator why they are/aren't wearing gloves. At all times ensure that you are working within best practice guidelines.
>
> **Alice Rowe, NQ RNMH**

Which gloves and when?

Table 22.2 outlines some issues and considerations frequently associated with glove selection. Note: some healthcare organisations have made the decision to only provide one type of examination glove

Table 22.2   Which glove: issues and considerations

Issue	Considerations
The activity to be performed	Be clear on why gloves are needed and select the appropriate glove type
Anticipated contact and compatibility with chemicals and chemotherapeutic agents (e.g. cytotoxic drugs or disinfectant solutions or wipes)	Are gloves required to protect the skin of staff? These should comply with the relevant EU standards to meet the Personal Protective Equipment Directive
Latex or other sensitivity	Alternative gloves should be available
Glove size required	Gloves should always be available in small, medium and large sizes
Local policies for creating a latex-free environment	Refer to local infection prevention and occupational health policies for further guidance

STEP-BY-STEP CLINICAL SKILL 22.3: WHEN TO REMOVE YOUR GLOVES AND WHY

☑ **Before you start**

Ensure you have undertaken an assessment to determine if gloves can be retained or should be changed.

☑ **Essential equipment**

Hand hygiene equipment (soap and water or hand sanitiser).

☑ **Field-specific considerations**

Mental health – gloves are infrequently used in mental health settings but may be required at times. Indications may include caring for incontinent patients, phlebotomy or dressing wounds. Differences may also be present in practice depending on whether you are working in an inpatient or community setting.

Learning disability – depending on the patients, glove-use need will vary. For those with physical needs, the indications for glove use are the same as for adult general nursing.

Child – indications for glove use in children's settings are the same as for adults, and this includes neonates. Newborn babies may look 'clean' but the same principles and risks apply.

CHANGING GLOVES

 When there is an indication for hand hygiene
Wearing gloves may afford you some protection but the patient remains vulnerable if you do not consider the risk of transfer of micro-organisms via gloves in the same way as hands

Whenever an indication for hand hygiene occurs, and gloves are being worn, these should be removed, hand hygiene performed and then clean gloves applied. This is particularly relevant when multiple care activities are undertaken on the same patient

 When glove integrity is breached or suspected
Gloves are not a complete barrier and defects may be present unknown to the wearer. Gloves reduce but do not eliminate risks

 When

a. **the actual or potential contact with blood, body fluids or mucous membranes is finished**
b. **contact with hazardous drugs or chemicals has finished**
c. **contact with a contaminated body site or device (e.g. infected wound, urinary catheter bag) has finished**

Once the activity is complete, gloves should be removed, disposed of and hand hygiene performed. This removes potential contamination from the hands of the nurse, protecting both them and the next patient

Source: Loveday et al. (2013); NICE (2012); RCN (2012)

for use by all staff (e.g nitrile) as a result of local risk assessment (for example, the need to deliver chemotherapy in multiple patient settings as opposed to dedicated chemotherapy suites).

Knowing when to use gloves appropriately, however, is only half the story. It is as important to understand when gloves need to be removed and either changed or disposed of. Clinical Skill 22.3 identifies when removal of gloves is required and explains why.

Glove use and hand hygiene compliance

As we have already discussed, gloves are not a substitute for hand hygiene and hand hygiene must be performed after gloves are removed, as the act of removing gloves can contaminate hands. Additionally, gloves may not provide a complete barrier to micro-organisms or chemicals (due to the presence of small breaches in glove integrity) and therefore hands may become contaminated during care activities. Most hand hygiene audits do not routinely collect data on glove use as a factor in determining hand hygiene compliance, and therefore this represents a gap in both our understanding of the extent of the issue and the available data on which to assess improvements in hand hygiene practice.

ACTIVITY 22.3: REFLECTION

There are many potential occasions when gloves may be required:

- Compile a list of occasions recently when you have determined it is necessary to wear gloves.
- Which of these were to protect the patient, and which to protect you?
- Now reflect on whether you wore gloves when perhaps they might not have been required – under what circumstances did this occur, and were you influenced by the behaviour of others to act in a similar way?

WHAT'S THE EVIDENCE?

Loveday et al. (2013) recommend that hand hygiene should be performed before and after donning gloves:

- Do you comply with this and have you seen other staff do this?
- What are the risks to you and the patient if you do not perform hand hygiene as recommended with gloves?
- Now read the guidelines and consider how you can best apply the recommendations to your practice.

ACTIVITY 22.4: REFLECTION

The promotion of patient hand hygiene and a culture of encouraging patients to challenge staff to perform hand hygiene remain core elements of many care organisations' local hand hygiene programmes. This is an extract from an article in the *Daily Telegraph*, from 18 July 2007:

Patients in hospital should challenge doctors and nurses to wash their hands before consultations, the Chief Medical Officer said yesterday. Good hand hygiene is the key to reducing hospital acquired infections such as MRSA and NHS staff are often too complacent, Sir Liam Donaldson said in his annual report. Patients on wards should be issued with their own alcohol hand gel and should ask doctors and nurses to use it before examinations and procedures, he said.

Estimates suggest that one patient is infected every two minutes in hospitals and one dies every two hours from healthcare-associated infections. Sir Liam said that even in the best hospitals compliance with hand hygiene rules is rarely above 60 per cent – yet up to three quarters of all patients do not feel comfortable challenging staff.

- What would your reaction be if you were challenged by a patient to wash your hands?
- Consider different patient groups in different settings – which groups of patients do you think might be at a disadvantage in challenging staff?
- How can this be overcome?

Skin health

In addition to placing patients at risk of infection, inappropriate (excessive) use of gloves can have a detrimental effect on the health of nurses' skin. Nurses are vulnerable to developing dermatitis due to a number of factors, including:

- exposure to a 'cocktail' of chemicals such as natural rubber latex or accelerators, disinfectant or detergent wipes, soap and alcohol hand sanitisers
- 'wet work' – where hands are frequently exposed to water, such as in bathing, showering or washing up
- frequent hand-washing or use of hand sanitisers.

Prolonged or frequent use of gloves can cause the skin to become over-hydrated and can also be a risk factor in the development of dermatitis. Combined, these potential factors place staff at risk of dermatitis on their hands (RCN, 2012), as shown in Figure 22.3.

Figure 22.3   Dermatitis and reddening of skin

Source: www.hse.gov.uk/skin/imagelibrary.htm. Copyright of HSE, contains public sector information published by the Health and Safety Executive and licensed under the Open Government Licence v1.0

WEBLINK:
SKIN
DISEASES
LIBRARY

CASE STUDY 22.2: IDRIS

Idris has just returned from placement on a neonatal care unit. He is about to start working on a children's oncology ward but the alcohol hand sanitiser is really stinging, so he has stopped using it. He can't wash his hands properly as his hands are so sore.

- What actions should Idris take and why?
- Do you think Idris should continue caring for patients if he can't perform hand hygiene?

What is dermatitis and why is it important?

Simply put, dermatitis is inflammation of the skin on the hands, a type of eczema. It may occur naturally or as a result of contact with substances which cause a reaction, known as 'contact dermatitis'. Different terminology is used to describe different types of dermatitis.

Not all dermatitis occurs as a result of work, and some factors associated with life outside of work, such as having children under the age of 5 or washing dishes by hand, can contribute to the risk of developing dermatitis.

Roles and responsibilities relating to occupational dermatitis

Both employers and employees have responsibilities when it comes to reporting and managing occupational dermatitis. Employers have a responsibility under health and safety laws to protect staff from illness caused as a result of work, and this incudes contact dermatitis. Healthcare workers (that's you) have a legal responsibility to cooperate with employers regarding health and safety matters. This includes following your organisation's policies and procedures (for example, those around standard precautions, skincare and the appropriate use of PPE), and reporting any incidences of hand dermatitis in a timely manner to your manager and occupational health department.

Always follow the glove good practice guidelines:

- Gloves are single-use items – which means wear for one task then take them off!
- Hand hygiene should be performed prior to putting gloves on.
- Hands should never be washed with gloves on.
- Wearing gloves is not a substitute for hand hygiene.
- Gloves can transmit micro-organisms capable of causing infection in the same way hands can.
- Gloves must only be used if necessary, following a risk assessment for both patient and nurse.
- Hand hygiene should always be performed after the removal of gloves.
- Gloves should not be routinely used for bed-making.
- Only powder-free gloves should be used.
- Always wear the correct glove size for you and report a lack of suitable glove types or sizes to the person in charge.
- Be aware of the signs of dermatitis and report any that occur.
- Never wear gloves 'just in case'.

YOUR RESPONSIBILITIES AS A WASTE PRODUCER

The production of waste as a result of healthcare activities is inevitable. The waste items we will cover in this chapter are healthcare waste and used linen.

While the management of waste may not strike you as a nursing responsibility, nursing accounts for approximately 70 per cent of the UK healthcare workforce and the production of waste is an unavoidable consequence of the role and the care tasks undertaken. The International Council of Nurses (ICN) states that 'nurses must understand the hazardous consequences of improper waste handling, the "cradle to grave" waste cycle and methods that mitigate the negative impact of waste on the environment' (ICN, 2009).

The principles of good waste management – the waste hierarchy

The waste hierarchy describes options that should be considered as part of an overall strategy for waste management, so it is not just applicable to healthcare organisations. The principle of the hierarchy is that waste production should be avoided wherever possible. The overall aim, as identified in Figure 22.4, is therefore to reduce the actual amount of waste that is generated for disposal, regardless of the end point, such as landfill or incineration.

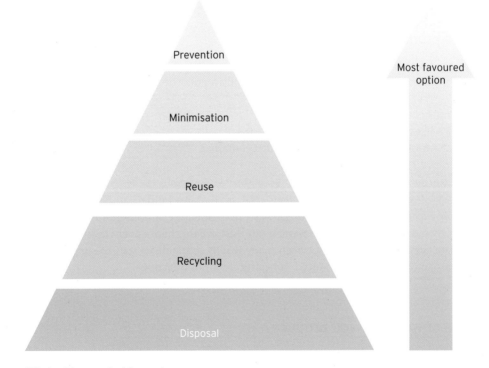

Figure 22.4   The waste hierarchy

Classification of healthcare waste

Many different types of waste are produced as a result of healthcare. Management of waste is governed by a multitude of regulations arising from both UK and EU requirements. Different types off wastes are produced, some harmful and some not. Types of waste include laboratory waste (including chemicals or growth media); human anatomical waste (e.g. limbs, used medical devices such as syringes, nebulisers); infectious waste; and household waste.

The RCN (2014) describes how the main types of waste may be classified simply into the following categories:

- clinical waste – most, but not all, of this is classified as hazardous waste. Sub-categories of clinical waste exist, such as infectious waste, medicinal waste and sharps. In healthcare, the term includes:
  - o waste which contains viable micro-organisms or their toxins which can cause disease in humans or other living organisms
  - o waste which contains or is contaminated with a medicine that contains a biologically active pharmaceutical agent, or is a 'sharp', or a body fluid or other biological material (including human tissue) containing or contaminated with a dangerous substance

- offensive waste (or hygiene waste) – this is best described as waste that is non-infectious but which may be deemed to be 'offensive' due to its contents (e.g. sanitary waste, soiled incontinence pads, etc.) and possibly smell
- municipal (household) waste – waste similar to that produced in your own home, e.g. waste packaging, dead flowers, etc.

The waste producer

The waste producer is the person who generates the waste (you), whether this is a sharp after you give an injection or packaging that you are disposing of. The producer of the waste is responsible for:

- assessing what type of waste they have generated
- placing the waste in the correct, colour-coded container.

Waste in healthcare is often 'over-classified' as clinical or infectious (RCN, 2011). The consequences of this is a lack of compliance with waste legislation and a huge burden on healthcare costs, as it is currently more expensive to dispose of clinical waste than offensive or household waste. This situation has arisen partly due to efforts to ensure waste is safe 'just in case', hence over-classification, or because offensive waste bags and bins have not been made readily available to staff to support their use. In reality, the vast amount of waste produced in healthcare is not infectious.

What type of waste do you produce?

It is important that the waste produced is assessed at the time of its production, separated correctly and placed in the right container. Nurses often note confusion about the classification of infectious and offensive waste. Table 22.3 offers advice on this.

Colour-coded segregation exists to help identify which type of waste is present in a container or bag. In this way, it is possible to identify sharps, medicinal waste, waste containing cytotoxic chemicals or offensive waste, which is important for the purposes of transporting waste to its final destination. This colour scheme can vary from country to country in the UK.

The main categories of bagged waste you are most likely to come across are illustrated in Figure 22.5. Always check your local policies for more detail.

Table 22.3 Classification of common waste according to 'infectious properties'

Waste contains	Proposed general classification	Examples of waste	Exceptions to this rule
Urine, faeces, vomit and sputum	**Offensive** (where risk assessment had indicated is present, and no other risk of infection exists)	Urine bags, incontinence pads, single-use bowls, nappies, PPE (gloves, aprons, etc.)	Gastrointestinal and other infections that are readily transmissible in the community setting (for example, *verocytotoxin*-producing *Escherichia coli* (VTEC), campylopacter, norovirus, salmonella, chicken pox/shingles)[1] Hepatitis B and C, HIV-positive patients – only if blood is present[1]
Blood, pus and wound exudates	**Infectious** unless assessment indicates no infection present. If no infection, and no other risk of infection, then offensive	Dressings from wounds, wound drains, delivery packs	Blood transfusion items Dressings contaminated with blood/wound exudates assessed not to be infectious Maternity sanitary waste where screening or knowledge has confirmed that no infection is present and no other risk of infection exists

Note: [1]Potential hazards from the use of cytotoxic and cytostatic medicines may also be relevant in some instances and with some drugs. This would also prevent the waste being considered offensive.

Source: RCN (2014)

Clinical waste   Infectious waste   Offensive waste   Household waste

Figure 22.5 Categories of bagged waste

Waste production in the community

Waste disposal as a result of nursing patients in their own homes poses some unique challenges and considerations.

Risk assessment of waste in community settings is the same as in hospital settings and the waste classification applies. The management of waste (storage, collection, etc.), however, is managed differently and will vary from one geographical area to another. This sometimes means nurses have to carry healthcare waste in their cars, or even take it with them on ferries in more remote communities. Use of the patient's waste bins is permissible for some waste produced, such as 'soft non-infectious waste', where the amount is comparable to what a patient would normally produce and has been deemed non-infectious (RCN, 2014). Infectious and sharps waste must be managed separately and must not be disposed of via the patient's home.

Waste management is just as important in the community as in hospital but the set-up and polices are just different. You would need to read and make yourself familiar with the policies when starting a new job.

Sarah Parkes, LD nursing student

ACTIVITY 22.6: REFLECTION

- Do you think community nurses should carry waste in their cars?
- Why do you think community nurses may have been asked to do this?
- Can you identify any improvements as to how healthcare waste is managed in the community?

Top tips for good waste management in all settings

If you follow these principles, it is possible to manage healthcare waste safely and effectively in all settings:

- Risk-assess all waste you produce, and segregate accordingly – do not be tempted to put everything in one bag regardless.
- In hospital and GP surgery settings, waste must be stored securely and separately to other items such as used linen.
- Waste bags should be removed, sealed and transferred to a storage facility when two thirds full – do not allow bags to overfill, otherwise they cannot be sealed safely, thus placing others at risk.
- Ensure different types of waste are segregated appropriately in the appropriate storage area.
- Label waste so the area where it originates can be identified. Tags should be available to use locally. Do not 'borrow' other areas' labels, as traceability is important should an issue be identified.
- Waste must not be allowed to accumulate in public areas – always use dedicated storage areas or move directly to large rigid containers.
- When handling waste, aprons and gloves should be worn; they should be removed immediately after the task is complete, followed by hand hygiene.
- Report issues with waste collection or storage immediately.

MANAGEMENT OF USED LINEN

The management of used linen includes handling and disposal and is mostly associated with hospital settings. Used linen is rarely implicated in outbreaks of infection, but it does pose risks to both other patients and staff on occasion.

Some units, such as neonatal or long-term care units, may have their own washing machines to enable them to wash patients' items locally. While these may seem convenient, they do pose risks, and outbreaks of infection have occurred that have been associated with washing machine use. Most used linen is processed via a central (usually off-site) laundry which has to comply with national standards for temperature controls and processes.

How to handle linen appropriately

When handling used linen, the following applies:

- Always wear a plastic apron for handling used linen to prevent contamination of your uniform.
- Do not routinely wear gloves for bed-making unless the patient is in isolation or being 'barrier nursed' with a risk of infection. Always perform hand hygiene after bed-making.
- Handle used linen carefully to avoid shaking it and disturbing skin cells and bacteria that will be present.
- Do not carry used linen through a ward or department. Always place it immediately into a linen skip and transfer to the storage area as soon as possible.
- Do not mix clean and used linen.

Segregation of used linen

As with waste, different colour coding applies to linen categories. The two main category codes are red and white bags:

- Red linen bags denote an infection risk and involve placing the linen in a red inner 'alginate' (water-soluble) bag before it is placed in a thicker plastic or cotton outer bag. This is because of the need to prevent laundry workers coming into contact with the linen (it is placed directly into the machine in the 'alginate' bag, which then dissolves). Linen should be segregated into red bags if a patient is being isolated with an infection or infectious condition, or if the linen is soiled with blood or body fluids.
- White linen bags are the most common type, used for uncontaminated linen.

Used linen bags should be sealed before they are overfull and stored appropriately at local level in a dedicated area.

CONCLUSION

This chapter identified the core infection prevention and control practices you need to develop to protect both patients and yourself, wherever you are on placement. Bacteria, viruses and fungi deserve the greatest respect at all times. Our challenge as nurses is to manage their presence in the context of care settings, wherever they may be.

It is fundamentally important for you to have a good understanding of the theoretical and practical aspects of hand hygiene. Think of your hands as tools that are used for work – they need to be clean, safe and cared for to maintain their use.

Hand hygiene on its own as an action to prevent infection will not be successful. It is one of a number of core practices that need to be undertaken together as a 'package' to protect both patients and staff in all care settings. In practice, hand hygiene is frequently combined with other practices, such as use of gloves, aprons and masks, plus aseptic technique. Glove use in particular is integral to hand hygiene, as gloves are also in direct contact with patients and can become contaminated through care activities.

Waste management is very costly for organisations and is environmentally important. While the management of waste may not strike you as a nursing responsibility, waste production is an unavoidable consequence of our role and the care tasks undertaken.

CHAPTER SUMMARY

- Preventing infection relies on an awareness and knowledge of all the factors that contribute to the complexity of decision-making regarding when to perform hand hygiene or wear gloves.
- Ensure that you are always able to identify both poor practice and positive role models for practice.
- Always reflect on incidents relating to poor infection prevention and control to enable you to improve your practice. It is important to know where to access infection prevention and control-related information and have the confidence to seek support from specialists.
- Ensure you develop and maintain an awareness of research findings, so the care you provide to patients has a sound evidence base.
- While the management of waste may not strike you as a nursing responsibility, the production of waste is an unavoidable consequence of our role and the care tasks undertaken.
- If you follow the principles, it is possible to manage healthcare waste safely and effectively in all settings.

CRITICAL REFLECTION

Holistic care

Infection prevention and control are important in providing holistic care for a patient. Review the chapter and note down all the instances where the care actions outlined can help you meet a patient's wider physical, psychological, social, economic and spiritual needs. Think of a variety of different patients across the fields, not just within your own field. You may find it helpful to make a list and refer back to it next time you are in practice, and then write your own reflection after your practice experience.

GO FURTHER

Books

RCN (2014) *The Management of Waste Arising from Health, Social and Personal Care*. London: RCN. This guidance represents the practical application of national guidance such as HTM 07-01 and applies it to nursing practice. It has been written in easy-to-read language and reflects the needs of care in a range of settings.

Wilson, J. (2006) *Infection Control in Clinical Practice*, 3rd edn. London: Elsevier. This book is an excellent reference source for further details of the microbiological aspects of infection prevention and control.

FURTHER
READING:
JOURNAL
ARTICLES

SAGE journal articles

Go to https://study.sagepub.com/essentialnursing2e for free online journal articles for this chapter. If you are using the interactive ebook, simply click on the book icon in the margin to go straight to the resource.

Lee, K. (2013) 'Student and infection prevention and control nurses' hand hygiene decision making in simulated clinical scenarios: A qualitative research study of hand washing, gel and glove use choices', *Journal of Infection Prevention*, 14(3): 96-103. This article describes how final-year nursing students and specialist IPC nurses verbalised their hand hygiene decision-making while working through clinical scenarios on a computer, to understand what factors they were taking into account in choosing to use hand-washing or alcohol-based hand-rub/gel or to wear gloves.

Nichols, A., Grose, G., Bennalick, M. and Richardson, J. (2012) 'Sustainable healthcare waste management: A qualitative investigation of its feasibility within a county in the south west of England', *Journal of Infection Prevention*, 14(2): 60-4. This article investigates the possibility of employing a sustainable 'reduce, reuse, recycle' philosophy in the management of waste within healthcare settings.

Other journal articles

Fuller, C., Savage, J., Hayward, A., Cookson, B., Cooper, B. and Stone, S. (2011) '"The dirty hand in the latex glove": A study of hand hygiene compliance when gloves are worn', *Infection Control and Hospital Epidemiology*, 32(12): 1194-9. This article describes observed hand hygiene and glove use across a mix of secondary care wards. The authors describe how gloves were often worn when not indicated, and vice versa.

Reilly, J., Price, L., Lang, S., Robertson, C., Cheater, F., Skinner, K. and Chow, A. (2016) 'A pragmatic randomized controlled trial of 6-step versus 3-step hand hygiene technique in acute hospital care in the United Kingdom', *Infection Control and Hospital Epidemiology*, 37: 661-6. This publication provides the first microbiological comparison of two techniques used to apply alcohol-based hand rub (AHBR). The 6-step technique was identified as a superior technique.

Weblinks

Go to https://study.sagepub.com/essentialnursing2e for weblinks related to this chapter. If you are using the interactive ebook, simply click on the book icon in the margin to go straight to the resource.

FURTHER READING: WEBLINKS

Health and Safety Executive (n.d.) Choosing the Right Gloves to Protect Skin: A Guide for Employers. Available at: www.hse.gov.uk/skin/employ/gloves.htm. This web page is a useful resource in helping students to gain a broader understanding of issues relating to gloves and guidance for employers. It applies to healthcare as well as other industries, such as hairdressing.

Loveday, H., Wilson, J., Pratt, R., Golsorkhi, M., Tingle, A., Bak, A., et al. (2013) 'EPIC 3: National evidence-based guidelines for preventing healthcare-associated infections in NHS hospitals in England', *Journal of Hospital Infection*, 86S1: S1-S70. Available at: www.his.org.uk/files/3113/8693/4808/epic3_National_Evidence-Based_Guidelines_for_Preventing_HCAI_in_NHSE.pdf. These guidelines were commissioned by the Department of Health and form the most up-to-date evidence-based IPC guidance available in the UK. They were developed after a systematic and expert review of all the available scientific evidence. Glove use and standard precautions are included.

National Institute for Health and Clinical Excellence (NICE) (2012) *Clinical Guideline 139, Infection: Prevention and Control of Healthcare-associated Infections in Primary and Community Care*. London: NICE. Available at: http://publications.nice.org.uk/infection-cg139. This guideline applies to all healthcare workers employed in primary and community care settings, including ambulance services, and should ensure safe practice is applied consistently. Much care is also delivered by informal carers and family members, and this guideline is equally applicable to them.

Royal College of Nursing (RCN) (2011) *Freedom of Information Report on Waste Management*. London: RCN. Available at: www.rcn.org.uk/professional-development/publications/pub-004108. This report highlights the significant variation in the classification of waste, with most waste disposed of via the 'infected' waste stream, although in reality only a small amount of waste produced by healthcare meets the infectious classification. The report identifies that significant financial savings could be made if waste was better segregated, and encourages better use of the offensive waste stream.

RCN (2012) *Tools of the Trade*. London: RCN. Available at: www.rcn.org.uk/professional-development/publications/pub-004242. Developed with experts and the Health and Safety Executive, this guidance explores glove use and its association with hand hygiene. It also addresses occupationally acquired dermatitis, which affects the hands of nurses in particular.

ACE YOUR ASSESSMENT

ONLINE
QUIZZES

Review what you have learned by visiting the book's online resources at: https://study.sagepub.com/essential nursing2e If using your interactive ebook, just click on the icon in the margin to go straight there.

- Test yourself with multiple-choice and short-answer questions.
- Revise key terms with the interactive flash cards.

REFERENCES

Ayliffe, G.A.J., Babb, J.R., Davies, J.G. and Lilly, H.A. (1978) 'Hand disinfection: A comparison of various agents in laboratory studies and ward studies', *Journal of Hospital Infection*, 11(3): 226–43.

Casewell, M.W. and Phillips, I. (1977) 'Hands as a route of transmission for *Klebsiella* species', *British Medical Journal*, 2: 1315–17.

Control of Substances Hazardous to Health Regulations (COSHH), The (2002, updated 2013). London: The Stationery Office.

Fuller, C., Savage, J., Hayward, A., Cookson, B., Cooper, B. and Stone, S. (2011) '"The dirty hand in the latex glove": A study of hand hygiene compliance when gloves are worn', *Infection Control and Hospital Epidemiology*, 32(12): 1194–9.

Health and Safety Executive (HSE) (2012) Selecting Latex Gloves. Available at: www.hse.gov.uk/skin (accessed 24 February 2015).

HM Coroner (2017) Regulation 28 Report to Prevent Future Deaths. Available at: www.judiciary.gov. uk/wp-content/uploads/2017/06/Haughey-2017-0116.pdf (accessed 4 June 2017).

International Council of Nurses (ICN) (2009) *Health Care Waste Management: Handbook for Nurses*. London: ICN.

Loveday, H., Wilson, J., Pratt, R., Golsorkhi, M., Tingle, A., Bak, A., et al. (2013) 'EPIC 3: National evidence-based guidelines for preventing healthcare-associated infections in NHS hospitals in England', *Journal of Hospital Infection*, 86S1: S1–S70. Available at: www.his.org.uk/files/3113/8693/4808/epic3_National_Evidence-Based_Guidelines_for_Preventing_HCAI_in_NHSE.pdf (accessed 19 March 2015).

National Institute for Health and Clinical Excellence (NICE) (2012, updated 2017) *Clinical Guideline 139, Infection: Prevention and Control of Healthcare-associated Infections in Primary and Community Care*. London: NICE. Available at: www.nice.org.uk/guidance/cg139 (accessed 28 March 2018).

Reilly, J., Price, L., Lang, S., Robertson, C., Cheater, F., Skinner, K. and Chow, A. (2016) 'A pragmatic randomized controlled trial of 6-step versus 3-step hand hygiene technique in acute hospital care in the United Kingdom', *Infection Control and Hospital Epidemiology*, 37: 661–6.

Royal College of Nursing (RCN) (2011) *Freedom of Information Report on Waste Management*. London: RCN. Available at: www.rcn.org.uk/__data/assets/pdf_file/0005/372308/004108.pdf (accessed 6 March 2018).

Royal College of Nursing (2012) *Tools of the Trade*. London: RCN.

Royal College of Nursing (2014) *The Management of Waste Arising from Health, Social and Personal Care*. London: RCN.

Sax, H., Allegranzi, B., Uckay, I., Larson, E., Boyce, J. and Pittet, D. (2007) 'My five moments for hand hygiene': A user-centred design approach to understand, train, monitor and report hand hygiene', *Journal of Hospital Infection*, 67: 9–21.

Taylor, L.J. (1978) 'An evaluation of hand-washing techniques', *Nursing Times*, 74(3): 108–10.

World Health Organization (WHO) (2009) WHO Guidelines on Hand Hygiene in Health Care. Available at: http://whqlibdoc.who.int/publications/2009/9789241597906_eng.pdf (accessed 6 March 2018).

ASEPTIC TECHNIQUE AND SPECIMEN COLLECTION

23

ROSE GALLAGHER

THIS CHAPTER COVERS

- Asepsis and aseptic technique
- Asepsis and your practice

- Specimen collection

REQUIRED KNOWLEDGE

- Before reading this chapter, it will be helpful to be aware of your local policies relating to aseptic technique and specimen collection.

It will also be helpful to have read Chapter 22 – Infection Prevention and Control; and Chapter 6 – Law.

> My name is Jo and I have a 3-year-old son called Sam. Sam had an accident and needs to have his wound dressed by the nurses every few days. This is painful as sometimes the dressing sticks and Sam now recognises when we are going to have it done and can be quite difficult. It's very upsetting to see him crying, but I know it's for the best.
>
> The nurse has a wonderful way with Sam and we always make sure he has had some pain medicine before we start. I help her by keeping his hands away from his dressing and together we make sure the wound is clean and securely bandaged afterwards. It takes time of course, but Sam is always so pleased to get his bravery reward when we have finished! Sam is very interested in what happens when his dressing is changed; he has learned the importance of asepsis – perhaps we have a future nurse in the making!
>
> **Jo, mother to Sam**

INTRODUCTION

Asepsis and aseptic technique are two commonly used terms associated with processes to avoid or eliminate contamination of normally sterile body sites or specimens. They are linked to a number of nursing skills, including the collection of patient specimens, and are fundamental to the delivery of quality care because if these skills are undertaken incorrectly the patient may suffer adverse effects such as infection or inaccurate laboratory results. The need to avoid contamination of specimens is crucial, given the importance of these as part of decision-making points for patient treatment. This is particularly relevant to antibiotic prescribing, the main driver of antimicrobial resistance (AMR). There are numerous reasons why specimens are requested, from assisting in the diagnosis of disease or infection, through monitoring a patient's recovery from illness, to requirements outside of 'traditional' care roles, for example as part of drug and alcohol testing in sport or as part of a police investigation. The role of the nurse extends to many health, social and public arenas in which they can be required to support any such scenarios. However, as an introduction, the context of this chapter is the healthcare environment.

ASEPSIS AND ASEPTIC TECHNIQUE

An aseptic technique process can be used in a variety of scenarios (e.g. invasive device insertion sites), wounds and specimens. Historically, the aseptic technique originated in operating theatres but today is performed in clinical and non-clinical areas (such as patients' own homes) using sterile equipment combined with other practices to prevent contamination entering the patient's body.

History

Historically, a number of individuals have contributed to our modern-day interpretation of asepsis and aseptic technique, including Joseph Lister (1827–1912) (use of carbolic acid as an antiseptic in operating theatres), Ignas Semmelweiss (1818–65) (hand-washing), Oliver Wendell Holmes (1809–94) (transmission of puerperal fever) and Louis Pasteur (1822–95) (pasteurisation and the germ theory). The work of these individuals and others has contributed to procedures we still use today in operating theatres to prevent infection in surgical wounds.

Asepsis and aseptic technique today, however, are used in and adapted to situations outside of operating theatres where control of the environment and equipment to reduce contamination is easier to achieve. This brings a number of practical challenges to reducing the risk of contamination of vulnerable body sites. A key challenge is the use of different terminologies/language to describe the aseptic technique, which can result in confusion. However, the biggest challenge is that there is no evidence to inform us *how* to best undertake an aseptic technique in non-theatre settings, including hospital and community situations. All we can consider is evidence of the impact of non-compliance with some elements of the process (Hopper and Moss, 2010). So, at best, aseptic technique has to be defined by 'best practice' or consensus agreement regarding principles with different interpretations, rituals, languages and preferences, all of which have contributed to its evolution over time.

Aseptic versus 'clean' technique

The term 'clean technique' describes a process or processes to meet the needs of different care settings (originally community settings, but this has expanded to potentially any area) which *reduces* contamination of vulnerable sites (for example, in the management of chronic leg ulcers which are already known to be heavily colonised with bacteria). This is, however, a good example of confusion regarding language, process and outcome expectations for both techniques (Flores, 2008; Gillespie and Fenwick, 2009), and in reality the two processes overlap.

How to perform an 'aseptic technique'

In practice, this issue has become a very contentious one, due to the need to move away from the traditional 'procedural approach' towards one that focuses on principles to avoid risks to vulnerable patient sites or devices. As a nurse, it is imperative to understand the fundamental principles, which you can then apply to any situation, rather than just being able to follow a procedure without the ability to customise it to meet patient or environmental demands.

It is important to apply the principles of asepsis to the chain of infection (see Figure 23.1). The chain of infection is a useful way of thinking about how different elements can combine to put patients at risk.

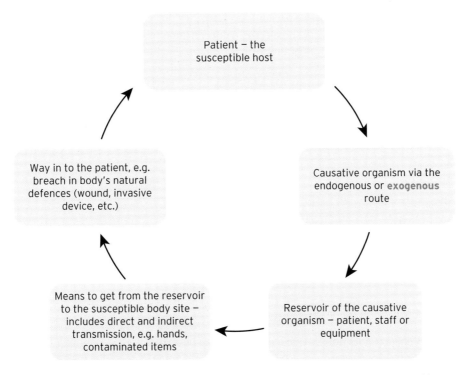

Figure 23.1   The chain of infection demonstrating where contamination can occur if an aseptic technique is not used

> It is important to understand and apply aseptic techniques as they prevent cross infection or worsening conditions of an existing wound. If we do not use these techniques we will risk further infection of the wounds, prolonged healing time, cross infection for the patient and ourselves and others.
>
> **Julie Davis, LD nursing student**

An aseptic technique, when performed correctly, will 'break' the chain of infection and by doing so protect the patient. However, procedures involving aseptic technique principles are frequently 'prescribed' within individual tasks, such as dressing a wound, inserting an intravenous cannula or administering intravenous drugs. There are potential problems with such an approach, as elements of ritual can find their way into practice and differences of opinion, and therefore variations in practice can develop which do not reduce the risk of contamination or produce benefit for the patient. Two examples relevant to current practice and debate are (1) whether it is necessary to wear gloves to perform an aseptic technique; and (2) if so, whether the gloves should be sterile or non-sterile. Another question is whether use of a dressing trolley is preferable to a tray in clinical settings.

The chain of infection

The 'chain of infection' (Figure 23.1) describes the necessary series of events that need to take place for infection to occur, regardless of whether this is caused by a virus, bacteria or fungi. For an infection to occur, all links in the chain must be present. As nurses, we prevent this from happening by putting in place procedures or techniques to 'break' the chain of infection. Always applying an appropriate aseptic technique is an excellent way of breaking the chain.

ACTIVITY 23.1: REFLECTION

Reflect on the aseptic techniques you have observed being carried out by the nurses you have been working with:

- Did they all do it the same way?
- What elements were common to all procedures observed?
- Did the option to use equipment such as gloves or a dressing tray/trolley require discussion? If so, how did you reach a decision regarding what was used?
- Do you think any elements of the chain of infection were broken?

ASEPSIS AND YOUR PRACTICE

Please note: this chapter does not provide a prescribed step-by-step procedure outlining how you should perform an aseptic technique, due to the issues previously highlighted. It does, however, present the important principles you need to consider (see Clinical Skill 23.1) and apply in the care you deliver to patients.

To start with I found aseptic technique quite difficult – you have to concentrate the whole time, being very self-aware about what you are touching. I had to really think hard about when I put gloves on to overcome the temptation to wear them all the time just in case. My practice educator helped me to gain confidence by assessing any risks for blood and body fluids in advance according to what procedure I was doing. I now practice confidently knowing I have safe clean hands and my patients and I are both protected in the right way without wearing gloves unnecessarily.

Charlie Clisby, NQN

Guidelines

There will be various local guidelines of which you must be aware when undertaking aseptic procedures. Remember never to undertake this care unless you are, or have supervision from, a trained, experienced and competent person. The types of guidelines you need to consider will be contained in:

- infection prevention and control policies
- local organisational policies, e.g. wound dressing formulary.

CASE STUDY 23.1: TOM

Tom is 15 and has a learning disability. He has a chronic wound on his leg which is very painful and smells offensive. Tom is very conscious of the smell and dislikes having his dressing changed. He expresses his anxiety through his behaviour, which can be perceived as aggressive at times, especially by people who do not know him.

Tom really enjoys bathing, because he finds it relaxes him and he loves playing with his collection of boats, and plastic dinosaurs.

To make Tom's dressing changes less stressful for him, your practice educator wants to use his bath as an opportunity to undertake his dressing change.

- What needs to be considered in order to prevent any contamination and support wound healing?

ACTIVITY 23.2: DECISION-MAKING

You and you practice educator are planning to dress a patient's wound while they are sitting in the living room of their home. The room is very unclean - there are six cats who live in the house and they have used the living room carpet as a litter tray. The facilities for you to wash your hands are poor, the sink is dirty and there is no hand towel, no hot water and only a trickle of cold.

- What actions would you take to reduce contamination of the wound?

My name is Jan. I was admitted to hospital because I had diarrhoea which wouldn't settle. Weeks I've had it. The docs think I might have an infection. I was given a foil container like a pie dish and told to do my business in it. How was I supposed to do that? And in a public toilet?

My nurse was wonderful. I didn't have to tell him I was embarrassed or ask how to use it. He explained everything and helped set up the toilet so all I had to do was use it as usual. It's a horrible thing to have to have somebody else handle your business but he was so professional and organised, there was no fuss and most of all I kept my dignity.

The results showed I did have an infection, and now I'm back to normal. I'm so grateful to him; I don't think I could have faced doing it by myself.

Jan, patient

STEP-BY-STEP CLINICAL SKILL 23.1: PRINCIPLES OF ASEPSIS

☑ Field-specific considerations

When caring for a patient with a learning disability, it is important to be mindful of their level of understanding, so that consent and cooperation for the procedure can be gained. You will need to allow time to explain what you are doing and consider whether it will cause discomfort or pain.

Patients who have impaired mental capacity may not understand why you need to undertake an aseptic procedure. They may therefore withhold consent and you may need to refer to local policies on presumed or assumed consent, which will reflect requirements of the Mental Capacity Act 2005 and best interest.

As younger children may not understand what you wish to do, you may need to modify your approach – it may be helpful to have the parents or carers present to assist.

☑ Care-setting considerations

Aseptic technique can be undertaken in any care setting, although you may need to think carefully about how best to manage the patient and the patient's environment.

☑ What to watch out for and action to take

While undertaking an aseptic procedure, you should also assess:

- the general condition of the patient; specific elements will vary according to the procedure being undertaken (e.g. respiratory rate for care of a chest drain)
- their neurological condition – are they alert and responsive? Are they agitated?
- any signs or complaints of pain or discomfort
- the patient's or relatives'/carers' views – for example, saying that their condition is 'not quite right' or they 'don't feel well'.

The information gained from these observations is additional to any assessment you make relating to, for example, the wound you are dressing and will enable you to fully assess the patient's condition and institute appropriate treatment as necessary, escalating care needs to senior nurses and the medical team.

☑ Helpful hints

- Do I wear gloves and an apron? Gloves and aprons must only be worn if contact with blood/body fluids/excreta is anticipated or the patient is in source isolation for IPC requirements.
- Hand hygiene must be performed before touching a patient, before clean/aseptic procedures, after body fluid exposure/risk, after removal of gloves and after touching a patient or the patient's immediate surroundings.
- Waste should be disposed of into the correct waste stream in line with a risk assessment.

ASEPTIC TECHNIQUE GUIDELINES

BEFORE YOU START

 Before commencing any care activity, introduce yourself to the patient, explain the procedure and gain their consent
Fully informed consent may not always be possible if the patient is a child or has impaired mental capacity or learning disabilities, but even in these circumstances, every effort should be made to explain what you are going to do in terms that the patient can understand. This is not only respectful of their individual human rights, but also helps to ensure that they will be more accepting of the treatment and that their anxieties are reduced
For patients who are unable to provide consent because they are unconscious, refer to local policies

 Assess the procedure and determine its complexity before you start, collecting all equipment that may be needed (and an assistant/chaperone if required)
Ensures you are fully prepared; also avoids you having to leave the patient or interrupt the procedure

 Consider what is going on around you – do you really need to do an aseptic technique now (even if planned)? Is the patient due to have other investigations that will cause you to rush, e.g. an x-ray?
Ensures that the environment is conducive to undertaking an aseptic technique – for example, there will be a negative environmental impact if bed-making or cleaning is being undertaken in close proximity to a large wound dressing being undertaken

 Ensure the patient is in a comfortable position where you can access the appropriate area
Ensure the patient has received appropriate analgesia as required
Promotes patient comfort

 Clear sufficient space within the environment, e.g. around the bed space, chair or treatment area
Ensure the area is private
Enables clear access for the patient and the nurse to work safely
Maintains patient privacy, dignity and comfort as required – patients will feel exposed if others can see the care they are receiving

 Transport equipment to the patient appropriately (consider a dressing trolley if available and appropriate)
Ensures all equipment is to hand
Maintains cleanliness of equipment and aids transport of all items safely

 Perform hand hygiene and apply non-sterile gloves only if required
Wearing apron and gloves is a standard infection prevention practice when dealing with body fluids or patients in isolation if they pose a risk of infection to others
Ensure your use of PPE is appropriate by considering the individual patient situation and the risk presented. Appropriate hand hygiene will assist in preventing and controlling infection

(Continued)

REMOVE AND DISPOSE

 If present, remove any soiled dressings, 'contaminated' or 'dirty' items and place in appropriate waste bag according to risk assessment
In preparation for dressing (etc.) change
Ensure soiled, contaminated or dirty items are disposed of appropriately in the offensive or infectious waste stream depending on risk assessment

 Remove gloves and perform hand hygiene
Appropriate hand hygiene will assist in preventing and controlling infection

CREATE A 'STERILE FIELD'

 If using a dressing pack, open sterile items and create your 'sterile field' by placing only sterile items within this area
Creating a sterile field avoids contamination through direct contact with non-sterile items. Remember, your hands are not sterile!

 Undertake procedure ensuring:

- only sterile items come into contact with the susceptible site
- sterile and non-sterile items do not come into contact with each other

In order to prevent and control infection

 Apply sterile or non-sterile gloves as required
A risk assessment will determine if sterile or non-sterile gloves are required

TO CONCLUDE

1 After completing the required care, ensure the patient is in a comfortable position, with drinks and call bells available as necessary
Promotes patient comfort and ensures they are well nourished and hydrated

2 Dispose of all waste and any single-use equipment, discard PPE (if used) and perform hand hygiene
Clean any equipment used as per the relevant policy every time it is used
Prevents cross-infection and maintains equipment in working order

3 Record the care provided in the patient's record
Maintains patient safety and accurate records

4 If any abnormal findings are observed, report to your practice educator or a registered nurse immediately
It is vital to report abnormal findings to a registered nurse immediately so they can ensure care is escalated; failure to do so can result in the patient's condition deteriorating and potentially preventable adverse outcomes

Source: Loveday et al. (2013); NICE (2017); WHO (2009)

SPECIMEN COLLECTION

Analysis of a specimen will determine important clinical decisions regarding a patient's condition or disease progress. Results also influence choices regarding ongoing or new treatment such as the prescribing of antibiotics. A specimen received at the laboratory in poor condition or taken inappropriately could therefore have profound implications for patient care, diagnosis and timeliness of any subsequent treatment. Therefore, the quality of a specimen is very important.

Nurses commonly take or handle specimens such as:

* wound swabs
* faeces
* urine
* blood (cultures or samples for analysis)
* sputum
* nasal and throat swabs (for detection of infection or screening for presence of clinically important bacteria, e.g. MRSA, Group A Streptococci).

As previously outlined, specimens are tested for a multitude of reasons, which can be summarised as:

* screening – for disease or the presence of micro-organisms such as malarial parasites, MRSA or Carbapenemase Producing Enterobacteriaceae (CPE)
* case finding – similar to screening but in a defined population such as blood tests for BRCA1 and 2 genes for breast cancer

- monitoring – for example, to reveal levels of drugs in the body, e.g. Gentamicin, Vancomycin
- diagnosis – to confirm or exclude the presence of disease.

I would discuss with the patient the reasons why we need to collect a specimen and gain consent. I would then discuss with them to see if they are happy to take their own nasal swab. If not I would explain what I need to do and collect the specimen as quickly and confidently as I could. Before collecting the specimen I would read up on the procedure and discuss with my practice educator, role playing it through with them if necessary.

Laura Grimley, adult nursing student

The importance of multi-disciplinary relationships

As mentioned previously, patient outcomes are directly influenced by the quality of specimens. The collection, transport, processing, analysis and results reporting of specimens all require efficient and reliable multi-disciplinary relationships to exist. Those involved in this process include nurses, porters (or transport drivers in community settings), laboratory reception staff, laboratory staff, technicians and biomedical scientists, plus doctors to interpret and communicate results. Each element of this relationship is of equal importance and a problem in any part has the potential to adversely affect the accuracy of the result of the specimen testing.

WHAT'S THE EVIDENCE?

Historically, evidence has developed to inform laboratory techniques and 'standard operating procedures', but these do not in themselves often reflect the patient experience. One example of where patient experience can be adversely affected is the contamination of blood culture specimens, for example when MRSA is identified as a result of poor technique due to skin contamination at the venepuncture site. If we think about what Jan said in his patient voice, however, he makes it very clear that patients value the support, advice and experience a nurse can offer to ensure that specimen collection is as simple and convenient as possible

Laboratory testing

As there are endless different ways in which a specimen can be analysed, a summary of common laboratory types and the tests they undertake are presented in Table 23.1. Not all healthcare providers will have all types of laboratory services: refer to your local provider's website for detailed information on what laboratory services are available.

Note: this chapter does not include the use of rapid diagnostic tests – use of these is subject to local policies and procedures in line with the manufacturer's guidance.

Principles common to the effective collection of all types of specimen

There are a number of principles which are applicable to the collection of all specimens.

Table 23.1   Types of laboratory and the tests they undertake

Laboratory type	General description of function
Microbiology	Function focuses on micro-organisms and their impact on human health. A number of departments may be present in hospitals or specimens may be referred to national or regional reference laboratories for further investigation or analysis
Biochemistry	Function focuses on chemical analysis of bodily fluids such as blood, plasma or urine. Includes common tests such as urea and electrolytes (U&E), liver function tests, tumour markers, drug levels (prescribed and illegal) and mineral levels, e.g. calcium, zinc
Pathology/Histopathology	The examination of human tissue. Specimens may be taken from live or deceased patients. Includes cytology
Haematology	Undertakes analysis of blood, including full blood count (FBC), Erythrocyte Sedimentation Rate (ESR), INR, Sickle cell screen, etc.

Guidelines

There are various national and local guidelines of which you must be aware when collecting specimens. Remember never to undertake collection of any type of specimen unless you are, or have supervision from, a trained, experienced and competent person. The types of guidelines you need to consider will be contained in:

- infection prevention and control policy
- local pathology policies/guidelines.

Once you are aware of these, you need to undertake a number of steps that will be common for the collection of all types of specimen (see Clinical Skill 23.2).

The usual procedures for collecting common specimens are described below, but remember that this should be read in conjunction with relevant local policies. At all times, complete the common steps (Clinical Skill 23.2) and ensure appropriate adjustments are made to suit the needs of the individual patient – local guidelines will be helpful for this.

ACTIVITY 23.3: CRITICAL THINKING

Tilly is three months old and has persistently loose, watery and offensive-smelling bowel motions. Her mother has been asked to collect a stool specimen so it can be tested, but is uncertain how she should do this.

- How would you explain the procedure?

STEP-BY-STEP CLINICAL SKILL 23.2: COMMON STEPS FOR THE COLLECTION OF ALL TYPES OF SPECIMEN

☑ **Essential equipment – depends on the specimen but is likely to include one or more of the following:**

- specimen container, specimen bag and laboratory form
- swabs as appropriate.

☑ **Field-specific considerations**

When collecting a specimen from a patient with a learning disability, it is important to know their level of understanding so that consent and cooperation can be gained. You will need to allow time to explain what you are doing, why you are doing it and whether it will cause discomfort or pain.

Patients who have impaired mental health may not understand why you need to collect a specimen. They may therefore withhold consent and you may need to refer to local policies on presumed or assumed consent, which will reflect requirements of the Mental Capacity Act 2005 and best interests.

Younger children may not understand why you need to collect a specimen. You will need to adopt an appropriate approach for consent. It may be helpful to have the parents or carers present to assist.

☑ **Care-setting considerations**

- Consideration must be given to any equipment needs, e.g. the refrigeration of viral transport media.
- Specimens can be collected in most care settings.

☑ **Key points to remember**

- There is a clear clinical need for the specimen.
- Explain the rationale to the patient and gain consent (refer to Chapter 6).
- The specimen must be obtained without contamination.
- The specimen must be stored appropriately or transferred to a laboratory as soon as possible.
- Check result and act on it accordingly.

☑ **Helpful hints**

- Gloves and aprons must be worn only if contact with blood/body fluids/excreta is anticipated or the patient is in isolation.
- Hand hygiene must be performed before touching a patient, before clean/aseptic procedures, after body fluid exposure/risk, after touching a patient and after touching a patient's surroundings.
- Waste should be disposed of in a waste bag if it is contaminated with blood/body fluids/excreta in line with risk assessment for waste, e.g. offensive or infectious waste.

SPECIMEN COLLECTION GUIDELINES

1 The first step of any procedure is to introduce yourself to the patient, explain the procedure and gain their consent

Fully informed consent may not always be possible if the patient is a child or has impaired mental health or learning disabilities, but even in these circumstances, every effort should be made to explain the procedure in terms that the patient can understand. This is not only respectful of their individual human rights, but also helps to ensure that they will be more accepting of the treatment and that their anxieties are reduced

For patients who are unable to provide consent because they are unconscious, local policies should be referred to

2 Ensure that it is an appropriate time to collect the specimen

The quality of the specimen can be affected by the time of collection and length of time before it reaches the laboratory. To make sure the specimen is of the best quality, ensure that it will reach the laboratory quickly once it has been collected and that it is the best time of day to collect the specimen. For example, it is best to collect a urine sample from the first voided urine in the morning for mycobacterial culture as this will contain the highest concentration of bacteria present

3 Gather the equipment required to collect the specimen; ensure this is clean and in working order

Reduces the chance of inaccurate results

All lids, containers and specimen bags should be checked to ensure there are no leaks or breaches which could result in spillage during transportation

Containers used for the collection and transportation of specimens should be CE-marked as this confirms that the container complies with essential requirements – only approved containers should contain specimens for laboratory analysis

This reduces the chance of infection and helps maintain the quality of the specimen

4 Clear sufficient space within the environment where the specimen is to be collected, for example around the bed space or chair

Enables clear access for the patient and the nurse to safely use the equipment required

5 Standard precautions should be used whenever there is a need to collect specimens

Wearing an apron and gloves as part of personal protective equipment (PPE) is a standard infection-control procedure when there is contact with body fluids or a patient is in isolation

Ensure your use of PPE such as gloves and disposable aprons is appropriate by considering the individual patient's situation and the risk presented. Do not use 'just in case'

6 Patients need to be in a private, comfortable and appropriate position and surroundings

Maintain patient privacy, dignity and comfort as required

To promote patient comfort and reduce anxiety

7 Complete the appropriate laboratory forms

The information provided on specimen or laboratory forms is very important. Incorrectly spelled or wrong patient names and identifying information could result in the wrong result being placed in a patient's notes. Alternatively, poorly completed forms could result in specimens being rejected by the laboratory, with significant implications for the patient

Some organisations use electronically generated specimen request forms and specimen labels to support laboratory tests. Always check local policies for more information

(Continued)

The laboratory request form must include the following information:

- patient surname and forename (care should be taken to avoid use of nicknames)
- date of birth
- gender
- NHS or hospital number – refer to local policies regarding patient unique identifiers and their use
- location of where specimen obtained (if relevant)
- requesting clinician or consultant in charge
- sample date and time
- name or initial of the person taking the specimen
- clinical information relevant to the specimen – this helps laboratory staff to interpret the clinical significance of specimen results. Examples include symptoms, possible or confirmed diagnosis, any current treatment (e.g. antibiotics) and other pertinent history such as foreign travel

Note: some NHS organisations are using barcoding technology to support procedures and trace specimens/equipment used to support patient care. If you are required to use this technology, ensure you have been trained on how to use this before undertaking procedures

Double-check to ensure the patient is correctly identified – ask the patient (where possible) to state their full name and date of birth. Use patient identifiers (e.g. wristbands) where possible to confirm

Prevents you from taking a specimen from the wrong patient. Never ask 'are you …?' Always ask the patient to state their name and date of birth

Some patients may not wear wristbands, e.g. neonates, those living in care homes or those with amputated limbs – check your local policies for alternatives to wristbands

Ensure specimen is collected in line with local policy

Using an aseptic technique reduces the risk of contaminating the specimen

Further details relating to taking the following specimens are available within the following:

Sample type	Details
Wound swab	Skill 23.3
Faecal specimen	SAGE edge
Urine sample	SAGE edge
Blood sample	p. 379
Sputum sample	Skill 23.4
Nasal swab	Skill 23.5
Throat swab	Skill 23.6

Specimens for microbiological investigation should ideally be taken before antibiotic therapy is commenced

If the patient is already on antibiotics before a specimen is taken, this may have a significant impact on identification of the causative organism (bacteria). The laboratory must be informed on the laboratory form of all therapy the patient is receiving or has recently received. Where sepsis is suspected, patients should have specimens taken if possible before commencing treatment, however this should not delay the administration of antibiotics

Specimens for viral investigation can require special transport media

Viruses are generally quite fragile and die easily

Examples include chickenpox (varicella), chlamydia, influenza, norovirus

Where specimens are taken directly from lesions, such as vesicles of herpes or chickenpox, then the swab must be placed inside special viral transport media to preserve any viral particles during transport to the laboratory. Viral transport media may require refrigeration and will have an expiry date

Refer to local policies for more information

Label container and seal in the specimen bag along with the laboratory request form, in line with local policy

Ensures the specimen and laboratory form are retained together and avoids loss of either during transport

Specimens should be transported to the laboratory and processed as soon as possible

Once a specimen is obtained, any micro-organisms present have been removed from their 'natural' habitat; therefore in order to preserve micro-organisms, transport to the laboratory should take place as soon as possible. If there is a delay in transportation, some specimens may be refrigerated in a designated refrigerator (do not put in a food fridge) until collection. This is preferable to leaving them at room temperature, which could interfere with the laboratory interpretation of results

For some specimens, delays of over 48 hours are considered unsatisfactory as the specimen will have deteriorated. Check local policy for further guidelines

14 **After collecting the specimen, ensure the patient is in a comfortable position, with drinks and call bells available as necessary**

Promotes patient comfort and ensures they are well nourished and hydrated

15 **Discard PPE, any single-use equipment and other used materials as per policy. Clean any equipment used as per the relevant policy and perform hand hygiene**
Prevents cross-infection and maintains equipment in working condition

16 **Document the specimen collection in the patient's notes**
Maintains patient safety and accurate records

Source: WHO (2009)

Collecting a blood sample

Nursing students in the UK would not take blood cultures or other blood specimens. However, knowledge of the process will enable you to support a patient when they are having a blood sample taken:

- Blood cultures are taken to determine the presence of bacteria or fungi in the blood (bacteraemia or fungaemia, respectively). Blood cultures should not be routinely taken, only when clinically indicated.
- Haematological investigations are undertaken to ascertain, for example, the patient's haemoglobin or platelet levels.
- Biochemical investigations are undertaken to ascertain, for example, the patient's potassium and sodium levels.

While blood cultures should be taken using a strict aseptic technique; there is less emphasis on this for routine blood tests (haematology or biochemistry). The other common steps and fundamental principles still apply, however, and there needs to be careful attention paid to prevent any sharps injuries. Many healthcare staff undertake venepuncture training but require additional knowledge and skills to be assessed as competent to provide this care.

ACTIVITY 23.4: CRITICAL THINKING

Jasmin is 3 years old and requires a blood sample to be taken:

- What might help Jasmin feel safe and comfortable so that the sample can be collected?
- Jasmin's mum is with her, and is very anxious and concerned about the blood test. How can you ensure that her worries do not impact on Jasmin's care?

STEP-BY-STEP CLINICAL SKILL 23.3: TAKING A WOUND SWAB

Wounds include surgical and traumatic wounds, burns, ulcers, folliculitis and invasive device insertion sites such as an intravenous cannula or wound drain.

☑ Indications for taking the specimen

Wound infection, cellulitis (in the presence of a break in the skin) and/or the presence of pus.

The presence of bacteria in a wound without signs and symptoms of infection reflects colonisation only, and is common in chronic wounds (such as leg ulcers in community settings).

WOUND SWAB GUIDELINES

Perform steps 1-8 of the common steps (see Clinical Skill 23.2)
To prepare the patient and yourself to undertake the task

Dip swab in transport media (if present with swab) or moisten with sterile saline
To preserve any bacteria present during transportation to the laboratory
Moisten swab to avoid **dessication** of any bacteria present

If pus is present, collect pus (via aspiration) or use a moistened swab
To preserve any bacteria present during transportation to the laboratory

Take swab from the part of the wound exhibiting symptoms of infection
This area will produce the best results

Using an aseptic technique, perform a 'zig-zag' motion while gently rotating the swab between the fingers
To ensure good contact by the swab with the wound

Place the wound swab immediately back into the container
To prevent contamination

Perform steps 10-16 of the common steps (see Clinical Skill 23.2)
To ensure that:

- the patient is safe and comfortable
- the specimen has been correctly collected and documented in the patient's records
- the equipment is clean and in working order

Source: PHE (2016a)

STEP-BY-STEP CLINICAL SKILL 23.4: COLLECTING A SPUTUM SAMPLE

☑ **Indications for taking the specimen**

Upper and lower respiratory tract infections, including pneumonia.

Micro-organisms normally present in the upper respiratory tract can contaminate the usually sterile lower respiratory tract and cause infection.

Green sputum does not necessarily mean the patient has an infection!

SPUTUM SAMPLE GUIDELINES

 Perform steps 1-8 of the common steps (see Clinical Skill 23.2)
To prepare the patient and yourself to undertake the skill

 The patient is required to expectorate in order to produce a specimen of sputum - saliva is not suitable
Patients who have difficulty coughing or expectorating may need a physiotherapist to help them produce a sample

 As necessary, place sample in specimen container, carefully avoiding contamination of the outside of the pot
A minimum of 1 ml of sputum is required

 Samples should be sent to the laboratory as soon as possible (sputum may be refrigerated for up to 2-3 hours)
Some bacteria die easily and overgrowth of other bacteria occurs quickly at room temperature, which will produce false results

 Perform steps 10-16 of the common steps (see Clinical Skill 23.2)
To ensure that:

- the patient is safe and comfortable
- the specimen has been correctly collected and documented in the patient's records
- the equipment is clean and in working order

Source: PHE (2016b)

STEP-BY-STEP CLINICAL SKILL 23.5: TAKING A NASAL SWAB

☑ **Indications for taking the specimen**

To detect clinically important bacteria in the nose, for example to determine if the patient is colonised with a bacteria such as meticillin-resistant *Staphylococcus aureus* (MRSA) or meticillin-sensitive *Staphylococcus aureus* (MSSA).

NASAL SWAB GUIDELINES

1 Perform steps 1–8 of the common steps (see Clinical Skill 23.2)
To prepare the patient and yourself to undertake the skill

2 Dip swab in transport media (if present with swab) or moisten with sterile saline
One swab can be used to swab both nostrils
To preserve any bacteria present during transportation to the laboratory
   Moisten swab to avoid dessication of any bacteria present

3 Swabs must be taken from the anterior nares of the nose (see Figure 23.2).

The swab should be inserted just inside the nostrils and then directed gently upwards back towards the tip of the nose and rotated to ensure gentle contact with the mucosal surface
The anterior nares are the external part of the nostrils (see Figure 23.2)

4 Perform steps 10–16 of the common steps (see Clinical Skill 23.2)
To ensure that:

- the patient is safe and comfortable
- the specimen has been correctly collected and documented in the patient's records
- the equipment is clean and in working order

Source: Dougherty and Lister (2015); PHE (2015a)

Figure 23.2   Nasal swab

STEP-BY-STEP CLINICAL SKILL 23.6: TAKING A THROAT SWAB

☑ **Indications for taking the specimen**

To detect a throat infection or carriage of clinically important bacteria, such as MRSA, or occasionally for screening in outbreak or contact situations with, for example, Group A Streptococci, *N. meningitides*.

THROAT SWAB GUIDELINES

 Perform steps 1–8 of the common steps (see Clinical Skill 23.2)
To prepare the patient and yourself to undertake the procedure

 Depress the tongue to expose the fauces of the tonsils (see Figure 23.3) and gently and quickly rub the swab over the affected or inflamed area
Ensure you have good lighting present to enable you to see into the throat
    The fauces or 'pillars of fauces' are two membranous folds which enclose the tonsils

Rubbing the swab over the affected area may make the patient gag, obstructing the view of the tonsils
    Avoid contact between the swab and other parts of the mouth (tongue and teeth) as this will contaminate the swab

 Perform steps 10–16 of the common steps (see Clinical Skill 23.2)
To ensure that:

- the patient is safe and comfortable
- the specimen has been correctly collected and documented in the patient's records
- the equipment is clean and in working order

Source: PHE (2015b)

CASE STUDY 23.2: MRS NEUMANN

Mrs Neumann is 58 and is undergoing a pre-operative assessment prior to a total hip replacement. As part of this, she requires a 'screen' for MRSA. This is local hospital policy. Mrs Neumann is very anxious about this and has read about 'superbugs' in the newspapers. She is worried that the fact she is having a screen means that she may have MRSA.

- How will you reassure Mrs Neumann regarding the need for an MRSA screen and gain her consent for the test (a nose swab)?
- What additional information can you provide for her while she awaits the result?

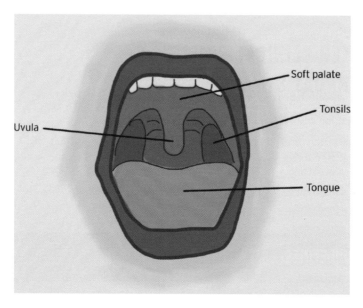

Figure 23.3   The fauces of the tonsils

Image © Robin Lupton

> Fully prepare the patient about what you need to do so they are relaxed and can cooperate. Ensure you have all the equipment needed and you are very familiar with the procedure you are carrying out. If you are unsure about anything ASK. Don't worry and relax, the patient is usually more anxious then you are.
>
> **Julie Davis, LD nursing student**

CONCLUSION

Maintaining asepsis and the accurate collection of specimens from patients are two skills fundamental to the role of the nurse.

It is most important when you are performing an aseptic technique to understand the principles, which you can then apply to any situation. This is a much safer way to work than just being able to follow a procedure without the ability to customise it to meet a patient's or their immediate environment's specific needs.

The 'chain of infection' describes a series of events that need to take place for infection to occur, regardless of whether this is caused by a virus, bacteria or fungi. For an infection to occur, all links in the chain must be present. An aseptic technique, when performed correctly, will 'break' the chain of infection and, by doing so, protect the patient.

There are numerous reasons why we would request a specimen from a patient, ranging from assisting in the diagnosis of disease or infection, through monitoring recovery from illness, to the need to take specimens outside of traditional healthcare settings, such as in professional sport. Always ensure that contamination is avoided whenever a specimen is collected, as this is critical to obtaining accurate results.

CHAPTER SUMMARY

- An aseptic technique protects the patient by preventing contamination of vulnerable body sites or contamination of specimens.
- Considerable confusion exists between the use of clean and aseptic techniques.
- It is important to understand the principles of asepsis, so you can apply them appropriately to the care required by patients.
- Specimens should only be sent when clinically indicated.
- Specimen or laboratory forms must be fully completed, with all relevant clinical information included.
- Storage, transport and time taken for specimens to reach the laboratory can impact on results.

CRITICAL REFLECTION

Holistic care

Maintaining asepsis and the appropriate and correct specimen collection are important in providing holistic care for a patient. Review the chapter and note down all the instances in which the care actions outlined can help you meet a patient's wider physical, psychological, social, economic and spiritual needs. Think of a variety of different patients across the fields, not just within your own field. You may find it helpful to make a list and refer back to it next time you are in practice, and then write your own reflection after your practice experience.

GO FURTHER

Books

Gould, D. and Brooker, C. (2008) *Infection Prevention and Control: Applied Microbiology for Healthcare*. Basingstoke: Palgrave Macmillan. This book uses microbiology as the foundation for supporting knowledge and learning relating to infection prevention and control.

Wilson, J. (2006) *Infection Control in Clinical Practice*, 3rd edn. London: Elsevier. This book provides generic information relating to all areas of infection control utilising good use of the current evidence base.

SAGE journal articles

Go to https://study.sagepub.com/essentialnursing2e for free online journal articles for this chapter. If you are using the interactive ebook, simply click on the book icon in the margin to go straight to the resource.

FURTHER
READING:
JOURNAL
ARTICLES

Knell, C., Pellow, C. and Potter, J. (2009) 'Long-term urethral catheter audit in patients' own home', *Journal of Infection Prevention*, 10(2): 62–5. This article describes risks associated with infection and indwelling urinary catheters. It acknowledges the importance of focusing on care in settings outside acute healthcare facilities and describes a programme of audit in order to improve the care that patients receive who have these devices **in situ**. Issues relating to urine specimen collection were identified as an area of practice to improve.

Jones, P. (1995) 'Pioneers of the transition from antiseptic to aseptic surgery', *Journal of Medical Biography*, 3: 201–6. This article describes the historical development of asepsis within the theatre context.

Other journal article

Flores, A. (2008) 'Sterile versus non-sterile glove use and aseptic technique', *Nursing Standard*, 23(6): 35–9. This article explores the evidence base for glove use in aseptic technique. It acknowledges the lack of evidence regarding the benefits of sterile versus clean gloves to achieve asepsis.

Weblinks

FURTHER READING: WEBLINKS

Go to https://study.sagepub.com/essentialnursing2e for weblinks related to this chapter. If you are using the interactive ebook, simply click on the book icon in the margin to go straight to the resource.

NHS Choices (2012) Report following Publication of 2012 HPA HCAI Prevalence Report. Available at: www.nhs.uk/news/2012/05may/pages/mrsa-hospital-acquired-infection-rates.aspx. This report provides an overview for patients and the general public on the estimated prevalence of HCAI in 2012 and the types of micro-organisms causing concern.

NHS Choices (2014) How to Collect and Store a Stool Sample. Available at: www.nhs.uk/chq/pages/how-should-i-collect-and-store-a-stool-faeces-sample.aspx. Part of the health questions series, this web page provides information for patients and the general public on stool specimens.

NHS Choices (2014) How Should I Collect and Store a Urine Sample? Available at: www.nhs.uk/chq/Pages/how-should-i-collect-and-store-a-urine-sample.aspx?CategoryID=69&SubCategoryID=692. This is useful information for patients and the general public on specimen collection and storage of urine samples, one of the most common samples requested.

National Institute for Health and Care Excellence (NICE) (2014) Clinical Knowledge Summaries: Urinary Tract Infection – Children. Available at: http://cks.nice.org.uk/urinary-tract-infection-children#!topicsummary. This link provides key points regarding urinary tract infection in children.

National Institute for Health and Care Excellence (NICE) (2014) Quality Standard QS 61: Infection Prevention and Control. Available at: www.nice.org.uk/guidance/qs61. This NICE Quality Standard describes ambitious standards that organisations should aim to meet to support ongoing improvements in IPC and reductions in associated HCAI.

—— ACE YOUR ASSESSMENT ——

ONLINE QUIZZES

Review what you have learned by visiting the book's online resources at: https://study.sagepub.com/essentialnursing2e If using your interactive ebook, just click on the icon in the margin to go straight there.

- Test yourself with multiple-choice and short-answer questions.
- Revise key terms with the interactive flash cards.

REFERENCES

Dougherty, L. and Lister, S. (2015) *The Royal Marsden Hospital Manual of Clinical Nursing Procedures*, 9th edn. Oxford: Wiley-Blackwell.

Flores, A. (2008) 'Sterile versus non-sterile glove use and aseptic technique', *Nursing Standard*, 23(6): 35–9.

Gillespie, B. and Fenwick, C. (2009) 'Comparison of the two leading approaches to attending wound care dressing', *Wound Practice and Research*, 17(2): 62–7.

Hopper, W. and Moss, R. (2010) 'Common breaks in sterile technique: Clinical perspectives and peri-operative implications', *AORN*, 91(3): 350–64.

Loveday, H., Wilson, J., Pratt, R., Golsorkhi, M., Tingle, A., Bak, A., et al. (2013) 'epic3: National evidence-based guidelines for preventing healthcare-associated infections in NHS hospitals in England', *Journal of Hospital Infection*, 86 (Suppl. 1): S1–70.

National Institute for Health and Clinical Excellence (NICE) (2017) *Prevention and Control of Healthcare-Associated Infections in Primary and Community Care*. Clinical Guideline 139. London: NICE. Available at: http://guideline.nice.org.uk/CG139 (accessed 30 May 2017).

Public Health England (2015a) Investigation of Throat Related Specimens. UK Standards for Microbiology Investigations. Bacteriology. B9 issue no 9. London: Public Health England. Available at: www.gov.uk/government/uploads/system/uploads/attachment_data/file/423204/B_9i9.pdf (accessed 30th May 2017).

Public Health England (2015b) Investigation of Nasal Samples. Bacteriology B5, issue 7.1. London: Public Health England. Available at: www.gov.uk/government/uploads/system/uploads/attachment_data/file/394716/B_5i7.1.pdf (accessed 30 May 2017).

Public Health England (2016a) Investigation of Skin, Superficial and Nonsurgical Wound Swabs. UK Standards for Microbiology Investigations. Bacteriology. B11 issue no 6.1. London: Public Health England. Available at: www.gov.uk/government/uploads/system/uploads/attachment_data/file/391745/B_11i5.2.pdf (accessed 30 May 2017).

Public Health (2016b) Investigation of Bronchoalveolar Lavage, Sputum and Associated Specimens. UK Standards for Microbiology Investigations. Bacteriology. B57 issue no. 3.2. Available at: www.gov.uk/government/uploads/system/uploads/attachment_data/file/580830/B_57i3.2.pdf (accessed 30 May 2017).

World Health Organization (2009) WHO Guidelines on Hand Hygiene in Health Care. Available at: http://whqlibdoc.who.int/publications/2009/9789241597906_eng.pdf (accessed 6 March 2018).

CLINICAL MEASUREMENT

VALERIE FOLEY

THIS CHAPTER COVERS

- Fundamental skills in the care of all patients
- Respiratory rate
- SpO$_2$ (peripheral oxygen saturation)
- Pulse rate
- Blood pressure
- Capillary refill time

- Temperature
- Early warning scoring systems
- Urine output
- Blood glucose
- Weight

REQUIRED KNOWLEDGE

- It will be helpful to have an understanding of the anatomy and physiology of the respiratory, cardiovascular and renal system before you start this chapter.

> I am nearly 12 and have Down's syndrome. I also have a heart that sometimes doesn't work properly and I have diabetes. This means that I visit my practice nurse very often and she always takes lots of recordings, of my pulse, temperature, weight and sugar levels. She is good at doing these, she makes it fun – but not everyone else is. Sometimes it hurts and that makes me cry.
>
> **Aoife, patient**

> A child has very good coping mechanisms and compensates extremely well when they are unwell. This leads to exhaustion and once they are exhausted and tired their deterioration is very quick and sudden. So any slight changes in clinical measurements can be an effective tool to determine if intervention for prevention of further deterioration is needed.
>
> **Alice Rowe, NQ RNMH**

INTRODUCTION

Many patients are used to having clinical measurements taken, either at GP surgeries, in hospital as part of routine monitoring or when they are ill, as outlined in Aoife's story above. Patients can also be taught how to monitor their own wellbeing and treatment by taking their own clinical measurements, such as blood pressure and blood glucose levels. As a nurse, taking, recording and acting on clinical measurements is a fundamental element of patient care that helps us to monitor a patient's physiological health. Clinical measurements, though, cannot be taken in isolation, as they are part of the skills and knowledge used by you as a nurse to complete a full clinical patient assessment. They combine the technological data available from clinical measurements with subjective data obtained from the patient through looking, listening and feeling (Smith, 2012). The interpretation of this combined data is key to identifying a patient's physiological condition and is particularly important in the care of children, who may deteriorate suddenly.

This chapter will provide you with a step-by-step guide to taking clinical measurements, while providing you with a baseline for abnormal results and what they may mean.

FUNDAMENTAL SKILLS IN THE CARE OF ALL PATIENTS

The underlying principles for taking essential clinical measurements will be similar for all types of patients. However, your approach to the patient, which measurements are required and when, and your interpretations of the measurements will vary based on individual patient need and response:

1. Respiratory rate
2. SpO_2 (peripheral oxygen saturation)
3. Pulse rate
4. Blood pressure
5. Capillary refill time (CRT)
6. Temperature
7. Early warning scoring systems
8. Urine output
9. Blood glucose
10. Weight

Respiratory rate, SpO_2, pulse, blood pressure and temperature are also often referred to as 'vital signs' or 'observations'. No matter which clinical measurement you are going to record or the care setting in which you are recording it, there are a number of issues and common steps you need to consider first.

Guidelines

There are various national and local guidelines of which you must be aware when monitoring clinical measurements. Remember never to undertake any of the following procedures unless you are, or have supervision from, a trained, experienced and competent person. The types of guidelines you need to consider will be contained in:

- infection prevention and control policy
- local organisational policies.

Once you are aware of these, you need to undertake a number of steps that will be common for all clinical measurement skills (see Clinical Skill 24.1 on the following page).

STEP-BY-STEP CLINICAL SKILL 24.1: COMMON STEPS FOR ALL CLINICAL MEASUREMENTS

☑ **Essential equipment**

Depends on skill but is likely to include one or more of the following:

- alcohol hand-rub
- fob watch with a second hand
- automated non-invasive blood pressure (NIBP) machine with oxygen saturation recording device (SpO$_2$), or a separate oxygen saturation recording device can be used
- aneroid sphygmomanometer with stethoscope
- thermometer (type depends on site to be used)
- blood glucose monitor and test strips
- clinical waste bag.

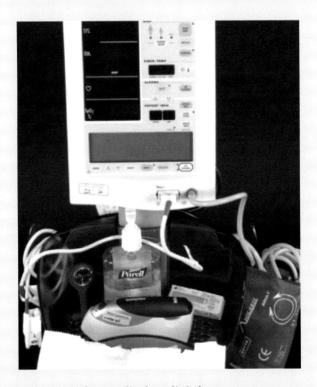

Figure 24.1   Essential equipment for monitoring vital signs

☑ **Field-specific considerations**

When caring for a patient with a learning disability, it is important to know their level of understanding so that consent for and cooperation with the measurement can be gained. You will need to allow time to explain why you are doing the measurements and whether they will cause discomfort or pain.

Patients who have mental health problems or those with a learning disability may not understand the relevance of why you need to take clinical measurements. They may therefore withhold consent to have their measurements taken and you may need to refer to the Mental Capacity Act 2005 and best interest.

Children's anatomy and physiology differ to adults' and vary from birth through to adolescence. You will need knowledge of paediatric anatomy and physiology to enable you to interpret the results. As younger children do not understand why you need to take measurements, this will determine your approach to taking the clinical measurements. It is usually helpful to have the parents or carers present to assist.

☑ **Care-setting considerations**

It is not always possible to have all the monitoring equipment available to undertake clinical measurements. For example, in a patient's home you may not have a sphygmomanometer with stethoscope and oxygen saturation probe; however, you can still monitor the patient's respiratory rate, heart rate and capillary refill time, which will give you a clear indication of the patient's physiological condition.

☑ **What to watch out for and action to take**

While monitoring a patient's clinical measurements, you should also observe and assess:

- the colour of the skin, lips and nail beds for signs of cyanosis
- the position of the patient
- their neurological condition – are they alert and responsive?
- any signs or complaints of pain or discomfort
- the patient's or relatives' views – for example, saying that their condition is 'not quite right' or they 'don't feel well'.

The information gained from these observations is additional to clinical measurements and will enable you to fully assess the patient's physiological condition, institute appropriate treatment as necessary and inform senior nurses and the medical team of the patient's escalated care needs.

☑ **Helpful hints**

- Gloves and aprons must be worn if contact with blood/body fluids/excreta is anticipated or the patient is in isolation.
- Hand hygiene must be performed before touching a patient, before clean/aseptic procedures, after body fluid exposure/risk, after touching a patient and after touching a patient's surroundings.
- Waste should be disposed of in a clinical waste bag if it is contaminated with blood/body fluids/excreta.
- Equipment must be cleaned as identified by the relevant policy every time it is used.

CLINICAL MEASUREMENT GUIDELINES

1 **The first step of any procedure is to introduce yourself to the patient, explain the procedure and gain their consent**
Fully informed consent may not always be possible if the patient is a child, has mental health problems or has learning disabilities; even in these circumstances, however, every effort should be made to explain the procedure in terms that the patient can understand. In the case of patients who are unable to provide consent because they are unconscious, advice should be sought from your practice educator or another registered nurse

 2 **Gather the equipment required (see individual skills for equipment required). Ensure these are clean and in working order**
Reduces the chance of abnormal readings
Reduces the chance of infection and maintains patient and nurse safety

 3 **Clear sufficient space within the environment, for example around the bed space or chair**
Enables clear access for the patient and the nurse to safely use the equipment required

 4 **Wash your hands with soap and water before you undertake clinical measurements. If taking vital sign recordings on more than one patient, use alcohol hand-rub between patients. Apron and gloves should only be worn if appropriate**
Consider the individual patient situation and the risk presented

5 **Ask the patient if they wish to have the curtains drawn for privacy or to be in a separate room**
Maintains patient privacy, dignity and comfort

6 **Patients need to be in a comfortable position, either sitting in a chair, resting on a couch or in bed. In an emergency**

situation where the patient has collapsed or is acutely unwell, vital sign observations should be taken wherever the patient is situated
Promotes patient comfort and reduces anxiety

 7 **If possible, the patient should refrain from physical activity for 20 minutes prior to taking measurements**
Strenuous activity can falsely elevate readings

 8 **Turn the monitoring equipment on and wait for it to go through its calibration checks**
Otherwise the results may be inaccurate

 9 **After performing the clinical measurements, ensure the patient is in a comfortable position, with drinks and a call bell available as necessary**
Promotes patient comfort and ensures they are well nourished and hydrated

 10 **Discard PPE, any single-use equipment and other used materials as per policy. Clean any monitoring equipment used as per the relevant policy and perform hand hygiene**
Prevents cross-infection and maintains equipment in working condition

 11 **Document findings on the patient's observation chart and/or in the patient's notes immediately**
Maintains patient safety and accurate records

 12 **If any abnormal readings are observed, escalate to senior nursing staff/your practice educator immediately**
It is vital to report abnormal findings to a registered nurse immediately so they can ensure care is escalated. Failure to do so can result in the patient's condition deteriorating, potentially leading to death

Source: Dougherty and Lister (2015); NICE (2014); Smith and Roberts (2011); Smith (2012); WHO (2009)

RESPIRATORY RATE (RR)

Respiratory rates are one of the most powerful predictors of respiratory dysfunction and significant indicators of a patient's deteriorating physiological condition (McQuillan et al., 1998; NICE, 2007), as they can be influenced by respiratory, cardiovascular and metabolic failure. Common clinical conditions that may cause respiratory failure are chest infections or pneumonia, pulmonary oedema (fluid in the lungs), chronic respiratory diseases and asthma; respiratory failure may also be secondary to other conditions such as strokes, muscular degenerative diseases and sepsis (severe infection).

I found the most difficult thing when doing observations is to get them done as quickly as possible, especially when a child is distressed – when they are distressed it takes longer and it is much more difficult, for example, to count respirations or feel for a pulse when they do not want to be touched. I try and do the things I find most difficult first. For example if a child is cuddled up with a parent/carer I will count their respiratory rate from a distance, ensuring the parents are aware of what I am doing. Before I try to take further observations I try to reassure them that what I am going to do is OK and will not hurt them, by demonstrating on the parents with consent, letting them feel the stethoscope or put the thermometer probe under their own arm. I find the small things make a big difference.

Alice Rowe, NQ RNMH

A&P LINK: RESPIRATION

Breathing movements are referred to as inspiration (breathing in) and expiration (breathing out). A normal adult breathing rate is about 12–18 breaths per minute (bpm); for a child, the normal rate can range from 12 to 60 bpm, depending on their age. The inhalation of oxygen and exhalation of carbon dioxide allow normal cellular function to take place in the body, meeting the body's cellular requirements for oxygen and energy and the removal of carbon dioxide.

Respiratory failure exists when oxygen levels are too low and/or carbon dioxide levels too high. When reviewing the patient's vital signs, you may find that the oxygen saturation level (SpO_2) is low, indicating hypoxia (low oxygen levels), and the respiratory rate is high. When the patient becomes exhausted, the respiratory rate can decrease, because they are becoming too tired to breathe.

Recording a patient's respiratory rate is the first 'vital sign', as it is a precise indicator of their condition. As with all vital signs, we need to ensure the result we obtain - in this case the respiratory rate - is accurate, so the steps outlined in Clinical Skill 24.2 need to be followed.

> I still find taking the respiration rate difficult. Throughout my training I was shown several methods that have proved helpful. It is worth trying different ways so you can find which way works best for you. Patients' talking certainly adds to the challenge of taking physical observations, so I will regularly ask if they can please not talk for the next short while whilst I carry out observations.
>
> Alice Rowe, NQ RNMH

CASE STUDY 24.1: VINCENT

Vincent is 8 years old and has cerebral palsy. He lives at home with his parents at weekends and attends a residential school during the week. Although he has a good level of understanding, he struggles to express his thoughts in speech. His parents and carers are able to interpret his expressions and therefore his needs.

He was admitted to the children's ward yesterday as he has a chest infection, which is not uncommon for him over the winter period.

A priority during Vincent's admission to hospital is to monitor his clinical measurements for signs of improvement in his condition or to detect early signs of deterioration, allowing timely interventions.

- How can you ensure that you count Vincent's respiratory rate accurately?
- What would you expect Vincent's respiratory rate and SpO_2 to be, taking into consideration that he has a chest infection?

ANSWER:
CASE STUDY 24.1

ACTIVITY 24.1: REFLECTION

Reflect on the answers you gave to Vincent's case study (24.1):

- Were the answers you gave correct?
- After having read more of the chapter, is there anything you would now do differently?

STEP-BY-STEP CLINICAL SKILL 24.2: COUNTING A RESPIRATORY RATE (RR)

☑ **What is normal?**

- Adult range: 12-18 breaths per minute (bpm)
- Child:

    o   infant (birth to 1 year): 30-60 bpm
    o   toddler (over 1 year to 3 years): 24-40 bpm
    o   preschool child (over 3 years to 5 years): 22-34 bpm
    o   school-aged child (over 5 years to 15 years): 18-30 bpm
    o   adolescent (over 15 years to 17 years): 12-16 bpm

☑ **Before you start**

Remember the common steps for all clinical measurements (Clinical Skill 24.1).

Other factors need to be considered when assessing a patient's respiratory function as it is not just the respiratory rate that detects abnormalities in breathing. As you approach the patient, observe for signs of hypoxia (a severe lack of oxygen) by observing for central cyanosis (a blue/purple tint around the lips, earlobes, nose and upper chest). Does the patient appear to be breathing fast or slow, are they making any noises when breathing in or out and does it look as though their breathing is laboured?

☑ **Essential equipment**

Fob watch.

☑ **Care-setting considerations**

Respiratory rates can be counted in any care setting, as long as the patient has not recently exercised and is not distressed or anxious.

☑ **What to watch out for and action to take**

If an abnormal respiratory rate is counted or any abnormalities in the respiratory function are observed, this must be reported to a qualified nurse immediately and recorded in the patient's notes.

Abnormal respiratory rates can sometimes be simply improved by altering the patient's position, ensuring they have adequate analgesia or increasing the amount of oxygen being administered to the patient. However, abnormal respiratory rates must always be reported and acted upon as they can be an early sign of a patient's physiological deterioration.

RESPIRATORY RATE GUIDELINES

 Perform steps 1-7 of the common steps (Clinical Skill 24.1)
To prepare the patient and yourself to undertake the skill

 Ask the patient to try and remain as quiet as possible - no moving or talking. Hold their wrist as though taking their pulse (see Figure 24.2)
Monitoring of a patient's respiratory rate and pulse is usually undertaken concurrently. By holding the wrist, the patient is less likely to be aware that you are counting their respiratory rate and will not alter their pattern of breathing while under observation

Figure 24.2 Respiratory rate and radial pulse

 Observe the patient's chest closely; count the number of breaths over one minute (60 secs) by watching the rise and fall of the chest. Each rise and fall of the chest counts as one respiration
To obtain an accurate rate and to monitor the respiratory pattern, respirations should always be counted for a full minute

 At the same time as counting the respiratory rate, note the depth of the respirations. Are they deep or shallow?

The depth of expansion of the chest gives an indication of the volume of air exchanged in each breath, which is known as the tidal volume. Shallow breathing is normally associated with a fast respiratory rate and can indicate a deteriorating respiratory condition, especially if the patient is at rest. Deep breathing may indicate a decreased level of consciousness

 Is the breathing pattern regular?
Irregular breathing patterns can indicate a neurological problem or be secondary to respiratory dysfunction

 Does the chest rise and fall equally on both sides (symmetry)?
If only one side of the chest is moving, the patient may have a **pneumothorax**, **consolidation** or collapse, a mucus plug or pleural fluid in one lung

 Is the patient using any accessory muscles, such as shoulders and abdominals?
Use of the accessory muscles is a sign that breathing is **compromised**, as they are not used in normal breathing. When pulmonary disease increases the work of breathing, the accessory muscles may be required to supplement the actions of the diaphragm and the external intercostal muscles

 Perform steps 9-12 of the common steps (Clinical Skill 24.1)
To ensure that:

- the patient is safe, comfortable and receiving the appropriate care
- results have been documented in the patient's records
- equipment is clean and in working order

Source: British Thoracic Society (2017); Dougherty and Lister (2015); Smith and Roberts (2011); Smith (2012)

PULSE OXIMETRY – SPO$_2$ (PERIPHERAL OXYGEN SATURATION)

Pulse oximetry is a device used to record a peripheral arterial blood oxygen saturation. Its function is to detect hypoxia (low oxygen levels), giving a non-invasive indication of a patient's cardio-respiratory status. Pulse oximetry has the ability to detect changes in oxygen levels rapidly, enabling us to identify problems before the patient is compromised. Although pulse oximeters provide good evidence of oxygen levels, they do not provide evidence of a patient's ability to expire carbon dioxide (CO_2). So, even if a patient has a normal SpO$_2$, their breathing pattern, rate or depth may not be adequate, and they may be retaining CO_2. This can only be determined by taking a sample of blood.

When recording vital signs, it is important at all times to be accurate. This includes not just the respiratory, pulse rate or blood pressure values which you are recording, but also the terms you use. Some things to remember around correct terminology for SaO$_2$ vs SpO$_2$ are:

Pulse oximetry in practice is often described as **SaO$_2$**. This is wrong, as **SaO$_2$** refers to arterial oxygen levels obtained by an actual sample of arterial blood.

SpO$_2$ is the correct term for the levels of peripheral arterial oxygen which have been obtained by a non-invasive pulse oximeter attached to a patient's periphery – their finger, for example.

The easy way to remember this is:

SaO$_2$ is the result obtained from an **a**ctual blood sample.

SpO$_2$ is the result obtained by the use of a non-invasive pulse oximeter attached to a patient's **p**eriphery.

It is always important to ensure that the precise term is used to describe how a vital sign has been obtained, because the normal ranges for these different methods may not be the same. Using inaccurate terminology could put a patient's life at risk.

A&P LINK: OXYGEN SATURATION

Oxygen is carried in the blood attached to haemoglobin molecules, referred to as oxyhaemoglobin. Oxygen saturation is a measure of how much oxygen the blood is carrying as a percentage (%) of the maximum it could carry.

One haemoglobin molecule can carry a maximum of four molecules of oxygen. So, if a haemoglobin molecule is carrying three molecules of oxygen, then it is carrying three quarters or 75% of the maximum amount of oxygen it could carry. However, we would be very concerned if a patient had an SpO$_2$ of 75%.

Due to the large number of haemoglobin molecules we have in our blood, the results of SpO$_2$ would normally be much higher than this. One hundred haemoglobin molecules could together carry a maximum of 400 (100 × 4) oxygen molecules. In normal healthy lungs, it is likely (Boore et al., 2016) that these 100 haemoglobin molecules would carry 380 oxygen molecules rather than the full amount of 400. So, they would be carrying 380 out of the maximum 400 molecules, which would give us a percentage of: (380/400) × 100 = 95%.

Hence, we would say that the patient is 95% saturated. This would be an acceptable result, as the normal range for SpO$_2$ in a healthy adult is 94-98%.

A pulse oximeter works by applying the principle of Beer's Law: 'the concentration of any substance can be determined by its absorption of light'. Thus, a pulse oximeter shines two different types of light, red and infrared, through the tissues of a patient's periphery, usually a finger or earlobe. The infrared light is absorbed by oxyhaemoglobin (haemoglobin carrying oxygen) and the red light by the de-oxygenated haemoglobin (haemoglobin not carrying oxygen).

The pulse oximeter is able to convert what it detects into a percentage, indicating the haemoglobin saturation. This is then displayed as a digital reading (95 per cent) or a waveform, or often both.

Figure 24.3 Pulse oximeter

The pulse oximeter measures light absorption over a number of pulse beats, which you can see as peaks in the waveform, so a patient needs to have a regular pulse in order for an accurate SpO_2 reading to be recorded.

It is important to check that the pulse oximeter shows you a good waveform, as this assures you that it is picking up the patient's pulse accurately. If this is not the case, and the waveform is poor, the pulse oximeter may not give you a correct reading. So, before recording the saturation value, make sure you have a good waveform.

Figure 24.4 How a pulse oximeter works

Pulse oximeters will often give inaccurate readings if the patient has cold peripheries, as this makes it difficult to obtain a good waveform. They can also be inaccurate if a patient has inhaled carbon monoxide or has an abnormal haemoglobin called methaemoglobin, as the pulse oximeter is unable to tell whether the haemoglobin is carrying molecules of oxygen or another substance.

(Continued)

Figure 24.5   Pulse oximeter probes

Note: Adapted from howequipmentworks.com

ACTIVITY 24.2: REFLECTION

Reflect on your experience of recording patients' vital signs:

- Have you heard other healthcare professionals talking about SaO_2 when they actually mean SpO_2?
- Next time you are on placement, listen out to hear if this is the case.

As we have already discussed, when recording any vital sign we need to ensure the results we obtain are accurate, so when measuring a patient's SpO_2 we must follow the correct procedure.

PULSE RATE (ALSO KNOWN AS HEART RATE = HR)

Monitoring a patient's pulse rate is a simple, non-invasive procedure that does not require any monitoring equipment, only the second hand of your watch. As a result, it can be undertaken wherever the patient is situated, such as in a bathroom on a ward, in a clinic or in their own home. It is a quick, reliable determinant of the patient's cardiovascular status.

Due to a number of physiological factors, normally accepted pulse rates vary significantly, from a rate of 180 beats per minute (bpm) in a newborn baby to 60 bpm in an adult.

A&P LINK: HEART RATE

A 'heartbeat' is caused by a contraction of the left ventricle of your heart. Each heartbeat results in oxygenated blood being ejected via the aorta into the arterial system. This causes a pressure wave that can be felt throughout the entire arterial system, and this is what we call the 'pulse'. This is best felt (or palpated) where an artery is near the surface of the body. The sites most commonly used by nurses are radial (especially in adults) or brachial (especially in children) (see Figure 24.7), although carotid and femoral sites can also be palpated.

Figure 24.6   ECG waveform

Figure 24.7   Radial and brachial pulse palpation sites

ACTIVITY 24.3: CRITICAL THINKING

Either find a picture or draw one which shows the location of:

• the carotid pulse palpation site
• the femoral pulse palpation site.

Write a list of the positive and negative aspects of using each of these sites, considering both children and adults.

ANSWER:
ACTIVITY 24.3

It is important never to be tempted to use automated monitoring equipment to measure pulse rates, even if you see others doing this. Automated equipment does not measure whether a pulse rate is regular or of good quality, which are both important factors to assess when measuring a patient's pulse. There are also further potential problems when using automated equipment, as the rate can be inaccurate if the pulse is irregular or if the patient has poor peripheral circulation, making the pulse weak and difficult to detect.

Measuring a patient's pulse accurately is a skill which, at first, may be difficult to master. Make sure you practise, applying the following 'top tips':

1. It may take you a few attempts to exert the right amount of pressure to enable the pulse to be felt. Too great a pressure and the pulse can be occluded, too little pressure and it will not be detected.
2. If it is difficult to feel the pulse at the radial or brachial artery, hyper-extend the hand or arm slightly so that the artery is nearer the skin (see Figure 24.? for this position).

STEP-BY-STEP CLINICAL SKILL 24.3: MEASURING A PULSE RATE (HR)

☑ What is normal?

- Adult range: 60-100 beats per minute (bpm)
- Child:

    ○ Neonate (birth to 28 days): 100-180 bpm
    ○ Infant (28 days to 1 year): 100-160 bpm
    ○ Toddler (over 1 year to 3 years): 80-110 bpm
    ○ Preschool child (over 3 years to 5 years): 70-110 bpm
    ○ School-aged child (over 5 years to 15 years): 65-110 bpm
    ○ Adolescent (over 15 years to 17 years): 60-90 bpm

☑ Before you start

Remember the common steps for all clinical measurements (Clinical Skill 24.1).

Most routine measurements of pulse rates are taken at the radial artery as this is easily accessible and does not compromise the patient's dignity.

For children under 1 year old, the brachial artery or the apex are the best sites to palpate a pulse as their wrists tend not to be well defined, so finding a radial pulse is difficult.

In emergency life-threatening situations and to confirm cardiac arrest, the carotid and femoral pulses are often used.

☑ Essential equipment

Fob watch.

☑ Field-setting considerations

When taking an infant or child's pulse, the apex (apical) or brachial site is frequently used.

☑ Care-setting considerations

Pulse rates can be counted in any care setting, so long as the patient has not recently exercised or is not distressed or anxious.

☑ What to watch out for and action to take

If an abnormal pulse rate is counted or if you suspect an abnormality in the regularity or volume of the pulse rate, this must be reported to a qualified nurse immediately and recorded in the patient's notes.

Abnormal pulse rates can sometimes be simply improved through adequate analgesia and encouraging the patient to drink more fluid. However, abnormal values must always be reported and acted upon as they can be an early sign of a patient's physiological deterioration.

PULSE RATE GUIDELINES

 Perform steps 1-7 of the common steps (see Clinical Skill 24.1)
To prepare the patient and yourself to undertake the skill

 Radial pulse
a. Ensure the patient's arm is resting on the chair arm, bed or couch. Place your second and third fingers over the inside of the wrist, in alignment with the thumb (see Figure 24.7)
b. Once a rhythmic beat is felt, count the number of times this occurs in 60 seconds (one minute)

 Brachial or apex pulse
a. If you are unable to palpate a radial pulse in an adult, the brachial artery is the next place to try as the artery is near to the heart and has a strong pulsation. The apex or brachial palpation site is usually the best position to measure a pulse in a child
b. The brachial pulse can be found at the bend of the arm on the inside edge. This is up from the radial pulse
c. The apex (or apical) pulse can be heard by placing a stethoscope at the fifth intercostal space (spaces between the ribs) on the chest, just left of the sternum
d. The same technique applies as taking a radial pulse

Brachial pulse

 Carotid pulse
a. Place your second and third fingers gently on the side of the neck approximately 5 cm down from the earlobe, slightly towards the throat
b. Once a rhythmic beat is felt, count the number of times this occurs in 60 seconds (one minute)

Carotid

 Femoral pulse
a. Place your second and third fingers in the groin approximately 10 cm inwards from the hip
b. Once a rhythmic beat is felt, count the number of times this occurs in 60 seconds (one minute)

Femoral

(Continued)

It is important to count the pulse rate for one minute as it is vital to assess whether the rhythm is regular and whether it has a good volume and quality. All of these factors can give you important information regarding a patient's cardiovascular status

 Perform steps 9-12 of the common steps (see Clinical Skill 24.1)
To ensure that:

- the patient is safe, comfortable and receiving the appropriate care
- the results have been documented in the patient's records
- the equipment is clean and in working order

Source: Dougherty and Lister (2015); Smith and Roberts (2011); Smith (2012)

3. Practise measuring pulse rates on friends and colleagues to understand where the pulses are located in a healthy person. Be careful if you are using the carotid site to palpate a pulse as too much pressure can cause adverse effects, such as faintness or even an irregular heartbeat.
4. It is possible for the presence or absence of a pulse to give you an indication of a patient's blood pressure.
5. If a radial pulse is present, then the systolic blood pressure is over 90 mmHg.
6. If a brachial pulse is present but *not* a radial one, this is a sign that the systolic blood pressure is low, at around 80 mmHg.
7. If the carotid is the *only* place a pulse can be palpated, the systolic blood pressure is extremely low, at around 60 mmHg.

Once you feel confident in accurately measuring the pulse rates of your friends and colleagues, follow the steps in Clinical Skill 24.3 to accurately measure the pulse rates of the patients for whom you are caring. Remember that it may be more difficult to find a pulse in patients who are sick than it has been to find a pulse in your friends and colleagues. If you are unable to find a pulse or are uncertain that you have accurately recorded a pulse, report this to your practice educator or another registered nurse straight away.

While we say that we are recording a patient's pulse, what we are actually recording is their heart rate, so the terms pulse and heart rate (HR) are frequently used interchangeably.

ACTIVITY 24.4: REFLECTION

Find and record your pulse at the radial, brachial, carotid and femoral sites:

- Reflect on how your pulse felt at these different sites.
- If you were asked to describe your pulse, what words would you use to do so?

When measuring a pulse, you need to take account of not just the rate but also the rhythm and quality, which are often referred to as the pulse characteristics. When considering the rhythm, we record whether the pulse beat is regular or irregular; quality, meanwhile, refers to the pressure we feel. The terms frequently used to describe a pulse and the reasons for these characteristics are outlined in Table 24.1.

A child's pulse can be difficult to take, not only because they can fidget quite a lot, sometimes their wrists and arms can be quite padded and it cannot be felt at all which presents a challenge in itself.

Siân Hunter, child nursing student

Table 24.1 Description of and reasons for pulse characteristics

Irregular pulse beat	Abnormal heart rhythm
Pulse > 100bpm	Tachycardia (fast heartbeat)
Pulse < 60bpm	Bradycardia (slow heartbeat)
Bounding pulse	Infection, fluid overload (too much fluid) Vasodilation (widening of blood vessels, which increases blood flow)
Weak, thready pulse	Shock, dehydration, cardiac abnormalities
No pulse (at radial artery)	Shock, collapse, dehydration, cardiac abnormalities, death

BLOOD PRESSURE (BP)

As we have discussed previously, pulse and blood pressure are very closely linked. A patient's blood pressure will depend on their age, gender, race, fitness level and pre-existing illnesses. It also varies according to the level of activity being undertaken and the time of day or night. Thus, it is normal to refer to a 'normal range' of blood pressure for an age range, rather than to a single precise value.

A&P LINK: BLOOD PRESSURE

Blood pressure is the force exerted by the blood on the walls of the arterial blood vessels. When the left ventricle contracts, it pushes blood into the aorta, causing an increase in pressure termed **systole**, which is the first measurement recorded when taking a blood pressure. **Diastole** is when the heart relaxes and the pressure in the blood vessels decreases.

Blood pressure is measured in millimetres of mercury (mmHg) and is recorded as, for example:

120 mmHg   - systole (the systolic figure is always higher than the diastolic one)

70 mmHg   - diastole

(Continued)

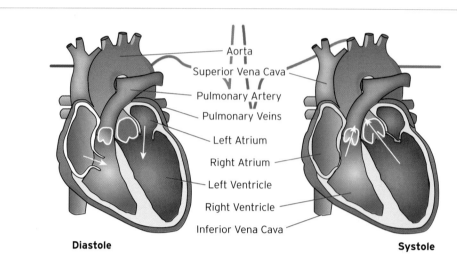

Figure 24.8   Ventricular blood flow

Blood pressure is ...

The blood pressure (BP) we measure in a patient is a result of both their cardiac output (CO), the volume of blood ejected into their aorta per minute, and their systemic vascular resistance (SVR), the tone of their arterial blood vessels:

$$BP = CO \times SVR$$

Cardiac output is ...

Cardiac output is a measurement of the volume of blood ejected into the aorta per minute. This volume is influenced by the patient's heart rate and their stroke volume (SV), the amount of blood ejected into the aorta by each heartbeat:

$$CO = HR \times SV$$

Systemic vascular resistance is ...

A patient's systemic vascular resistance (SVR) depends on the diameter (tone) of the arterial blood vessels, which is the main factor determining resistance to blood flow. When the blood vessels narrow, the SVR is increased and we say that the patient's circulation is 'vasoconstricted'. When the blood arterial vessels dilate, the SVR is decreased and we say the patient's circulation is 'vasodilated'.

While you are on placement, you will see blood pressure being measured using both automatic machines and manual sphygmomanometers.

Automated blood pressure machines tend to be the most commonly used method, although there is a current trend to return to manual sphygmomanometers due to the inaccuracy of automated machines in certain conditions. To ensure it is safe to use an automated machine to measure blood pressure, always palpate the patient's radial or brachial pulse to ensure their pulse rate is regular. If the pulse is regular and palpated at the radial artery, their blood pressure can be measured using an automated device.

STEP-BY-STEP CLINICAL SKILL 24.4: MANUAL BLOOD PRESSURE MEASUREMENT (BP)

☑ **What is normal?**

Refer to 'Automated blood pressure measurement (BP)' at https://study.sagepub.com/essentialnursing2e

☑ **Before you start**

Refer to 'Automated blood pressure measurement (BP)' at https://study.sagepub.com/essentialnursing2e

AUTOMATED BP
MEASUREMENT

☑ **Essential equipment**

Aneroid sphygmomanometer with stethoscope.

☑ **Care-setting considerations**

Manual blood pressure measurements can be taken in any care setting.

☑ **What to watch out for and action to take**

Refer to 'Automated blood pressure measurement (BP)' at https://study.sagepub.com/essentialnursing2e

Figure 24.9 Aneroid sphygmomanometer

Figure 24.10 Different sizes of BP measurement cuffs

(Continued)

BLOOD PRESSURE GUIDELINES

1 Perform steps 1-8 of the common steps (see Clinical Skill 24.1)
To prepare the patient and yourself to undertake the skill

AUTOMATED BP MEASUREMENT

2 Perform steps 1-6 in 'automated blood pressure measurement' (see https://study.sagepub.com/essentialnursing2e)
To ensure the patient is comfortable and correctly positioned, with a cuff of the appropriate size to enable accurate BP measurement

3 Position the sphygmomanometer no more than 1 metre away from the patient, upright, on a flat surface with the centre of the gauge at your eye level
To ensure the measurement is as accurate as possible

4 Check that your stethoscope is turned to the diaphragm side and working by tapping it with your finger
To ensure your stethoscope is working and ready for use

Check diaphragm side

5 Palpate the patient's brachial artery (see Figure 24.7), ensure that the valve is closed and then start pumping air into the cuff using the bulb. At the point when the pulse can no longer be felt, this provides a systolic estimation. The cuff should now be deflated
By palpating the brachial pulse, the correct position for the stethoscope can be located

6 Deflate the cuff completely and wait 15-30 seconds
This provides an approximate value of the systolic blood pressure
Allows venous congestion (dilated blood vessels due to the constriction caused by the cuff) to resolve

7 Place the diaphragm of the stethoscope over the brachial artery where the pulse is palpable
Ensure the valve on the bulb attached to the cuff is closed firmly, but not so tightly that it cannot be deflated easily

Brachial BP

Inflate the cuff again to 20-30 mmHg above the predicted systolic blood pressure, as identified in step 6
While observing the sphygmomanometer, slowly release the valve, at an approximate rate of 2-3 mmHg per pulsation, until the first thudding sounds are heard
So you can listen for the sounds that will indicate the blood pressure
You will need to be able to manipulate the valve to inflate and deflate the cuff
Inflating the cuff will cause venous congestion
This is to compensate for an auscultatory gap and to ensure accuracy of measurement
These first thudding sounds are called the first **Korotkoff sound** and indicate the value for the systolic blood pressure
You need to note the pressure reading on the sphygmomanometer when you hear this sound

Continue to slowly release air from the valve, deflating the cuff. Listen carefully to the Korotkoff sounds until they disappear
The disappearance of the Korotkoff sound is the value for the diastolic blood pressure - known as the Fifth Korotkoff sound. Again, you need to note the pressure reading on the sphygmomanometer when the Korotkoff sounds disappear

 Continue to slowly deflate the cuff another 20-30 mmHg, until you are completely sure that all of the sounds have disappeared, then rapidly deflate the cuff

To ensure your measurement is accurate
If the BP needs to be rechecked immediately, because the measurement is not what was expected or is too low or too high, wait for 1-2 minutes before proceeding

 Perform steps 9-12 of the common steps (see Clinical Skill 24.1)
To ensure that:

- the patient is safe, comfortable and receiving the appropriate care
- results have been documented in the patient's records
- equipment is clean and in working order

Source: British Hypertension Society (2009); Dougherty and Lister (2015); Smith and Roberts (2011)

If the patient has an irregular pulse, or it is weak and thready radially, measure blood pressure using a manual sphygmomanometer (NICE, 2011) as outlined in Clinical Skill 24.4, because an automated device may not give you an accurate measurement.

WHAT'S THE EVIDENCE?

National Institute for Health and Clinical Excellence (NICE) (2011) *Hypertension in Adults: Diagnosis and Management*. London: NICE. Available at: www.nice.org.uk/CG127 (updated Nov. 2016).
The NICE (2011: 4) **hypertension** guidelines state:

WEBLINK: NICE

High blood pressure (hypertension) is one of the most important preventable causes of premature morbidity and mortality in the UK. Hypertension is a major risk factor for stroke, myocardial infarction, heart failure, chronic kidney disease, cognitive decline and premature death.

British and Irish Hypertension Society (n.d.)

The clinical management of hypertension is one of the most common interventions in primary care.

Blood pressure is **normally distributed** in the population and there is no natural cut-off point above which 'hypertension' definitively exists and below which it does not. Hypertension is remarkably common in the UK and the prevalence is strongly influenced by age. With ageing, systolic hypertension becomes a more significant problem, as a result of progressive stiffening and loss of compliance of larger arteries. At least one quarter of adults (and more than half of those older than 60) have high blood pressure.

- Next time you are measuring patients' blood pressure, reflect on this NICE guidance, the accepted blood pressure ranges and how many of the patients you are caring for would be described as being hypertensive.

CASE STUDY 24.2: BARBARA

Barbara, aged 83, is visiting the GP practice where you are working to have her routine six-monthly blood pressure check. She normally takes an anti-hypertensive medication to maintain her blood pressure within a normal range. Last year, she had two falls and has lost her confidence in going out, so she now mobilises outside with a mobility walking aid.

Barbara looks pale and when you touch her hand she feels cool to the touch. Her daughter, who is with her, says she doesn't seem right today, a bit 'muddled'.

You decide to take a set of vital signs. The readings are:

Respiratory rate: 20

SpO_2:   94% on air

Heart rate: 105, weak, thready and irregular

Blood pressure: 102/62 mmHg

Temperature: 38.2°C

- Calculate the NEWS.
- Which physiological parameters are you concerned about?
- Is the systolic blood pressure normal for Barbara?
- In this situation, would you use an automated sphygmomanometer or a manual sphygmomanometer?
- Consider the cause of the abnormal heart rate.
- What action should you take?
- What do you think might be causing Barbara's abnormal vital signs?

ANSWER: CASE
STUDY 24.2

CAPILLARY REFILL TIME (CRT)

In a similar manner to monitoring a patient's pulse rate, measuring their CRT is a simple non-invasive procedure that does not require any equipment. This means it can be undertaken in any setting and wherever the patient is located – in a bathroom, in a clinic or in bed. The test is a measurement of the time taken from the release of pressure on a nail bed or superficial soft tissue (sufficient to cause 'blanching of the area', which means the normal skin colour becomes white) until normal colouration returns. If this takes longer than two seconds, it can be an indication of reduced peripheral circulation. So CRT helps to determine the patient's cardiovascular status.

I found the CRT very useful, especially when a child had just come back from theatre with a full arm plaster cast. This was an excellent way to establish how good the blood flow was after surgery.

Alice Rowe, NQ RNMH

TEMPERATURE

Body temperature is a measure of the body's ability to produce and lose heat; it represents the balance of metabolic processes taking place and helps to maintain homeostasis. A healthy body will maintain its temperature within a narrow range using thermoregulation mechanisms.

A&P LINK: THERMOREGULATION

Signals arrive at the thermoregulatory centre, in the hypothalamus of the brain, from the sensory receptors in the skin and organs. Responses, such as vasodilation, vasoconstriction and the activation of sweat glands, are instigated to maintain **core body temperature** within the homeostatic range (Clancy and McVicar, 2009; McCallum and Higgins, 2012).

If the temperature is high, it is an indication that the metabolic rate is faster than normal and also that the body has an increased need for fuel to feed the tissues, in the form of oxygen and glucose. If the temperature is low, it indicates that metabolism is slowing down (Smith and Roberts, 2011).

Different areas of the body have different temperatures. Core body temperature, which is the highest, is found in the blood-supplying organs such as the brain and those within the thoracic cavity and abdomen. Lower peripheral temperatures are recorded in tissues such as the skin (McCallum and Higgins, 2012).

As children and infants have a large surface area relative to their body mass, they lose more heat from their skin than adults.

Measuring a patient's temperature therefore provides us with essential information indicating whether their body is functioning effectively. Temperature ranges and how they are interpreted are outlined in Table 24.2.

Table 24.2 Temperatures and interpretations

Normal 36.0–37.00 C	Hypothermia <35°C	Pyrexia 37.5–38.5° C	Hyperthermia >38.5°C
All bodily functions able to occur effectively within the most conducive temperature range	Ageing	Fever or infection	Heat stroke
	Cold environment	Post-op	Septic shock
	Alcohol or drug abuse	Post-**MI**	Drug induced
	Shock	**Post-partum**	Hypothalamic injury
	Diabetes	Ovulation	
	Overwhelming infection	Warm environment	

It is possible to record a patient's temperature using a number of different sites. The oral, tympanic, temporal and axilla sites are used most frequently. Oral thermometers used to be very popular, but because of a lack of accuracy and safety concerns their use is declining.

STEP-BY-STEP CLINICAL SKILL 24.5: MEASURING BODY TEMPERATURE (T)

☑ What is normal?

Normal adult range: 36.0–37.0° C.

Normal child range: 36.6–37.7° C.

☑ Before you start

Remember the common steps for all clinical measurements (Clinical Skill 24.1).

☑ Essential equipment

The correct thermometer for the site you are using. A number of different types are available: oral, tympanic, temporal and axilla are the sites most often used.

☑ Field-setting considerations

You need to carefully consider which site is the most appropriate to use to measure your patient's temperature. For example, you would not use an oral thermometer if you were concerned that the patient might bite it, or if they had difficulty breathing through their nose. Tympanic thermometers are thought to be the most accurate and are used very frequently, but you would not use this site if a patient had wax or an infection in their ear canal or was younger than three months old.

Do not take a child's temperature immediately after they have had a bath or been wrapped in blankets, as this will not give an accurate recording.

☑ Care-setting considerations

Temperature can be measured in any care setting.

Consider the environmental temperature's effect on the patient. It may feel warm to you, but the patient may be immobile and ill, so will need more clothing to keep them warm.

If the patient's temperature is raised, consider removing excess clothing.

☑ What to watch out for and action to take

Assessing your patient's temperature involves observation and feeling, as well as measurement. If the patient's temperature is elevated, they may appear flushed and sweaty. When you are feeling their forehead or hands, they may feel hot to the touch. Alternatively, if they are cold they may be shivering, wrapped in clothing or blankets and look pale, and their peripheries may feel cold to the touch.

TEMPERATURE GUIDELINES

 Perform steps 1–7 of the common steps (see Clinical Skill 24.1)
To prepare the patient and yourself to undertake the skill

 Oral
Digital or disposable thermometers can be used to take oral temperatures
   Attach the disposable probe cover and place the thermometer in the patient's mouth, positioned under their tongue, posteriorly into the sublingual pocket. Ask the patient to close their lips around the thermometer
   Leave in this position for the specified amount of time
   Read the temperature displayed
   Dispose of the probe cover by pressing the RELEASE or EJECT button while holding over a clinical waste bag

 Tympanic
This is the most commonly used method of measuring temperature in adults as it is quick, minimally invasive and gives a rapid indication of a change in core temperature as the tympanic membrane is close to the hypothalamus
   Remove the thermometer from the base unit. Check that the probe tip is clean and intact
   Press the probe tip into the disposable probe cover without touching the cover
   Gently pull the pinna (top of the ear) backwards so that the ear canal is straightened
   Gently insert the thermometer into the ear canal until it is sealed
   Press the scan button on the thermometer and wait for it to beep

Tympanic

   Gently remove the thermometer from the ear canal and read the temperature displayed
   Dispose of the probe cover by pressing the RELEASE or EJECT button while holding over a clinical waste bag
   Return to base unit

 Temporal
The temporal artery thermometer is held over the forehead to sense infrared emissions radiating from the skin
   Hold in this position for the specified amount of time
   Read the temperature displayed

 Axilla
Digital or disposable thermometers can be used to take axilla temperatures
   Place in the centre of the axilla and hold the arm close to the chest wall
   Leave in this position for the specified amount of time
   Read the temperature displayed
   Dispose of the probe cover by pressing the RELEASE or EJECT button while holding over a clinical waste bag

 Oral
Factors affecting accuracy include the recent ingestion of food or fluid, a respiratory rate of greater than 18 bpm and smoking. Ensure the patient can breathe through their nose and is not at risk of biting the thermometer

 Tympanic
Avoid using this site if there has been a recent ear infection or there is wax in the ear canals as this can affect readings. Ask patients to remove any hearing aid if there is one in the ear to be used
   Use the same ear for readings as anatomical differences can account for a 1° difference
   If the ear canal is not straightened, the reading will not be accurate

 Temporal
Is quick to use but it has been shown to underestimate temperature

(Continued)

Axilla
Not as reliable as tympanic measurements for estimating core temperature as there are no main blood vessels around the axilla
   Environmental temperature and perspiration can affect accuracy

 Perform steps 9–12 of the common steps (see Clinical Skill 24.1)
To ensure that:

- the patient is safe, comfortable and receiving the appropriate care
- the results have been documented in the patient's records
- the equipment is clean and in working order

Source: Clancy and McVicar (2009); Dougherty and Lister (2015); Jevon (2010); McCallum and Higgins (2012); Smith and Roberts (2011)

ACTIVITY 24.5: REFLECTION

Reflect on an example of patient care in which you have been involved in taking vital sign recordings:

- Why were you taking the vital sign observations?
- How often were the vital signs being recorded?
- What was the reason for this frequency of recording?
- How did you explain what you were doing to the patient?

EARLY WARNING SCORING SYSTEMS

The use of routinely measured vital signs is a fundamental aspect of Early Warning Scoring Systems (EWSS) and Paediatric Early Warning Scoring Systems (PEWS). These are known as physiological track-and-trigger scoring systems that provide early recognition of potential or established acute illness. There are several variations of the scoring systems in use, including the 'Patient at Risk Score', 'Modified Early Warning Score' (MEWS), 'Early Warning Scoring System' (EWSS) and 'National Early Warning Score' (NEWS).

The National Early Warning Score (NEWS), was first produced in 2012 and updated in December 2017. NEWS2 has now received formal endorsement from NHS England and NHS Improvement to become the national early warning system for identifying acutely ill patients - including those with sepsis - in hospitals in England. This provides a system wide standardised approach for assessing the severity of patients' acute illnesses which can be used both in hospitals and in pre-hospital assessments, such as in primary care and the ambulance service. The NEWS system has been proven to improve the care given to patients as it is used as a surveillance system for all patients, tracking their condition, alerting the healthcare team to any deterioration and triggering a timely response. The NEWS trigger system assists those caring for patients by not only outlining how urgently the patient requires clinical intervention to improve their deteriorating condition, but also identifying who this care needs to be provided by.

Measuring NEWS

The NEWS is based on a simple aggregate scoring system in which a score is allocated to physiological measurements, already recorded in routine practice on a standardised clinical observation chart (Chart 2 below) when patients present to, or are being monitored in hospital. Six simple physiological parameters form the basis of the scoring system:

1. respiration rate
2. oxygen saturation
3. systolic blood pressure
4. pulse rate
5. level of consciousness or new confusion*
6. temperature

A score is allocated to each parameter as they are measured, with the size of the score reflecting how extremely the parameter varies from the norm. The score is then aggregated and uplifted by 2 points for people requiring supplemental oxygen to maintain their recommended oxygen saturation. (Chart 1 below)

Chart 1: The NEWS scoring system

Physiological parameter	3	2	1	score 0	1	2	3
Respiration rate (per minute)	≤8		9-11	12-20		21-24	≥25
Spo₂ scale 1 (%)	≤91	92-93	94-95	≥96			
Spo₂ scale 2 (%)	≤83	84-85	86-87	88-92 ≥93 on air	93-94 on oxygen	95-96 on oxygen	≥97 on oxygen
Air or oxygen?		Oxygen		Air			
Systolic blood pressure (mmHg)	≤90	91-100	101-110	111-219			≥220
Pulse (per minute)	≤40		41-50	51-90	91-110	111-130	≥131
consciousness				Alert			CVPU
Temperature(°c)	≤35.0		35.1-36.0	36.1-38.0	38.1-39.0	≥39.1	

NEWS key	FULL NAME	
0 1 2 3	DATE OF BIRTH	DATE OF ADMISSION

	DATE																DATE
	TIME																TIME

A+B Respirations Breaths/min	≥25							3								≥25
	21-24							2								21-24
	18-20															18-20
	15-17															15-17
	12-14															12-14
	9-11							1								9-11
	≤8							3								≤8

A+B SpO₂ Scale 1 Oxygen saturation (%)	≥96															≥96
	94-95							1								94-95
	92-93							2								92-93
	≤91							3								≤91

SpO₂ Scale 2† Oxygen saturation(%) Use Scale 2 if target range is 88-92%, eg in Hypercapnic respiratory failure	≥97 on O₂												3												≥97 on O₂
	95-96 on O₂												2													95-96 on O₂
	93-94 on O₂												1													93-94 on O₂
	≥93 on air																									≥93 on air
	88-92																									88-92
†Only use Scale 2 under the direction of a qualified oilnilation	86-87												1													86-87
	84-85												2													84-85
	≤83%												3													≤83%

Air or Oxygen?	A=Air																									A=Air
	O₂ L/min												2													O₂ L/min
	Device																									Device

C Blood pressure mmHg Score uses systolic BP only	≥220												3													≥220
	201-219																									201-219
	181-200																									181-200
	161-180																									161-180
	141-160																									141-160
	121-140																									121-140
	101-120												1													101-120
	91-100												2													91-100
	81-90																									81-90
	71-80												3													71-80
	61-70																									61-70
	51-60																									51-60
	≤50																									≤50

C Pulse Beats/min	≥131												3													≥131
	121-130												2													121-130
	111-120																									111-120
	101-110												1													101-110
	91-100																									91-100
	81-90																									81-90
	71-80																									71-80
	61-70																									61-70
	51-60																									51-60
	41-50												1													41-50
	31-40												3													31-40
	≤30																									≤30

D Consciousness Score for NEW onset of confusion (no score if chronic)	Alert																									Alert
	Confusion																									Confusion
	V												3													V
	P																									P
	U																									U

E Temperature °c	≥39.1°												2													≥39.1°
	38.1-39.0°												1													38.1–39.0°
	37.1-38.0°																									37.1–38.0°
	36.1-37.0°																									36.1–37.0°
	35.1-36.0°												1													35.1–36.0°
	≤35.0°												3													≤35.0°

NEWS TOTAL																								TOTAL

Monitoring frequency																							Monitoring
Escalation of care Y/N																							Escalation
Initials																							Initials

NEWS trigger levels

There are three 'trigger levels' that indicate that the patient is unwell or has the potential to deteriorate, requiring a clinical response (see Table 24.4). It is these triggers that determine the urgency of the clinical response and the clinical competency required in the responder(s).

Table 24.4   NEWS trigger levels

Chart 2: NEWS thresholds and triggers

NEW score	Clinical risk	Response
Aggregate score 0-4	Low	Word-based response
Red score Score of 3 in any individual parameter	Low-medium	Urgent word-based response*
Aggregate score 5-6	Medium	Key threshold for urgent response*
Aggregate score 7 or more	High	Urgent or emergency response**

*Response by a clinician or team with competence in the assessment and treatment of acutely ill patients and in recognising when the escalation of care to a critical care team is appropriate.

**The response team must also include staff with critical care skills, including airway management.

NEWS and the nurse

When a patient has 'triggered' a NEWS or has abnormal vital signs, it is part of the nurse's responsibility to ensure the abnormal result, presumed cause and action taken are documented in chronological order in the patient's notes (Chart 4). This provides evidence of a response to a patient who is or has the potential to become acutely unwell, which will ensure that they receive the right care in the right place at the right time.

Clinical Response to the NEWS trigger thresholds

Chart 4: Clinical response to the NEWS trigger thresholds

NEW score	Frequency of monitoring	Clinical response
0	Minimum 12 hourly	• Continue routine NEWS monitoring
Total 1-4	Minimum 4-6 hourly	• Inform registered nurse, who must assess the patient • Registered nurse decides whether increased frequency of monitoring and/or escalation of care is required
3 in single parameter	Minimum 1 hourly	• Registered nurse to inform medical team caring for the patient, who will review and decide whether escalation of care is necessary
Total 5 or more Urgent response threshold	Minimum 1 hourly	• Registered nurse to immediately inform the medical team caring for the patient • Registered nurse to request urgent assessment by a clinician or team with core competencies in the care of acutely ill patients • Provide clinical care in an environment with monitoring facilities
Total 7 or more Emergency response threshold	Continuous monitoring of vital signs	• Registerd nurse to immediately inform the medical team caring for the patient – this should be at least at specialist registrar level • Emergency assessment by a team with critical care competencies, including practitioner(s) with advanced airway management skills • Consider transfer of care to a level 2 or 3 clinical care facility, ie higher-dependency unit or ICU • Clinical care in an environment with monitoring facilities

ACTIVITY 24.6: RESEARCH ACTIVITY

- Does the NEWS accurately reflect all patients' risk of acute illness?

> As you record observations you will start to see patterns emerging throughout the hours and days. Obs can alter due to medication, environment, the patient's activity level, etc. But if the patient starts to deteriorate you need to be able to notice what is happening and seek medical assistance. That is where the EWSS can be very useful – it indicates the level of urgency and severity at which the patient is deteriorating. My hospital now uses an electronic system where we record the obs on a hand-held device; if the patient's NEWS score is increasing the device will offer medical advice to the user and even alert a doctor if needed.
>
> Charlie Clisby, NQN

URINE OUTPUT

One of the first signs indicating that a patient may be at risk of acute kidney injury (AKI) is poor urine output, defined as *oliguria* (a fall in urine output to less than 0.5 ml/kg/hour). Consequently, it is important that a reduced or falling urine output is identified and treated as soon as possible.

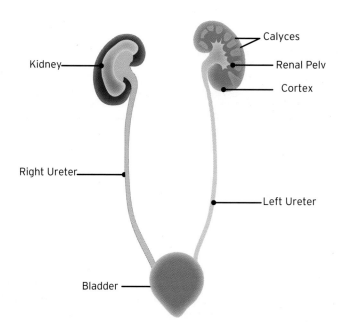

Figure 24.11   The renal system

A&P LINK: RENAL FUNCTION

The kidneys are one of the main organs that control homeostasis of body fluid composition and volume. Other kidney functions include the regulation and elimination of **electrolytes** and the waste products of metabolism (such as urea and creatinine). The kidneys also play an important role in regulating blood pressure.

Normal renal function (see Figure 24.11) is reliant on the kidneys receiving approximately 20 per cent of the body's cardiac output to sustain filtration of the plasma and the high oxygen demands of kidney cells (Clancy and McVicar, 2009). Two important elements affect the kidneys' ability to function efficiently: a reduced blood supply due to inadequate volume/blood pressure and a lack of oxygen. A fall in blood flow leads to poor perfusion pressure to the kidneys and risk of acute kidney injury.

In order to ensure our body remains sufficiently hydrated, to ensure it can function effectively, it is important that there are enough fluids taken in to balance those being lost. Table 24.5 shows how much fluid we need to take in on a daily basis to balance what we lose.

As you can see from Table 24.5, adults need a minimum of 2500 ml of fluid each day to balance the amount lost by our normal bodily processes, to ensure that the fluids going into our body balance those coming out. If we do not take sufficient fluids in, we will become dehydrated.

Table 24.5   Daily fluids

Fluid (water) input (ml per day)		Fluid (water) output (ml per day)	
Oral/enteral/IV	1500	Urine	1400
Food	800	*Evaporation:*	
		Lungs	500
		Skin	400
Metabolic production*	200	Faeces	200
Total	**2500**		**2500**

Note: *Mainly produced when glucose is broken down into carbon dioxide and water during respiration.

Source: Clancy and McVicar (2009)

ACTIVITY 24.7: CRITICAL THINKING

The values provided in Table 24.5 relate to a healthy adult. What effect do you think the following would have on a patient's fluid balance?

- being pyrexic (having a high temperature)
- having diarrhoea and vomiting
- being a child.

ANSWER:
ACTIVITY 24.7

Measuring fluid balance

A doctor or registered nurse will decide as part of the patient's clinical management plan how a patient's hydration status should be assessed and, if required, how often to measure and record a patient's fluid balance, with the frequency depending on the patient's condition. This can be hourly for acutely ill patients, and 2-, 4-, 12- or 24-hourly for patients who are less unwell. If fluid balance measurement and recording are required, an input/output chart is used (see Table 24.6), where all fluid that an individual has taken in over a 24-hour period, and fluid he or she has passed out over the same period, is documented. An overall balance, termed cumulative balance, will indicate if the patient is in an equal fluid balance, or has a fluid deficit or fluid overload. This important non-invasive tool is part of a fluid balance and hydration assessment that includes clinical assessment, blood chemistry results and body weight to guide clinicians in clinical decisions.

For a record of fluid balance to be useful, it needs to be accurate. The volume of fluid the patient takes in must be documented in mls, the same measurement as the output. All fluid intake (oral, IV, drugs) plus all fluid output (diarrhoea, drains, blood, vomit, stoma, nasogastric tube losses) need to be documented.

The easiest and most efficient way to monitor urine output accurately is via a urinary catheter, which is frequently used in the sickest patients. The urinary catheter chamber is either measured or emptied hourly into the receptacle bag or, if the measurement is required less frequently, the amount is recorded on the fluid chart at the time, measured and divided by the number of hours since it was last measured to gain an estimation of hourly measurement.

If the patient does not have a urinary catheter, ask them to urinate into a bottle or a bedpan, or in the case of an infant weigh their nappy. The volume of fluid can be measured in a jug or alternatively weighed (1 ml weighs 1 g), but remember to take off the weight of the bottle, bedpan or nappy. When emptying urine, as well as recording the volume it is important to observe the colour and smell, as these can also indicate problems with the renal system. In normal renal function, urine should be pale yellow with no odour, whilst in dehydrated patients it can be dark and concentrated.

ANSWER:
ACTIVITY 24.8

ACTIVITY 24.8: CRITICAL THINKING

Review the information presented in Table 24.6 (the fluid balance chart):

- What is the patient's name?
- How much fluid has he taken orally during the 24 hours covered by the fluid balance chart?
- What was his urine output for the 24 hours covered by the fluid balance chart?
- Is he in positive or negative fluid balance for the 24-hour period?
- How would you explain to the patient what this means?

Whenever you are caring for a patient, remember the following 'top tips' and ensure you are aware of the fluid input and output of all patients you are responsible for:

- Ask the patient if they feel thirsty as this is a good sign of hydration status. Thirst can be the first sign of dehydration, so if the patient is able to drink, encourage and assist them to have some fluid. Apply this with caution to elderly people as they can have an impaired response to dehydration and will not always feel thirsty, even though they are dehydrated.
- Assess the patient's tongue and mouth mucosa for signs of dehydration. If the patient is dehydrated, their tongue and mouth mucosa will look dry.

Table 24.6 A fluid balance chart

Urine output monitoring: 1 hourly   2 hourly   3 hourly   (Circle one)

Permitted Oral Fluids: Free fluids   Reason for Monitoring: Sepsis & post-op

Previous Day Balance +/-: +68   Date: 12.12.17   Ward:

Name: IVOR WELL

Address:

Hospital Number: J666666

Date of Birth: 01.01.1996

NHS Number:

Input (MLS)

Time	Oral	Enteral/ parenteral	NG/ PEG Flush	Other	IV 1 N/ SALINE	IV 2 DRUGS	Running Total In	Urine
07.00					84			65
08.00	150				84			50
09.00					84			45
10.00	200				84	20	706	30
11.00	100				84			110
12.00					84			50
13.00	150				84			35
14.00					84	20	1312	40
15.00	50				84			30
16.00					84			90
17.00	150				84			110
18.00	50				84		1898	85

Output (MLS)

Time	Running Total Urine	NG/ Vomit	Bowels/ Stoma	Drain	Total	Running Other Losses	Running Total Out	Running Total Balance	Reg Nurse Signature
07.00									
08.00									
09.00									
10.00	190			20	20	300	510	+196	
11.00									
12.00									
13.00									
14.00	425				20		745	+567	
15.00									
16.00									
17.00									
18.00	740				20		1060	+838	

(Continued)

	Input (MLS)								Output (MLS)							
Time	Oral	Enteral/ parenteral	NG/PEG Flush Other	IV 1 N/ SALINE	IV 2 DRUGS	Running Total In	Urine	Running Total Urine	NG/ Vomit	Bowels/ Stoma	Drain Total	Running Other Losses	Running Total Out	Running Total Balance	Reg Nurse Signature
19.00				84			45					200			
20.00	200			84			50								
21.00				84			35								
22.00				84	40	2474	60	930			20		1450	+1024	
23.00				84			75								
24.00				84			25								
01.00				84			45								
02.00				84		2810	50	1125			20		1645	+1165	
03.00				84			95								
04.00				84			35								
05.00				84			40								
06.00	150			84	40	3186	30	1325			20		1995	+1191	

- Ask the patient if they have passed urine in the past 6 hours. If they haven't and they are able to drink, encourage them to have a full glass or cup of fluid.
- Look at the colour of the patient's urine. If it is dark and concentrated, this is a sign of dehydration and you need to investigate further.
- If the patient has a urinary catheter that is not draining any urine, the first thing to do is to check if it is blocked, either due to the patient's position or debris.
- Bladder scans are quick and easy to perform and provide an estimate of the amount of urine in the bladder.

An alternative method of measuring fluid status – especially in chronic conditions, such as for patients with heart failure, renal failure and liver failure – is to weigh them daily. This is further discussed later in this chapter.

ACTIVITY 24.9: REFLECTION

Billie is 27 years old and has a moderate learning disability. She lives with her mother and father, is independent in terms of her personal care needs, can prepare simple meals for herself and works eight hours per week at her local supermarket. Billie is an insulin-controlled diabetic and has been feeling generally unwell for the last five days with pyrexia and loss of appetite, so she has been admitted to an acute hospital for investigations. Your mentor has asked you to record Billie's blood sugar level. When you ask her if you can do this, she says: 'No. You are not doing it – the nurses make it hurt lots more than it does when I do it at home.'

- How would you manage this situation?

ANSWER:
ACTIVITY 24.9

BLOOD GLUCOSE

Monitoring blood glucose provides information about how effectively the body is controlling its glucose metabolism. For patients with diabetes, a long-term illness, this is a vitally important part of assessing their wellbeing. Other patients who are acutely sick may also need their blood glucose monitored to provide information on the body's metabolism. As with all the other clinical measurements, you need to ensure that you achieve accurate results.

WEIGHT (WT)

Weighing patients in any care setting is not solely done to assess nutritional status and body mass index (BMI): many drugs/interventions are calculated on weight. In paediatrics especially, most drugs and treatments are prescribed on the basis of weight rather than age. Weight can also determine how much fluid a patient is retaining, which is especially useful when assessing patients with long-term heart or renal failure.

CONCLUSION

Taking, recording and acting on clinical measurements are fundamental elements of care that help to monitor a patient's physiological health. Clinical measurements are part of the care of all patients, no matter the field of nursing. While the principles are the same, the approach to the patient, which measurements are recorded and how frequently, plus the care setting, may well differ greatly.

Before taking any clinical measurements, it is important that you are, or have supervision from, a trained, experienced and competent person, to ensure the results obtained are accurate. Abnormal findings must always be reported immediately to a registered nurse, so that the patient can be given the correct care required.

While it is important when recording clinical measurements to be precise and undertake the skill accurately, communicating effectively with the patient and their relatives or carers is also a fundamental aspect of care.

CHAPTER SUMMARY

- Detecting early deterioration in a patient's physiological condition is an essential skill for all nurses.
- Effective communication skills are of fundamental importance while taking clinical measurements.
- Attention to detail when performing clinical measurements is vital to ensure accurate results.
- An understanding of the relationship between anatomy/physiology and clinical measurements is key to monitoring a patient's wellbeing.
- Clinical measurements can be recorded in all fields of nursing and your skills need to be adapted to the context.
- Appropriate responses to the findings of clinical measurements are central to ensuring a patient receives effective care.
- Performing clinical measurements requires a combination of skill and knowledge that can be life-saving for a patient.

CRITICAL REFLECTION

Holistic care

This chapter has highlighted the importance of having knowledge of anatomy and physiology to underpin the accurate taking of clinical measurements, plus the vital nature of ensuring your recordings are correctly interpreted. Review the chapter and note down all the instances in which monitoring a patient's vital signs is part of providing holistic care. Think of a variety of different types of patients you may work with, not just within your own field. You may find it helpful to make a list and refer back to it next time you are in practice, and then write your own reflection after your experience in placement.

GO FURTHER

Books

Dougherty, L. and Lister, S. (2015) *The Royal Marsden Hospital Manual of Clinical Nursing Procedures*, 9th edn. Oxford: Wiley-Blackwell. An outstanding reference guide on how to carry out a wide range of nursing procedures.

Smith, J. and Roberts, R. (2011) *Vital Signs for Nurses: An Introduction to Clinical Observations*. Oxford: Wiley-Blackwell. A practical and accessible guide that provides an in-depth resource for the theory and practice of clinical observations.

National Patient Safety Agency (2007) *Recognising and Responding Appropriately to Early Signs of Deterioration in Hospitalised Patients*. London: NPSA. Available at: www.nrls.npsa.nhs.uk. Guidelines on the prevention, detection and management of acute kidney injury.

Royal College of Nursing and National Patient Safety Agency (2007) *Water for Health: Hydration Best Practice Toolkit for Hospitals and Healthcare*. London: RCN. Available at: www2.rcn.org.uk/__data/.../Hydration_Toolkit.

Journal articles

Boulanger, C. and Toghill, M. (2009) 'How to measure and record vital signs to ensure detection of deteriorating patients', *Nursing Times*, 105(47): 10-12. Practical advice on using essential observations to monitor patients, including two case studies.

Elliott, M. and Coventry, A. (2012) 'Critical care: The eight vital signs of patient monitoring', *British Journal of Nursing*, 21(10): 621-5. Clinical issues to be considered when measuring vital signs in acute settings.

Eyikara, E. and Baykara, Z.G. (2018) 'Effect of simulation on the ability of first year nursing students to learn vital signs', *Nurse Education Today*, 60: 101-106. A research paper outlining how simulation assists in learning vital signs.

Kaba, A. and Beran, T.N. (2016) 'Impact of peer pressure on accuracy of reporting vital signs: An interprofessional comparison between nursing and medical students', *Journal of Interprofessional Care*, 30(1): 116-122.

An interesting research paper highlighting how peer pressure can influence accuracy of vital signs reporting.

McGloin, S. (2015) 'The ins and outs of fluid balance in the acutely ill patient', *British Journal of Nursing*, 24(1): 14-18. Fluid physiology and the importance of accurate fluid balance measurement to evaluate an individual's fluid status, thereby guiding appropriate fluid management in the acute care setting.

Van Kuiken, D. and Huth, M.M. (2013) 'What is "normal?" Evaluating vital signs', *Paediatric Nursing*, 39(5): 216-24. A systematic review to define the normal vital signs in children aged 1-5 years.

Weblinks

Go to https://study.sagepub.com/essentialnursing2e for weblinks related to this chapter. If you are using the interactive ebook, simply click on the book icon in the margin to go straight to the resource.

www.ncepod.org.uk – NCEPOD's purpose is to improve standards of medical and surgical care by reviewing the management of patients. The reports can be accessed through this site and provide an understanding of the experiences of patients and the quality of care.

www.nice.org.uk/CG50 – key recommendations regarding performing and monitoring patients' vital signs. This NICE clinical guideline describes how patients in acute hospitals should be monitored to help identify those whose health has become worse and how they should be cared for if this happens.

www.nursingtimes.net/nursing-practice/clinical-zones/educators/-measuring-vital-signs-an-integrated-teaching-approach/5032313.article – how a holistic, integrated approach can help you to learn how to measure vital signs and appreciate their importance from the outset.

FURTHER READING: WEBLINKS

Video links

Have a break from the text and go to https://study.sagepub.com/essentialnursing2e for useful videos related to this chapter. If you are using the interactive ebook, simply click on the lightbulb icon in the margin to go straight to the resource.

VIDEO LINKS

ACE YOUR ASSESSMENT

Review what you have learned by visiting the book's online resources at: https://study.sagepub.com/essential nursing2e If using your interactive ebook, just click on the icon in the margin to go straight there.

- Test yourself with multiple-choice and short-answer questions.
- Revise key terms with the interactive flash cards.

REFERENCES

Boore, J., Cook, N. and Shepherd, A. (2016) *Essentials of Anatomy and Physiology in Nursing Practice.* London: SAGE.

British Hypertension Society (2009) How to Measure Blood Pressure. Available at: www.bhsoc.org/resources/measure-blood-pressure (accessed 28 March 2018).

British and Irish Hypertension Society (n.d.) *Hypertension Management.* Available at: https://bihsoc.org/guidelines/hypertension-management

British Thoracic Society (2017) 'BTS guideline for oxygen use in adults in healthcare and emergency settings', *Thorax; BMJI* 72 (Suppl. 1): 11–190.

Clancy, J. and McVicar, A. (2009) *Physiology and Anatomy for Nurses and Healthcare Practitioners: A Homeostatic Approach*, 3rd edn. London: Hodder Arnold.

Dougherty, L. and Lister, S. (2015) *The Royal Marsden Hospital Manual of Clinical Nursing Procedures*, 9th edn. Oxford: Wiley-Blackwell.

Jevon, P. (2010) 'How to ensure patient observations lead to effective management of patients with pyrexia', *Nursing Times*, 106(1): 16–18.

McCallum, L. and Higgins, D. (2012) 'Measuring body temperature', *Nursing Times*, 108(45): 20–2.

McQuillan, P., Pilkington, S., Allan, A., Taylor, B., Short, A., Morgan, G., et al. (1998) 'Confidential enquiry into quality of care before admission to intensive care', *British Medical Journal*, 316: 1853–8.

National Institute for Health and Clinical Excellence (NICE) (2007) *Acutely Ill Patients in Hospital: Recognition and Response to Acute Illness in Adults in Hospital.* Guideline 50. London: NICE.

National Institute for Health and Clinical Excellence (NICE) (2011) *Hypertension in Adults: Diagnosis and Management.* London: NICE. Available at: www.nice.org.uk/CG127 (updated Nov. 2016; accessed 18 June 2017).

National Institute for Health and Care Excellence (NICE) (2014) *Acutely Ill Patients in Hospital.* Available at: http://pathways.nice.org.uk/pathways/acutely-ill-patients-in-hospital (accessed 6 March 2018).

Royal College of Physicians (RCP) (2012) *National Early Warning Score (NEWS): Standardising the Assessment of Acute-illness Severity in the NHS.* London: RCP. Available at: www.rcplondon.ac.uk/projects/outputs/national-early-warning-score-news-2 (accessed 23 April 2018).

Smith, G. (2012) *ALERT. Acute Life-threatening Events, Recognition and Treatment: A Multi-professional Course in Care of the Acutely Ill Patient*, 3rd edn. Portsmouth: Institute of Medicine. Available at: www.alert-course.com (accessed 6 March 2018).

Smith, J. and Roberts, R. (2011) *Vital Signs for Nurses: An Introduction to Clinical Observations.* Oxford: Wiley-Blackwell.

World Health Organization (WHO) (2009) WHO Guidelines on Hand Hygiene in Health Care. Available at: http://whqlibdoc.who.int/publications/2009/9789241597906_eng.pdf (accessed 6 March 2018).

PAIN MANAGEMENT

ANN KETTYLE

25

THIS CHAPTER COVERS

- Introduction
- An understanding of types of pain
- Assessment of pain
- Ensuring your pain assessment is effective
- Importance of communication skills
- General strategies to manage pain
- Management of acute pain

- Management of persistent or cancer-related pain
- Pain and you
- Further considerations…
- Antidepressants for chronic non-cancer pain in children and adolescents

---

REQUIRED KNOWLEDGE

- It will be helpful to have a clear understanding of the anatomy and physiology of pain before you start this chapter.

> " My name is Jenny and I have suffered from painful arthritis for the last 60 years but it was only when the nurse asked whether there was anything he could do to help me manage my pain, listened to my answer and offered me some help that I realised that there was something else that could be done for me. It was so good to have someone listen to me and actually understand how much the pain affected me. He even made some sensible suggestions about some gadgets that I could get to help me with my cooking so now I can bake cakes for my grandchildren again.
>
> **Jenny, patient** "

> " The importance of pain management in nursing seems obvious – pain is an uncomfortable and unpleasant sensation for everyone. The inadequate management of pain not only influences patient recovery and therapy **concordance**, but also has a profound impact on loved ones who witness the suffering endured when it is not controlled effectively.
>
> Effective pain management is one of the most important skills a nurse can have as the rewards are almost instant.
>
> **Ashley Lee, nursing student, adult field** "

INTRODUCTION

Everyone has experienced some form of pain and you can find many definitions of pain, ranging from the technical explanation of the physiological process of how pain is felt to the person-centred approach which identifies the psychological perception and impact of pain. Pain experts agree that pain is both subjective and individual. The International Association for the Study of Pain (IASP) (1992) states on its website that pain is 'an unpleasant sensory and emotional experience associated with actual or potential tissue damage or described in terms of such damage'.

While this defines pain from a biological perspective, it does not consider the individual experiencing the pain, which is why many healthcare professionals approve of McCaffery and Beebe's (1989: 7) definition: 'Pain is whatever the experiencing person says it is and occurs whenever and wherever that person says it does'.

Whichever definition you choose, pain experts all agree that pain is experienced in different ways by different individuals; you may have heard people say they have a high pain threshold, for instance. But what is most important in nursing is the relevance of the pain, what it is telling us. Some pains tell us that our body has had enough (such as cramp in the leg of a runner), that our body has been injured (think about the pain experienced when a bone is broken, for instance) or that there is something wrong in our body (for example, the pain associated with tissue damage to the heart or joint pain when someone has degenerative changes in their joints). Whatever the reason for the pain, the individual should be believed and actions taken until the pain is managed or addressed to that individual's satisfaction.

This chapter will outline the role of the nurse in understanding a patient's pain and how we can manage it. We will initially look at how pain is experienced by a patient and its impact on them. We will then describe how to undertake a holistic pain assessment, and finally we will consider what you, as a nurse, can do to assist a patient in managing their pain, including medication and alternative therapies and strategies.

AN UNDERSTANDING OF TYPES OF PAIN

In order to manage pain effectively, first it is necessary to consider the different types of pain:

- **organic** (sometimes referred to as **somatogenic** pain) – this is where there is a physical cause for the pain, e.g. injury/trauma, surgery or disease
- **psychogenic** (often referred to as functional pain) – this is where no physical reason can be found to exist for the individual to have pain but the individual still experiences pain. Melzack and Wall (1988) found that this type of pain is often associated with tissue damage which, although healed, still generates pain. A good example of this is the pain that someone experiences after they have had a limb amputated (phantom limb pain).

While it is good to be able to categorise pain so effectively, it is also important to remember that there is always a degree of overlap, and that within each category we also have to consider the duration of the pain and identify whether it is acute or chronic:

Acute pain is short term (less than six months) and is reversible. Commonly, it is experienced suddenly (as in the case of a heart attack or appendicitis) with a physical reason for its existence and, with appropriate interventions, is reversible.

Chronic pain is pain that has lasted for longer than six months and that is related to an initial injury or disease but that persists long after the initial cause has been treated. McCaffery (1983) indicates that at this stage the pain has become the dominant disease. You may wonder why treatment cannot be given to remedy the cause of the pain; there are many reasons for this, such as the actual cause of the pain being unidentified, the pain being masked by another condition or the impact of the treatment being life-threatening or detrimental to the wellbeing of the individual. The experience of ongoing chronic pain can often lead to depression due to individuals feeling restricted by their pain, having to make adjustments (sometimes detrimental) to their life in order to cope, feeling under pressure all of the time to carry on, or because they are unable to maintain any physical activity.

CASE STUDY 25.1: RAPHAEL (ACUTE)

Raphael is aged 48 and is an experienced nurse who has worked in Accident and Emergency (A&E) departments for 12 years.

Following a serious car accident, he experienced severe shoulder pain with limitations to his mobility and strength, along with head and neck pain. Raphael had to adapt his physical movements to ensure that he did not exacerbate the severe, sharp shoulder pain which progressed to include reduced strength in his hand. Following review by a shoulder specialist, he learnt that he needed an operation which, when completed, resolved the shoulder pain and increased his mobility and strength. Although the resolution of the shoulder pain was effective, Raphael then started to realise that the head and neck pain was more acute than he had previously perceived.

Following consultation with a neurosurgeon, Raphael learnt that the initial car accident had resulted in damage to the cervical discs, which was trapping the nerves resulting in the pain. Due to the serious nature of any operation in the cervical region, he could not have surgery until the effects of the injury were having a more detrimental effect. It took nearly six years for his condition to worsen, during which time Raphael had to change his job as he was no longer able to carry out fundamental nursing duties. At this important time, he began to feel inadequate and experienced mild depression. Fortunately, Raphael was under the care of a pain specialist team and was commenced on anti-depressants which not only helped the depression but also helped with the pain itself.

- How many changes had Raphael been forced to make to his lifestyle due to the physical pain he was experiencing?
- What do you think was the underlying cause(s) of Raphael's depression?

Summary of the physiology of pain

Injury or disruption to tissue as a result of trauma, surgery or inflammatory disease will result in a physiological response throughout the body, as summarised in Figure 25.1.

A&P LINK: THE PHYSIOLOGY OF PAIN

The most important part of this process is related to the nerve endings (stage 4 of Figure 25.1) which carry stimuli to the cortex of the brain. There are three different nerve fibres that are important in

(Continued)

Figure 25.1   A summary of the physiology of pain

A delta fibres are the ones that react quickly and get us out of trouble. They transmit their message quickly, resulting in a reflexive reaction. Think about if you touched a hot iron or pricked your finger on a pin, you would react quickly, withdrawing your hand. You don't consciously do it and you experience instant pain which is felt at the site of injury – this is the type of sensation carried by the A delta fibres and is usually called 'first' or 'fast' pain.

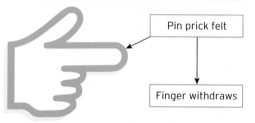

C fibres are associated with 'second' pain and conduct the impulses more slowly than the A delta fibres. This results in the individual complaining of dull, burning, aching or throbbing pain which is felt over a larger area. C fibre pain or 'second' pain is usually well managed by the administration of opioids.

The third important nerve fibre to consider is the **A beta fibres** and although they are not linked with passing on the pain message, they are important when we consider pain management. This is because their stimulation can be used to distract the individual from the perception of pain, such as a mother's kiss when a child hurts itself. The A beta fibres are the largest of all three fibres and are concentrated mainly in the skin; they do not cross over to the other side of the spinal cord but they still send a message to the brain quickly from the same side of the spinal cord that they enter. These fibres are activated by touch and sensation that is not perceived as painful, for instance the touch of a feather.

Figure 25.2   Nerve fibres important when considering pain

transmitting the stimuli (see Figure 25.2) and these are classified according to the type of message being conveyed, the rate of conduction and their size. A delta fibres (myelinated) and C fibres (unmyelinated) transmit painful sensations and A beta fibres transmit other sensations, such as warmth and touch.

All three fibres enter the dorsal horn of the spinal cord at the same point, but while the A beta fibres convey the message from the same side, the A delta and C fibres cross the dorsal horn before travelling up to the brain.

ASSESSMENT OF PAIN

We can only achieve effective pain management if the pain is assessed accurately using the most appropriate pain assessment tool. Casual enquiries as to whether a patient has pain may not give you an accurate answer, as they may feel you are not listening properly or, if it is in a busy environment, they may feel embarrassed to talk about their pain.

A full pain assessment should be undertaken at the time of admission or consultation and should be considered to be part of the admission procedure or review, especially if the patient has indicated that they have pain or their condition is likely to cause pain.

It is this initial assessment that provides a baseline for comparison and gives the nurse an opportunity to discuss any pain experienced and how the patient has previously managed their pain.

However, there are many obstacles to undertaking an accurate pain assessment, which are outlined in Table 25.1.

Table 25.1 Obstacles to undertaking an accurate pain assessment

- Patient misconceptions – for example, fear of addiction to the medication, fear of having to take medication, fear of showing weakness, fear of identifying pain and having to stay in hospital or receive treatment for a long period of time
- Previous experiences of pain, especially if it was not managed adequately
- Communication barriers – for example, the patient may
  - ○ not understand or speak English
  - ○ have a visual, speech or auditory impairment
  - ○ have a cognitive impairment, e.g. dementia, head injury, sedation
  - ○ be in so much pain that they have completely withdrawn and are uncommunicative
  - ○ have a learning disability that prevents them from communicating their pain
  - ○ have a mental health illness that prevents them from communicating their pain, e.g. depression, catatonia or paranoid thoughts
- The patient's age – younger people may not be able to communicate their pain, while older people tend to 'hide' their pain, believing that it is something that is to be expected and tolerated
- If the patient has a learning disability, they may not just experience communication difficulties but also actually not perceive pain in the same way as would be expected
- If the patient has mental health concerns, they may feel that they won't be believed or they may not be able to communicate their feelings accurately
- Cultural background – some cultures believe that it is inappropriate to express pain, while some believe that it is acceptable to be expressed verbally and behaviourally in a vigorous manner. Davidhizar and Giger (2004) propose that subtle genetic differences suggest that individuals from different cultures will experience pain and respond to analgesia in different ways
- Gender – some men may feel that it is a sign of cowardice to say they are in pain
- Environment – there may be a lot of noise or lack of privacy which prevents the patient from identifying pain-associated factors
- The nurse's preconception of how the patient should feel
- The nurse's lack of understanding of appropriate pain assessment and pain management

ACTIVITY 25.1: REFLECTION – OBSTACLES TO UNDERTAKING AN ACCURATE PAIN ASSESSMENT

Reflect on the experience you have had in observing nurses undertake an assessment of a patient's pain:

- Were any of the obstacles identified in Table 25.1 evident?
- How did the nurse deal with these obstacles?
- Do you feel the patient's pain was effectively assessed?

ENSURING YOUR PAIN ASSESSMENT IS EFFECTIVE

The most effective method of assessing pain holistically is for the nurse to observe and communicate with the patient, whilst using an appropriate pain assessment tool.

When observing a patient, especially if there are communication barriers, you may be able to identify some non-verbal signs (clues) (Table 25.2).

Table 25.2   Non-verbal clues

- Facial expression – crying, tears in their eyes, looking alarmed, clenching teeth, screwing up their eyes, have increased or decreased eye contact
- Verbal – they may be crying out loud, moaning, calling out for help, grunting, sighing, their voice may be high or low pitched, they may swear or be unable to talk at all
- Body language – they may be staying very still, moving less or moving awkwardly; they may be adopting an abnormal position or protecting (guarding) parts of the body; they may be restless, rocking
- Distancing – some people prefer to be alone and become withdrawn, quiet and uncommunicative
- Emotional – many people become emotional when they are in pain and may look worried, angry or sad; it might simply be that their mood changes and they become 'snappy' or tearful
- Appearance – the impact of pain can also lead to individuals losing interest in what is going on around them, losing their appetite and being unable to sleep. They may appear uncared for or look tired or exhausted. Your senses of observation and smell may also help here as people who are in pain often do not have the ability, or inclination, to maintain their own personal hygiene or the cleanliness of their home.

As part of the assessment, you may also observe physical indicators of pain such as changes in limb size, change of colour of the skin, change of temperature of the skin, neurological changes (reduced strength) or muscle spasm. You may also identify physiological changes when you record the patient's vital signs – the blood pressure may go up or down, you may observe changes in the pulse or respiratory rate, the patient may be sweating, be pale or complain of nausea.

IMPORTANCE OF COMMUNICATION SKILLS

Whilst your observational skills can enhance your assessment of someone's pain, the most effective tool you can have is good communication skills. If you are going to complete a comprehensive pain assessment, you need to inform the patient of the reason for the assessment, which would be to effectively manage their pain. You need to listen to the answers they give to your questions without being judgemental and then work with them to identify appropriate interventions, including how they would like to manage their pain. Within all of this, you will need to manage any communication barriers and the patient's own fears and preconceptions, as well as educating them on all possible strategies and interventions.

If the patient is uncommunicative – they may, for example, be a child or someone who has a learning disability or mental illness – you may need to elicit information from family members, carers or friends. When eliciting information from the patient or others, remember the key aspects set out in Table 25.3.

Table 25.3   Key aspects when eliciting information

- What words are commonly used by the patient to identify they are in pain?
- Are there any verbal or behavioural cues that the patient uses to express pain?
- What do the carers or parents do when the patient has pain?
- What do the carers or parents not do when the patient has pain?
- What works best for the patient in relieving the pain?
- Where is the pain and what are the characteristics of it (site; severity; character of pain as described by the patient or others, e.g. sharp, burning, aching, stabbing, shooting, throbbing)?
- How did the present pain start (was it sudden/gradual)?
- How long has the pain been present (duration since onset)?
- Where is the pain (single/multiple sites)?
- Is the pain disturbing the patient's sleep/emotional state?
- Is the pain restricting the patient's ability to perform normal physical activities (sit, stand, walk, run)?
- Is the pain restricting the patient's ability/willingness to interact with others, and their ability to play or continue with their daily living?

You may think that by asking the questions in Table 25.3 you have covered everything you need to know, however nurses need to be able to evaluate the severity of the pain and the effect of pain management strategies in a repeatable, objective and patient-centred way.

This is done through the use of an appropriate pain assessment tool which provides a pain score and can be repeated accurately by anyone trained to use it. Pain assessment tools are integral to the

Figure 25.3   Visual analogue scale

[1]If used as a graphic rating scale, a 10 cm baseline is recommended.
[2]A 10 cm baseline is recommended for VAS scales.

reliable management of pain and will allow healthcare professionals to consistently gauge the level, type and location of the pain. There are many pain assessment tools available, such as:

- the Visual Analogue Scale or a simple descriptive and numerical scale (Figure 25.3) – these scales can be used by asking the patient to rate their pain on a score of 1 to 10 or pointing to the line or word that reflects their pain level
- the short-form McGill pain questionnaire (Figure 25.4), which is more comprehensive and asks for further explanation or indication from the service user as to their experience of their pain – this tool is only suitable for those patients who are able to communicate effectively

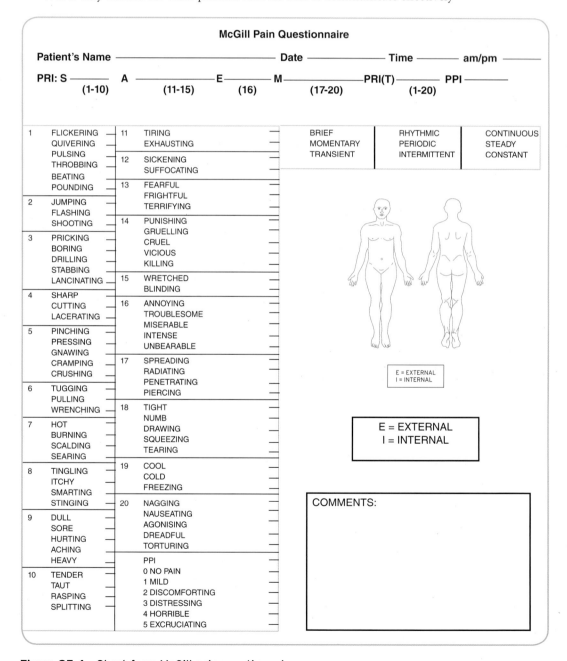

Figure 25.4   Short-form McGill pain questionnaire

- the Wong-Baker faces pain scale (Figure 25.5) – this is appropriate for those who are unable to communicate effectively, e.g. young children, those with a learning disability, individuals who are withdrawn or have a language barrier

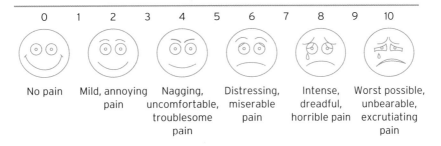

Figure 25.5   Wong-Baker faces pain scale

- the Riley infant pain scale (Figure 25.6) – this is appropriate for very young children.

SCORE	FACIAL EXPRESSION	SLEEP	MOVEMENTS	CRY	TOUCH
0	Neutral, smiling, calm	Sleeping quietly	Moves easily	None	
1	Frowning Grimaces	Restless	Restless body movements	Whimpering	Winces with touch
2	Clenched teeth	Intermittent	Moderate agitation	Crying	Cries with touch Difficult to console
3	Crying expression	Prolonged with periods of jerking or no sleep	Thrashing flailing	Screaming, highpitched	Screams when touched Inconsolable

Figure 25.6   Riley infant pain scale

Source: Schade, J.G., et al. (1996) 'Comparison of three preverbal scales for post-operative pain assessment in a diverse pediatric sample', *Journal of Pain Symptom Management* 12(6): 348-59

These are only a representative sample – there are many other assessment tools available and you may find that the area where you work has developed its own tool.

ACTIVITY 25.2: REFLECTION – USING A PAIN ASSESSMENT TOOL

Review an experience you have had of using a pain assessment tool with patients. Reflect on how you communicated with the patients:

(Continued)

✓

ANSWER:
ACTIVITY 25.2

- Were there any barriers?
- Did you gain sufficient information?
- Whom did you share that information with?

Now read Clinical Skill 25.1 and reflect on your experience and consider whether you might do anything differently next time you undertake a pain assessment.

GENERAL STRATEGIES TO MANAGE PAIN

ACTIVITY 25.3: REFLECTION – HOW DO YOU MANAGE YOUR PAIN?

Reflect on the last time you experienced pain – for example, when you 'stubbed' your toe, cut your finger, or had a headache:

- What did you do to make the pain better?
- Did you take any medication?
- Did you use any non-medication measures to reduce your pain?

As may have been evident in the experience of pain you considered in Activity 25.3, do not think of just administering medication to manage pain. In the first instance, you should ask the patient, their family or carer what interventions they would usually undertake to manage this type of pain. This does not mean that you should leave the individual in pain, but you should identify whether other strategies can be used to assist with pain relief or until pain relief is administered and becomes effective.

The following section identifies some alternative strategies that can either be used as an adjunct to medication, or chosen by some patients instead of medication. These are not presented in any specific order and nor is this an exhaustive list.

Reassurance and education

Explaining what is happening and reassuring anyone is essential to an effective therapeutic relationship so you should always keep people informed. If a patient presents to you in pain, you will need to reassure and educate them as you manage their pain. Similarly, if a patient is going to have a procedure where pain might be expected, they should be informed of what to expect and how the pain will be managed; this, in turn, will reduce anxiety and enhance communication (Gilmartin and Wright, 2007).

Always take into account that when people are stressed, anxious or distressed, they may not remember everything you tell them, so you need to repeat your education and reassurance frequently. You may also be able to provide some form of written information to which they can refer.

Consider the environment the patient is being cared for in. Simple measures can often be useful, for example a sense of calm and reassurance can be promoted by keeping noise and light to a minimum. This can be particularly helpful when caring for young children, neonates or those with a learning disability or dementia.

Support

Emotional

Sadly, patient experiences highlight that many healthcare professionals forget that the presence and physical/psychological support of friends, families, loved ones and carers can help a patient to express their pain and to tolerate the pain and the interventions more effectively. This should be considered when caring for all patients who may be distressed because they are in pain, in an unfamiliar environment and with people they do not know, but becomes even more important when caring for a child or a patient with a learning disability or dementia.

Environmental

Enabling the provision of home adaptations or aids to daily living can frequently benefit a patient.

CASE STUDY 25.2: MAUD (COMMUNITY)

Maud was reviewed by her GP four times over the summer months as she kept feeling unwell and fainting. During her fourth consultation, Maud told the doctor that she thought maybe she was feeling unwell and fainting because she did not drink enough fluids. The reason for this was because climbing the stairs to use the toilet caused her a great deal of pain, even though she took her analgesia as often as it was prescribed.

The doctor reviewed her analgesia and following a home visit by a community nurse and social worker, Maud had a downstairs toilet installed.

Three months later, the community nurse visited Maud again, at which time Maud declared herself very happy with her new toilet and stated that her new medication was working very well.

- Identify the ways in which Maud's case demonstrates how her quality of life has improved because a holistic approach was applied to her care.

Financial

Some patients may not take their medication as prescribed if they find it difficult to pay for their prescriptions. A simple review of their case by their GP may identify whether they are entitled to free prescriptions, or referral to a social worker may provide them with assistance to access relevant benefits.

STEP-BY-STEP CLINICAL SKILL 25.1: UNDERTAKING A PAIN ASSESSMENT

☑ **Before you start**

If the patient notes are available, review them in order to gain as much information about the patient and their current situation as is possible.

Your assessment should not just focus on the pain itself but also on whether the pain is new, re-occurring or persistent. It is helpful to ask the patient what medication they normally take for the pain and whether they have taken or done anything to alleviate the pain and, more importantly, whether it helped at all.

Gather the appropriate assessment tool and a pen. Make sure that you have something to rest on!

☑ **Essential equipment**

An appropriate pain assessment tool.

☑ **Field-specific considerations**

When caring for a patient with a learning disability, it is important to know their level of understanding. You will need to allow time to explain what you are doing. It may be helpful to have the patient's family or carers present.

Patients who have mental health needs may not understand the relevance of what you are doing. Ensure you spend sufficient time explaining this. It may be helpful to have the patient's family or carers present.

Children, younger ones especially, may not understand what you are doing. It is often helpful to have the parents or carers present to assist.

☑ **Care-setting considerations**

A pain assessment can be undertaken in any care setting.

Always ensure that you have the most appropriate assessment tool available, however you may start with one type to provide appropriate care as soon as possible and then return with a more appropriate assessment tool at a later time or date. For example, in a hospital ward it may be possible to have a variety of assessment tools to hand, however if a patient is being assessed in their own home then you may not have the most appropriate tool.

Comprehensive questions will provide you with an understanding of what pain is being experienced and this will indicate the most appropriate tool to be used on the next visit.

If you feel that the assessment was incomplete, then you should arrange to return as soon as is convenient.

In an acute, hospital-based setting and once a full assessment has been completed, it is easier to provide medication or implement alternative strategies to help alleviate the pain; it is also easier to monitor the effects of the interventions as you see the patient more frequently. Outside of the acute setting, this becomes more difficult as you may only see the patient once a week or even less, however visiting their home will give you the opportunity to observe how they cope with their pain, especially if it is chronic or persistent pain.

Reviewing a patient in their home setting affords you not only the opportunity to establish whether their normal medication is being taken as prescribed, but also whether there is anything else that you can do for them, such as home adaptations.

☑ **What to watch out for and action to take**

Whilst undertaking a pain assessment, you should also observe for non-verbal cues which may support the patient's answers (see Table 25.2) or provide you with further information.

You should always ask to view the site of the pain and observe for signs of:

- discolouration - any bruises, pale or reddened areas
- open areas or wounds and whether there is any **exudate** or bleeding - see Chapter 26 on skin integrity for further details relating to the care required

- swelling or inflammation around the site of the pain
- the temperature of the skin around the site of the pain
- any potential concerns – if you are undertaking an initial pain assessment, you also need to consider whether the 'story' around the pain being described is alerting you to a safeguarding concern – see Chapter 20 on safeguarding for further details relating to the care required or whether it is identifying a possible life-threatening condition, e.g. central chest pain may indicate serious heart damage
- any changes – if you are undertaking a subsequent pain assessment, make sure that you are able to review, compare and discuss any changes in the pain score provided by previous pain assessments with the service user and other healthcare professionals.

☑ Helpful hints

- Gloves and aprons must be worn if contact with blood/body fluids/excreta is anticipated or the patient is in isolation.
- Hand hygiene must be performed before touching a patient, before clean/aseptic procedures, after body fluid exposure/risk, after touching a patient and after touching a patient's surroundings.
- Waste should be disposed of in a clinical waste bag if it is contaminated with blood/body fluids/excreta.

UNDERTAKING A PAIN ASSESSMENT

BEFORE YOU START

1 **The first step of any procedure is to introduce yourself to the patient, explain the procedure and gain their consent**
Fully informed consent may not always be possible if the patient is a child, has mental health needs or learning disabilities; but even in these circumstances, every effort should be made to explain the procedure in terms that the patient can understand. This is not only respectful of their individual human rights, but also helps to ensure that they will be more accepting of the treatment and that their anxieties are reduced
See Chapter 6 for further information relating to why consent must be gained

2 **Ask the patient whether it is acceptable to them for the assessment to be undertaken where they are**
If the patient wishes the assessment to be undertaken in a different area, find an appropriate location
Ensure you maintain patient privacy, dignity and comfort at all times. See Chapter 12 for further information relating to promoting dignity in all aspects of care

3 **Identify whether the patient is able to communicate with you or whether they want someone with them, such as an interpreter, a family member or carer, to assist or support the assessment**
Ensures that the service user is supported and their answers are communicated accurately in a timely manner. See Chapters 15 and 16 for further information relating to the importance of effective communication in all aspects of care

4 **Prepare the environment, which includes making sure that the patient is able to see you, that they are as comfortable as possible (you may need to help them get into a comfortable position) and that the conversation is private**
Ensure that you position yourself at eye level with the service user without risk to yourself
To promote patient comfort and reduce anxiety
Making sure that the conversation is taking place in a suitable environment will demonstrate respect for the patient and ensure that they feel able to communicate freely

(Continued)

Throughout the assessment, observe for non-verbal and visual signs of pain, e.g. sweating, grimacing, guarding (see Table 25.2)

Enables you to identify whether the patient is 'holding back' or experiencing pain when they are unable to communicate with you. This is especially important in those with a learning disability or mental health need, where English is a second language, the elderly infirm or young children

 Talk to the patient in a gentle and unhurried manner; do not talk too loudly but do make sure that you can be heard

Effective communication is demonstrated and you are showing respect for the patient's feelings and experience

 Work through the assessment tool and listen to the patient's answers – if you are unclear, ask them to elaborate or explain further

Enables a comprehensive understanding of the patient's feelings and experience and the impact of their pain

 Document answers on the pain assessment tool and in patient notes

Accurate documentation allows for review of the efficacy of interventions and the identification of further interventions

See Chapter 18 for further information relating to record keeping

 If a patient identifies that they are in pain or you observe them to be in pain during the assessment, do not complete a full assessment but instead complete a primary assessment:

Where is the pain?
How long have they had it?
Have they had this pain before?
Have they taken anything for it? If so, did it work at all?
Are they allergic to anything?
Do they have any other conditions or take any other medication?

Other than give medication, is there anything else they would like you to do to help relieve the pain?

Administer medication and monitor effectiveness

This primary assessment ensures that the patient is not left in pain for an unacceptable length of time

Do not delay in obtaining appropriate pain relief – if the patient is in pain now, you need to act efficiently to ensure that they are treated as quickly as possible. Approach a doctor or nurse prescriber immediately to obtain directives for analgesia, or if you are in the patient's own home ask them what they would like to take and whether you can get it for them

You can return later, when the patient is more comfortable, to complete the assessment

To ensure appropriate pain control

 On completion of the pain assessment and if there are any previous assessments documented, compare and discuss with the patient the effect of any interventions previously provided or undertaken by themselves and identify the need for analgesia

Pain assessments should be undertaken whenever the patient's vital signs are recorded See Chapter 25 for further details or whenever the patient complains of pain. Comparison with previous pain assessments should be undertaken and review of the efficacy of any interventions to identify whether further strategies need to be implemented

 If any changes are noted, report the findings to your practice educator, the doctor or senior nurse in charge and obtain a medication review as soon as possible

This ensures that changes are addressed and that the patient's pain is controlled or that the patient is not on unnecessary medication

 Before leaving the patient, ensure they are in a comfortable position with drinks and call bells available as necessary

Promotes patient comfort and ensures they are well nourished and hydrated. See Chapter 32 for further information relating to nutrition and hydration

Source: NICE (2013)

Positioning

Positioning or re-positioning, for example raising an injured leg on a pillow and footstool, or, if someone has back pain, laying them flat, or, if someone has chest pain, sitting them upright, can alleviate pain. These strategies not only help with the immediate pain but also assist in improving the patient's condition, for instance by reducing swelling or improving chest expansion. It may also be helpful to consider using a splint to help with the positioning of a limb, such as hard or soft resting splints for someone with osteoarthritis (Masiero et al., 2007).

Massage

Relating to the physiology of pain (Figures 25.1 and 25.2), by stimulating the A beta fibres the pain gate can be closed – this is because the stimulation of the A beta fibres can prevent the pain impulses from the C fibres reaching the central nervous system.

This is why firm but gentle massage of the foot, hand or arm can effectively relax, and distract, the patient until analgesia takes effect. The massage can be done by a family member or carer, adding further support for the patient, and may also assist the family member or carer to feel less helpless.

Relaxation

Pain causes stress and anxiety which leads to tension and more pain so it is helpful to break this cycle by encouraging the patient to relax. Relaxation is not simply a case of directing the patient to relax and nor is this helpful. To use relaxation effectively, you need to develop an understanding of some relaxation techniques that you can explain and encourage the patient to use. You will often see healthcare professionals encouraging patients to take a deep breath or count to ten slowly while they focus on their breathing – these are relaxation techniques and can be very effective if used properly. It is also possible that listening to, and concentrating on, music can help in managing pain (Vaajoki et al., 2012).

Distraction

This is a strategy that individuals use to focus on something pleasant rather than the pain. They may listen to music, watch TV or read a book, whatever they want to do to help them cope with the pain. For babies, being in the arms of their mother, sucking on a pacifier may help to distract them from pain. Evidence shows that if a neonate is given a dummy sprinkled with sucrose, the pain response is significantly reduced; Kracke, Uthoff and Tobias (2005) suggest that the sucrose stimulates the release of endorphins.

Many people who experience chronic pain are very adept at using distraction to help them cope with their pain. However, for any patient, when the pain becomes more intense or they have a different, acute pain, they may forget or be unable to use distraction to help them.

Heat/Cold

You may have experienced the comfort of a warm bath or a soothing hot-water bottle or heat pad – this relief may be as a result of the stimulation of the A beta fibres which closes the 'gate' and reduces the perception of the pain. The warmth is also reassuring and the reduced perception of pain helps us to feel less anxious. The application of heat to the damaged tissue can also enhance the healing process by increasing the metabolic rate, improving the circulation (vasodilation) and reducing swelling. It is important to remember, however, that heat should never be applied immediately following the initial injury as this will increase the swelling.

In contrast, cold therapy, although not as pleasant, can be helpful in reducing the perception of pain in the same way. An example of the effect of cold therapy is the use of a refrigerated spray to help relieve the pain experienced on insertion of a cannula.

'Relieve the problem'

This is a simple statement but it may not always be quite so easy to achieve. Think carefully when you are caring for a patient in pain, identify the problem and work out if there is any way it can be relieved, even if only partially. For example, applying a splint to a broken limb or inserting a nasogastric tube for abdominal distension are both measures which will reduce pain. Although these interventions may well be identified as required by the medical team, the expediency of their application is in the control of the nurse.

You

It is fundamentally important to remember that you are the main component in making any form of pain management effective. You must never ignore someone who is in pain, even if you find it uncomfortable to deal with or do not have the knowledge or experience to do so – find someone that does.

Table 25.4   Further complications

- Compromised respiratory function, reluctance to cough or breathe deeply which can lead to a chest infection or even collapse of the lung.
- Tachycardia and hypertension which increase the risk of myocardial infarction (MI), especially if the service user has a history of heart disease.
- Increased platelet adhesion which in turn, increases the risk of deep vein thrombosis (DVT) and pulmonary embolism (PE).
- Increased metabolic rate which leads to immunosuppression and this in turn leads to an increased risk of infection.
- Compromised gastrointestinal function increasing the risk of ileus (reduced gut motility).
- Sleep disturbance which results in fatigue, which can result in the patient having less energy in the daytime and lead to a risk of reduced movement, apathy and loss of appetite. Lack of sleep can also increase the risk of depression or mood disturbance.
- Resultant inactivity increases the risk of chest infection, pressure ulcers, DVT and PE. There is also muscle wasting or loss of muscle tone, changes in gait which, particularly in the elderly, can lead to an increase in the risk of a fall and resultant injury.
- Uncontrolled pain is also associated with postoperative nausea and vomiting which, when it occurs, can increase pain. If the patient is nauseous or vomiting, they can quickly become dehydrated which delays recovery. The associated abdominal movement also increases the risk of postoperative haemorrhage.
- Depression can develop as a result of uncontrolled pain, even if it is of short duration.
- And finally, the consequences of pain and the delayed recovery can include personal financial hardship, increased burden on family or carers as well as an increased cost to the National Health Service.

You must never tell a patient that pain is to be expected or normal, ignore their complaints of pain, change the subject or jolly them along. It is essential that you identify the physical, psychological and social impact of pain in order to reduce the stress and impact of the pain itself. It is accepted that this may take time that you feel could be used to undertake other elements of care but in the long term you will save time as you will be able to identify appropriate, effective interventions in a timelier manner and provide better holistic patient-centred care.

Effective management of a patient's pain will reduce the risk of further complications outlined in Table 25.4.

ACTIVITY 25.4: CRITICAL THINKING – INEFFECTIVE PAIN MANAGEMENT

- Considering the potential further complications highlighted in Table 25.4, how many of a patient's bodily systems could be compromised by ineffective pain management?
- What effect is it likely that ineffective pain management will have on the time it takes for a patient to recover from illness?

MANAGEMENT OF ACUTE PAIN

Acute pain is expected after surgery or serious injury such as trauma or a burn, but it can also be experienced in times of infection (appendicitis, ear infection or dental abscess) or in acute conditions (myocardial infarction) or certain diseases. Even though we are aware that, in these situations, the patient will experience pain, research shows us that more than 50% of patients continue to experience pain due to ineffective pain management (Faculty of Pain Medicine of the Royal College of Anaesthetists, 2015).

Since 1990, all major hospitals have been recommended to introduce an Acute Pain Service (APS) to facilitate the management of acute pain (Royal College of Surgeons and College of Anaesthetists, 1990). The APS usually consists of an anaesthetist, an acute pain clinical nurse specialist, a pharmacist, a physiotherapist and, possibly, a clinical psychologist, although they may not provide 24-hour cover.

The APS is responsible for ensuring efficient pain management following surgery and, in cases of trauma, the production of pain management protocols, the effective monitoring of efficacy of the method of pain management chosen and the education of all staff. However, as previously mentioned, the most important member of the extended APS team is you, as you will work closely with patients and be the first to observe that they may be in pain.

Whilst many care environments use pain management protocols identified by the APS, it is essential for you to understand the general pharmacological approaches for pain management. Commonly used analgesics are available in a range of preparations, so they can be delivered by a number of different routes, for example tablets, injection, liquid suspension, cream, sublingual preparations, effervescent solutions, suppository, patch or lozenge. Table 25.5 identifies some commonly used analgesics for the management of acute pain in adults and children.

Table 25.4 Commonly used analgesics

Level of pain	Indications	Type	Sub-type	Examples	Preparations	Other uses	Side-effects	Other notes
Mild to moderate pain – acute and persistent pain	Headache, transient musculo-skeletal pain and dysmenorrhoea, post-operative pain	Non-opioid analgesics	Compound analgesics	Aspirin	Tablets, dispersible tablets, suppositories	Aspirin - anti-inflammatory, antiplatelet, anti-pyretic	Aspirin - gastric irritation	Can be combined with other analgesics to increase their effect
				Paracetamol	Tablets, capsules, soluble tablets, paediatric soluble tablets Intravenous injection, oral suspension (paediatric), suppositories	Paracetamol - to reduce pyrexia	Are rare but can include rash, blood disorders, hypotension, headache, if taken regularly, and, most importantly, liver damage in over dosage	Not recommended for children
				Co-codamol (a combination of codeine phosphate + paracetamol)	Tablets, dispersible tablets, capsules			
				Co-dydramol (a combination of dihydrocodeine tartrate and paracetamol)	Tablets and forte tablets			Caution when using for elderly - reduced dose recommended
				Co-proxamol (a combination of dextropropoxyphene and paracetamol)	Tablets			Not recommended for children and adults under 18 years
	Dental pain Transient musculo-skeletal pain Dysmenorrhoea Pain associated with secondary bone tumours			Non steroidal anti-inflammatory (NSAIDs), e.g. aspirin, ibuprofen	Tablets, topical preparations		Highly toxic if maximum dose exceeded. Not to be given to those with active peptic ulcer disease and should be used with caution in asthma, renal impairment and coagulation disturbances	Treatment of pain and inflammation associated with chronic disease as it reduces swelling, muscle tenderness and joint stiffness Can be given with opioid analgesics to increase their effect and reduce need to increase opioid dose

Level of pain	Indications	Type	Sub-type	Examples	Preparations	Other uses	Side-effects	Other notes
Severe pain	Postoperative pain, palliative care, chronic non-malignant pain	Opioids	Weaker opioids:	Codeine phosphate	Tablets, syrup, injection	Diarrhoea	Nausea Vomiting Constipation Drowsiness Larger doses produce respiratory depression	Can be given with paracetamol and/or NSAIDS to enhance pain relief Some people cannot metabolise opioids, resulting in ineffective pain management If administered, Naloxone should be available at all times Not effective for sharp pain and some chronic pain syndromes do not respond effectively
				Dihydrocodeine tartrate	Tablets, tablets forte, oral solution, injection (subcutaneous or intramuscular)			
				Tramadol	Tablets, capsules, orodispersible tablets, and injection (intramuscular and intravenous)			
	Moderate to severe pain, peri-operative analgesia, post-operative analgesia, obstetric analgesia		Stronger opioids:	Morphine	Injection (subcutaneous, intramuscular or intravenous, patient-controlled analgesia) – appropriate for children over 1 year, oral suspension, modified release tablets, suppositories		As above, plus can cause respiratory depression, hypotension and urinary retention Facial flushing, dry mouth, sweating, headache, vertigo, bradycardia,	Should not be used in acute respiratory failure, acute alcoholism, head injury, raised intracranial pressure and if there is a risk of paralytic ileus
				Fentanyl	Lozenges, patches	Beneficial for breakthrough pain if already receiving opioid analgesia or having chronic intractable pain	tachycardia, palpitations, postural hypotension, hypothermia, mood changes, dependence, itching, hallucinations Patches can cause local irritation to the skin	
				Pethidine	Injection (subcutaneous or intramuscular), tablets			Can be given intravenously if diluted to at least 10 ml with water for injection
				Buprenorphine	Sublingual tablets, injection (intramuscular or intravenous), patches			Beneficial for those with opioid dependence but can result in mild withdrawal symptoms

ACTIVITY 25.5: REFLECTION – INCREASING YOUR KNOWLEDGE OF DIFFERENT ANALGESICS

As is made clear by Table 25.4, there are a large number of analgesics which are commonly used. To care effectively for patients who are experiencing pain, you need to develop an understanding of these. Reflecting on your most recent placement:

- were any of the patients you cared for taking analgesics?
- If so:

    o   which analgesic?
    o   why had it been prescribed?
    o   was it effective?
    o   did the patient experience any side-effects?

It is often easier to understand how drugs work by remembering the patients you have cared for who were taking them. When you go to your next placement, start to compile your own 'directory of analgesics', by keeping a note of the answers to the questions above. Remember the importance of confidentiality and that you must not include any names of patients or other identifying details in your analgesic directory.

One of the common myths related to opioids is that people will become addicted to, or dependent on, the drug. However, this is highly unlikely if the patient is appropriately monitored and supported (Benyamin et al., 2008). Unfortunately, it is this misperception that results in patients declining medication or nurses being reluctant to administer opioid analgesics, resulting in poor pain management and increased risk to the patient. The nurse's misperception is usually based on the experience of seeing patients exhibiting withdrawal symptoms when their medication has been significantly reduced or stopped abruptly and is not related to any form of dependence. Opioids can be very effective in pain management although their side-effects should also be managed effectively in order to provide optimum care.

Considering the physiology of pain again, it is important to note that the A delta fibres do not have opioid receptors on their surface, so they will not respond to opioid analgesia such as morphine. This is an important nursing consideration as someone receiving an opioid analgesia will still be able to perceive 'first' or 'fast' pain; it is a natural protective measure that the body uses to reduce the risk of further damage. This means that if you give a morphine-type analgesic to someone with an inflamed appendix, you will make them feel more comfortable but if, for example, their abdomen is palpated as part of the doctor's examination, they will still complain of pain.

As we have discussed previously, analgesia must never be withheld to allow for further assessment as this causes unnecessary distress. This is, however, a common misperception, with patients being told that analgesia cannot be given until they are reviewed by a doctor, so that they can describe the pain when they are examined.

Further investigation must always be carried out if the situation arises where a patient has been receiving analgesia which they identify as controlling their pain and then they complain of further pain. It is possible that this could indicate an alteration in their condition.

If the initial analgesia is ineffective, pain specialists recommend a graduated approach, adding in further medication until effective pain relief is achieved, as indicated in Figure 25.7.

Figure 25.7   A graduated approach

If a patient is receiving analgesia for moderate or severe pain, you must ensure that it is administered regularly, as if analgesia is only given intermittently it may allow the pain to become uncontrolled. This, in turn, makes it more difficult to manage or control the pain overall. If a patient's pain continues, despite the administration of prescribed medication, you should review the patient, re-assess the pain and administer other medication, as appropriate, for example an anti-emetic. However, you should also consider whether the type of pain or symptoms being experienced would benefit from the addition of further medication. Table 25.5 outlines the medication frequently added to analgesics in order to improve pain management (adjuvant therapy).

Table 25.5   Adjuvant therapy

Adjuvant Therapy	Example (Drug)	Notes
Muscle spasm	Baclofen or Diazepam	Should be taken regularly and only stopped under the direction of a doctor
Gut spasm or colicky pain	Hyoscine Butylbromide (Buscopan)	
Ischaemic pain which tingles and shoots	Gabapentin	
Ischaemic pain which burns	Amitriptyline	

MANAGEMENT OF PERSISTENT OR CANCER-RELATED PAIN

In 1986, the World Health Organization (WHO) developed the three-step 'ladder' to ensure effective pain relief for adults with cancer (see Figure 25.8).

Figure 25.8   Three-step 'ladder'

Source: WHO (1986)

WHO advises the use of medication on a regular basis (every 3 to 6 hours) rather than as required, as this provides more effective pain control and in palliative care any concern over addiction should not influence the provision of much-needed pain relief.

Since its development, the three-step 'ladder' approach has been effectively used in conditions other than cancer which result in chronic or persistent pain. However, this approach does not ignore the possibility of other interventions, such as surgery on appropriate nerves to reduce or remove the perception of pain.

In the case of persistent pain in children with a medical illness, WHO (1986) recommends a two-step ladder (see Figure 25.9).

Figure 25.9   Two-step 'ladder'

Source: WHO (1986)

PAIN AND YOU

If assessment identifies that a patient is experiencing pain, it is important for you to support them in gaining some form of pain relief. In the instance of a patient experiencing new acute pain, a pain assessment, review and referral to a doctor must be undertaken immediately; if you are visiting them in their own home, liaison with their own GP is recommended, however it may be necessary to call an ambulance.

If the pain is one that they have experienced before, you need to ask the patient how they normally deal with their pain and help them to access their medication or intervention safely; you are not, as a student nurse, administering their medication but assisting them in self-administration. However, a safe medication administration procedure must be adhered to (NMC, 2008). See Chapter 29 for further details relating to medicine administration. In the acute setting, the nurse is ideally placed to be able to provide medication when the patient requires it, to ask for a medication review if the initial analgesia is found to provide inadequate pain relief, and to monitor the effects of any pain management strategies implemented.

When giving any analgesia, you should check whether the patient is on any other medication and review them for risk of interactions, over dosage or allergy.

Other strategies to manage pain that may be considered are:

• Acupuncture

This involves a trained professional placing fine solid needles into the skin at specific points (energy pathways called meridians) and impacting on the 'gate control'. Although this technique is not fully understood, it is thought that the acupuncture needle stimulates sensory nerves in the skin and muscles which send a message to the spinal cord and midbrain. As a result of this stimulation, there is a release of endorphins and an increased release of serotonin and noradrenaline into the central nervous system which results in an alteration in the pain felt (Mann and Carr, 2009).

Acupuncture has been found to be an effective treatment option for children with chronic pain, however it must be used with caution and undertaken by a trained professional and, preferably, with the agreement of the supervising medical staff (Vas et al., 2006). Acupuncture could also be preferable to aid the management of chronic pain for those individuals on medication that restricts the use of some analgesics, for example in drug dependency or some mental health illnesses such as schizophrenia or depression where pain medication may interact with regular medication.

- Acupressure

This relates to the application of finger or hand pressure over specific points on the body, producing similar effects to acupuncture. Only those trained professionals in acupressure should apply this intervention. Research has shown that acupressure can be effective in the management of postoperative nausea and vomiting in adults and children (Streitberger et al., 2006).

- Physical manipulation

This is a commonly used therapy for chronic pain in adults and children which should always be undertaken by a trained professional (chiropractor, osteopath or physiotherapist). Interestingly, this therapy exists despite the limited evidence to support its use.

- Entonox

This is commonly referred to as 'gas and air' as it contains a 50% mixture of oxygen and nitrous oxide. Nitrous oxide is an effective analgesic that has a fast onset and wears off quickly. The patient controls how much they take by holding the mask themselves and breathing in, and triggering the release of, the mixture.

Frequently, it is used during childbirth but is also offered by the ambulance service as it provides immediate pain relief in traumatic injuries, such as dislocated joints or fractures. Because of its immediate pain relief and short duration, it can be used with good effect when undertaking painful dressing changes or other painful procedures. However, it should not be used with patients who have a suspected or proven pneumothorax, bowel obstruction, severe head injury, decompression sickness or middle ear or sinus disease. Nitrous oxide (50%) has been proven an effective analgesic for children when having lacerations repaired as it is short acting and gives the child something else to focus on (Burton et al., 2008).

- Transcutaneous nerve stimulation (TENS)

This consists of a small, battery-operated device which delivers an electrical impulse to the skin surface of the affected area. The touch and stimulus of the impulses gently overwhelm the pain-sensing nerves and block, or reduce, the pain signals going to the spinal cord, acting on the A beta fibres and closing the 'gate'. Using a TENS machine on a low frequency setting can also stimulate the body to release pain-relieving hormones called endorphins. TENS machines are commonly used for women in labour and, although there is limited evidence to support its use, some people find it beneficial for alleviating chronic pain. TENS can be used by any adult or child and the most commonly reported side-effect is a mild reaction to the adhesive on the electrodes.

- Spinal cord stimulation

This is a long-term treatment for chronic pain and should only be implemented where there is an appropriate infrastructure for ongoing surveillance and support in place. For this intervention, electrodes are surgically implanted over the dorsal column of the spine and once activated they produce an electrical field which activates the pain-inhibiting mechanisms. Although recommended by both the National Institute for Clinical Excellence and the British Pain Association, further research is required to fully understand its potential.

FURTHER CONSIDERATIONS...

Another factor to consider when managing pain is the environment in which the patient is cared for. You may think that the best place to manage a service user's pain is in the acute setting due to the access to a variety of medication and the speed in which it can be administered. But think of the strange environment and, if you do not understand what is happening around you, the distress that someone may experience, especially if they are a young child or someone with a learning disability or mental health needs.

Distress can intensify the experience of pain and prove a difficult obstacle in its management. You need to adopt a calm and reassuring approach combined with excellent communication skills in order to overcome such a difficult obstacle. However, if the patient is critically ill and furthermore being nursed in an intensive care, high dependency or cardiac care unit, their distress is likely to be magnified by their reduced ability to communicate, especially if they are sedated, intubated and on a ventilator (Azzam and Alam, 2013).

Whilst hospital is considered to be the best place for someone experiencing acute pain, for those with chronic or persistent pain it has been found that effective pain management in their home setting improves quality of life as well as maintaining their mental wellbeing (Skevington et al., 2001). Although the value of caring for a patient in their home setting is proven, there may be times when a patient's pain is such that they need to be admitted for improved pain management. The goal for this, however, should be enhanced quality of life and supported discharge home as soon as possible.

WHAT'S THE EVIDENCE?

FURTHER
READING:
PAIN IN
THE ICU

Azzam, P. and Alam, A. (2013) 'Pain in the ICU: A psychiatric perspective', *Journal of Intensive Care Medicine*, 28: 140-50.

In this analytical review, Azzam and Alam found that care providers do not demonstrate adequate understanding of the emotional and cognitive components of pain to provide adequate management of pain in the intensive care unit.

Reflect on an episode of care you were involved in with a patient who was experiencing pain:

- How did the nurse seek to understand the patient's pain?
- Were there any additional questions you would have asked?
- What other strategies could the nurse have applied to gain an even better understanding of the patient's pain?

Now read the article and identify the actions you can implement in your nursing care.

ANTIDEPRESSANTS FOR CHRONIC NON-CANCER PAIN IN CHILDREN AND ADOLESCENTS

For many years, healthcare professionals thought that children would forget the pain they were in and therefore it did not need to be treated as effectively as in adults. Fortunately, viewpoints have changed and effective, proactive pain management is recognised as essential. In 2017, a systematic review by Cooper et al. was undertaken to assess the efficacy of pain management for children and adolescents with non-cancer pain.

ACTIVITY 25.6: RESEARCH TASK

Cooper, T.E., Heathcote, L.C., Clinch, J., Gold, J.I., Howard, R., Lord, S.M., et al. (2017) 'Anti-depressants for chronic non-cancer pain in children and adolescents', *Cochrane Database of Systematic Reviews*, 5 August.

- Review the article at: http://onlinelibrary.wiley.com/doi/10.1002/14651858.CD012535.pub2/full
- Identify how the findings of this systematic review have shaped pain management for this service user group.

Answer

The research has finally enabled healthcare professionals to understand that children and adolescents can be treated as adequately as adults with similar conditions. More importantly, this service user group can have their pain managed effectively. The review has started the process of a more defined effective pain management service for adolescents and children that will improve their quality of life and reduce complications. You may see this in your clinical areas as increased acceptance of the need to provide adequate pain control, use of adjuncts to achieve optimum pain control and more holistic service delivery.

CONCLUSION

As a nurse it is fundamental to remember that you are the key to making any assessment or form of pain management effective. Even if you find it uncomfortable to deal with a patients' pain, or do not have the knowledge or experience to do so, find another person who does. Pain is never to be expected or normal, so do not tell patients this, or ignore their complaints of pain, change the subject or 'jolly' them along. You role is to identify the physical, psychological and social impact of pain in order to reduce the stress and impact of the pain itself.

When assessment shows that a patient is experiencing pain you need to support them to gain some form of pain relief. If it is the case that the patient is experiencing new, acute pain, an assessment of the pain, review and referral to a doctor must be undertaken immediately. If you are not in an acute hospital you need to liaise with the patient's GP, or it may be necessary to call an ambulance.

When the initial analgesia administered to a patient is ineffective, a graduated approach needs to be used, adding in further medication, until effective pain relief is achieved.

It is important to remember that distress will intensify the patient's experience of pain and can prove a very difficult obstacle in pain management. You need to be calm and reassuring, plus use excellent communication skills to overcome this.

—————————— **CHAPTER SUMMARY** ——————————

- Being able to undertake an effective pain assessment is key to managing a patient's pain.
- In order to undertake an effective pain assessment you need to be familiar with the stages in this clinical procedure.
- There are many potential strategies you can use to manage a patient's pain. In order to be able to apply the correct one you need to understand how they differ.
- The provisions of effective analgesia will ensure that the patient can continue to undertake their activities of daily living independently.
- Always ensure that whilst caring for a patient and managing their pain you maintain their dignity, promote independence and ensure they are safe.

—————————— **CRITICAL REFLECTION** ——————————

Holistic care

This chapter has outlined the pain assessment process and identified aspects to be considered when providing holistic pain management. Review the chapter and write down the key physical, emotional, social, economic and spiritual aspects that you think need to be considered when:

- undertaking an holistic pain assessment
- supporting a patient to manage their pain.

Try to think of a variety of patients across the fields and identify further considerations that you would include the next time you undertake a pain assessment and support a patient to manage their pain. The next time you are in practice, return to this list of considerations and write a reflection on your experience.

—————————— **GO FURTHER** ——————————

Books

Mann, E. and Carr, E. (2009) *Pain: Creative Approaches to Effective Pain Management*, 2nd edn. London: Palgrave MacMillan. An essential read for all nurses to aid in the provision of strategies to manage pain effectively in conjunction with, or instead of, medication.

Toates, F. (2007) *Pain*. New York: Oxford University Press. A more comprehensive overview of pain perception and management.

SAGE journal articles

Doody, O. and Bailey, M.E. (2017) 'Interventions in pain management for persons with an intellectual disability' *Journal of Intellectual Disabilities*. Available at: http://journals.sagepub.com/doi/abs/10.1177/1744629517708679

This is a useful resource to better understand and provide pain management for individuals with an intellectual disability.

FURTHER
READING:
JOURNAL
ARTICLES

Go to https://study.sagepub.com/essentialnursing2e for free online journal articles for this chapter. If you are using the interactive ebook, simply click on the book icon in the margin to go straight to the resource.

Other journal articles

Davidhizar, R. and Giger, J. (2004) 'A review of the literature on care of clients in pain who are culturally diverse', *International Nursing Review*, 51: 47–55. This article will help you to further develop your understanding of the cultural influences on pain perception and management.

Gilmartin, J. and Wright, K. (2007) 'The nurse's role in day surgery: A literature review', *International Nursing Review*, 54(2): 183–90. Although this article is about caring for patients following day surgery, you will find that you can apply the principles to any setting. The article will help you to understand the importance of communication and education in the assessment and management of pain.

Skevington, S.M., Carse, M.S. and Williams, A.C.D.C. (2001) 'Validation of the WHOQOL-100: Pain management improves quality of life for chronic pain patients', *The Clinical Journal of Pain*, 17(3): 264–75. A useful article to aid you in understanding the benefits of effective pain management on the simplest aspect of someone's life.

Weblinks

Go to https://study.sagepub.com/essentialnursing2e for weblinks related to this chapter. If you are using the interactive ebook, simply click on the book icon in the margin to go straight to the resource.

FURTHER READING: WEBLINKS

www.iasp-pain.org/AM/Template.cfm?Section=Pain_Definitions – this is an excellent International Association for the Study of Pain (IASP) resource for nurses to better understand the evidence behind effective pain management.

www.who.int/cancer/palliative/painladder/en – this web page will give you a better understanding of the Pain Ladder; it was developed by WHO for cancer pain relief.

www.rcn.org.uk/__data/assets/pdf_file/0018/518130/004393.pdf – the RCN's better medicines management advice for nursing staff and patients.

www.nmc-uk.org/Documents/NMC-Publications/NMC-Standards-for-medicines-management.pdf – the NMC standards for medicine management, required by all nursing staff.

www.evidence.nhs.uk/search?q=Acute%20Pain%20Guidelines – the main portal to review the evidence supporting methods and guidelines to enhance pain management within a variety of conditions.

Video links

Have a break from the text and go to https://study.sagepub.com/essentialnursing2e for useful videos related to this chapter. If you are using the interactive ebook, simply click on the lightbulb icon in the margin to go straight to the resource.

VIDEO LINKS

ACE YOUR ASSESSMENT

Review what you have learned by visiting the book's online resources at: https://study.sagepub.com/essential nursing2e If using your interactive ebook, just click on the icon in the margin to go straight there.

ONLINE QUIZZES

- Test yourself with multiple-choice and short-answer questions.
- Revise key terms with the interactive flash cards.

REFERENCES

Azzam, P. and Alam, A. (2013) 'Pain in the ICU: A psychiatric perspective', *Journal of Intensive Care Medicine*, 28: 140–50.

Benyamin, R., Trescot, A., Datta, S., Buenaventura, R., Adlaka, R., Sehgal, N., et al. (2008) 'Opioid complications and side effects', *Pain Physician*, Opioid Special Issue, 11: S105–S120.

Burton, J., Auble, T. and Fuchs, S. (2008) 'Effectiveness of 50% nitrous oxide/50% oxygen during laceration repair in children', *Academic Emergency Medicine*, 5(2): 112–17.

Cooper, T.E., Heathcote, L.C., Clinch, J., Gold, J.I., Howard, R., Lord, S.M., et al. (2017) 'Antidepressants for chronic non-cancer pain in children and adolescents', *Cochrane Database of Systematic Reviews*, 5 August.

Davidhizar, R. and Giger, J. (2004) 'A review of the literature on care of clients in pain who are culturally diverse', *International Nursing Review*, 51: 47–55.

Faculty of Pain Medicine of the Royal College of Anaesthetists (2015) Core Standards for Pain Management Services in the UK. Available at: www.rcoa.ac.uk/system/files/CSPMS-UK-2015-v2-white.pdf (accessed 1 December 2017).

Gilmartin, J. and Wright, K. (2007) 'The nurse's role in day surgery: A literature review', *International Nursing Review*, 54(2): 183–90.

International Association for the Study of Pain (IASP) (1992) IASP Taxonomy. Available at: www.iasp-pain.org/Taxonomy#Pain (accessed 6 December 2017).

Kracke, G., Uthoff, T. and Tobias, S. (2005) 'Sugar solution analgesia: The effect of glucose on expressed Mu opioid receptors', *Anaesthesia and Analgesia*, 101: 64–8.

McCaffery, M. (1983) *Nursing the Patient in Pain*. London: Harper Row.

McCaffery, M. and Beebe, A. (1989) *Pain: A Clinical Manual for Nursing Practice*. St Louis, MO: C.V. Mosby.

Mann, E. and Carr, E. (2009) *Pain: Creative Approaches to Effective Management*. Houndmills: Palgrave Macmillan.

Masiero, S., Boniolo, A., Wasserman, L., Machiedo, H., Volante, D. and Punzi, L. (2007) 'Effects of an educational–behavioural joint protection program on people with moderate to severe rheumatoid arthritis: A randomized controlled trial', *Clinical Rheumatology*, 26(12): 2043–50.

Melzack, R. and Wall, P.D. (1988) *The Challenge of Pain*. London: Penguin Books.

National Institute for Clinical Excellence (NICE) (2011) Knee Pain Assessment. Available at: http://cks.nice.org.uk/knee-pain-assessment (accessed 19 December 2017).

National Institute for Clinical Excellence (2013) Neuropathic Pain: The pharmacological management of neuropathic pain in adults in non-specialist settings. Available at: http://guidance.nice.org.uk/CG/Wave0/629 (accessed 19 December 2017).

Nursing and Midwifery Council (NMC) (2008) *Standards for Medicine Management*. London: NMC.

Royal College of Surgeons and College of Anaesthetists (1990) *Report of the Working Party on Pain after Surgery*. London: HMSO.

Schade, J.G., et al. (1996) 'Comparison of three preverbal scales for post-operative pain assessment in a diverse pediatric sample', *Journal of Pain Symptom Management* 12(6): 348–59.

Skevington, S.M., Carse, M.S. and Williams, A.C.D.C. (2001) 'Validation of the WHOQOL-100: Pain management improves quality of life for chronic pain patients', *The Clinical Journal of Pain*, 17(3): 264–75.

Streitberger, K., Ezzo, J. and Schneider, A. (2006) 'Acupuncture for nausea and vomiting: An update on clinical and experimental studies', *Autonomic Neuroscience*, 129(1/2): 107–17.

Vaajoki, A., Pietilä, A., Kankkunen, P. and Vehviläinen-Julkunen, K. (2012) 'Effects of listening to music on pain intensity and pain distress after surgery: An intervention', *Journal of Clinical Nursing*, 21(5–6): 708–17.

Vas, J., Perea-Milla, E., Mendez, C., et al. (2006) 'Efficacy and safety of acupuncture for chronic uncomplicated neck pain: A randomised controlled study', *Pain*, 126: 245–55.

World Health Organization (WHO) (1986) Pain Ladder. Available at: www.who.int/cancer/palliative/painladder/en (accessed 19 December 2017).

SKIN INTEGRITY

IRENE ANDERSON

THIS CHAPTER COVERS

- The skin
- Caring for a patient with a wound
- Pressure ulcers
- Leg ulcers

- Diabetic foot ulcers
- Surgical wounds
- Traumatic wounds
- Wound assessment and management

REQUIRED KNOWLEDGE

- It will be helpful to have a clear understanding of the structure and function of the skin and to have read Chapters 22, 23 and 25 before reading this chapter.

> My name is Gerald and I like to think of myself as an active 73 year old! I have had a venous leg ulcer on my left ankle for 18 months now. I have no idea how the ulcer occurred, but I do have lots of trouble with my legs, with varicose veins and previous ulcers, plus a clot a little while ago. The District Nurse is trying a new dressing underneath the bandages to get the ulcer healed and when she redressed it this morning there did seem to be some improvement. It is still painful if I stand for too long, but having to wear the tight bandages all the time, especially when it is hot, is the worse bit. They really do not make me look 'cool' when I am in my shorts!
>
> **Gerald, patient**

> Caring for wounds is something we do often, whether these are big surgical wounds, pressure ulcers or the 'wound' caused by us inserting an IV line in to a patient. There is lots to learn about the care required, but I think the most important thing to remember is to ensure the patient has had adequate analgesia before you attempt to do anything to their wound.
>
> **Betty, child student**

Visit https://study.sagepub.com/essentialnursing2e to access a wealth of online resources for this chapter – watch out for the margin icons throughout the chapter. If you are using the interactive eBook, simply click on the margin icon to go straight to the resource.

INTRODUCTION

Maintaining and promoting skin integrity is an important nursing role in relation to many of the patients for whom we care. The condition of our skin and the systemic conditions we experience determine our ability to withstand physical and environmental challenges. This chapter aims to highlight the most common types of wounds (breaches in the integrity of the skin) that patients suffer and to consider the effects this can have.

To make rational and effective clinical decisions about the management of skin integrity, it is important to understand how normal wound healing occurs and how patient-related factors may disrupt this process. Once these processes are understood, it becomes easier to understand how wounds occur and how decisions are made about caring for a patient with a wound.

THE SKIN

Skin matures from birth; the epidermis of an infant is about 30 per cent thinner than adult skin. Neonates and infants have immature skin which has a reduced bacterial barrier function, putting them at higher risk of infection and trans-epidermal moisture loss (evaporation of moisture through the skin and dehydration), and reduced sebum (oil) production (high immediately following birth; then reduces until adolescence, when it increases again).

Advancing age results in decreased sebum production, which can cause dryness and itching. The older person's skin gradually thins and there is a weakening of the adhesion between the dermis and epidermis, making the skin more susceptible to shearing forces. This results in blistering and other types of skin damage as the layers of skin are pulled away from each other; this is particularly likely to develop when, for example, the skin drags on a bed because of poor patient handling.

A&P LINK: SKIN

To effectively assess and care for a patient's skin, you need to understand how it should look and what its normal functions are.

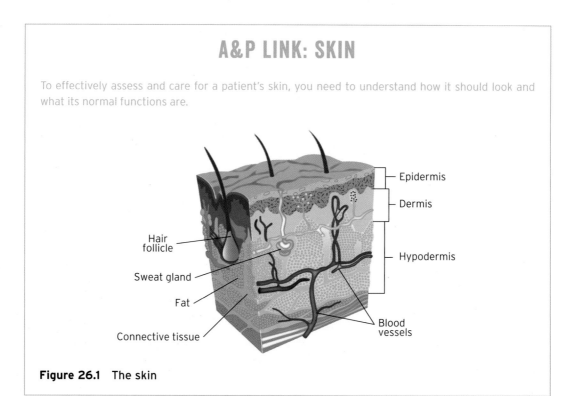

Figure 26.1 The skin

The skin provides a barrier between the dry external environment and the fluid environment of bodily cells, as shown in Figure 26.1. Skin covers the body, contains numerous sensory nerve endings, is an excretory organ, assists temperature regulation and protects the internal organs.

The epidermis is composed of dead cells which originate from the dermis. These cells are continuously replaced as they are constantly being rubbed off.

The dermis is made up of living cells and contains tiny sweat glands which end in ducts on the skin surface. These aid cooling because sweat evaporates on the surface of the skin which helps to maintain body temperature.

Hairs grow from follicles in the dermis which contain groups of specialised cells called sebaceous glands. These secrete sebum into the hair follicle and onto the skin surface, which keeps the skin soft, flexible and waterproof. Sebum also contains lysozymes, a chemical substance which kills micro-organisms, protecting the body.

The sensory nerve endings in the dermis can be stimulated by pain, touch and temperature. The main skin functions are:

- protection – by covering the internal organs and acting as a barrier against micro-organisms and other harmful substances; sensory nerve endings react by reflex action to unpleasant or painful stimuli, preventing further injury
- vitamin D formation – ultraviolet light causes a fatty substance (7-dehydrocholesterol) in the skin to be converted into vitamin D, which is used in bone formation and maintenance
- temperature regulation – the optimum temperature for bodily chemical reactions is 36.8°C (98.4°F). To maintain this temperature, there must be a balance between the heat produced by the body and that lost to the environment.

How do wounds heal?

Very superficial wounds affecting only the epidermis (see Figure 26.1) generally heal without scarring: how many paper cuts and minor abrasions have you experienced that have left no mark on your skin?

Wounds affecting layers deeper than the epidermis heal by a process of repair described in four stages: haemostasis, inflammation, proliferation and maturation (see Figure 26.2). While there are four stages in this sequence of events, it is important to remember that the process is a dynamic one, so some of the four stages may overlap. This process of repair leaves an enduring mark on the skin once the wound has healed and is the same in children and adults, although wounds in younger people generally heal quicker than those in their elders.

Stage 1: Haemostasis

This is a newly sustained wound which may be bleeding and painful for the patient.

When the skin integrity is breached, bleeding occurs and platelets aggregate (clump together) to form a clot over the damaged area of the blood vessel.

Clots mainly consist of fibrin, which creates a scaffold to support new migrating cells (see stage 2).

Figure 26.2   The four stages of wound healing

Stage 2: Inflammation

This stage can start as soon as the wound is sustained and can last up to five days.

The clot begins to break down and the surrounding capillaries dilate, making them more permeable, which causes fluid to leak into the wound site. White cells (neutrophils, macrophages and lymphocytes) are activated. Neutrophils 'wash' through the site for up to three days to destroy bacteria (by phagocytosis), then reduce in number unless there is infection. Macrophages also destroy bacteria and initiate the next stage of healing.

As part of the inflammatory process, mast cells release histamine and other substances.

The wound bed may have:

- yellow, cream or brown tissue called slough, which consists of old fibrin and destroyed bacteria
- dead tissue called necrotic tissue, which can appear dark brown or black and may be moist or hard and leathery.

Dilated capillaries will mean the area surrounding the wound will be red or flushed (inflamed) and fluid leaking from the capillaries will cause swelling around the wound (oedema). This oedema will increase pressure in the tissues and may be painful.

Stage 3: Proliferation

This may last for days or weeks depending on the extent of the injury. The space that has resulted from the wound fills up with granulation tissue, a structure composed of various cells including fibrin, keratin, collagen and glycoproteins.

The swelling will be subsiding and the wound will be filling with red, moist, shiny granulation tissue. There will be evidence of new tissue at the wound edges (epithelialisation). The epithelialisation will appear paler than the original skin because it is new.

Macrophages in the previous stage have stimulated the production of fibroblasts, which now enable the growth of new blood vessels. Elastin is also produced, which gives the new tissue resilience and elasticity.

Once the wound is filled with new granulation tissue, a process of re-epithelialisation occurs, starting at the wound edges and from any epithelial cells in the wound bed (found in the hair follicles). The epithelial cells cover the surface of the wound while fibroblasts and myofibroblasts (types of cells) contract to pull the wound edges together.

Stage 4: Maturation

Although the wound is covered by epithelial tissue, healing is continuing. The wound will appear healed but remains vulnerable to damage.

Collagen in the new tissue is initially immature and disorganised, but gradually matures and comes to lie in a more organised way. Although the wound appears healed, it may take several months, perhaps up to a year, for the tissue strength to reach an optimum level, and even then it may only be about 80 per cent of the original tissue's strength. Therefore, healed tissue is always at increased risk of further breakdown.

CARING FOR A PATIENT WITH A WOUND

While knowledge of the stages of wound healing is important, being able to relate this knowledge to patient care is fundamental in ensuring you provide effective care. Following the steps outlined in the step-by-step clinical guide 'Principles of caring for a patient with a wound' (Clinical Skill 26.1) will assist you in doing this.

ACTIVITY 26.1: REFLECTION

Using the information in Clinical Skill 26.1, reflect on the care you have been involved in delivering to patients with wounds:

- What stages of healing were these wounds at?
- How were the principles outlined in the table evident in the care you delivered?

Mechanisms of wound healing

There are two mechanisms of wound healing. One is primary intention where the edges of the wound are brought together and sutured, clipped or glued. The wound healing process then continues underneath the closed skin. The other type is secondary intention; in this situation, it is not possible to bring the edges together, so the wound has to fill with granulation tissue, which is then covered by epithelial tissue and there is contraction from the wound edges (as described in Clinical Skill 26.1). Healing by secondary intention is more visible, will take longer depending on the size of the wound and is more susceptible to delay because it is exposed to damage and infection. In general wounds, healing by secondary intention is more significant because there may have been tissue loss and the injury usually occurs in less than ideal circumstances. For instance, a patient can have a large wound

STEP-BY-STEP CLINICAL SKILL 26.1: PRINCIPLES OF CARING FOR A PATIENT WITH A WOUND

☑ Essential equipment

This will depend on patient need and the type of care being undertaken but is likely to include some of the following: analgesia, dressings and equipment to clean the wound aseptically.

Always ensure any equipment is clean and in working order before you use it.

☑ Field-specific considerations

When caring for a patient with a learning disability, it is important to know their level of understanding so that consent for and cooperation with the wound-related care can be gained. You will need to allow time to explain what you are doing and whether your actions will cause discomfort or pain.

Patients who have mental health problems may not understand the relevance of what you are doing. Ensure you spend sufficient time explaining this. It may be helpful to have the patient's family or carers present.

Younger children may not understand why you need to perform wound-related care; this will determine your approach to undertaking the procedure. It is usually helpful to have the parents or carers present to assist.

☑ Care-setting considerations

Wound-related care can be performed in both hospital and community care settings as long as the equipment required is available.

☑ What to watch out for and action to take

While delivering wound-related care, you should also use your observations to assess the patient's condition. For example, it is possible to assess:

- the colour of the skin, lips and nail beds for signs of cyanosis
- the patient's positioning and how they are moving
- their neurological condition – are they alert and responsive?
- any signs or complaints of pain or discomfort
- the patient's or relatives' views – for example, saying that their condition is 'not quite right' or they 'don't feel well'.

The information gained from these observations is additional to the wound care procedure but enables you to fully assess the patient's condition and institute appropriate treatment as necessary, escalating any concerns to senior nurses and the medical team.

☑ Helpful hints

- Gloves and aprons must be worn if contact with blood/body fluids/excreta is anticipated or the patient is in isolation.
- Hand hygiene must be performed before touching a patient, before clean/aseptic procedures, after body fluid exposure/risk, after touching a patient and after touching a patient's surroundings.
- Waste should be disposed of in a clinical waste bag if it is contaminated with blood/body fluids/excreta.
- Equipment must be cleaned as identified by the relevant policy every time it is used.

WOUND CARE GUIDELINES

The first step of any procedure is to introduce yourself to the patient, explain the procedure and gain their consent

Fully informed consent may not always be possible if the patient is a child or has mental health problems or learning disabilities, but, even in these circumstances, every effort should be made to explain the procedure in terms that the patient can understand. This is not only respectful of their individual human rights, but also helps to ensure that they will be more accepting of the treatment and that their anxieties are reduced

For patients who are unable to provide consent because they are unconscious, advice should be sought from your practice educator or another qualified nurse

Gather any equipment required. Ensure this is clean as appropriate and in working order

Reduces the chance of infection and maintains patient and nurse safety

Clear sufficient space within the environment, for example around the bed space or chair

Enables clear access for the patient and the nurse to safely use the equipment required

Wash your hands with soap and water. Apron and gloves should only be worn if appropriate

Wearing an apron and gloves as part of personal protective equipment (PPE) is a standard infection-control procedure when dealing with body fluids or patients in isolation

Ensure your use of PPE such as gloves and disposable aprons is appropriate by considering the individual patient situation and the risk presented

Close the curtains or take other appropriate measures to maintain the patient's privacy

Maintain patient privacy, dignity and comfort as required

Using the information provided in Figure 26.2, identify the healing stage of the wound

Identifying the healing stage of the wound will enable you to provide the most effective care

Ensure the care you deliver focuses on the priorities identified

Stage 1: Haemostasis

In order for the wound healing process to start, the bleeding has to stop. To do this, elevate the limb affected (where possible) and apply localised pressure to start the clotting process

The patient may be shocked and in pain so it is important they are reassured, basic first aid principles are applied and appropriate help is sought

If the patient is in pain, this must also be treated as a priority

Stage 2: Inflammation

Slough and necrotic tissue needs to be removed from the wound (debridement) as it can delay healing by causing a barrier to cell movement, and can potentially harbour infection

Pain relief, immobilisation and protection of the wound site are necessary

The use of antiseptics should be avoided unless there is a risk of infection, because the presence of inflammation is normal at this stage of the wound healing process. Wounds which have occurred in 'dirty' conditions (e.g. trauma) may need immediate antimicrobial therapy, but this should not be a matter of routine

Patient-related factors may reduce the inflammatory response needed for optimum wound healing. For example, patients on long-term steroid therapy or with poorly controlled diabetes, cardiovascular disease or an inflammatory condition such as rheumatoid arthritis will not experience a full inflammatory response. This will result in a reduced inflammation phase of healing, so the wound care provided must take all of these factors into account

(Continued)

Stage 3: Proliferation

At this stage, the wound requires warmth, moisture and protection from damage
The patient will require regular pain assessment and management, as well as reassurance about the progress of the wound

Pale granulation tissue (rather than healthy red) may indicate a lack of tissue oxygen (ischaemia), which is possible if the patient has a cardiac condition. Granulation tissue that is dark red and/or bleeding spontaneously may indicate infection

If granulation is allowed to dry out, due to prolonged exposure of the wound to air or an inappropriate dressing, then the cell activity may slow down and healing will be delayed. In very exceptional circumstances, a dry wound may be preferred (e.g. necrotic fingers or toes in a patient with diabetes), but normally the wound should be moist and warm

Children or patients with cognitive impairment may need extra support to protect delicate granulation tissue from harm through scratching or other damage

Stage 4: Maturation

The patient needs to be educated that healing is still continuing although signs may not be obvious

Although the wound has repaired, there will be scar tissue. The patient, family or carers may be anxious about the appearance of the scar tissue, which may be red and standing proud of the surrounding skin. Normally, over time, this will become paler and flatter. However, in some cases there may be abnormal scarring, where the tissue remains red and raised (hypertrophic). A less common type of scarring is keloid, where scar tissue remains prominent and may spread beyond the boundaries of the original wound. Scarred areas should be protected from injury, sun damage and excessive dryness as part of a good skincare regime, and scratching should be particularly avoided as this will damage newly healed skin

 After performing wound-related care, ensure the patient is in a comfortable position, with drinks and call bells available as necessary
Promotes patient comfort and ensures they are well nourished and hydrated

 Discard PPE, any single-use equipment and other used materials as per policy. Clean any equipment used as per the relevant policy every time it is used and perform hand hygiene
Prevents cross-infection and maintains equipment in working condition

 Document the care provided, and if necessary any findings, on the patient's observation chart and/or in the patient's notes
Maintains patient safety and accurate records

 If any abnormalities are observed, escalate to senior nursing staff/your practice educator immediately
It is vital to report abnormal findings to a registered nurse immediately so they can ensure care is escalated. Failure to do so can result in the patient's condition deteriorating, potentially leading to death

Source: Dougherty and Lister (2015); Trott (2012); WHO (2009)

from a surgical incision, but this will have occurred in a theatre with a controlled environment and appropriate instruments; a patient who has suffered an injury in a road traffic incident, meanwhile, will have sustained their injury in a manner which results in multiple contaminants and uncontrolled tissue damage.

In addition to this, a patient with a long-term or chronic condition may have sustained their injury because of their compromised tissue integrity. Examples of this would include a patient who develops pressure ulceration resulting from ischaemic tissue, a foot ulcer from the complications of diabetes or a venous leg ulcer from prolonged lower limb venous disease. It is very unusual for these wounds to heal in a manner other than secondary intention due to the extent of the tissue damage. While an acute wound generally follows a normal healing process (unless complicated by infection or further trauma), a chronic wound is likely to take longer to heal because of the patient's underlying condition. Often, the wound healing process becomes disrupted; chronic wounds can experience a prolonged inflammatory process (stage 2), which can result in more tissue damage, and then do not move into the proliferative phase (stage 3), so granulation tissue is slow to form and very weak. This leaves the wound site vulnerable to infection and further skin breakdown.

Wound types

Patients can experience many types of wounds, including surgical wounds, traumatic wounds and those caused by cancers and skin conditions. When caring for patients, it is highly likely that you will meet patients with both acute and chronic wounds, which are healing by primary or secondary intention.

The three types of chronic wounds you are most likely to see are pressure ulcers, leg ulcers and diabetic foot ulcers.

These three forms of ulcer affect at least 1 million adults at a cost of over £5bn, although this figure is likely to be an underestimate and it does not include children under 18 years of age. In addition to these costs is the inconvenience for patients, their families and carers that is caused by the wounds, especially in relation to the impact on their ability to go to work; the need for extra resources such as laundry, specialist equipment and prescriptions; and, most importantly, any negative impact on their quality of life (Guest et al., 2015).

CASE STUDY 26.1: KAMAL

Kamal is 6 years old and has presented at the minor injuries department. He tripped and fell on a path with sharp stones and gravel one hour ago. His outer malleolus has a 6 cm by 1 cm wound which has subcutaneous tissue visible. It is bleeding and Kamal is in pain.

- What are the two immediate priorities for Kamal?
- What must be ensured before wound closure takes place, and why?
- Is this an acute or a chronic wound?
- Is there likely to be a scar, and why?
- What information should Kamal's parents or carers be given about adverse events to look out for?

CASE STUDY 26.2: MISS MCDOUGAL

Miss McDougal is 60 years old and tripped and fell on a path of sharp stones and gravel seven weeks ago. She has been dressing the wound herself with simple dressings but there is a lot of fluid coming out of the wound and it is bleeding. She has ankle oedema and prominent varicose veins visible on her lower leg. The skin around the wound appears red and shiny. The district nurse has been asked by the general practitioner to see Miss McDougal.

(Continued)

- From the presenting signs and symptoms, why do you think Miss McDougal has ankle oedema?
- What might be the cause of the increasing exudate from the wound?
- In the absence of trauma, why might the wound be bleeding?
- What are the two immediate priorities in the management of Miss McDougal's wound?
- Is this an acute or a chronic wound?
- What will be involved in the ongoing management of this wound and what support is Miss McDougal likely to need?

PRESSURE ULCERS

A pressure ulcer is defined as 'localized injury to the skin and/or underlying tissue usually over a bony prominence, as a result of pressure, or pressure in combination with shear' (European Pressure Ulcer Advisory Panel (EPUAP), 2014) and has four categories:

- non-blanchable erythema
- partial thickness
- full-thickness skin loss
- full-thickness tissue loss.

Additional categories of 'unstageable' and suspected deep tissue injury are used where the actual depth of the ulcer is not visible due to thick slough (unstageable) or there is a localised area of purple or maroon discolouration or blood-filled blister due to the damage of underlying soft tissue from pressure and/or shear (suspected deep tissue injury).

ACTIVITY 26.2: REFLECTION

When you are next on placement, find the pressure-ulcer-related documentation used in the area:

- What risk assessment scale is used?
- How often are patients assessed?
- What pressure redistribution equipment is used to assist with pressure area care?
- Is any reference made to the EPUAP (2014) pressure ulcer guidelines on prevention and treatment?

All patients, regardless of age, are potentially at risk of pressure ulcers. The level of risk determines the preventative action to be taken and will be governed by local policy. A person's risk may change throughout one episode of healthcare, for instance if they are fasting, unconscious, or have a nutritional status that is changed for any length of time.

When we have been still for too long, we move our position to feel more comfortable; any pressure our skin has been subjected to is removed and any skin redness will quickly resolve. Any patient who has an altered consciousness level, paralysis or a lack of sensation is likely to need help to move. If this help is not given on a frequent basis, there will be prolonged pressure over bony areas which can damage underlying tissue, indicated by reddening of the skin which does not resolve (non-blanching erythema). If this pressure is prolonged and complicated by other factors, including illness and malnutrition, the tissue experiences ischaemia. This will result in ulceration involving the skin and underlying tissue, perhaps even down to the bone (full-thickness tissue loss).

If a patient can move and has cognitive impairment or uncontrolled movements (such as spasm), they may also incur damage. For instance, there may be repeated rubbing of their head, heels or elbows on a bed or chair, leading to abrasion or blistering of the skin. Patients may also be subjected to poor manual handling techniques when being moved and lifted, or may slip down in a bed or chair due to incorrect positioning. These can all result in shearing forces within the tissues, causing 'tearing' of underlying tissue and deep tissue injury. In addition to this, skin which is poorly hydrated or over-moist will add to the risk of injury.

This is why the NICE guidelines (2014) state that patients should have a pressure ulcer risk assessment within six hours of admission and regularly thereafter. Adults should be helped to reposition at least every 6 hours and neonates and infants at least every 4 hours.

Ulceration which does not occur over a bony prominence and is associated with constantly wet skin (such as in the case of incontinence) may be a moisture lesion rather than a pressure ulcer (Ousey et al., 2012). It is important to differentiate causes of skin damage because using pressure-reducing equipment would be a costly intervention if the actual problem was caused by inadequate continence management and skincare. Likewise, managing continence and skincare would not be enough if there was also prolonged pressure on bony areas. In reality, both causes can be present at the same time, which highlights the importance of treating a patient holistically and not just homing in on one problem.

Damage can be caused by low pressure over a long time, or high pressure for a very short time, therefore skin inspection is important as is immediate action where risk is identified. Patients, their families and carers all need to be involved in pressure ulcer prevention and identification.

In 2012, a UK initiative was launched with a target of zero avoidable pressure ulcers. This was part of a campaign related to the Safety Thermometer (DH, 2012). This focused attention on the maintenance of skin integrity, with careful analysis of the care provided to patients as a way to identify training needs for staff (McDonagh, 2013). Many patients can participate in their own harm-reduction actions in this area, but many more rely on nurses to assess their risk and take appropriate action to protect skin integrity.

There are a range of risk assessment tools available. The most well-known is Waterlow (2005) although there are many others, including Braden (1997) and Norton (Schoonhoven et al., 2002). There are also tools specifically for neonates and children (Willock et al., 2009). While risk assessment tools are a means of achieving a structured approach to assessing a patient, clinical judgement is also vital to ensure that the correct preventative strategies are put in place. The key priorities in preventing pressure ulcers are:

- regular repositioning
- careful moving and handling techniques
- use of special mattresses and cushions to help redistribute pressure.

All of these need to be based on the level of risk the patient presents with.

Apply what you have learned about caring for a patient with pressure ulcers by reading Mrs Amhed's case study, at https://study.sagepub.com/essentialnursing2e.

CASE STUDY: MRS AHMED

ACTIVITY 26.3: REFLECTION

Reflect on the pressure area care you have been involved in delivering:

- Were the key priorities evident in this care?
- Can you make any recommendations to improve pressure area care in your most recent placement area based on these key priorities?

LEG ULCERS

Leg ulceration affects up to 3 per cent of the population and most people with leg ulcers are in community settings. They may however be admitted to hospital for ulcer-related or other health reasons. The most common type of leg ulcer is a venous ulcer (Anderson, 2009; Guest et al., 2015).

Venous leg ulceration can be very painful and this can be made worse by eczema and oedema causing discomfort and heaviness of the legs, all of which impact on quality of life. For people of working age, it can have a profound effect on their jobs and income.

The treatment of venous ulceration involves elevating the limb when sitting or lying, exercise (walking and other ankle exercises) to keep the calf pump moving and, most importantly, compression therapy using bandages, hosiery or compression wrap systems. Compression therapy applies high external pressure to the leg, which maximises the action of the calf muscle pump, squeezes the veins to help prevent backflow of blood and allows fluid to flow from the tissues back into the capillaries, thereby reducing oedema and enabling the ulcer to heal.

A&P LINK: VEINS AND VALVES

In healthy individuals, the calf muscle squeezes the leg veins to enable the return of blood to the heart, with valves in the veins preventing blood flowing back down the leg. If the valves are damaged, perhaps through trauma or **deep vein thrombosis**, they cannot prevent the backflow of venous blood (Figure 26.3). This results in excess blood pooling in the capillaries in the lower leg. This excess volume of blood makes the capillary swell, which allows red cells and plasma to leak out in the tissues. If this situation is not corrected, the swelling becomes chronic and eventually the veins become permanently dilated (Anderson, 2009).

There are visible signs of venous backflow in the leg. Small broken veins are visible at first, and then varicose veins become evident. The leakage of red cells into the tissues causes permanent staining in the skin as red or brown discolouration (hyperpigmentation). The plasma which leaks into the tissues results in ankle oedema. Initially, this oedema resolves when the feet are elevated but eventually the oedema becomes more chronic and does not reduce on leg elevation. The extra pressure in the veins is called chronic venous hypertension and causes changes to the integrity of the skin, which becomes dry and flaky. The skin may become itchy and more prone to

Figure 26.3   Venous backflow

acute flare-ups of varicose eczema. Eventually, the skin becomes less elastic and appears indurated (like the bark of a tree) because the underlying tissue has become fibrosed and hardened. This skin change, together with the colour change, is called lipodermatosclerosis. The shape of the leg changes over time, with the calf becoming hardened and enlarged, often referred to as an inverted champagne bottle shape. The leg can appear red, which can be mistaken for infection and lead to patients having unnecessary antibiotic therapy. It is important to recognise lipodermatosclerosis because in this case the skin is extremely prone to injury – even a seemingly minor scratch may result in prolonged ulceration.

Leg ulceration can also be due to other causes, such as arterial disease. Narrowing of arteries causes ischaemia in the tissues. Injury to the lower leg may result in a non-healing or slow-healing wound which is often extremely painful. Treatment is through lifestyle changes such as stopping smoking and increasing exercise tolerance, and possibly surgery where appropriate. Symptom management and psychosocial support are also important, especially where surgery is not an option. Many patients have a mixture of venous and arterial disease, especially as they become older.

Venous ulceration treatment by compression therapy is very effective but could seriously compromise arterial flow if arteries are narrowed or blocked; therefore, it is very important that the correct diagnosis is made so that the patient is managed safely. A full patient assessment plus evaluation of the arterial flow by the use of a hand-held Doppler is essential to help diagnose whether the ulcer is venous or arterial. If there is some arterial disease but also venous disease, a reduced amount of compression may be indicated. If there is significant arterial disease, then no compression would be used. It is vital that any practitioner involved in leg ulcer assessment and compression therapy is appropriately trained and competent in such procedures. All nurses have a role to play in support of the patient, prevention of further damage and good cleansing and skincare.

Young people can experience leg ulceration, especially when they have congenital problems with veins, or poor calf muscle function. People with conditions such as sickle cell anaemia can also experience ulceration at an early age, and intravenous drug users who inject into their legs can also experience ulceration and extensive tissue destruction (Devey, 2010).

WHAT'S THE EVIDENCE?

Scottish Intercollegiate Guideline Network (SIGN) (2010) SIGN Guideline: Venous Leg Ulcers. Available at: www.sign.ac.uk/assets/sign120.pdf (accessed 18 May 2018).

Read SIGN's guidelines for venous leg ulcer management and consider whether the care you provided was in line with them:

- Reflect on a placement you have attended where you were involved in caring for patients with venous leg ulcers.
- What wound-related care activities did the patient receive?

CASE STUDY 26.3: JACK

Jack is 19 years old and has been homeless for 18 months. He injects crack cocaine, mostly into his femoral vein. He was treated for a deep vein thrombosis in the same leg a year ago.

An outreach worker at the needle exchange centre had noticed malodour and staining on the leg of Jack's trousers, and that he was limping. Although at first reluctant to discuss it, Jack admitted that he has a large wound on his inner ankle which has been present for about seven weeks and was often so wet he had to pad it with newspaper. The wound was extremely painful and injecting drugs gave him some relief from the pain.

Jack was persuaded to attend the outreach clinic. On examination, ankle flare was visible and there was ankle oedema. He also had signs of varicose eczema. The nurse used a hand-held Doppler ultrasound device to assess Jack's arterial flow and was satisfied that after a full assessment the presenting signs and symptoms indicated venous disease with no evidence of arterial problems. There did not appear to be any systemic signs of infection but the wound was malodorous and getting wetter and more painful.

The wound was shallow, approximately 20 cm², and the wound bed was 80 per cent slough and 20 per cent granulation tissue.

- What signs on Jack's leg would make you suspect that this is a venous ulcer?
- Why would compression therapy be a good treatment option for Jack?
- What could be done to encourage Jack to attend the outreach clinic for management of his wound?

DIABETIC FOOT ULCERS

Almost three million people in the UK have diabetes (Diabetes UK, 2017) and in addition to this an unknown number is yet undiagnosed. A major complication of diabetes is foot ulceration, which is a high risk for both infection and amputation. In addition to this, those who have had amputations due to ulceration are much more likely to die prematurely.

Diabetes has a number of complications, including neuropathy and peripheral arterial disease. These can result in neuropathic ulcers or neuro-ischaemic ulcers where arterial disease and neuropathy are combined. The Diabetes UK (2012) Feet First campaign sought to raise awareness amongst patients, members of the public and healthcare workers of the complications of diabetes and to reduce ulceration and amputation rates.

Neuropathy leads to altered sensation (sensory neuropathy) and reduced sweating (autonomic neuropathy). The altered sensation in the foot can mean that pain from trauma – perhaps a stone in the shoe – is not noticed until there is a significant injury to the foot. It is often assumed that people with diabetic neuropathy do not feel pain, but there is sufficient evidence to doubt this assumption.

WHAT'S THE EVIDENCE?

Bengtsson, L., Jonsson, M. and Apelqvist, J. (2008) 'Wound related pain is underestimated in patients with diabetic foot ulcers', *Journal of Wound Care*, 17(10): 433-43.

The findings of this small Swedish study indicated that over 50 per cent of people with neuropathic ulcers experience significant pain, with many patients reluctant to discuss their pain as they were afraid that amputation would be their only option:

- How can your knowledge of the findings of this study improve the care you give to patients with diabetic foot ulcers?
- What principles of the care you deliver to patients with diabetic foot ulcers can be transferred to the care of all patients?

Because the neuropathic foot does not sweat normally, the skin becomes very dry and the skin can develop fissures which could potentially become infected. Areas such as the ball of the foot or the heel may build up layers of hard skin (callus) which press on underlying tissue every time the person stands or walks, causing deep ulceration. A wound can easily go unnoticed under the callus as it is not immediately visible, with the patient becoming extremely unwell because of a wound infection or osteomyelitis (bone infection) before anything untoward is noticed. Due to the patient's diabetes, the response to infection may be depressed, so the wound or bone infection can quickly become life- or limb-threatening.

Motor neuropathy leads to the wasting of the small foot muscles and toe deformities; the toes retract into a claw shape which means the upper aspect of the toes is more likely to be damaged by footwear, causing toe ulcers. A rarer complication is destruction and demineralisation (breaking down) of bone in the foot, causing deformity (Charcot foot), and altered pressure points in the foot leading to ulceration from pressure damage.

Most patients with ulcers of the foot are older and have had their disease for a long time. Key to diabetic foot ulcer management is reducing pressure, infection prevention and control, wound debridement, regular foot inspection and clear wound treatment objectives. It is vital therefore that all patients with diabetes are helped from the time of diagnosis to look after their feet, have regular foot checks, wear sensible footwear and control their weight. As the number of children who are obese is increasing, early intervention and health promotion are vital in maintaining skin integrity and preventing amputations (Rhodes et al., 2012).

Apply your understanding of neuropathic foot ulcers by reading Mr Owusu's case study, at https://study.sagepub.com/essentialnursing2e.

CASE STUDY:
MR OWUSU

SURGICAL WOUNDS

Most surgical wounds heal effectively. However, there may be complications, such as infection, abscess or wound dehiscence (breakdown). Surgical site infections may be due to a number of factors, such as surgical technique or materials, environment or patient-related factors: for instance, malnourished patients, or those with significant or advanced disease, or where emergency surgery has been necessary. Dehiscence is mainly due to an abscess or infection but may also be caused by excessive wound tension, exacerbated by obesity or surgical technique (Sandy-Hodgetts et al., 2013).

ACTIVITY 26.4: COMMUNICATION

Polly is 11 and is visiting hospital for a pre-operative assessment, as she is due to have planned bowel surgery:

- What information would you share with Polly during this visit about her surgical wound and the care this will require?
- How could you give Polly this information in a way she will understand, and encourage her to ask questions and share her worries?

Most surgical wound sites are superficially healed within 48–72 hours but require patient support, pain relief and careful monitoring for infection. All wound dressings need to be selected very carefully, considering the condition of the surrounding skin. Adhesive dressings are most commonly used, but would be unsuitable for fragile or sensitive skin. Simple gauze-type materials should be avoided in wound care because they are likely to adhere to the wound, causing trauma on removal, and when exudate wets the dressing the risk of infection increases. Table 26.1 identifies the wide range of modern wound dressings available and why they would be applied.

A full patient and wound assessment must be carried out before setting specific treatment objectives and making dressing choices. Additional important factors also need to be addressed, such as nutrition, fluids, infection control, pressure redistribution and patient choice, before finally deciding on a dressing.

No dressing?

Some surgical wounds are left open for a time before closure or allowed to heal by secondary intention, especially if there is a risk of foreign body material in the wound, a high risk of infection or extensive excision of tissue that does not allow wound edges to be brought together. In these cases, skilled wound care is necessary to ensure the wound is protected, exudate and other fluids (such as bowel content) are not allowed to damage the skin around the wound and granulation is promoted. Patients with this type of wound will require constant monitoring and may need return visits to theatre for wound debridement. Topical negative pressure wound therapy is increasingly used for this type of wound in adults and children as it seals the wound, promotes granulation tissue and removes excess exudate in a closed system that also reduces the risk of infection.

TRAUMATIC WOUNDS

Many of us experience relatively minor traumatic wounds that cause anxiety and pain at the time, but heal and cause no further problem. Traumatic wounds may result from accidents such as road traffic incidents, a fall or a slip using a knife. These wounds can often result in a foreign body or other contaminants in the tissues, which can cause infection or poor healing. There can also be substantial tissue

Table 26.1 Wound dressings

Dressing type	Primary or secondary dressing	Exudate level	Main treatment objective	Additional information
Film	Primary or secondary May be used over a hydrogel to increase moisture in the wound, e.g. for debridement, or used over a hydrofibre or alginate which will absorb excess exudates	Low if used as a primary dressing Moderate if used as a secondary dressing to cover absorbent material	Wound covering for superficial wounds or to hold primary dressing in place	Skin must be suitable for an adhesive dressing
Foam	Primary or secondary (as above)	Low to moderate. Some versions have extra absorbency	Absorbency, wound protection, debridement	Adhesive and non-adhesive versions available
Hydrocolloid	Primary or secondary	Low (thin versions); low to moderate (standard versions)	Absorbency, debridement, waterproofing, bacteria barrier	Standard or extra-thin versions available Thinner versions may be suitable for fragile skin
Silicone	Primary	Some are silicone meshes and others are foam-type dressings with a silicone adhesive which is suitable for fragile skin	Absorbency, debridement, protection	Low adherence for fragile skin
Hydrogel	Primary – requires a secondary dressing unless a sheet hydrogel is used	Low	Adding moisture to a dry wound, debridement	Sheet hydrogels are available which can help reduce wound pain
Hydrofibre	Primary – requires a secondary dressing	Moderate to high	Absorption of excess exudate, debridement	Hydrofibre will adhere to the wound if there is a low level of exudate (also applied to alginates below)

(Continued)

Dressing type	Primary or secondary dressing	Exudate level	Main treatment objective	Additional information
Alginate	Primary - requires a secondary dressing	Moderate to high	Absorption of excess exudate, debridement	Generally used for short time periods (no more than 14 days at a time)
Antimicrobial (silver/honey/ iodine/PHMB - polyhexamethylene biguanide)	All primary. Some versions require a secondary dressing, some are complete dressings	Moderate to high	Used for prevention of infection in high-risk wounds or for locally infected wounds	Frequent monitoring of the wound is essential to reduce the risk of deterioration. Where appropriate, the patient must also have systemic antimicrobial therapy
Larvae (maggots)		Low to moderate	Wound debridement	Short-term treatment. Patient requires full explanation of the treatment and support throughout
Topical negative pressure wound therapy		Moderate to high	Wound debridement, infection management, control of excess exudate, management of large, deep, complex wounds	

loss or jagged wound edges, making suturing or other types of wound closure impossible. In this case, the wound will need to heal by secondary intention. The patient may require wound debridement to ensure the granulation tissue can form without impediment and skin grafting may be necessary once there is sufficient granulation tissue in the wound.

Cognitive or mental health issues can contribute to traumatic injury, with potential injuries including bites, scratching or head/limb banging. Accidental traumatic injuries, such as burns, can occur during seizures or blackouts. It is also possible for traumatic injury to be due to deliberate self-harm. This mostly affects younger people, with the deliberate harm an attempt to release deep psychological stress. It used to be common for patients presenting with self-harm injuries to be dismissed or treated harshly by practitioners (Friedman et al., 2006) but, thanks to a better understanding, more research and national guidelines (NICE, 2013) (from 8 years of age to adult), the experience of those who self-harm should now be more positive and supportive. A key issue in self-harm that involves repeated wounding is the effect on skin integrity. Each time a wound heals, the tissue loses some of its original strength. If the same place is continually cut, it eventually loses a significant amount of its resilience and ability to heal, which may result in chronic ulceration at the wounded site.

Iatrogenic injury

Traumatic injury can also occur due to medical intervention – for instance, a compression bandage which is too tight or inappropriately applied, a medical device such as a urinary catheter or nasal cannula for oxygen causing pressure damage or extravasation due to an intravenous infusion.

Making every effort to protect patients from such harm (known as iatrogenic injury) is an important nursing role.

WOUND ASSESSMENT AND MANAGEMENT

Understanding wound aetiology and how patient-related factors impact on wound healing helps in setting treatment objectives. A thorough assessment of the patient and their environment is vital. The first step is recognising what is happening in the wound bed and what intervention there needs to be – often referred to as wound bed preparation. As well as wound assessment, the skin surrounding the wound needs to be assessed for damage from excessive exudate or potential trauma caused by inappropriate dressings. Patient-related factors become very important here, especially in the very young, the very old and others likely to have fragile skin. People who are confused or are unable to articulate their wound experience clearly may suffer additional harm. In order to have a positive impact on the wound, specific treatment objectives need to be set. The TIME framework (Schultz and Dowsett, 2012) can be a useful tool to highlight key wound considerations (see Table 26.2).

ACTIVITY 26.5: CRITICAL THINKING

You will meet Precious again in Chapter 28, where you will manage the initial first aid aspect of her wound. In this activity, we are going to concentrate on the longer-term care of her wound.

Precious is a 21-year-old woman who suffers with an anxiety disorder. Along with this she has a history of self-harming behaviour. You are on a placement with a mental health team and have been

(Continued)

asked to help support Precious while you are on this placement. You note that she has become quite withdrawn after a verbal altercation with one of the other patients. You go to check on Precious and you find that she has cut herself quite badly with the broken edge of a toothbrush which she has embedded in her forearm. Precious goes to pull the toothbrush out of her arm as you approach her.

Because you read Chapter 30 very carefully, you managed the initial first aid care of her wound effectively, and are now considering the longer-term care of her wound.

- How might Precious's mental health problems affect her recovery from this injury?
- What care would you deliver to Precious in order to assist her wound to heal as effectively as possible?

WHAT'S THE EVIDENCE?

Webster, J., Osborne, S., Rickard, C.M. and New, K. (2010) 'Clinically indicated replacement versus routine replacement of peripheral venous catheters'. *Cochrane Database of Systematic Reviews*, 17(3): CD007798. [Updated 2013]

This Cochrane review by Webster et al. recommended that IV catheter sites should be inspected on every shift to ensure there are no signs of inflammation. This is especially important for children and babies, who are more at risk because their veins are smaller and more fragile than adults'. Patients who are restless are also at risk because the IV catheter may irritate the vein or be completely pulled out.

If a vein is irritated, it will become inflamed (thrombophlebitis), increasing the risk of infection and causing considerable pain. Signs of thrombophlebitis include tautness of the skin, oedema or fluid leaking from the site. Pressure, elevation and pain relief may be necessary and the infusion will need to be stopped and a new cannula sited if therapy is to continue. Infection following thrombophlebitis may present as heat, redness and swelling, perhaps with frank pus. The patient is at high risk of septicaemia and will require antibiotics.

- Reflect on a placement you have attended where patients frequently had IV catheters in situ.
- How often were these patients' IV catheters checked for signs of thrombophlebitis, infection or extravasation?
- Now read the Webster et al. article and consider how you can apply the findings to your practice.

Discomfort, pain and distress

When caring for adults and children, especially those who are confused or restless, it is not unusual to experience them removing their wound dressings. Using adhesive dressings can be problematic as they might try to rip the dressing off, causing significant skin trauma. In such cases, it is important to question whether the patient is trying to remove the dressing because it is uncomfortable or because they are unhappy with the unfamiliar object. We need to be alert to non-verbal signs of discomfort, pain and distress. Always ensure that patients are given as much information as possible and are offered appropriate options regarding how their wounds are managed. If a patient constantly removes a dressing, the safer option would be to apply one that is not going to cause trauma if removed prematurely, and to be prepared to dress the wound more often. Pain must always be anticipated and treated as a priority.

Table 26.2   The TIME framework

T is for tissue	Necrotic and sloughy tissue needs to be debrided, otherwise it will impede granulation tissue and will encourage the multiplication of bacteria, which may lead to infection. Debridement with dressings (autolytic) is a slower process than sharp or surgical debridement but may be more appropriate for the patient if they are not suitable for surgery or the necessary expertise is not available for sharp methods. If the necrotic or sloughy tissue is dry, then dressings which increase moisture in the wound will stimulate the enzymes in the wound fluid to debride the dead tissue (see Table 26.1). If the wound is wet, a dressing which absorbs the excess exudate but preserves a moist wound will aid the debridement process. Simply having gauze or padding materials as primary wound dressings is not suitable because the material dries out, causing adherence and trauma, and also holds wet dressing against intact skin, which will cause tissue damage.
I is for inflammation or infection	Inflammation is a vital part of the wound-healing process. However, chronic inflammation can cause tissue destruction. Wound infection is also characterised by inflammation and will delay healing, cause pain and possibly result in wound deterioration. Signs of infection are not always obvious. Patients with a reduced immune response may not exhibit the classic signs of infection, such as the area being red, hot, swollen and painful. Infection may cause a wound to deteriorate or stop healing, so if all other reasons for this have been excluded infection may be present, or at least a state of 'critical colonisation' where the signs of infection are more subtle. Where appropriate, antibiotics will be used to treat infected wounds, but topical antimicrobial dressings may also be used (see Table 26.1).
M is for moisture	Wound exudate is vital in the healing process as it contains enzymes and growth factors, and moist granulation tissue allows cells to move across the wound. However, excess exudate can make the surrounding skin wet, having a detrimental effect on skin integrity. The key to wound moisture is balance. If the wound is too wet, management options involve the absorption of fluid and skin protection. If the wound is dry, then moisture needs to be added by using a dressing that promotes the production of exudate such as a hydrogel or occlusive dressing such as a film or hydrocolid. Silicone barrier creams and sprays can also be very useful in protecting the surrounding skin.
E is for edge	New epithelial cells grow from the wound edges; therefore, it is important that they are protected. Decisions here will depend on the treatment objectives for the wound and the condition of the patient's skin. For instance, in a healthy adult or child the use of an adhesive dressing can be useful, because the dressing can act as a waterproof/bacterial barrier and stay on for several days. However, if a dressing needs to be removed frequently, perhaps because the wound is wet or infected, then repeated removal of adhesives will damage the skin and make it sore. So, a non-adherent dressing held in place by paper tape, tubular netting or a light retention bandage would be preferable. If the skin is fragile, because the patient is very elderly or young or because of long-term steroid use, adhesive dressings must be avoided.

CASE STUDY 26.4: KERRY

Kerry is 4 years old and is in hospital following a bout of pneumonia. She is small for her age and is underweight. She has cystic fibrosis and has been on a prolonged course of oral corticosteroids. Kerry has been very unwell and has been having oxygen therapy via a nasal cannula which caused a wound above her left ear, extending onto her cheek.

The wound is 3 cm long, narrow and superficial; it oozes exudate and the dressing often leaks and is itchy, which results in Kerry pulling her dressing off. There is no evidence of wound infection and the wound is improving. The wound is dressed daily but Kerry and her mother both find this distressing.

(Continued)

- What type of wound is this and what could have been done to prevent it?
- What should be the key considerations when selecting an appropriate dressing for Kerry, especially as it is often removed?
- How could Kerry be involved in her wound care?

Skincare

Skin integrity is enhanced by good skincare and self-management of skin should be encouraged where possible. Part of this involves monitoring the condition of the skin and the products that are used on it. The skin of patients with chronic conditions such as venous disease can become increasingly sensitive and many products, even those targeted at babies and young children, contain perfumes and other additives that could cause sensitivities, especially if the skin is already damaged. Where possible, water-soluble soap substitutes should be used for vulnerable skin and emollients kept as bland as possible. Emollients and other substances should be applied in the direction of hair growth to avoid irritation of hair follicles (folliculitis). Careful washing and drying of skin is very important to maintain skin integrity.

CONCLUSION

In order to make rational and effective clinical decisions about the management of skin integrity, it is important to understand how normal wound healing occurs and how patient-related factors may disrupt this process.

Patients can experience many types of wounds, including surgical wounds, traumatic wounds and those caused by cancers and skin conditions. When caring for patients, it is highly likely that you will meet patients with both acute and chronic wounds, which are healing by primary or secondary intention.

A full patient and wound assessment must be carried out before setting specific treatment objectives and making dressing choices. Additional important factors also need to be addressed, such as nutrition, fluids, infection control, pressure redistribution and patient choice, before finally deciding on a dressing.

We always need to be alert to non-verbal signs of discomfort, pain and distress. If we personally had a dressing that was uncomfortable or painful, we would remove it, and patients have the right to do this too. Always ensure that patients have as much information as possible and are offered appropriate options on how their wounds are managed. If a patient constantly removes a dressing, the safer option is to apply one that is not going to cause trauma if removed prematurely and to be prepared to dress the wound more often.

Whenever you care for patients with a wound, pain must always be anticipated and treated as a priority.

CHAPTER SUMMARY

- Pain management is a priority in caring for a patient's wound.
- Any decision about wound care needs to consider all of the patient's needs, not just their wound.
- Recognising the type of tissue in the wound, the stage of wound healing and the factors that may adversely affect healing are fundamentally important when setting realistic and achievable treatment objectives.

- All wound-care-related treatment should, where possible, be discussed with the patient.
- If a patient is malnourished and/or dehydrated, this must be addressed or it will negatively impact on healing.
- Any patient at risk of pressure damage has to be nursed using pressure-redistributing devices, and manual handling must be carefully carried out to avoid harming their skin.
- Always consult relevant guidance and protocols to ensure that patients benefit from a consistent approach and evidence-based decisions.

CRITICAL REFLECTION

Holistic care

This chapter has highlighted the importance of providing holistic care for your patient when delivering wound-related care. Review the chapter and note down all the instances where you think in caring for a patient's wound you would also need to meet their wider physical, psychological, social, economic and spiritual needs. Think of a variety of different patients across the fields, not just within your own field. You may find it helpful to make a list and refer back to it next time you are in practice, and then write your own reflection after your practice experience.

GO FURTHER

Books

Dealey, C. (2012) *The Care of Wounds*, 4th edn. Oxford: Wiley-Blackwell. This book addresses all aspects of holistic wound management, outlining current research and evidence-based practice. It includes chapters on the physiology of wound healing, general principles of wound management, wound management products and the management of patients with both acute and chronic wounds.

Wounds UK (2012) *Best Practice Statement: Care of the Older Person's Skin*, 2nd edn. London: Wounds UK. A very useful pocket guide.

SAGE journal articles

Go to https://study.sagepub.com/essentialnursing2e for free online journal articles for this chapter. If you are using the interactive ebook, simply click on the book icon in the margin to go straight to the resource.

FURTHER READING: JOURNAL ARTICLES

Gardner, S., Blodgett, N., Hillis, S., Borhart, E., Malloy, L., Abbott, L., et al. (2014) 'HI-TENS reduces moderate-to-severe pain associated with most wound care procedures: A pilot study', *Biological Research for Nursing*, 16(3): 310-19. This study examined pain associated with wound care procedures and evaluated the effectiveness of high-intensity transcutaneous electrical nerve stimulation (HI-TENS) in reducing this pain. The findings demonstrate that pain during wound care procedures is a significant problem and although nurses appropriately administer analgesics, these are not sufficient. Using HI-TENS may further reduce pain, particularly in patients experiencing severe wound care procedure pain.

Guo, S. and DiPietro, L.A. (2010) 'Factors affecting wound healing', *Journal of Dental Research*, 89(3): 219-29. Available at: www.ncbi.nlm.nih.gov/pmc/articles/PMC2903966/pdf/10.1177_0022034509359125.pdf. This article reviews the recent literature on the most significant factors that affect cutaneous wound healing and the mechanisms involved.

Meissner, M. (2014) 'Venous ulcer care: Which dressings are cost effective?', *Phlebology*, 29: 174. Healed or open venous ulcers may be present in up to 1 per cent of western populations and consume a large amount of healthcare resources. A number of specialised wound dressing products are now available, although there is little solid evidence to guide the choice of primary dressings.

Weblinks

FURTHER READING: WEBLINKS

Go to https://study.sagepub.com/essentialnursing2e for weblinks related to this chapter. If you are using the interactive ebook, simply click on the book icon in the margin to go straight to the resource.

www.diabetes.org.uk/Guide-to-diabetes/Complications/Feet – a very useful web page with information relating to the footcare required by patients with diabetes.

www.stopthepressure.com/path – the Stop the Pressure campaign (NHS Midlands and East) has an excellent site with a range of relevant information relating to preventing pressure ulcers.

www.nice.org.uk/guidance/cg74 – a web page which includes a range of resources relating to the prevention and treatment of infection following surgery.

http://ewma.org/it/what-we-do – the European Wound Management Association (EWMA) was founded in 1991 to promote the advancement of education and research into native epidemiology, pathology, diagnosis, prevention and management of wounds of all aetiologies.

www.nes.scot.nhs.uk/media/705715/dermatology_guide__amended_may_2012_.pdf – a very useful web page explaining common skin conditions.

Video links

VIDEO LINKS

Have a break from the text and go to https://study.sagepub.com/essentialnursing2e for useful videos related to this chapter. If you are using the interactive ebook, simply click on the lightbulb icon in the margin to go straight to the resource.

ACE YOUR ASSESSMENT

ONLINE QUIZZES

Review what you have learned by visiting the book's online resources at: https://study.sagepub.com/essential nursing2e If using your interactive ebook, just click on the icon in the margin to go straight there.

- Test yourself with multiple-choice and short-answer questions.
- Revise key terms with the interactive flash cards.

REFERENCES

Anderson, I. (2009) 'What is a venous leg ulcer?', *Wound Essentials*, 4: 20–9.

Bengtsson, L., Jonsson, M. and Apelqvist, J. (2008) 'Wound related pain is underestimated in patients with diabetic foot ulcers', *Journal of Wound Care*, 17(10): 433–43.

Braden, B.J. (1997) 'Risk assessment in pressure ulcer prevention', in D. Krasner and D. Kane (eds), *Chronic Wound Care*. Wayne, PA: Health Management Publications.

Department of Health (DH) (2012) *Delivering the NHS Safety Thermometer CQUIN 2012/13: A Preliminary Guide to Delivering 'Harm Free' Care*. London: DH. Available at: www.gov.uk/ government/uploads/system/uploads/attachment_data/file/216534/dh_134329.pdf (accessed 19 November 2014).

Diabetes UK (2012) State of the Nation 2012. Available at: www.diabetes.org.uk/Documents/Reports/State-of-the-Nation-2012.pdf (accessed 24 February 2015).

Diabetes UK (2017) New Diabetes Prevalence Figures for England. Available at: www.diabetes.org.uk/about_us/news/new-diabetes-prevalence-figures-for-england (accessed 10 November 2017).

Devey, T. (2010) 'Using an outreach service to meet the needs of users of intravenous drugs with leg ulceration', *Nursing Times*, 106(20): 10–14.

Dougherty, L. and Lister, S. (eds) (2015) *The Royal Marsden Hospital Manual of Clinical Nursing Procedures*, 9th edn. London: Blackwell Science.

European Pressure Ulcer Advisory Panel (EPUAP) (2014) Quick Guide: Pressure Ulcer Prevention. Available at: www.npuap.org/wp-content/uploads/2014/08/Quick-Reference-Guide-DIGITAL-NPUAP-EPUAP-PPPIA.pdf (accessed 17 September 2017).

Friedman, T., Newton, C., Coggan, C., Hooley, S., Patel, R., Pickard, M. and Mitchell, A.J. (2006) 'Predictors of A&E staff attitudes to self-harm patients who use self-laceration: Influence of previous training and experience', *Journal of Psychosomatic Research*, 60: 273–7.

Guest, J.F., Ayoub, N., McIlwraith, T., Uchegbu, I., Gerrish, A., Weidlich, D., et al. (2015) 'Health economic burden that wounds impose on the National Health Service in the UK', *BMJ Open*, 5: e009283.

McDonagh, V. (2013) 'Sustaining pressure ulcer prevention in practice', *Nursing Times*, 109(15): 12–16.

National Institute for Health and Clinical Excellence (NICE) (2013) Quality Standard QS34. Available at: www.nice.org.uk/guidance/qs34 (accessed 10 December 2017).

National Institute for Health and Clinical Excellence (NICE) (2014) Pressure Ulcers: The Management of Pressure Ulcers in Primary and Secondary Care. Available at: www.nice.org.uk/guidance/cg179 (accessed 17 September 2017).

Ousey, K., Bianchi, J., Beldon, P. and Young, T. (2012) 'The identification and management of moisture lesions', *Moisture Lesions Supplement*. London: Wounds UK.

Rhodes, E.T., Prosser, L.A., Hoerger, T.J., Lieu, T., Ludwig, D.S. and Laffel, L.M. (2012) 'Estimated morbidity and mortality in adolescents and young adults diagnosed with type 2 diabetes mellitus', *Diabetic Medicine*, 29: 453–63.

Sandy-Hodgetts, K., Carville, K. and Leslie, G.D. (2013) 'Determining risk factors for surgical wound dehiscence: A literature review', *International Wound Journal*, 12: 265–75.

Schoonhoven, L., Haalboom, R., Buskens, E., et al. (2002) 'Prognostic ability of risk assessment scales', *EPUAP Review*, 4(1): 17–18.

Schultz, G. and Dowsett, C. (2012) 'Wound bed preparation revisited', *Wounds International*, 3(1): 25–9.

Scottish Intercollegiate Guideline Network (SIGN) (2010) SIGN Guideline: Venous Leg Ulcers. Available at: www.sign.ac.uk/guidelines/fulltext/120/index.html (accessed 6 March 2018).

Trott, A.T. (2012) *Wounds and Lacerations: Emergency Care and Closure*, 4th edn. London: Elsevier.

Waterlow, J. (2005) The Waterlow Pressure Ulcer Prevention Manual. Available at: www.judy-waterlow.co.uk/the-waterlow-manual.htm (accessed 6 March 2018).

Webster, J., Osborne, S., Rickard, C.M. and New, K. (2010) 'Clinically indicated replacement versus routine replacement of peripheral venous catheters', *Cochrane Database of Systematic Reviews*, 17(3): CD007798. [Updated 2013]

Willock, J., Baharestani, M.M. and Anthony, D. (2009) 'The development of the Glamorgan paediatric pressure ulcer risk assessment scale', *Journal of Wound Care*, 18(1): 17–21.

World Health Organization (WHO) (2009) WHO Guidelines on Hand Hygiene in Health Care. Available at: http://whqlibdoc.who.int/publications/2009/9789241597906_eng.pdf (accessed 17 September 2017).

SAFE HANDLING OF PEOPLE

DIANNE STEELE

> " Hi folks! I have just celebrated my 14th birthday and my family and friends bought me a new wheelchair, which is 'cool'. I have Duchenne Muscular Dystrophy and so I have to rely on my mum, dad and carers to look after me. I spend more time in bed because my muscles are getting weaker and need help to change my position, not just because I have to look after my skin, but also it does get hugely boring looking at the same wall.
>
> **Charlie, patient** "

> " I thought turning a patient in bed would be an easy skill to learn; however, when working in the community I realised moving anyone is complex, as many elements of care have to be considered. My practice educator helped me to understand safe handling techniques, however I now appreciate that dignity and safety for the patient are crucial, plus the importance of learning safe handling techniques so I remain healthy too.
>
> **Frances, child nursing student** "

INTRODUCTION

This chapter outlines the importance of safe manual handling of people in community and hospital settings. As highlighted in the student voice, we will review how you and others can maintain safe working postures when moving patients to achieve optimal musculoskeletal health, which is the basis of good back care.

Within this chapter, it is not possible to cover all elements of safe handling of people, so we will focus on providing the requisite knowledge for you to ensure that your handling practice is safe and effective, making it unlikely that you will injure yourself or others.

THE PRINCIPLES OF SAFE PATIENT MOVING AND HANDLING

At the beginning of your nursing programme, you will receive theoretical guidance for safe manual handling practices from your university to comply with current UK and European Community legislation, the Health and Safety at Work Act 1974 (HSE, 1974) and Manual Handling Operations Regulations (HSE, 2004). This theory will then be applied to patient care through simulated practice. The opportunity to practise and rehearse skills to assist people to move provides a sound foundation for safe manual handling of people.

The handling of people is a complex science, posing several challenges. Humans are unpredictable in their movement and sometimes present challenging behaviour; they have joints which are unstable – indeed, the human shape is a difficult one to move. Further to this, people have differing underlying diseases and pain, plus physical and cognitive abilities all vary with age and individual backgrounds. Fluctuations in the wellbeing of the individual will also impact on the way you support and assist them to move, in order to maintain their independence. Therefore, the principles of 'risk assessment' are applied to the individual person to be moved each time they are moved. The principles of safe handling of people apply to all groups of patients, be they children or adults, including support for people with learning disabilities or mental health illness and any equipment you may need to move.

The importance of posture

The implementation of the Manual Handling Operations Regulations (HSE, 2004) is intended to improve the health and wellbeing of all workers. Health workers frequently refer in their care plans to risk assessment models and specialist equipment to assist people to move. During the introduction to your nursing programme, you will receive instruction on safe working postures and ways to avoid musculoskeletal injury. Thus, you are introduced to the importance of maintaining your health, preventing injury and promoting safe working systems even before you embark on your first placement.

ACTIVITY 27.1: CRITICAL THINKING

To safely move equipment and patients, you require knowledge of how the anatomical structures listed below relate to movement and back posture:

- bones of the vertebral column
- structure of the lumbar vertebra, including the intervertebral disc

- muscles supporting the pelvic girdle
- muscles of the back, abdomen and legs.

Produce notes explaining the roles that each of these structures play in posture and movement.

Good posture

Good posture means the balance and alignment of the bony joints and the action of muscles to maintain this without causing discomfort or pain, allowing the body to move with maximum efficiency against the force of gravity. So, any act of movement requires force and energy.

> Understanding good posture helps as it enables you to maintain a stable base – a stable base allows you to move quickly and safely, ensuring the safety of not only yourself but also the patient.
>
> Alice Rowe, NQ RNMH

Poor posture can lead to stress around the joints and, if persistent, will lead to joint malfunction with intermittent or persistent pain. Achieving postural awareness as a nursing student is important and relates to being aware of the tensions and stresses whenever you are pulling, pushing, carrying, or lifting loads, but also includes activities such as standing, sitting, lying and kneeling. Figure 27.1 identifies a variety of frequent postures, with the arrows identifying where stress will be placed on the musculoskeletal system.

| Sway back | Lumbar lordosis | Thoracic kyphosis | Forward head | Good posture |

Poor posture   **Good posture**

Figure 27.1   Poor and good posture

Your spine

Your spinal column has natural curves (Figure 27.2) which form an 'S' shape and act as a spring to compress and accelerate movement.

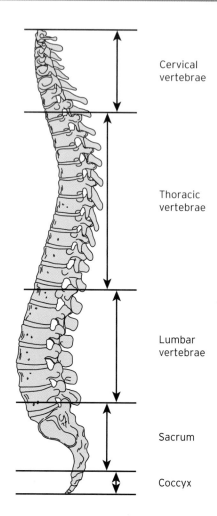

Cervical
vertebrae

Thoracic
vertebrae

Lumbar
vertebrae

Sacrum

Coccyx

Figure 27.2   Natural curved 'S' shape of the spinal column

Good
posture

Figure 27.3   Maintaining the 'S' shape

In a standing position to maintain these natural curves:

- your head position should be aligned in neutral, neither in extension or flexion; eyes and chin should be level
- shoulders are relaxed and level with weight to the floor, not towards the neck
- arms hang evenly by the sides of the trunk with palm of hands facing inwards against sides of the thighs
- hips level, aligned with shoulders and legs, with kneecaps facing forwards
- feet straight with weight balanced between heel and toes
- muscles should support without fatigue, movement or alteration in position.

ACTIVITY 27.2: REFLECTION

Ask a fellow nursing student, friend or family member to observe your standing posture for five minutes and give you feedback, which could include taking photographs of what happens to your posture over this time:

- Read the following section, 'Standing', and reflect on whether you adopted any of the postures described during the activity.

Standing

While standing, you are likely to shift your weight, resulting in a slouched position which moves the spinal column out of its neutral position. You will start to collapse forwards as the muscles fatigue and eventually you will start to walk or attempt to sit. This is normal, because our bodies are not designed to adopt fixed postures, so when our muscles start to fatigue we become uncomfortable. This uncomfortable feeling is known as musculoskeletal fatigue. This physiological response of muscle discomfort occurs when a muscle contracts for a prolonged period, causing blood supply to the muscle to be interrupted and resulting in ischaemia, where oxygen transmission to muscle cells becomes restricted and the exchange of rising carbon dioxide results in the build-up of lactic acid (Marieb, 2013). The pain this causes makes you adjust your posture to one which increases blood flow to the muscles, so the pain disperses. This signal of discomfort is actually very useful and one you need to be aware and take notice of, as it indicates that you are adopting an unsafe posture which you must adjust to prevent injury, and that you may need to consider an alternative technique to achieve the result you require.

ACTIVITY 27.3: REFLECTION

- Draw a diagram of what you would describe as an optimal sitting position.
- Then, and with permission, observe someone sitting and draw a diagram of the position adopted by the person you observe. Make a note of what you think is good and not so good in their sitting posture.
- Finally, refer to Figure 27.4 to review the sitting posture you observed.

(Continued)

Figure 27.4   Sitting posture

As is shown in Figure 27.4, to achieve an optimal sitting posture, it is not just postural alignment (as shown by the lines) but also the type of seating and individual leg length which are important.

To maintain standing posture, your body relies on the muscles arising from the pelvic girdle, 'transverse abdomens' and deep back muscles called 'multifidus' – you will have identified these in Activity 27.1. These act together as your core muscles, often referred to as a 'girdle' or 'corset' because they stabilise the lumbar spine, maintaining alignment of the vertebra by preventing any shearing forces when the body is required to engage in activity. The function of your core muscles when adopting working postures is to act as stabilisers and levers, so body balance and safety are achieved. Other groups of muscles play an important part in movement; most tighten and shorten when contracted and lengthen and relax when returning to a neutral position. The way you use your muscles will depend on your posture, which itself is dependent on your body weight, fitness, nutrition, hydration and lifestyle. Inherited disorders of the musculoskeletal system and underlying disease will all also impact on your movement.

A&P LINK: INTERVERTEBRAL DISC MECHANISMS

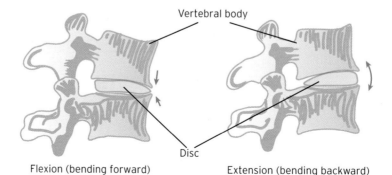

Flexion (bending forward)   Extension (bending backward)

Figure 27.5   The intervertebral disc

Image © Robin Lupton

To understand the principles of movement, it is necessary to further explore the anatomy and functions of the intervertebral disc (Figure 27.5). This will further develop the knowledge of the anatomical structure of the vertebral disc that you acquired in Activity 27.1.

Nucleus pulpous
Annulus fibrosus
Vertebral end plate

Figure 27.6   Facet joints in motion

Image © Robin Lupton

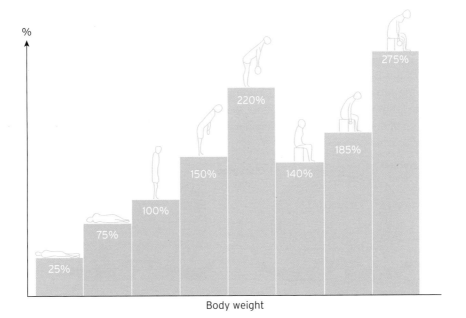

Figure 27.7   Disc pressures

(Continued)

The intervertebral discs comprise two distinct structures – the inner nucleus pulposus and the outer annulus fibrosus, both constructed of cartilage. The outer annulus contains fibrous rings plus fibres lying in different directions, making a strong and pliable structure which facilitates movement forward and lateral flexion plus extension. The inner annulus contains a softer gelatinous tissue known as the nucleus pulposus, which also assists with movement because it can change shape more readily than the outer annulus. Discs act as 'spacers' between the bony vertebral body of the spinal column, including the facet joints, which assist with movement of the vertebrae, sliding as the back bends and twists. The facet joints (Figure 27.6) protect the spinal column from any excessive movement and maintain alignment.

Discs also act as shock absorbers when your body is moving. For example, when you are walking, the 'S' shape of the spinal column compresses and flexes as your heel is placed on the floor and then lifted during the motion of walking. The pressures exerted on the intervertebral discs will alter according to the activity undertaken. Figure 27.7 shows the variations in disc pressures when different postures are adopted (Nachemson, 1992).

The numbers in Figure 27.7 represent a percentage of your body weight. So, when standing upright, your third and fourth lumbar discs are loaded with all of your body weight. Lying posture will reduce the disc loading: in both lying postures, the percentages are under 100. It is important to understand that as soon as you adopt postures in forward flexion (leaning forwards), either when sitting or standing, the pressure on discs increases – interestingly, the pressure is higher when seated than standing.

Remember these figures when you are working out how to position yourself when preparing to move patients, when you are leaning over beds and when seated while communicating with patients.

Care for your discs

The intervertebral disc, being made of cartilage, has no blood supply and is reliant on the movement of fluid and nutrients through the cells to maintain hydration and health. When standing, the fluid within the disc is forced out, and this increases further if the worker engages in poor posture and lifting loads. This causes the disc to compress and become thinner, eventually resulting in a reduction of your height during and after a work phase. If loading on the discs persists and is excessive, the vertebral joints are affected, however the effects may not become apparent for many months or years. This is known as the cumulative effect. The spinal ligaments become slack, which predisposes the person to

Figure 27.8   Disc disruption

injury as the spine is more mobile. If you continue to adopt poor working postures, you become more likely to disrupt your intervertebral discs, which will cause chronic back pain (Adams et al., 2012). Disc disruption (herniation) results from the inner nucleus pulposus erupting through the outer annulus fibrosus (see Figure 27.8). Discs are subject to the ageing process in the same way as the remainder of the body. The spine will become less flexible and more prone to damage over time. When you rest by lying down, fluid and nutrients replenish the discs, plumping them up and restoring them to their pre-work level of health.

> Nursing can be strenuous on both your body and mind, especially when working on a busy ward. It is very important to take regular breaks to rest – it is easy to focus so much on caring for patients that you forget to care for yourself. Treat yourself holistically as you do with your patients. Everything is interlinked – if you're dehydrated your concentration will be poor and you will be more likely to make mistakes and less aware of aspects like your posture and positioning, in turn meaning you are more likely to hurt yourself.
>
> Charlie Clisby, NQN

REMAINING HEALTHY

Case study 27.1 shows a correlation between lifestyle and work-related stresses. The aim of ensuring people remain healthy resulted in the government undertaking a review of Britain's working-age population, *Working for a Healthier Tomorrow* (Black, 2008). Black's findings noted that employers must be proactive in improving the health and wellbeing of their employees and prevent illness or injury in the workplace. Further findings by Koppelaar et al. (2013) suggest that the behaviour of nurses within healthcare settings – including their reluctance to use lifting devices, especially in hospital settings – has a clear influence on their health and wellbeing. This is one of the reasons why you are introduced to manual handling skills before commencing your first placement.

CASE STUDY 27.1: PINJA

Pinja is 56 and has worked in healthcare for 35 years. Initially, this was in Estonia, her home country, but she now works part-time in the UK while raising her three children. She enjoys her job and commutes to work by car, which is a total journey of one hour.

Pinja used to work in the community, but after ten years has returned to work on an acute ward at her local NHS Trust. Pinja is required to work shifts, including three night shifts per month, which she detests. Pinja never sleeps well when she is working on night shift, which leaves her feeling tired and unsure of when and what to eat, and she finds the shifts too long. She misses the interaction of her colleagues on day duty and feels there are insufficient staff on night duty to provide proper care to all patients. Pinja is very keen to reduce her night shifts, especially as these make it more difficult for her to care for her mother, who has osteoporosis.

Today, Pinja attended a well women's clinic at her local health centre and is feeling upset because the screening results show she is overweight (but not obese) and she was told she should stop smoking. Pinja states she has little time for recreational exercise and feels that caring for her family and

(Continued)

working part-time demonstrate she is active. Pinja thinks she has reached the menopause which, combined with her work, makes her feel physically tired while she often experiences backache in the lumbar region by the end of her working shift, although it disperses after a period of rest.

ANSWER: CASE
STUDY 27.1

- Make a list of what you think are Pinja's work and lifestyle risk factors, identifying how these may contribute to her history of lower back discomfort.
- What would you suggest to Pinja in order to enable her to improve her musculoskeletal health?

WHAT'S THE EVIDENCE?

FURTHER
READING:
APPLIED
ERGONOMICS

Heiden, B., Weigl, M., Angerer, P. and Muller, A. (2013) 'Association of age and physical job demands with musculoskeletal disorders in nurses', *Applied Ergonomics*, 44(4): 652-8.

Heiden et al. found that there is a correlation between increasing age and physical job demands, which result in musculoskeletal disorders amongst nurses, but age alone is not the only risk factor – time employed is also important.

- Reflect on the 'safe handling of people' procedures you have taken part in while on placement. Have you observed nurses finding the physical demands of their role difficult?
- What support is available to assist nurses who suffer from musculoskeletal disorders?
- Now read the article and consider how you can apply the findings to your practice.

The Black Report (2008) notes that where workers become ill or injured, employers need to implement an intervention to ensure adjustments are made. The Boorman Review (2009), carried out in relation to the health and wellbeing of NHS staff, noted that those employers who invested in wellbeing services for their staff showed better work productivity and performance and less sickness absence, retained staff in the workforce and, most importantly, saw improvements in patient care.

Safe moving and handling principles

Before moving any patient, it is always important to review their manual handling risk assessment, with the plan recorded in the patient's notes. The aim of risk assessment is to reduce harm to you and the patient and improve wellbeing, thus maintaining health for all. To make it simple, we should ascertain the best way of moving the patient and consider any risks to nurses to reduce injury. Guidance is provided by The Manual Handling Operations Regulations 1992 (HSE, 2004) and the Management of Health and Safety at Work Regulations 1999 (HSE, 2000).

The foundation for defining manual handling risk assessment is derived from the science of ergonomics, which is the study of people and their interface with the workplace. Where ergonomics are disrupted, harm is likely to occur.

The process of risk assessment relating to the moving of humans may seem to lack the 'caring' aspect of nursing; however, you need to transpose the professional guidance on such matters as consent, privacy and dignity detailed in the Code (NMC, 2015) to any situation involving patient care. The skill of the nurse is to apply appropriate safe handling methods, select the best equipment for this and ensure that her or his patients participate in their mobility to assist them to maximise their independence. The nurse is required to assist with patients' mobility, but this assistance will vary depending on the individual's wellbeing. Thus, a plethora of health professionals are employed to assist in safe handling practices and these include physiotherapists, occupational therapists and manual handling advisors employed to provide specialist advice. Effective risk assessment within the patient's care plan to ensure best handling practice is based on the following principles:

- **AVOID** – refrain from manual handling activities where practicable
- **ASSESS** – the risk where the task of manual handling cannot be avoided
- **REDUCE** – the risk to a minimum in order to avoid injury to you and your patient
- **REVIEW** – reconsider the care required at regular intervals and when circumstances change.

Risk assessment is completed in hospital and community areas using specific assessment tools and the information is documented in the patient's records. There is no standard risk assessment tool; however, some examples can be found in Smith (2011), HSE (2004), Welsh Assembly (2003) and Scottish Government (2014).

ACTIVITY 27.4: REFLECTION

When you are next on placement, review a manual handling risk assessment tool used.

Try to identify how the assessment categories are based on the principles of the following five categories, often referred to as **TILEE** (HSE, 2004):

- **T**ASK – identifies what is to be achieved during the handling task
- **I**NDIVIDUAL CAPABILITY – identifies the functional capability of the worker: for example, would any harm occur to you because of your height?
- **L**OAD – refers to what is being moved, be it a bed or a person: does it pose a potential hazard to you?
- **E**NVIRONMENT – identifies potential hazards such as constricted working space
- **E**QUIPMENT – selection of appropriate equipment, used and maintained correctly.

CASE STUDY 27.2: CHARLIE

You met Charlie at the beginning of the chapter, so you may want to re-read his story to help you remember. Charlie needs assistance to turn in his bed every two hours and prefers to be moved on a slide sheet. He has a height-adjustable bed, one side of which is placed against the wall. A ceiling track hoist to move between his bed and the bathroom is fitted, starting above his bed. The floor covering is carpet. The free floor space is about 2 m × 1 m 40 cm, and this is the space in which the carers work. Charlie's personal space and belongings are organised by him, so family and carers must gain his permission to change his environment.

- Using the TILEE risk assessment criteria to help you, identify as many possible risk factors as you can that would be associated with turning Charlie.

ANSWER:
CASE STUDY 27.2

STEP-BY-STEP CLINICAL SKILL 27.1: EFFICIENT MOVEMENT PRINCIPLES

☑ **Care-setting considerations**

For your health and safety, you must always apply efficient movement principles in all care settings (see movement guidelines, below).

MOVEMENT GUIDELINES

 Ensure you establish a stable base

Figure 27.9   An unstable base

The body is not designed to take this stance because it needs to be alert and ready to move

The body's balance is enhanced when the feet are placed further apart, but to a degree remains unstable if a force is applied laterally

Figure 27.10   A wider base

For almost all manual handling manoeuvres, one foot should be placed forwards and the other behind and with the leg bent at the knee as this provides a stable base

The stride stand is the start of movement. It allows the body to move by bending the knee, allowing the worker to flex at the hips while maintaining the 'S' shape of the spine

Figure 27.11   A stable base: stride stand

This maintains a natural relaxed posture. Always remember that feet control a stable base and allow movement, so ensure you consider how you can best achieve this when working around beds, chairs, baths, low surfaces and confined working spaces, especially those in the community setting

Knees and hips – these must be slightly flexed
To assist in free movement and enable the individual to be relaxed

Spinal column – the spine should not be in tension but should maintain the natural 'S' shape, with little flexion, lateral bending or trunk torsion
Adopting a 'C' shape in the spine suggests increased hip and lumbar flexion, which will result in you adopting a stooping posture, as shown in Figure 27.1 – thoracic kyphosis

Head alignment

Arms – your hand placement must be non-invasive and must neither grip nor cause discomfort to the patient
Holding the load close reduces the amount of effort required and increases control of the load

Figure 27.12   Head position

Ensure you avoid extension, flexion or twisting of the neck

Source: HSE (2000, 2004); Marieb (2013); NMC (2015); Polak (2011); Smith (2011)

EFFICIENT MOVEMENT PRINCIPLES

For your body to move efficiently, you have to ascertain the body's centre of gravity. The centre of gravity alters as the body adopts different postures, so without constant adjustments to our posture as different muscles engage we become unstable, predisposing us to a fall or an injury. Following the principles identified in Clinical Skill 27.1 each time you move equipment or assist a patient to move will help you remain injury-free.

STEP-BY-STEP CLINICAL SKILL 27.2: A SAFE WAY OF WORKING WHEN MOVING A PATIENT

☑ **Before you start**

Ensure you perform a thorough risk assessment.

☑ **Essential equipment**

This will depend on patient need and type of move being undertaken but is likely to include some of the following: hoist, sling, stand and turn aids, transfer aids, glide sheets. Always ensure any equipment is clean and in working order before you use it. Refer to local policy and manufacturers' instructions.

☑ **Field-specific considerations**

When caring for a patient with a cognitive impairment, it is important to know their level of understanding so that consent for and cooperation with the move can be gained. You will need to allow time to explain what you are doing and whether your actions will cause discomfort or pain.

Patients who have mental health needs may not understand the relevance of what you are doing. Ensure you spend sufficient time explaining this. It may be helpful to have the patient's family or carers present.

Younger children may not understand why you need to move them; this will determine your approach to undertaking the move. It is usually helpful to have the parents or carers present to assist.

☑ **Care-setting considerations**

With sufficient care and planning, safe moving and handling can be performed in both hospital and community care settings as long as the equipment required is available.

☑ **What to watch out for and action to take**

While moving a patient, you should also use your observation skills to assess the patient's condition. For example, when moving a patient, it is possible to assess:

- the colour of the skin, lips and nail beds for signs of cyanosis
- their previous position
- their neurological condition – are they alert and responsive?
- any signs or complaints of pain or discomfort
- the patient's or relatives' views – for example, saying that their condition is 'not quite right' or they 'don't feel well'.

The information gained from these observations is additional to the safe handling procedure but enables you to fully assess the patient's condition and institute appropriate treatment as necessary, escalating any concerns to senior nurses and the medical team.

☑ **Helpful hints**

- Gloves and aprons must be worn if contact with blood/body fluids/excreta is anticipated or the patient is in isolation.
- Hand hygiene must be performed before touching a patient, before clean/aseptic procedures, after body fluid exposure/risk, after touching a patient and after touching a patient's surroundings.
- Waste should be disposed of in a clinical waste bag if it is contaminated with blood/body fluids/excreta.
- Equipment must be cleaned as identified by the relevant policy every time it is used.

MOVEMENT GUIDELINES

1 **The first step of any procedure is to introduce yourself to the patient, explain the procedure and gain their consent**
Fully informed consent may not always be possible if the patient lacks understanding, but even in these circumstances every effort should be made to explain the procedure in terms that the patient can understand. This is not only respectful of their individual human rights, but also helps to ensure that they will be more accepting of the treatment and that their anxieties are reduced

For patients who are unable to provide consent because they are unconscious, advice should be sought from your practice educator or another qualified nurse

2 **Gather the equipment required. Ensure this is clean and in working order**
Reduces the chance of infection and maintains patient and nurse safety

3 **Clear sufficient space within the environment, for example around the bed space or chair**
Enables clear access for the patient and the nurse to safely use the equipment required

4 **Wash your hands with soap and water Apron and gloves should only be worn if appropriate**
Wearing an apron and gloves as part of personal protective equipment (PPE) is a standard infection-control procedure when dealing with body fluids or patients in isolation

Ensure your use of PPE such as gloves and disposable aprons is appropriate by considering the individual patient situation and the risk presented

5 **Close the curtains or take other appropriate measures to maintain the patient's privacy**

Maintain patient privacy, dignity and comfort as required

6 **Position yourself comfortably close to any equipment you are using and adjust the height of beds where possible**
To apply efficient movement principles (see Clinical Skill 27.1)

7 **The person nearest the head of the patient will lead the move The move lead must ensure all those in the team understand the requirements of the move and, if not, individuals must acknowledge this and step aside**
The move lead takes this position because they can see and communicate with the patient

Moving patients is not just a physical activity but includes interpersonal interaction and is a two-way process between the nurse/ move team and the patient to ensure the move is safe and coordinated

8 **All of those involved in moving the patient must be familiar with the handling manoeuvre and agree verbal team commands**
Team members must verbally acknowledge to the leader that they are ready, or indeed if they are not

Verbal instructions should include three distinct commands:

'Ready' – allows those involved to prepare a secure starting posture
'Steady' – allows those involved to confirm if they are ready to proceed or not
'Move' – the movement is undertaken

9 **After performing the move, ensure the patient is in a comfortable position, with drinks and call bells available as necessary**
Promotes patient comfort and ensures they are well nourished and hydrated

(Continued)

Discard PPE, any single-use equipment and other used materials as per policy
Clean any moving and handling equipment used as per the relevant policy every time it is used and perform hand hygiene
Prevents cross-infection and maintains equipment in working condition

 If any abnormalities are observed, escalate to senior nursing staff/your practice educator immediately
It is vital to report any abnormal findings to a registered nurse immediately so they can ensure care is escalated. Failure to do so can result in the patient's condition deteriorating, potentially leading to death

 Document the move and, if necessary, any findings on the patient's observation chart and/or in the patient's notes
Maintains patient safety and accurate records

Source: HSE (2000, 2004); Marieb (2013); NMC (2015); Polak (2011); Smith (2011)

 Understanding good posture is important as it enables you to maintain a stable base. Having a stable base allows you to move quickly and safely, ensuring the safety of not only yourself, but also the patient.

Siân Hunter, child nursing student

So how do we move a load?

Having considered the moving principles, these need to be applied to all handling activities and adapted to the work environment. If we consider the handling of people from an ergonomic perspective, the working environment should be designed to fit the worker. This happens to a degree – for example, the use of adjustable beds allows workers to raise or lower the bed to the comfort of the worker and not the patient – but in some environments, it is the worker who has to adapt, for example in working around a non-adjustable bed in a patient's home, thus increasing the risk of musculoskeletal injury (Kumar, 2001, 2007). Clinical Skill 27.2 identifies a safe way of working when moving a patient, regardless of the environment.

CASE STUDY:
ABEEKU

Apply your understanding of moving people safely by reading Abeeku's case study, at https://study.sagepub.com/essentialnursing2e.

CONCLUSION

The handling of people is a complex science which poses a number of challenges. Therefore, the safe handling of people involves applying a 'risk assessment' to the individual person and to each move before you start. In addition to this, to move equipment and patients safely you also require knowledge of how your anatomical structures relate to movement and back posture.

The principles of safe handling of people apply to all groups of patients, be they children or adults, and include support for people with learning disabilities or mental health problems. Safe working postures must be maintained when moving patients or equipment in order to maintain optimal musculoskeletal health, which is the basis for good back care.

In order for you to remain healthy throughout your nursing career, it is fundamentally important to care for your back by applying safe moving and handling principles to ensure that you move efficiently, taking adequate rest and adapting any environment as best you can to the move you intend to perform.

Always remember that moving patients is not just a physical activity; it also includes interpersonal interaction and is a two-way process between the nurse/move team and the patient.

CHAPTER SUMMARY

- The safe handling of people is a complex procedure.
- A risk assessment must be undertaken for all people who require assistance with their mobility.
- You need to understand how your anatomical structures relate to movement and back posture in order to ensure you do not injure yourself.
- Always consider the principles of movement and posture when assisting people to move.
- Utilise the principles of movement to work around beds, trolleys and couches in hospital and community settings.
- Moving patients is not just a physical activity – ensure you listen to the views of the patient and the team involved in the move.
- Health professionals currently follow Smith (2011) *The Guide to the Handling of People: A Systems Approach*, to ensure they plan effective mobility care.

CRITICAL REFLECTION

Holistic care

Helping a patient with their mobility needs is clearly linked to providing holistic care. Review the chapter and note down all the instances where you think assisting a patient with their mobility needs can help meet their wider physical, psychological, social, economic and spiritual needs. Think of a variety of different patients across the fields, not just within your own field, and in a range of different healthcare settings. You may find it helpful to make a list and refer back to it next time you are in practice, and then write your own reflection after your practice experience.

GO FURTHER

Books

Marshall, P., Gallacher, B., Jolly, J. and Rinomhota, S. (2015) *Anatomy and Physiology for Nurses*. Bloxham: Scion Publishing.

Smith, J. (ed.) (2011) *The Guide to the Handling of People: A Systems Approach*, 6th edn. Teddington: Backcare.

SAGE journal article

FURTHER
READING:
JOURNAL
ARTICLES

Go to https://study.sagepub.com/essentialnursing2e for free online journal articles for this chapter. If you are using the interactive ebook, simply click on the book icon in the margin to go straight to the resource.

Kay, K., Glass, N. and Evans, A. (2014) 'It's not about the hoist: A narrative literature review of manual handling in healthcare', *Journal of Research in Nursing*, 19(3): 226-45.

Other journal articles

Alamgir, H., Drebit, S., Li, H.G., Kidd, C., Tam, H. and Fast, C. (2011) 'Peer coaching and mentoring: A new model of educational intervention for safe patient handling in health care', *American Journal of Industrial Medicine*, 54(8): 609-17.

Kneafsey, R., Ramsay, J., Edwards, H. and Callaghan, H. (2012) 'An exploration of undergraduate nursing and physiotherapy students' views regarding education for patient handling', *Journal of Clinical Nursing*, 21(23/24): 3493-503.

Weblinks

FURTHER
READING:
WEBLINKS

Go to https://study.sagepub.com/essentialnursing2e for weblinks related to this chapter. If you are using the interactive ebook, simply click on the book icon in the margin to go straight to the resource.

www.hse.gov.uk
www.nationalbackexchange.org
www.nursingtimes.net/nursing-practice/clinical-zones/educators/improving-training-and-education-in-patient-handling/5031007.article#

Video links

VIDEO
LINKS

Have a break from the text and go to https://study.sagepub.com/essentialnursing2e for useful videos related to this chapter. If you are using the interactive ebook, simply click on the lightbulb icon in the margin to go straight to the resource.

GREAT FOR
REVISION

ONLINE
QUIZZES

ACE YOUR ASSESSMENT

Review what you have learned by visiting the book's online resources at: https://study.sagepub.com/essential nursing2e If using your interactive ebook, just click on the icon in the margin to go straight there.

- Test yourself with multiple-choice and short-answer questions.
- Revise key terms with the interactive flash cards.

REFERENCES

Adams, M.A., Bogduk, N., Burton, K. and Dolan, P. (2012) *The Biomechanics of Back Pain*, 3rd edn. Edinburgh: Churchill Livingstone.

Black, C. (2008) Working for a Healthier Tomorrow. Available at: www.dwp.gov.uk/docs/hwwb-working-for-a-healthier-tomorrow.pdf (accessed 23 August 2017).

Boorman Review (2009) Final Report, August. Available at: http://webarchive.nationalarchives.gov.uk/20130103004910/http://www.dh.gov.uk/en/Publicationsandstatistics/Publications/PublicationsPolicyAndGuidance/DH_108799 (accessed 23 August 2017).

Health and Safety Executive (HSE) (1974) Health and Safety at Work Act 1974. London: HMSO. Available at: www.hse.gov.uk/legislation/hswa.htm (accessed 23 August 2017).

Health and Safety Executive (2000) *The Management of Health and Safety at Work Regulations 1999.* Sudbury, Suffolk: Health and Safety Executive Books.

Health and Safety Executive (2004) *Manual Handling: Manual Handling Operations Regulations 1992* (as amended). Guidance on Regulations L23, 3rd edn. Sudbury, Suffolk: Health and Safety Executive Books.

Heiden, B., Weigl, M., Angerer, P. and Muller, A. (2013) 'Association of age and physical job demands with musculoskeletal disorders in nurses', *Applied Ergonomics*, 44(4): 652–8.

Koppelaar, E., Knibbe, J., Miedema, H.A. and Burdoff, A. (2013) 'The influence of individual and organisational factors on nurses' behaviour to use lifting devices in healthcare', *Applied Ergonomics*, 44(4): 532–7.

Kumar, S. (2001) 'Theories of musculoskeletal injury causation', *Ergonomics*, 44(1): 17–47.

Kumar, S. (2007) 'Selected theories of musculoskeletal injury causation', in S. Kumar (ed.), *Biomechanics in Ergonomics*, 2nd edn. London: Taylor & Francis. pp. 3–39.

Marieb, N.E. (2013) *Human Anatomy and Physiology*. Boston, MA: Pearson.

Nachemson, A. (1992) 'Lumbar mechanisms as revealed by lumbar intradiscal pressure measurements', in M. Jayson (ed.), *The Lumbar Spine and Back Pain*, 4th edn. Edinburgh: Churchill Livingstone. pp. 157–71.

Nursing and Midwifery Council (NMC) (2015) *The Code: Professional Standards of Practice and Behaviour for Nurses and Midwives*. London: NMC.

Polak, F. (2011) 'Mechanics and human movement', in J. Smith (ed.), *The Guide to the Handling of People: A Systems Approach*, 6th edn. Teddington: Backcare. pp. 53–61.

Scottish Government (2014) *The Scottish Manual Handling Passport Scheme*. Edinburgh: Scottish Government. Available at: www.gov.scot/Publications/2014/08/8582 (accessed 23 August 2017).

Smith, J. (ed.) (2011) *The Guide to the Handling of People: A Systems Approach*, 6th edn. Teddington: Backcare.

Welsh Assembly (2003) All Wales NHS Manual Handling Training Passport and Information Scheme. Version 2.1 (January). Available at: www.wales.nhs.uk/documents/NHS_manual_handling_passport.pdf (accessed 23 August 2017).

World Health Organization (WHO) (2009) WHO Guidelines on Hand Hygiene in Health Care. Available at: http://whqlibdoc.who.int/publications/2009/9789241597906_eng.pdf (accessed 23 August 2017).

EMERGENCY CARE

28

CHRIS MULRYAN

THIS CHAPTER COVERS

- Defining first aid
- The ABCDE of resuscitation

- Medical emergencies

REQUIRED KNOWLEDGE

Before reading this chapter, it would be helpful to refresh your anatomical knowledge of:

- the upper airway – www.youtube.com/watch?v=v6jirfdWAGs
- the respiratory system – www.youtube.com/watch?v=x5x19lwPnbo

- the heart and the circulatory system.

VIDEO
LINK:
FIRST AID

My name is Ameet. I am 12 years old and I have learning difficulties. Because of this I have seizures quite often. When I have a seizure I lose consciousness, become tense and my muscles shake. When I wake up I am very disorientated and it can be quite frightening, especially if I have injured myself. Having a nurse around who knows how to keep me safe during my seizures and who can help me recover is very reassuring.

Ameet, patient

I was on placement in a small community hospital when a patient was brought in by their relative after collapsing. There was only me and one trained nurse on shift in the nearest department. The patient had no pulse. Having the knowledge of CPR and the confidence of performing chest compressions in an A&E department previously made me feel confident to deal with the situation. When the crash team showed up and an ambulance did arrive, there was more disorder than in an A&E resus environment. The ambulance crew that arrived had technicians, not paramedics, which meant that they would not be able to administer drugs. There was no one leading the times of the rounds of CPR. Therefore I took up the role of timing the rounds of CPR, stating when to check for a pulse and when to shock. I felt comfortable doing this as I knew how important this was, but when there were highly trained medical staff present, I thought it more important that they take over the physical care of the patient.

Laura Grimley, adult nursing student

INTRODUCTION

Have you ever heard the question 'Is there a nurse or a doctor in the house?' The presence of a nurse at a time when a person is sick or injured can be tremendously reassuring for members of the public. Indeed, one of the fundamental expectations of the public is that a nurse is able to care and provide first aid when someone is taken ill and manage that patient safely and effectively until such a time that the patient has recovered or been handed over to more definitive emergency care providers. The ability to 'cope' when someone becomes seriously sick or injured may well appear to be an impressive endowment, though in reality the effective management of a sick or injured person really involves nothing more than having an ability to remain calm and a knowledge of what to do. Knowing what to do is what enables you to remain calm in the face of an emergency.

This chapter will introduce you to the 'what to do' when faced with an emergency. It will enable you to recognise individuals whose health is at risk and then safely initiate care in an effective manner. Doing this will provide you with a structured system through which you can approach all health-related emergency situations. This system, the 'ABCDE of resuscitation', will remain with you throughout your career and will be built on as you progress through your nursing degree and into your professional life. It is this system that is common to all emergency care, from the most basic of first aid to the most advanced life support techniques, with each one striving to ensure a clear airway, effective breathing and a competent circulation: the requisites for life.

DEFINING FIRST AID

The International Liaison Committee on Resuscitation First Aid Task Force has defined first aid and the characteristics that should be expected from a first aid provider: 'First Aid is the helping behaviours and initial care provided for an acute illness or injury' (Zideman et al., 2015). In this same guideline, the Committee asserts that first aid can be initiated by anyone in any situation. This is a point which is also supported by the Resuscitation Council UK (2015a) which not only emphasises but also encourages the use of automated external defibrillators by an individual with no prior training in an emergency situation. Zideman et al. (2015) state that 'A First Aid Provider is defined as someone trained in first aid who should:

recognise, assess and prioritise the need for first aid

provide care using appropriate competencies

recognise limitations and seek additional care when needed.'

These characteristics are supported by the goals of first aid which are to:

1. Preserve life
2. Alleviate suffering
3. Prevent further illness or injury, and promote recovery.

Preserving life is concerned with those first aid activities which can be directly life-saving. These activities include things like clearing an obstructed airway, performing cardiopulmonary resuscitation and defibrillation or stopping catastrophic bleeding. The alleviation of suffering involves activities such as providing compassionate reassurance, or keeping a person warm, as well as responding to those who may be experiencing a panic attack or another acute deterioration in their mental health. Preventing further illness or injury involves protecting the safety of the patient yourself and those around them as well as activity that aims to stabilise a person; cleaning and dressing a wound to prevent infection or keeping a person's head still after a car accident in order to prevent any aggravation of possible spinal injury sustained by the individual are each examples. Promoting recovery is concerned with minimising the effects of an illness. In the initial moments after an injury or illness, it can be difficult to immediately see what actions are associated with promoting recovery; simple acts are needed, like arranging appropriate ongoing care, such as referral to an acute stroke centre for a person who has a suspected stroke.

WHAT'S THE EVIDENCE?

St John Ambulance (2010) Dramatic Numbers Dying. Available at: https://www.theguardian.com/society/2010/apr/12/first-aid-skills-deaths

According to the St John Ambulance charity, dramatic numbers of people are dying due to a lack of first aid knowledge, and up to 150,000 people a year **could be given a chance to live if** more people knew first aid. People die each year in situations where first aid could make a difference, including:

Nearly 900 people who choke to death
2,500 who asphyxiate from blocked airways
29,000 who die from heart attacks.

- Would you feel competent in your ability to help a patient who was choking, had a blocked airway or was having a heart attack?
- Now visit the web page to read the full article and devise a plan to enable you to deliver appropriate first aid to any patient who requires it.

FURTHER READING: FIRST AID SKILLS

In reality, there is a large degree of crossover between first aid interventions and it can be difficult to define one intervention as fitting into one or other of the goals distinctly; the exact distinction will often depend on the patient's condition and the circumstances in which the care is provided. Rather, it is probably more helpful to think about the goals as a cohesive whole that can be used in an emergency situation to guide your thought process about what the current presenting priorities are and how best to respond to them.

THE ABCDE OF RESUSCITATION

The ABCDE (Airway, Breathing, Circulation, Disability and Exposure) of resuscitation provides a focus for all your first aid activities. The term 'resuscitation' can be a little misleading, as it can conjure up an idea that the ABCDE system is only relevant in cardiac arrest situations – this is not the case. Resuscitation, in its wider sense, means returning or restoring a person to their previous state of health. Accepting this broader definition of resuscitation gives the ABCDE system relevance in a much wider range of circumstances. This appreciation of the principles of resuscitation will serve to improve the care of those who are sick or injured by making consideration of the ABCDE a central aspect of the care delivered. This is fundamentally important: many deaths occur needlessly when simple aspects of care – which relate to protection of the airway, support for breathing or circulation – do not occur in the first few minutes after an accident or illness.

In the context of first aid, the ABCDE system can be expanded to 'Drs ABCDE', with the D representing danger, R the response from the patient and S a shout for help from you to engage the assistance of others.

Dangers: Assessing for and making safe (Drs ABCDE)

In emergencies in or out of hospital, you should be acutely aware of any present or emerging dangers that may pose a threat to the health or safety of yourself, any other rescuers and, finally, the sick or injured patient. On encountering an emergency situation, it is mandatory to stop and think what has caused this person to be in need of help, and what dangers exist or could exist in this situation that can cause a threat to health or safety.

While it is easy to forget this aspect of responding to casualties in the hospital setting, where the dangers present are often more limited, in the out-of-hospital setting there is a diverse range of dangers. Always remember that danger can be present in any setting, for example consider the case described in Activity 28.1.

ACTIVITY 28.1: CRITICAL THINKING

You are in university on your way to lunch after the morning's session on emergency care. You come across a man who is lying face down with his torso in a cupboard. The man is wearing overalls.

- What potential dangers might you anticipate in this situation?
- What clues might you find to potential dangers?
- How could you manage the dangers presented by this situation?

ANSWER:
ACTIVITY 28.1

Consideration of dangers is essential if you are to be useful and not further complicate or compromise the rescue of sick or injured patients. There have been numerous occasions in which well-meaning rescuers have fallen into peril by not considering the dangers. The action that you can take when faced with a dangerous situation will depend on a number of factors, including what the danger is, the resources available to you and the level of threat that the danger presents. It is certainly not possible to provide you with a comprehensive and detailed list of the actions that you should take when faced with a dangerous situation, as each situation will be unique and will require careful and ongoing assessment if you are to safely manage the situation.

There are several dangers you could encounter while trying to give first aid you have to be aware of: Having a car being moved in a small space in order that more people and equipment could get to the patient needing CPR. Maintaining a barrier between the member of staff, patient and car. Also thinking of things like the patient's hands, which can get trodden on easily in an emergency situation. When I was assisting with CPR, there was also concern for the patient's dignity as it was in a public space. At the time there were members of the public filming, and barriers were needed along with staff to ask them to stop.

Laura Grimley, adult nursing student

You should centre your activities on identifying the dangers and taking actions to make the situation as safe as possible. Where the threat from an incident is serious – say, in a situation involving chemicals or fire – your emergency care may not extend beyond summoning help from the professional rescue services and keeping yourself and others at a safe distance from the incident. In other incidents where the level of harm is reduced and the risk to your own safety is less, you can consider taking action to reduce the risk of further injuries occurring, for example by stopping traffic or removing sharp objects from the immediate vicinity of the patient and other rescuers.

While on the subject of dangers, it is important to mention infection prevention and control. In many emergency situations, fluids that have the potential to transmit infections may be released from the body into the environment. As such, it is important to follow standard precautions when dealing with emergency situations to prevent onward transmission.

Checking for a response (Drs ABCDE)

Once you are sure it is safe to approach the casualty, the next thing you want to establish is whether the person is responsive. To do this, ask the patient loudly: 'Are you alright?' If you get a response to this question, you know that they are conscious. If there is no response, repeat the question more loudly and give a command such as: 'Are you alright? Open your eyes, stick out your tongue!' Again, if you get a response you know that your casualty is able to understand what you are saying and can obey simple commands, although they may not be fully conscious. If there is still no response, place a hand on the person's forehead to hold the head still and give them a gentle shake, again asking: 'Are you alright? Open your eyes, stick out your tongue!' Figure 28.1 demonstrates this. Remember though that children should not be shaken.

It is important to remember a baby cannot verbalise, so when checking for awareness check if they respond to your voice, your touch, are they making sounds? What type? Are they moving at all in response to what you are doing?

Julie Davis, LD nursing student

'Is the patient responsive?' is not a simple yes-or-no question. Rather, a person's level of responsiveness is measured on a continuum ranging from fully alert to unresponsive. The AVPU scale in Table 28.1 is used to describe, in a very simple way, the level of response gained from the patient. In a first aid situation, the AVPU scale is a simple way of communicating the level of responsiveness to other care providers in a clear and understandable way. As you progress through your nursing programme, you will learn about more detailed methods that can be used to assess a person's level of consciousness, such as the Glasgow Coma Scale (GCS).

It is so important to reassure your patients and try your best to keep them calm, especially if you are concerned about their condition. In my experience anxiety and panic will exacerbate the patient's symptoms/condition; their respiration rate will increase and blood pressure and heart rate will increase.

Charlie Clisby, NQN

Figure 28.1 Assessing a patient for a response

Table 28.1 The AVPU scale

A = Alert

The person is able to interact with their surroundings; they are aware of things going on around them

V = Responds to Voice

The person only responds when there is a coaching verbal stimulus

P = Responds to Pain

The person only responds when a painful stimulus is applied, such as squeezing of the trapezius muscle in the neck or pressure applied over the supraorbital ridge in the eyebrow

U = Unresponsive

The person shows no response at all even when a painful stimulus is applied

Top tip – AVPU

One of the deficiencies of the AVPU scale is that it does not record subtle changes in a person's mental state, which may be an early sign that a person's health is deteriorating. There is quite a significant difference between a person who is alert and a person who is only responsive to voice. Any agitation or new confusion should also signal a need to fully reassess the patient's overall stability and, as such, should be commented on

If the person responds, try to keep them still and attempt to stop any bleeding if necessary. Summon help from other emergency care providers as appropriate. Make sure you provide reassurance to the individual and try to keep them warm using coats or blankets. Observe them very closely for changes in their condition which might signal your need to provide additional care, as described in the following sections in this chapter. Be mindful of any changes in the situation that might also pose a threat to the health and safety of you or the casualty.

Shout (Drs ABCDE)

If the patient does not respond or does not respond fully, you should initially shout for help as you continue your assessment of the patient. When help arrives, you need to ask them to summon the emergency services, whether this be an ambulance if you are out of hospital or the resuscitation team if you are in a hospital setting. If assistance is not forthcoming, continue your assessment while shouting for help; this will help you to both provide the most suitable care for the patient and summon the most appropriate form of help.

Assessing and supporting the airway (Drs ABCDE)

After you have established the individual's level of responsiveness, the next step is to assess and, if necessary, support the individual's airway. The human airway is quite simply the passageway that air uses to enter and leave the body en route to and from the lungs, as is shown in Figure 28.2. Gas exchange takes place in the lungs so that oxygen, necessary for life, can be absorbed into the body and waste carbon dioxide can be excreted. A clear airway is therefore a prerequisite for both effective breathing and, as such, life – as without the ability to breathe, an individual will soon die.

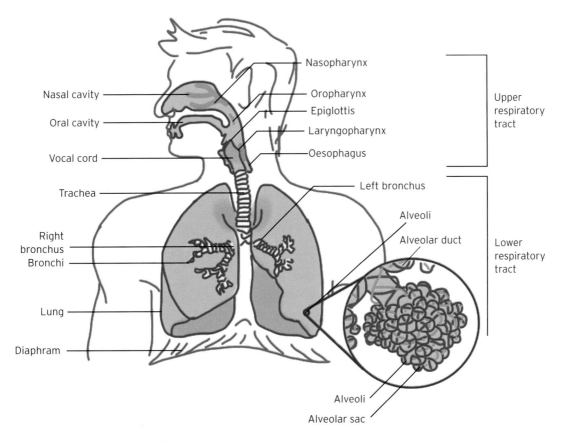

Figure 28.2   The human airway

Image © Robin Lupton

In a healthy patient, a number of protective mechanisms serve to keep the airway clear. At the time of illness or severe injury, these protective mechanisms can be lost and the illness state itself may lead to a change in the anatomy of the airway. Vomiting or the presence of secretions in the airway can make it difficult to maintain a clear airway. A patient therefore becomes dependent on support from rescuers if their life is to be saved. All too often, airway management is an area of care that is overlooked and not given sufficient consideration; the consequence of this is needless deaths. It is essential that, in the acutely ill patient, you ensure that constant attention is paid to care of the airway in order to anticipate potential problems and provide appropriate care when problems present.

Assessing the airway

Key to airway care is your vigilance and your ability to recognise potential or actual airway problems so that you can take action to correct these problems as soon as they occur. In the seriously ill patient, the airway situation can quickly change from one in which it is clear to one in which the airway is obstructed. Ideally, if the number of rescuers allows, you should explicitly delegate to one person specific responsibility for caring for the airway. In doing this, any changes to the integrity of the airway should be immediately recognised, allowing for appropriate care to be provided promptly. Your responsibility will then be to make sure that the person charged with responsibility to care for the airway carries out that role and does not become distracted by other activities. Where a specific rescuer is not available to maintain the airway, ensure that you are mindful of reassessing this often or when the patient's condition changes.

To assess the airway, you need to:

- *Look*: look at the person. If they are anything other than alert, then the airway should be considered at risk. Is there any injury to the neck or anything tightly around it that needs to be removed? Open the mouth and look in (see Figure 28.3a): are there any objects in the mouth – loose teeth, vomit, pieces of food, pen tops, etc.? You must only ever remove items you can see, being careful not to push items deeper into the airway where they may cause a more serious obstruction. Never undertake a 'blind sweep' of a patient's airway to check whether anything you can't see is lodged in it. You may need to roll a person onto their side to remove liquids from the airway. Look for abnormal see-saw movements of the chest and abdomen (not moving in tandem with each other), as this can indicate an obstructed airway.
- *Listen*: listen for any added sounds – normal breathing is relatively quiet. Any snoring, snorting, bubbling or wheezing sounds indicate that the airway is not intact.
- *Feel*: feel for air moving in and out of the mouth. The best way to do this is to perform a 'head-tilt, chin-lift' manoeuvre, and then place your cheek close to the patient's mouth and look towards the chest (see Figure 28.3b).

This sequence is illustrated by Figure 28.3.

(a)

(b)

Figure 28.3 Assessing the airway

Open the mouth and look inside to see if there are any obvious obstructions to the airway. Remove these if possible. Place your head close to the patient, looking along the line of the chest. Can you hear the patient breathing? Can you hear any sounds such as wheezes or bubbling which indicate the airway is obstructed? Can you feel any air moving on your cheek?

The information that you gain from this 'look, listen and feel' assessment of the patient's airway will enable you to form an overall impression of the integrity of their airway. From this you can decide whether the airway is currently safe, at risk or obstructed.

Causes of airway obstruction

These can include anything which causes a physical obstruction to normal air movement in or out of the lungs:

- flaccid tongue and epiglottis
- vomit
- secretions and mucus plugs
- food and other foreign objects
- blood
- swelling of the airway
- strangulation
- trauma
- inhalation burns
- asthma (inflamed airways limit airflow)
- chronic obstructive pulmonary disease (flaccid airways trap air in the lungs on expiration)
- tumour growth inside the airway.

Managing the airway

Thankfully, in many cases the airway can be maintained using simple techniques alone, without any equipment. No matter how simple or complex, airway care is always a solution-focused endeavour. That is to say, you must ask yourself: has the action you have performed relieved the airway problem? If the answer is yes, then carry on with that care and continue to monitor the airway. If the answer is no, then you will need to try alternative methods to secure the airway. It is at this point that you may need skilled help to provide assistance to manage the airway. A further value of applying the Drs ABCDE approach is that you know such help is on its way to you, in order to provide additional assistance to the patient.

The head-tilt, chin-lift

The simplest of all the airway techniques to perform is the 'head-tilt, chin-lift' manoeuvre. This should be the first technique that you attempt when trying to open an airway (Figure 28.3b):

1. Place the head in line with the body.
2. Place two fingers under the chin.
3. Place your hand on the forehead.
4. Lift the chin and at the same time tilt the head back, taking care not to overstretch the neck.
5. Assess to see if this has relieved the airway problem. If so, maintain the position. If the airway is not cleared, you should again shout for help. Try alternative methods and telephone for definitive help.

Jaw-thrust

The jaw-thrust manoeuvre is an alternate method for opening the airway. The jaw-thrust is slightly more difficult to perform than the head-tilt, chin-lift manoeuvre and requires practice to perform correctly. It suffers from the additional disadvantage that once you start to perform a jaw-thrust you are committed to maintaining the position, as should the jaw-thrust be removed, the airway will no longer be held in the open position. The jaw-thrust can also be difficult to maintain even for short periods of time, as it is quite demanding on the hands of the individual performing it. To perform a jaw-thrust manoeuvre, follow the instructions in Figure 28.4.

1.

Position yourself at the head of the patient

Place the tips of your fingers under the angle of the jaw

2.

Place your thumbs on the jaw slightly below the mouth

Pull your fingers up towards you to lift the jaw

3.

Push your thumbs downward towards the patient's feet to open the mouth

Assess to see if this has relieved the airway problem

Figure 28.4   Performing a jaw-thrust manoeuvre

Both the jaw-thrust and the head-tilt, chin-lift manoeuvres open the airway by lifting flaccid airway structures such as the tongue and epiglottis away from the posterior wall of the airway, creating space for air to flow. While these manoeuvres are very effective, they do little to protect the airway from the risk of inhalation of vomit, blood or other secretions. If your patient is breathing normally and you are concerned that their airway is at risk from inhalation of vomit or another substance, then the patient should be placed on their side in the recovery position. If your patient is at imminent risk of cardiac arrest or they are seriously injured, it may not be appropriate to move the patient (Zideman et al., 2007).

Recovery position

The recovery position is a position into which the patient can be placed which allows for the drainage of vomit and secretions from the airway. Many different recovery positions have been described over the years, but important features of any recovery position have been identified by the European Resuscitation Council (Koster et al., 2010), which acknowledges that any recovery position should:

- be stable
- be as close to true lateral position as possible (the patient is on their side)
- have the head dependent (angled downwards)
- have no pressure on the chest which could impair breathing.

The recovery position should be used in spontaneously breathing patients where the need to maintain the airway takes priority over any other injuries that the individual might have. There is evidence that suggests that for patients who are placed in the recovery position, if they should stop breathing there can be delays in recognising this; so if you place a person in the recovery position, continue to check that they are breathing regularly. To place a person in the recovery position, you should follow the instructions in Clinical Skill 28.1.

Care of the cervical spine

When considering airway management, it is also necessary to consider the integrity of the cervical spine. In patients with cervical spinal injuries, movement of the neck can aggravate and in some cases worsen cervical injuries. That notwithstanding, the risk of aggravating cervical injuries historically associated with airway care has probably been overstated. Unstable cervical spinal injuries are rare but deaths from untreated airway obstruction are common. As such, airway care should take precedence, but if there is reason to suspect cervical spinal injury you should only move patients sufficiently to open the airway. The mechanisms of injury that are most commonly associated with cervical spinal injuries include road traffic accidents, falls from a height, rugby scrum collapses and lightning strikes. If spinal injury is suspected, then the jaw-thrust may be theoretically safer than the head-tilt, chin-lift manoeuvre, as the jaw-thrust is considered to produce the least movement of the neck. The priority, however, remains opening the airway.

Assessing and supporting breathing (Drs ABCDE)

Once you have established a clear airway, your next priority is to assess the adequacy of breathing and provide care for any breathing problems that may have developed. Again, use an approach where you look, listen and feel (see Figure 28.3). Ask yourself: is this person breathing normally? This means that they are breathing regularly, moving sufficient air to sustain life. Occasional gasps of breath should be treated as if the person is not breathing, as this is common in the early stages of cardiac arrest and can be misinterpreted as normal breathing. Compare your own breathing pattern with the patient's to estimate if the patient is breathing normally.

   If the person is unconscious and not breathing, or is only making occasional gasps, then you should assume that the person has suffered a cardiac arrest. At this stage, if your shouts for help have been unsuccessful you should telephone for the emergency services yourself. If you have a mobile phone, you can do this without leaving the patient; using the speaker phone option will allow you to talk to the operator while keeping both hands free to provide care. If you do not have a mobile phone, leave

STEP-BY-STEP CLINICAL SKILL 28.1: THE RECOVERY POSITION

☑ **Before you start**

Perform a risk assessment to ensure your safety.

☑ **Field-setting considerations**

You would not put a baby under 1 year old in the recovery position; instead, you would simply hold them with their head tilted downwards, as shown in Figure 28.5.

☑ **Care-setting considerations**

A patient can be nursed in the recovery position in any setting.

Figure 28.5   Recovery position for babies under 1 year old

RECOVERY POSITION GUIDELINES

 Perform a head-tilt, chin-lift airway manoeuvre and confirm a clear airway and that the patient is breathing

To ensure the patient is breathing normally

 Remove any glasses and place the arm nearest to you bent at the elbow out to the side – the so-called 'How position'

To make it easier to roll the patient

3 Place the patient's hand (from the opposite side of the body to which you are located) against the patient's face with the palm facing outwards; place your palm against the patient's

To support their head

4 Lift the leg on the opposite side of the body to which you are located at the knee, keeping the foot on the ground

To assist you to roll the patient

5 Grasp the patient's hip on the opposite side of the body and roll the patient towards you until they are on their side; use your knees to control their body movements and your hand to support the head

Remember to remove any spectacles and any sharp objects from the pockets on the side the person is being rolled on to, to avoid the risk of pressure ulcers developing

6 Position the bent leg so that the knee and hip are at right angles, which acts as a support

Source: Mulryan (2011); Zideman et al. (2015)

To reduce the risk of the patient rolling on to their front, which can impair breathing

7 Tilt the head backwards to ensure that the airway remains open; using the palm as a support, position the head downwards so that secretions or vomit will drain from the airway

To ensure the airway remains clear

8 Get help if this has not already been done and monitor the patient's condition; specifically check that the person is still breathing regularly

The patient is now in the recovery position

9 Ensure the incident is reported to a senior nursing staff/your practice educator if they are not already aware
It is vital to report any abnormal incident to a registered nurse immediately so they can ensure care is escalated. Failure to do so can result in the patient's condition deteriorating, potentially leading to death

10 Document the incident in the patient's notes as appropriate
Maintains patient safety and accurate records

the patient to make the call. While leaving the patient might not feel like the correct action, it is what you must do, because an unresponsive patient is likely to be seriously unwell and you will quickly need skilled assistance to help you manage. If this help is not on its way to you at an early stage, the chances of your patient surviving will be reduced. The only exception to this would be if your patient was a child or if the patient has been a victim of drowning: this will be considered later in the chapter. After specialist help has been telephoned for, you should follow the ABCDE action plan described later, which will involve starting chest compressions and using an automated external defibrillator.

If the person shows signs of life but is not breathing as well as you would like, you can support their breathing using mouth-to-mouth ventilations or a pocket mask. These techniques are illustrated in Figure 28.6. In the in-hospital setting, anyone who is being supported in breathing should also receive supplemental oxygen attached to the device being used to breathe for them.

(a) Mouth-to-mouth expired air resuscitation

(b) Mouth-to-mouth mask expired air resuscitation

Figure 28.6 Methods of supporting breathing

In the patient who is breathing

If the patient is breathing, go on to consider other signs which might indicate that the person is having difficulty with breathing. Ask yourself if the person is using the accessory muscles of the neck or abdomen to assist them with breathing. Does the person have a blue tint to the skin of their face, lips, tongue or chest? This blue discolouration is called cyanosis and is a clear sign that there is a significant reduction in the amount of oxygen in the individual's blood.

Look at the person's chest. Does the chest seem to be moving symmetrically and normally as the person breathes? The chest should move equally upwards and outwards on both sides of the chest as a person inhales, and should fall as the person exhales. If this is not the pattern of movement, then the chest movements are abnormal. Count the respiratory rate. For an adult, the respiratory rate should be 12–20 breaths per minute; any deviation from this is a marker of severe illness. The respiratory rate in children is faster and changes with age (see Table 28.2). Listen to the sounds created by the person's breathing. There may be secretions in the chest which create a bubbling or gurgling sound, or a wheeze occurring on inspiration or expiration, and possibly both. If any of these signs of abnormal breathing are present, you should summon help urgently, as breathing problems can quickly become life-threatening.

In the first aid setting, you are quite limited in terms of the number of interventions you can provide to support breathing. Loosen any tight or constricting clothing across the neck and chest and around the abdomen. Sitting the person up can also assist with and make breathing easier, although do not do this in the case of an individual with multiple injuries or those with a severe allergic reaction (anaphylaxis), as in this context you could worsen the situation. If the person has any prescribed medication, such as an asthma inhaler, you should assist them with taking this.

Table 28.2 Normal respiratory rates in children by age

Age	Respiratory rate per minute
Infant (birth to 1 year)	30-60
Toddler (over 1 year to 3 years)	24-40
Preschool (over 3 years to 5 years)	22-34
School-aged children (over 5 years to 15 years)	18-30
Adolescents (over 15 years to 17 years)	12-16

In the in-hospital setting, you will use pulse oximeters to assess how much oxygen is in the blood bound to haemoglobin, and if this becomes low you will be able to initiate oxygen therapy when trained to do so.

Assessing and supporting circulation (Drs ABCDE)

If the person is not breathing normally, is making occasional gasps or is not breathing at all, you should immediately start external chest compressions. If an automated external defibrillator (AED) is available, you should ensure that this is brought to the patient's side so that the person can be defibrillated if the machine advises. Many shopping centres, train stations, airports, gyms, schools and universities now have AEDs available for public use in the case of an emergency; send someone to find one in such a setting.

To perform external chest compressions, place the heel of one hand in the centre of the patient's chest, place the other hand directly on top of the first hand and interlock your fingers. Lift your fingers clear of the chest so that only the heel of your hand is in contact with the breastbone. Position your shoulders directly above the patient's chest and, with your elbows locked so that your arms are completely straight, push downward at least 5 cm (in the case of an adult casualty). After each compression, release the pressure so that the chest returns to its original shape, then repeat the compression, aiming for a rate of 100–120 per minute. The correct technique for performing chest compressions is shown in Figure 28.7.

(a)   (b)

Figure 28.7 Correct position for chest compressions

(a) Shoulders directly above the patient's chest with your arms completely straight and locked at the elbow.
(b) Hands placed in the centre of the chest with only the heel of your hand in contact with the chest.

When you have delivered 30 chest compressions, you should ideally give the patient two 'rescue' breaths if you are trained and able to do so. To perform mouth-to-mouth, you should pinch the patient's nose closed and open your mouth as if you are about to take a bite of a big apple. You then seal your lips around the patient's lips and blow into the patient's mouth just enough to see the chest rise; take about one second to deliver the breath. Alternatively, a pocket mask provides a physical barrier between you and the patient. If such a device is available, you can use this technique to perform mouth-to-mask resuscitation. This is illustrated in Figure 28.6.

After the first breath is delivered, move your head away from the patient, take a breath of fresh air and then deliver a second breath to the patient. Immediately after this breath is given, start cycles of 30 chest compressions interspaced with two breaths. Continue this until an automated defibrillator is available or medical help arrives and takes over. If you decide that you do not want to deliver rescue breaths or you are not able to make the chest rise with the breaths that you deliver, then perform chest compressions continuously. You should stop resuscitation only when the patient starts to show signs of life – that is, they start to breathe normally – or you become too exhausted to continue. When an automated external defibrillator becomes available, you should attach this to the person with as little interruption to chest compressions as is possible.

Automated external defibrillation

Defibrillation is the definitive treatment for certain types of cardiac arrest. For defibrillation to be most effective in terminating cardiac arrest and restoring a normal heart rhythm, it must be applied as soon as possible after cardiac arrest occurs, as chances of success diminish with every second that passes. To facilitate early defibrillation, automated external defibrillators (AEDs), which talk you through the process of defibrillation, have been developed. These AEDs have massively simplified the process of defibrillation, meaning that defibrillation can be provided by literally anyone. Even those without formal training can safely and effectively defibrillate using an AED. There are many examples of

1 Turn the AED on. Remove clothes from the patient's chest. Aim to interrupt chest compressions as little as possible

2 Open the defibrillator pads and apply these to the patient's chest as illustrated on the pads

3 If not already connected, connect pads to the defibrillator. Push the analyse button if present and follow the instructions given by the AED

4 If instructed to do so ensure everyone is clear of the patient including yourself and push the shock button

5 Restart chest compressions as soon as the shock is delivered. Carry on following the instructions from the AED until the patient recovers or help takes over the patient's care

Figure 28.8   Procedure for using an AED

members of the public, cabin crew, swimming pool lifeguards, police and security guards having used AEDs successfully and saved lives. As such, nurses, including nursing students, should be trained and empowered to use AEDs should the need arise. Where an AED is available, you should make every effort to use such a device as soon as possible, as the impact of early defibrillation is life-saving. The basic procedure for using an AED is illustrated in Figure 28.8.

My first experience as a student nurse in a medical setting with a cardiac arrest was in A&E. The patient had been in majors and needed to go to resus. The patient was elderly and frail. I was asked to be ready to do chest compressions. Just as I was about to do this further news of the patient's history and relatives' wishes was received. CPR was stopped. I found this experience particularly challenging after the event, as it was the first death I had experienced since my father two months earlier. Luckily I had an understanding practice educator, who allowed me to take my break and decompress after the event. I had the events and reasoning behind decisions explained to me. I feel that compartmentalising and mindfulness are important for dealing with difficult situations. I find CPR on frail and terminally ill patients difficult. If you are successful in reviving the patient, the patient's prospect isn't good. My greatest fear is breaking ribs, or equally not performing efficient CPR.

Laura Grimley, adult nursing student

Resuscitation in children

Cardiac arrest in children is, thankfully, a rare event; however, when a child needs resuscitating, this is one of the most challenging situations that you will ever face. Children's bodies are obviously smaller than those of adults; their physiology is slightly different and the reasons why they become so sick as to require resuscitation are often quite different from the causes seen in adults. As such, the techniques required to resuscitate children are slightly different from those which are used on adults. That said, however, the principles of resuscitation for children mimic those for adults and, with a few simple modifications, the procedures described in this chapter can be applied to children.

All too often, people withhold necessary resuscitation in children as a result of fear that they may injure a child. This fear, however, is not borne out in the evidence. You should remember that some resuscitation is better than no resuscitation! It is perfectly safe to apply the adult procedures described in this chapter with the following modifications:

- Use either the head-tilt, chin-lift or jaw-thrust manoeuvre to open the airway. However, do not tilt the head too far back or apply pressure to the fleshy part of the chin or neck, as this can obstruct the airway.
- Give five initial rescue breaths at the start of resuscitation to fully oxygenate the lungs – many cardiac arrests in children are caused by a lack of oxygen. In babies and very small children, you can seal your mouth around both the nose and mouth. In older children, you will need to pinch the nose closed and seal around the mouth, as in the case of adults. Paediatric pocket masks are available.
- To compress the chest: in infants under 1 year of age, use the tips of two fingers in the centre of the chest. In older children, use the heel of one hand on the lower half of the breastbone. In children with a larger build, around puberty, compress the chest as described for adults.
- You should aim to compress the chest by at least one third of its depth at a ratio of 15 chest compressions to two breaths.

- If you are on your own, you should consider performing one minute of resuscitation before leaving the child to call for help, as this may help to improve the outcome.
- If a child is not breathing and has no pulse, you can use an AED. Some AEDs are supplied with special paediatric pads or a paediatric mode. If these are present then use them, but adult defibrillators should be used if no other device is available.

Circulation assessment in the person who shows signs of life

If the person shows signs of life, then you should think about how you can help to prevent and limit the impact of shock on the patient. A patient in shock would have a low blood pressure and a slow capillary refill time (CRT). One of the most common causes of shock is blood loss, so you need to know how to manage bleeding.

Control of external haemorrhage

As external bleeding is one of the major causes of shock, being able to competently control this is a fundamentally important skill in the prevention and treatment of shock. External bleeding can occur for a range of reasons and the exact method of bleeding control will depend on the type of injury that has occurred. Some bleeding may be torrential and spurting in pulses from a wound, this can quickly become life-threatening; you should aim to stop this as a priority and possibly before attending to the airway. Think catastrophic haemorrhage first! Blood which is pulsing out indicates arterial bleeding in a person who still has a heartbeat. Once the blood is lost, it cannot easily be replaced. Prioritise bleeding control in such circumstances, especially if the patient is talking or crying out. Blood which is trickling from a wound suggests venous bleeding and oozing suggests capillary bleeding. While oozing may appear less dramatic with smaller volumes lost, if there is a large area of oozing or multiple small sites of oozing, the comparatively small amount of blood lost from each of these sites quickly adds up to a large volume and as such they should not be ignored, though in these circumstances the standard DRs ABC system is likely the most appropriate way to proceed.

When you are faced with a patient who is bleeding from a wound, make a rapid assessment of the wound itself; consider if there are any foreign objects embedded in the wound or whether there are fractures protruding from the wound. Also, consider the degree of bleeding and the colour of the blood that is being lost; arterial blood is likely bright red with venous and capillary blood a darker red. If the wound is free from embedded objects, your first objective is to firmly apply direct pressure over the wound. Ideally, use a sterile, absorbent dressing pad, though in an emergency any absorbent, clean material will suffice. The amount of pressure that you apply should be proportionate to the amount of blood lost. If bleeding can be controlled with light pressure, this is sufficient; increase the amount of pressure that is applied until the bleeding is controlled. Apply a bandage so that pressure is applied over the wound and the edges of the dressing pad are sealed. If no absorbent material is available, ask the patient to apply direct pressure to the wound themselves using their own hand. If the patient is not able to do this, then you or an assistant will need to apply the pressure, for which you should wear protective gloves and eye protection if blood is spurting from the wound. If the bleeding comes though the dressings you have applied, then apply a second and increase the amount of pressure applied by manually pressing over the dressed wound. The pressure will need to be applied in a sustained manner rather than in short bursts; resist the tendency to release pressure to see if the wound has stopped bleeding. If blood has ceased coming through the dressing, then your interventions are effective and you should continue doing this until help arrives. If the bleeding still comes through the second dressing, you should assume it has not been controlled by the direct pressure alone. Do not remove any of the dressings that you have already applied as this will disrupt any clotting that has managed to occur, and continue to apply firm pressure to the wound and proceed to the next section.

Bleeding not controllable by direct pressure

Where the bleeding has not responded to direct pressure alone, there are two first aid options available for treatment – the application of a tourniquet or a haemostatic dressing. A tourniquet is a band of material with a plastic bar which is placed around a limb; the plastic bar is then used to tighten the band to such a degree that arterial blood is prevented from entering the entire limb, hence preventing further blood loss. Commercially available tourniquets are available and these are preferable to improvised devices which can be fashioned from belts or bandages and a rigid object – the latter should be used only when haemorrhage is not controllable by any other means. Ideally, training in the use of a tourniquet should be undertaken as its use in uncontrolled bleeding can be life-saving. Whenever you apply a tourniquet, note down the time of its application and hand this information over to the emergency services.

Haemostatic dressings are specialised dressings which contain a material which promotes blood clotting. They come in the form of both impregnated gauzes and granules. They are particularly useful in controlling haemorrhage from wounds which are not amenable to tourniquet placement, such as a wound high up on the thigh or in non-compressible haemorrhage like a penetrating wound into the abdomen. Again, the use of these should be supported by specific training but you should know about these and where you can locate them in an emergency.

If there is an object embedded in the wound, then pressure should be applied at the edges of the wound, not over the embedded object as this can push it in, making the wound worse. As soon as is practicable after this, a dressing should be built up around the object embedded in the wound to both stem the bleeding and support the object. You must never remove objects from a wound as this can make bleeding from the wound significantly worse. This is certainly a situation where tourniquets and haemostatic dressings have a role.

Disability (Drs ABCDE)

Once the Drs ABC have been assessed and treated as necessary, you should move on to consider if there is any impairment to the neurological functioning of the patient. In simple terms, here you are seeking to establish if there are any problems with the functioning of their brain and nervous supply.

Establishing the level of consciousness that a patient is able to maintain is a fundamental part of establishing the level of disability. The AVPU scale (see Table 28.1) assists in this, but the level of consciousness can be established more reliably using, for example, the Glasgow Coma Scale (GCS).

As well as the level of consciousness, you should specifically consider any other factors that can impact on the health of the brain and associated nerves. In a first aid emergency situation, this can be simplified to establishing if the individual has any pain, if their blood glucose is lower than usual or if there are any signs and symptoms of the person having suffered a stroke. You can use the FAST test for this: is the 'Face' drooping? Can they lift their 'Arms' and keep them in the air? Is their 'Speech' slurred at all? 'Test' all three and it is time to call for help if any factor is present.

Exposure (Drs ABCDE)

Once you have dealt with any immediately life-threatening conditions, you can go on to look for any other injuries that the person may have. They may not be immediately aware of these due to a reduction in their level of consciousness, or the presence of another distracting injury which is causing the individual so much pain that they have not actually noticed the additional injuries. This step is called 'exposure', as in the hospital setting it would mean removing the patient's clothes and exposing them so that a thorough examination can be made in order to search for any signs of injury that they may have. In the out-of-hospital setting, it may not be appropriate to remove all of a person's clothes; rather, a systematic 'trauma sweep' of the body can be performed. You must ensure you maintain a patient's privacy and dignity when you do this.

CASE STUDY 28.1: PRECIOUS

Precious is a 21-year-old woman who suffers with an anxiety disorder. Along with this, she has a history of self-harming behaviour. You are on a placement with a mental health team and have been asked to help support Precious while you are on this placement. You note that she has become quite withdrawn after a verbal altercation with one of the other patients. You go to check on Precious and you find that she has cut herself quite badly with the broken edge of a tooth brush which she has embedded in her forearm. Precious goes to pull the tooth brush out of her arm as you approach her:

ANSWER: CASE
STUDY 28.1

- How would you manage this situation?
- What type of pressure would you apply to the wound?
- Could a tourniquet be used safely in this situation? Give the reasons for your answer!

To perform a trauma sweep, start at the patient's head and gently but firmly sweep your hands across each surface of the head, face, neck, chest wall, abdomen, pelvis and legs, not forgetting to return to check the arms in the same way. The assessment must be from head to toe and front to back. As you do this, look to see if it causes the patient any pain and ask them to tell you if it does. Check to see if there is any blood or other fluid loss by looking at your gloves for any signs of contamination after you assess each body area. Feel for the integrity of every structure as you inspect them: are there any abnormal protrusions, or areas of the body that feel softer than expected when compared to the adjacent structures?

ABCDE summary action plan

Clinical Skill 28.2 contains a summary of the actions that you should take in an emergency situation.

Putting it all together

Use the ABCDE summary actions to help you decide how you would act if you were involved in the care of David and Malick (Activity 28.2).

ANSWER:
ACTIVITY 28.2

MEDICAL EMERGENCIES

While the Drs ABCDE approach provides a good foundation for all emergency care, there are two further topics which deserve special mention – seizure and choking – as there are additional care activities that you can deliver in order to enhance patients' care and outcomes.

Seizure

The term 'seizure' requires some clarification, as this is often poorly understood. Seizures formally represent abnormal electrical activity within the brain. A seizure can take many forms, ranging from a partial seizure – where the individual experiences a period of absence from understanding – through to a generalised seizure, where there is likely to be a loss of consciousness and loss of muscle control, which may manifest as a loss of muscle tone or uncoordinated involuntary muscle contractions. It is not uncommon for an episode of incontinence to occur during a seizure and people may also injure themselves. Secondary to the loss of consciousness and muscle control, there may be problems maintaining the patient's airway and breathing.

Seizures can be a feature of many disease processes which interrupt the normal function of the brain. They can occur in conditions as diverse as epilepsy and stroke through to complications of low blood glucose and pregnancy. As such, the definitive management of a seizure will be dependent on the underlying condition which has resulted in the seizure. While simple partial seizures require little first aid care, generalised seizures that result in loss of consciousness and convulsions can benefit significantly from first aid care.

In the individual with a generalised seizure, the priority of first aid care is to establish a clear airway and protect the individual to reduce the risk of them causing injury to themselves. In the hyperacute phase, during which a person may be actively convulsing, definitive management of the airway may be difficult given the resources available to you as a part of the first aid response. Ideally, you will want to place the person in the recovery position; however, you should wait for the convulsions to subside before doing this. While you are waiting for the seizure to subside, you should attempt to prevent physical injury to the person by placing soft padded items between the patient and any surfaces with

STEP-BY-STEP CLINICAL SKILL 28.2: ABCDE SUMMARY ACTIONS

☑ **Before you start**

Perform a risk assessment to ensure your safety.

☑ **Field-setting considerations**

You can apply Drs ABCDE to any patient in any field.

Cardiac arrest in children is a very rare event. Children's bodies are obviously smaller than those of adults, their physiology is slightly different and the reasons why they become so sick and require resuscitation are often moderately different from the causes seen in adults. The techniques required to resuscitate children are different from those which are used on adults. That said, however, the principles of resuscitation for children mimic those for adults and with a few simple modifications, as described in this chapter, can be applied to children.

☑ **Care-setting considerations**

You can use Drs ABCDE in any care setting.

DRS ABCDE GUIDELINES

Danger
Ensure you are not putting yourself in any danger
You will not be able to assist the injured person if you also become injured

Response
Assess responsiveness
To ascertain whether there is anything seriously wrong with the patient, check whether they can respond to you
    Ask the patient loudly: 'are you alright?'

Shout
Shout for help
You will need help in caring for the patient if they are seriously ill, so you need to shout for help and then telephone for either an ambulance or the hospital resuscitation team as soon as you know that your patient is seriously ill

Airway
Assess the airway
If a patient does not have a patent airway, their body will not be able to receive the oxygen it needs, and they will soon die
    Assess their airway by looking for obstruction, listening for sounds and feeling for movement of air

Breathing
Assess the breathing
If a patient is not breathing regularly, they will not be receiving sufficient air to sustain life
    Assessment of the patient's airway in the previous step using the 'look, listen, feel' approach will have provided you with information relating to the patient's breathing. Ask yourself: is this person breathing normally? This means that they are breathing regularly, moving sufficient air to sustain life. If the person is not breathing normally, is making

occasional gasps or is not breathing at all, then you should assume that the patient is in cardiac arrest and call for immediate help, start chest compressions and ensure that an AED is being located and brought to the patient's side

Circulation
Assess the circulation
A patient needs effective cardiac circulation in order to supply their bodily organs with oxygen and nutrients, and then to remove waste products, in order to function effectively

If trained and experienced to do so, check whether the patient has a carotid pulse **at the same time** as assessing their breathing. If a patient is not breathing, it is highly unlikely that they will have a pulse. If the patient does not have a pulse, then you should start external chest compressions

Disability
Assess the neurological system
A patient needs a fully functioning brain and nervous system for the body to function effectively
Establishing the level of consciousness that a patient is able to maintain is a fundamental part of establishing the level of disability

Exposure
Assess for other injuries
Once you have dealt with any immediately life-threatening conditions, you can go on to look for any other injuries that the person may have. They may not be immediately aware of these, due to their level of consciousness being reduced or the presence of another distracting injury which is causing them so much pain that they have not actually noticed the additional injuries

Source: Mulryan (2011); Resuscitation Council (UK) (2015a)

which they may be making contact. At no point should you ever attempt to restrain a person who is having a seizure. Likewise, do not place anything in the individual's mouth. Patients will commonly bite their tongue during a seizure and this may cause bleeding in the mouth, although it is usually only minor; depending on the size of the injury, however, it has the potential to block the airway.

If a person who is known to have epilepsy has a seizure, then it may be that this is a self-limiting event and they will recover without any intervention. You should time the seizure: if it lasts for longer than five minutes, the person takes a long time to recover or they have a second seizure without first fully recovering, then you should call an ambulance or the hospital medical emergency team. If a person without a diagnosis of epilepsy has a seizure, then you should immediately call an ambulance or the hospital medical emergency team, as the cause of this needs to be investigated. Be alert to the fact that the onset of a seizure may signal the onset of a cardiac arrest in some patients; as blood flow to the brain is suddenly reduced, a seizure can occur.

CASE STUDY 28.2: AMEET

You meet Ameet, whose patient voice started the chapter, while you are on a placement at a school for children with learning disabilities. You are sitting at a table with Ameet helping him to practise his spelling when he lets out a loud cry, his muscles become rigid, he slides to the floor and his muscles start to contract. You notice that there is some blood mixed with saliva draining from his mouth. A fellow nursing student comes across to help you and insists that you place some rolled-up gauze in Ameet's mouth to prevent him from biting his tongue further.

(Continued)

ANSWER:
CASE STUDY
28.2

- What is your immediate priority in this situation?
- What actions should you take to help keep Ameet safe?
- Should you use the gauze to prevent Ameet from biting his tongue further?
- What medical care may Ameet need to help terminate his seizure and stabilise his condition?

Choking

Choking – or foreign body airway obstruction, as it is more formally known – is the obstruction of the airway caused by an object which is introduced into the airway. Choking is essentially an airway problem and normally occurs suddenly in the conscious individual who is eating. However, it should not be forgotten that a complete airway obstruction can quickly lead to unconsciousness resulting from hypoxia, and an individual who is found unconscious may well be the victim of choking. By far the most common cause of choking is a bolus of food, although other inhalable objects can also be responsible.

Like many medical emergencies, choking ranges from the most serious type, complete airway obstruction, through to the less serious partial airway obstruction, which may still develop into complete airway obstruction. No matter the degree of airway obstruction, experiencing an episode of choking can be extremely frightening and it is important to recognise this and take firm control of the situation.

When managing a person who is choking, the first priority is to establish if the patient actually is choking. This may seem simple, but patients who are choking can present in an inconsolable state without obvious cause – if the airway is completely obstructed, they will not be able to communicate verbally. If you are caring for a person whom you suspect is choking, it is important that you adopt a confident, firm but caring manner. This is needed in order to quickly gain the trust of the individual who is choking, which is necessary as successful management of choking often requires cooperation from the patient. You should suspect choking in a person who suddenly starts coughing or who is silent and clutching or pointing to their neck. Certain factors, such as the person being engaged in eating at the onset of the episode, are potential clues.

Clinical Skill 28.3 identifies the correct steps to take in order to effectively manage choking.

Figure 28.9   Managing a patient who is choking

As Figure 28.9 shows, encourage the person to cough and then follow the A–E steps:

A—B: Perform up to five back slaps with the heel of your hand in the centre of the patient's back, with the patient leant slightly forwards, using your free hand to support the patient's chest. If back slaps fail to dislodge the obstruction, perform an abdominal thrust, or a chest thrust in children and pregnant women.

C: Make a fist and place it thumbside in towards the patient's abdomen halfway between the belly button and the base of the breastbone.

D: Reach around the patient and grasp your fist from the opposite side.

E: Pull inwards and upwards up to five times to try and dislodge the object. If this is unsuccessful, alternate five back slaps with five abdominal thrusts until the object is dislodged. If the patient loses consciousness at any time, start CPR and call for medical help if you have not yet done so.

Summoning help

In the vast majority of medical emergencies, you will need to summon help. If you are working in the community or in a non-acute hospital setting, it is likely that you will be calling for help from the ambulance service. If you are in an acute hospital setting, then you are likely to have a number of sources of help to select from – this may include the ward or an on-call doctor, critical care outreach services and/or the medical emergency and resuscitation teams. In each setting in which you are working, you should be familiar with the sources of medical help available to you and how you can contact them. Never forget the importance of remembering to call for help: it is always better, for both the patient and yourself, for help to arrive that you don't need, rather than trying to deal with a complex medical emergency alone.

I don't really know what happened. I was babysitting my little niece Ellie. It was about a week after her first birthday and she was sitting on the floor munching on some dry cereal. One must have gone down the wrong tube. I had never been so scared in my life. She started choking. Then she wasn't making any noise at all. Her eyes got huge. I am so glad I took a CPR class before she was born. At first I was worried I was going to hurt her but after a few back blows she spat out the cereal and started crying. That's when I knew she was going to be okay. I never thought I would be so relieved to hear her cry. I was terrified to tell her mum. I am not sure she is going to ever let me babysit again!

Robin, Ellie's very nervous auntie

Apply your understanding of caring for a person who is choking by reading Marjory's case study, at https://study.sagepub.com/essentialnursing2e.

STEP-BY-STEP CLINICAL SKILL 28.3: MANAGEMENT OF CHOKING

☑ **Before you start**

Perform a risk assessment to ensure your safety.

☑ **Field-setting considerations**

If the patient who is choking is a child, there are two differences in the procedure. First, the force of any actions should be reduced. Second, abdominal thrusts are unsafe in infants under 1 year of age and chest thrusts should be used in place of abdominal thrusts. Babies can be picked up and placed with their head positioned downwards, supported on your arm. Larger children can be draped across your knee if you are in a stable sitting position. This again will enable the child's head to be positioned downwards.

☑ **Care-setting considerations**

Choking can be managed in any setting.

CHOKING GUIDELINES

1 **Ask the conscious person: 'are you choking?' If the person confirms this, carry on. If not, look for an alternative cause**
To ensure the person is choking

2 **Assess the severity of the episode. If the person has an effective cough, then the incident is likely to be less severe. Encourage the person to cough: this should be sufficient to clear the obstruction**
If the person can cough, you need to remain with them offering reassurance, but encouraging them to cough is the most effective way of clearing the obstruction. Closely monitor the person for signs of the cough becoming ineffective

3 **If there is no coughing or the cough does not appear to be effective, then you will need to perform back slaps. If possible, and if the person is not already in a standing position, stand them up and lean them forwards**

The person requires your assistance to clear the obstruction
This is an effective position for delivering back slaps

4 **Stand at the side of the patient and place one hand on their chest to support them**
To ensure the patient is safe

5 **Then slap them firmly between the shoulder blades using the heel of your hand. Do this up to five times or until the obstruction is cleared**
The procedure for performing back slaps is illustrated in Figure 28.9

6 **If the airway obstruction persists after you have performed five back slaps, then you will need to proceed to perform abdominal thrusts. Stand behind the patient and make a fist using your right hand. Place**

your fist thumbside first, halfway between the patient's belly button and the base of the rib cage

Reach around the patient from the opposite side with your left hand and grasp your fist. Next, pull sharply inwards and upwards while at the same time bending the person forwards. Again, repeat this up to five times or until the obstruction is released. Keep your head to one side of the patient's, so their head does not hit you as it comes back

The procedure for performing abdominal thrusts is illustrated in Figure 28.9

Chest thrusts present an alternative to abdominal thrusts when abdominal thrusts are not possible or are unsafe. Obesity in the patient makes abdominal thrusts difficult to perform and pregnancy makes abdominal thrusts unsafe. You would also never perform abdominal thrusts on a child under 1 year of age. Chest thrusts are performed in a similar way to abdominal thrusts, the principal differences being that chest thrusts are performed in the middle of the chest and the force applied is inwards more than inwards and upwards, as is the case in abdominal thrusts

7 **If, after you have completed the five abdominal thrusts, the airway remains obstructed, continue to repeat cycles of**

five back slaps with five abdominal/chest thrusts until the airway obstruction is relieved or the patient loses consciousness. If the patient losses consciousness, then immediately start cardiopulmonary resuscitation, starting with chest compressions

This in itself may be effective in clearing the obstruction

8 **Any patient who has undergone either abdominal or chest thrusts should be evaluated by a doctor**

Both of these first aid interventions can cause injury to the individual. This is the case even if the immediate airway compromise has been completely relieved

9 **Document the incident in the patient's notes as appropriate**

Maintains patient safety and accurate records

10 **Ensure the incident is reported to a senior nursing staff/your practice educator if they are not already aware**

It is vital to report any abnormal incident to a registered nurse immediately so they can ensure care is escalated. Failure to do so can result in the patient's condition deteriorating, potentially leading to death

Source: Mulryan (2011); Resuscitation Council (UK) (2015b)

ACTIVITY 28.3: REFLECTION

Much of this chapter has focused on the recognition of and response to individuals who become seriously ill or injured. The interventions described in this chapter have largely assumed that the individual's condition is reversible. However, in the case of a significant number of individuals, both in hospital and the community, resuscitative interventions cannot rectify their underlying diseases. In such cases, there is the potential for significant harm to be created should inappropriate resuscitation efforts be pursued.

- Reflect on circumstances in which resuscitation efforts may be considered inappropriate.
- Discuss with a fellow nursing student and then an experienced nurse how you might best address situations where resuscitation may be inappropriate.

(Continued)

- How could you potentially manage a situation where a patient's relative tells you that they forbid the performance of resuscitation on their loved one?

The *Decisions Relating to Cardiopulmonary Resuscitation* document, published jointly by the British Medical Association, The Resuscitation Council (UK) and the Royal College of Nursing (2016), will assist you in reflecting on these questions.

CONCLUSION

The ability to deliver appropriate first aid interventions in a wide range of situations, both in and out of a hospital setting, is an important skill that all nursing students need to acquire. It is possible to apply the Drs ABCDE approach to all situations, and to use it as a guide to ensure you correctly provide the care necessary. There is no secret ingredient in the ability to 'cope' when someone becomes seriously sick or injured – it is applying the Drs ABCDE approach that enables you to remain calm in the face of an emergency.

In essence, there are three things you need to remember whenever you become involved in an emergency situation. First, never place yourself or the patient in further danger; second, apply the Drs ABCDE approach; and third, call for help from skilled emergency care providers as soon as you think it might be required.

CHAPTER SUMMARY

- The goals of first aid are to preserve life, limit worsening of the condition and promote recovery.
- The Drs ABCDE approach is helpful in all emergency situations.
- To achieve the priorities of first aid, pay attention to ensuring a clear airway and effective breathing and circulation.
- Early good-quality cardiopulmonary resuscitation and defibrillation offer the best chance of survival for a patient who suffers a cardiac arrest.
- External bleeding can often be controlled by applying direct pressure to a wound. If there are objects in the wound, pressure at the side of the wound should be applied, while tourniquets and hemostatic dressings may be helpful.
- Never forget to call for help as soon as you realise you might need it.

CRITICAL REFLECTION

Holistic care

This chapter has highlighted the fundamental importance of first aid when providing care for patients. However, while it is necessary to correctly deliver the skills of first aid, doing this in a holistic manner is of equal importance. Review the chapter and note down all the instances in which you think that when performing first aid actions you could also meet the patient's wider physical, psychological, social, economic and spiritual needs. Think of a variety of different patients across the fields, not just within your own field. You may find it helpful to make a list and refer back to it next time you are in practice, and then write your own reflection after your practice experience.

GO FURTHER

Books

Mulryan, C. (2011) *Acute Illness Management*. London: SAGE. *Acute Illness Management* expands on this chapter, providing greater detail about the physiology of acute illness as well as guidance on the medical management of the airway, breathing and circulation, including the use of equipment that is commonly found in ambulances and hospitals.

St John Ambulance, St Andrew's First Aid and the British Red Cross (2016) *First Aid Manual*. London: Dorling Kindersley. This is the authorised first aid manual of all three of the major voluntary first aid organisations that operate in the UK. While this book is aimed at lay individuals undertaking a first aid course, the text is authoritative and is a useful read for those learning about first aid for the first time.

SAGE journal article

Go to https://study.sagepub.com/essentialnursing2e for free online journal articles for this chapter. If you are using the interactive ebook, simply click on the book icon in the margin to go straight to the resource.

FURTHER
READING:
JOURNAL
ARTICLES

Ketilsdottir, A., Albertsdottir, H.R., Akadottir, S.H., Gunnarsdottir, T.J. and Jonsdottir, H. (2014) 'The experience of sudden cardiac arrest: Becoming reawakened to life', *European Journal of Cardiovascular Nursing*, 13(5): 429–35. A study describing the experiences of survivors of sudden cardiac arrest and resuscitation.

Other journal articles

British Thoracic Society (BTS) (2017) 'BTS guideline for oxygen use in adults in healthcare and emergency settings', *Thorax*, 72: i1–i90. Oxygen therapy is an important part of care for people who develop a problem with breathing that is severe enough to compromise their oxygen saturation when measured by a pulse oximeter. This BTS guideline describes how oxygen should be administered and titrated against the individual's response. This is a very important read for anyone involved in the administration of oxygen.

Devi, W. R. (2017) 'Effectiveness of video assisted teaching on CPR (cardiopulmonary resuscitation) for children among student nurses', *International Journal of Nursing Education*, 9 (3): 37. An interesting study investigating how much knowledge nursing students have on CPR for children

Kenny, G., Bray, I., Pontin, D., Jefferies, R. and Albarran, J. (2017) 'Original research: A randomised controlled trial of student nurse performance of cardiopulmonary resuscitation in a simulated family-witnessed resuscitation scenario', *Nurse Education in Practice*, 2421–26. This randomized controlled trial, conducted in a UK University nursing department, compared student nurses' performance during a simulated cardiac arrest. The results are very interesting!

Weblinks

Go to https://study.sagepub.com/essentialnursing2e for weblinks related to this chapter. If you are using the interactive ebook, simply click on the book icon in the margin to go straight to the resource.

FURTHER
READING:
WEBLINKS

International Federation of Red Cross and Red Crescent Societies (2016) International First Aid and Resuscitation Guidelines 2016. Available at: www.ifrc.org/Global/Publications/Health/First-Aid-2016-Guidelines_EN.pdf. One of the first documents to analyse the evidence base for many of the first aid interventions which are undertaken. It highlights a number of areas where there is little evidence base for historic practice and provides new and clear guideline statements where these are needed.

Royal College of Physicians (RCP) (2012) *National Early Warning Score (NEWS): Standardising the Assessment of Acute-illness Severity in the NHS*. London: RCP. Available at: www.rcplondon.ac.uk/sites/default/files/documents/national-early-warning-score-standardising-assessment-acute-illness-severity-nhs.pdf. Early warning scoring systems are a helpful adjunct to the recognition of deteriorating patients. This paper describes the recently introduced National Early Warning (NEW) scoring system which overcomes some of the problems which have been traditionally associated with such scoring systems.

www.nhs.uk/conditions/accidents-and-first-aid/Pages/Introduction.aspx – information on accidents, first aid and treatments by NHS Choices.

www.resus.org.uk – the website of the Resuscitation Council for the UK. Here you can find evidence-based information about resuscitation, including guidelines not only for clinical practice but also training standards, equipment provision and medico-legal issues, as well as information relating to the ethics of resuscitation and how decisions relating to the appropriateness of resuscitation in a given case can be found. You will also find here 'Lifesaver', an interactive emergency simulation which you can go through online.

www.sja.org.uk – the website of St John Ambulance, a UK-based first aid charity which offers first aid advice and training courses.

www.nice.org.uk/cg50 – this NICE guideline, *Acutely Ill Patients in Hospital*, examines the issues that surround the early recognition of acutely ill patients and provides guidance on the minimum standards of care that should be provided in order to recognise the acutely ill patient. It also details the systems and structures that should be in place to ensure that the needs of patients identified as being acutely ill are responded to appropriately.

www.survivingsepsis.org – the website of the Surviving Sepsis campaign provides evidence-based guidelines on the definition of the sepsis syndromes, assessment of the severity of sepsis and care bundles that together serve to improve the outcome of an individual with sepsis.

Video links

VIDEO
LINKS

Have a break from the text and go to https://study.sagepub.com/essentialnursing2e for useful videos related to this chapter. If you are using the interactive ebook, simply click on the lightbulb icon in the margin to go straight to the resource.

————— ACE YOUR ASSESSMENT —————

ONLINE
QUIZZES

Review what you have learned by visiting the book's online resources at: https://study.sagepub.com/essential nursing2e If using your interactive ebook, just click on the icon in the margin to go straight there.

- Test yourself with multiple-choice and short-answer questions.
- Revise key terms with the interactive flash cards.

REFERENCES

British Medical Association, Resuscitation Council (UK) and Royal College of Nursing (2016) *Decisions Relating to Cardiopulmonary Resuscitation*. London: Resuscitation Council UK.

Koster, R.W., Baubin, A.M., Bossaert, L.L., Caballero, A., Cassan, P., Castrén, P., et al. (2010) 'European Resuscitation Council Guidelines for Resuscitation 2010 Section 2: Adult basic life support and use of automated external defibrillators', *Resuscitation*, 81(10): 1277–92.

Mulryan, C. (2011) *Acute Illness Management*. London: SAGE.

Resuscitation Council (UK) (2015a) *Resuscitation Guidelines 2015*. London: Resuscitation Council (UK).

Resuscitation Council (UK) (2015b) Prevention of Cardiac Arrest and Decisions about CPR. Available at: www.resus.org.uk/resuscitation-guidelines/prevention-of-cardiac-arrest-and-decisions-about-cpr (accessed 6 December 2017).

St John Ambulance (2010) Dramatic Numbers Dying. Available at: www.theguardian.com/society/2010/apr/12/first-aid-skills-deaths

Zideman, D.A., De Buck, E.D.J., Singletary, E.M., Cassand, P., Chalkias, A.F., Evans, R., et al. (2015) 'European Resuscitation Council Guidelines for Resuscitation 2015 Section 9: First aid', *Resuscitation*, 95: 278–87.

MEDICINES ADMINISTRATION

CAROL HALL

THIS CHAPTER COVERS

- Medicine optimisation and holistic person-centred care
- Administering medicines
- Calculating the right dose

REQUIRED KNOWLEDGE

- It is essential to have a basic understanding of pharmacology, including how medicines act on the body, and an awareness of commonly used groups of medicines, such as analgesics, antipyretics, antihistamines, steroids, antibiotics and medicines used in cardiac arrest.

> " I am 10 and I have asthma and eczema – I am allergic to everything! To stop my skin from itching, I have to have a lot of creams and for my asthma I have inhalers. I can do these myself now, which is good because I need to have them at school. Last month I had a bad asthma attack and ended up in hospital again for three days and had lots of inhalers and medicines, and my mum stayed with me.
>
> **Cheng Lei, patient** "

> " Cheng is 10 years old now and has been a patient since he was a baby. He has to take a lot of medication. When he was a little boy, we taught his mum to give him his medicines and worked with the community nursing team so that he could be managed at home. Cheng's mum is great – she has learned how to manage his care holistically and flexibly at home and to recognise the signs of an asthma attack so they can take action quickly. We still give him his medicines if he is admitted to hospital and he is very unwell, but as his condition improves we are working with Cheng and his family to support him as he learns to manage his condition more independently.
>
> **Martin, registered child nurse** "

Visit https://study.sagepub.com/essentialnursing2e to access a wealth of online resources for this chapter – watch out for the margin icons throughout the chapter. If you are using the interactive eBook, simply click on the margin icon to go straight to the resource.

INTRODUCTION

Cheng's story outlines the wide-ranging care you will provide as a nurse to ensure your patients receive their medicines optimally. His story identifies that you may work in a hospital or in the community, possibly as a school nurse or in a community outreach service. Cheng's story also illustrates one example of the changing relationship which you may have with your patients, depending on whether they are assessed as independent and able to self-medicate, need some assistance or are completely dependent on nursing care. This may be due either to the medication to be administered or to your patient's capacity to manage independently, because of their developmental stage or their mental capacity.

This chapter intends to focus on the core skills surrounding the administration of medicines as this remains an essential of nursing practice through which students begin their clinical learning in the area of medicines management. Registrants of nursing will need to take further many concepts of medicine management by the time they reach registration and these additional components will be introduced in this chapter, with reading signposted to support further learning.

Medicine administration is identified by the Nursing and Midwifery Council (NMC) as:

> an important part of the professional practice of persons whose names are on the Council's register. It is not solely a mechanistic task to be performed in strict compliance with the written prescription of a medical practitioner (or independent or supplementary prescriber). It requires thought and the exercise of professional judgement. (NMC, 2004, cited in NMC, 2007: 3)

This concept is critically important, as the media-inspired perception of nurses as focused on giving out pills, liquids and injections is often evident when people are asked what it is they think that nurses do. However, it may be that the full extent of this role – the knowledge required to effectively enable and evaluate treatment and to be able to fully integrate medicines holistically within a person's life – is not fully appreciated. In the future, newly qualified nurses may require the knowledge and skills to be ready to prescribe medicines and this will require further development of your understanding of the whole arena of medicines management.

This chapter will help you to understand your fundamental role as a nursing student in supporting medicines assessment and administration, and prepare you to achieve the NMC requirements for registration as you progress through your studies. The complementary element of nurse prescribing will be introduced and resources will be signposted to assist in your learning. However, it must always be remembered that, as a nursing student, you must never administer or supply medicinal products without direct supervision (NMC, 2007). Throughout this chapter, you will be guided to consider what medicine administration means to patients and their families or carers, exploring your role and appreciating how it changes as your knowledge increases and you become a registered nurse.

MEDICINE OPTIMISATION AND HOLISTIC PERSON-CENTRED CARE

As individuals, patients will have personal preferences and it is important for you to use your knowledge about their medication to be able to empower them. For example, your patient may want to take their medicine before breakfast each morning. This may be possible, but could become more complicated if one of their prescribed medicines includes the instruction 'take *after* food' in order to protect the stomach lining. You may be able to suggest that they take their tablets with a glass of milk in this case, but this would need to be considered in respect of all other treatments if they are taking more than one, because another prescription might require administration before food. This illustrates how a clear understanding of the fundamental principles of pharmacology is a prerequisite for administering medicines. Clearly, if you can work together with a patient to find a routine which suits their lifestyle and the medicines they are taking, you will be better able to optimise both the effects of the medicines and the likelihood that the patient will take them as intended, thus reducing the risk of harm. The above example describes a situation relating to medicines management which involves managing the medicinal treatment and the outcome. This is identified by NICE (2015) as 'medicines optimisation'.

In nursing, you always aim to find solutions through partnership with patients. However, the concept of medicines optimisation also includes compliance with prescription as an outcome, and sometimes negotiation is impossible if your patient will not accept the required prescription. This is challenging, as it involves patient rights and their capacity to consent to or refuse treatment. The outcome of such a situation may differ depending on the field of nursing in which you are practising:

- For capable adults, the choice to refuse ultimately belongs to the patient and the most you could do would be to ensure that the patient is aware of the implications of their choice.
- For children, individuals with a learning disability or those with mental health concerns, however, you may have more considerations.

It is also your role in all areas to understand the patient's viewpoint, to assess their capability for informed consent and to explore the options for those who refuse a prescribed treatment with medicines.

CASE STUDY 29.1: JULIA [COMMUNITY]

Julia is 25 and has recently been diagnosed as having episodes of psychotic behaviour. Following a period in hospital, she is now being cared for in her own home and the community mental health team visit twice a week. It is imperative that Julia receives her medication to manage her psychosis, but she is currently refusing any treatment, as she says that she is better and does not need it any more.

- What would be your priority?
- What specific additional assessments and actions would you perform to ensure Julia's safety?
- What steps could the community mental health team take if Julia continues to refuse treatment?

Your role in medicines administration

Medicines administration practice occurs in the period after an order for a medicine (prescription) has been made. In respect of prescription, this chapter focuses mostly on patient-specific directions (PSD) – which refers to only those prescriptions and medicines orders written specifically for one patient; it is important to know that the administration of medicines may also use patient group directions (PGD) where medicines may be prescribed to a group of patients. Medicines may also be prescribed today by a range of professionals (both medical and non-medical staff, including nurses, midwives and other health practitioners who have met strict criteria for prescribing) and your course of study is likely to include learning in this as you progress towards registration as a nurse.

There are three aspects of medicines administration, which are:

- ensuring the safe and effective storage and administration of medications to patients (or the support of patients or their carers to self-medicate)
- evaluating the impact and effectiveness of the medication given and assessment of any untoward effects
- recording the administration and the outcome.

These may seem quite simple when summarised, but the rest of this chapter will show you that medicine administration is a complex process which requires considerable knowledge and skills to achieve effectively. Your role as a nurse is also a small component of a bigger role undertaken for your patients by the multi-disciplinary team, which is called medicines management.

Medicines management

While medicine administration is mostly subject to professional requirements (NMC, 2007), many of the wider aspects of 'medicines management' are bound by law (MHRA, 2013). As a registered nurse, administering medicines within the wider context of medicines management, it is your role to understand how the complementary parts are bound by core pieces of legislation. These laws are grouped together with other regulations under the umbrella of the Medicine Regulations (2012):

- **1968 Medicines Act** – governs the manufacture, sale and supply of medicines. Medicines can be categorised as:
  - General Sales List (GSL), which can be purchased in retail outlets such as supermarkets
  - Pharmacy Only (P), which can only be purchased in a pharmacy
  - Prescription Only (POM), which must be prescribed by a health professional who is authorised to prescribe
- **1971 Misuse of Drugs Act** – defines medicines within schedules which are restricted further through their danger in public use
- **2001 Nurses and Midwives Act** – enabled nurses (and midwives) to prescribe drugs
- **2006 The Health Act and the Controlled Drugs (Supervision of Management and Use) Regulations** – changed the requirements for controlled drug management.

Storage and supply of medicines

Medicines should always be kept in locked drug cabinets or fridges. The only exception to this is medications required in an emergency, such as during a cardiac arrest. To enable rapid access to these, they are normally kept in a special container (or drug box) that is sealed with a band or easily cut tag. Individual prescriptions and patients' own medications may be kept within a locked cabinet beside a patient's bed or within the ward trolley or cabinet. When not in use and therefore away from continuous attendance, drug cabinets and trolleys should be locked and secured to a wall so that they cannot be removed. Keys should be the responsibility of the nurse in charge of the area, who should know where they are at all times. It is your role in practice to ensure the medicines that patients receive are stored safely. This is to protect the patient and other people. For example, it is important to keep insulin in a locked fridge. Doing this protects the insulin from deteriorating, as it must be kept cool; it also protects patients or others from taking the medication inappropriately (for example, in children's areas) and ensures a regular supply is available, as supplies are likely to be maintained by the pharmacy.

ACTIVITY 29.1: CRITICAL THINKING

You and your practice educator have moved the drug trolley to the middle of a patient area and are administering the 18.00 drugs to patients you have been helping him care for. The cardiac arrest bell goes off and you hear a staff member call for help in the next room.

- What should your practice educator do?

Controlled medicines

For some medicines, controlled under the Misuse of Drugs Act 1971 schedules, there are strict rules around storage and administration in accordance with the Controlled Drugs (Supervision of Management and Use) Regulations 2006. In all nursing fields in acute (hospital) settings, it is necessary to have an identified accountable officer and a set of standardised operating procedures (SOPS) to which practitioners must adhere. This practice is regularly audited and should be managed in accordance with the latest guidance (NICE, 2016).

The SOPS include exact details of processes to which you must adhere. For example, controlled medicines must be transported in a specially sealed pack and the seals must remain intact until the destination is reached. Once delivered to a patient care area, controlled medicines must be counted by an authorised practitioner and kept in a special locked cabinet within a locked drug cupboard. Controlled medicines must be counted daily and on each occasion that any medicine is either supplied by the pharmacy or taken from the cupboard to be used. When a controlled medicine is administered, the record made must include the patient's name and the amount given. If any medication is to be wasted, then the amount discarded must also be recorded. All activities must be completed by an authorised and specifically prepared practitioner, and be witnessed.

I have never been in a community setting and encountered patients holding on to lots of old and out of date medication but if I did I would ask the person if they knew they had a lot of old medication in their home or if it was medication that was no longer needed I would want to know if they were still taking it. I would want to get the permission of the individual to dispose of the medication safely and to go through with them what they are taking and what they are for. I would also want to assess whether the individuals are able to continue to administer their own medication or whether a medipack may be more suitable.

Samantha Vanes, NQ RNMH

Community settings

In community care, where patients are being cared for in their own homes, the rules are different since the medicines are the patient's own prescriptions, but those involved in care should still adhere to NICE guidelines (2016). Nevertheless, it remains part of the nurse's role to ensure that the medicines are optimally stored so that they do not deteriorate, and kept safely away from children or those who may abuse them. A large part of your role will involve educating the patient about using the prescriptions they have been given properly, and making sure they are not stockpiling medicines. This is done for two reasons. The first is to ensure patient safety, because medicines do deteriorate. There may also be an increased risk of misuse or unsafe use of medicines; for example, in patients where there is a suicide risk or where children may easily access medicines. The second reason is that it is wasteful.

FURTHER
READING:
MEDICINES
OPTIMIZATION

WHAT'S THE EVIDENCE?

National Institute for Health and Care Excellence (NICE) (2015) Medicines Optimisation: The safe and effective use of medicines to enable the best possible outcomes. Available at: www.nice.org.uk/guidance/ng5live.

A scoping exercise undertaken by NICE (2015) found the following:

The cost of waste prescription medicines in primary and community care in England is estimated to be £300 million a year, with up to half of that figure likely to be avoidable. An estimated £90 million worth of unused prescription medicines are retained in people's homes at any one time.

Patients and their carers often have inadequate information about their medicines. Up to half of all patients may not be taking their medicines as recommended by the prescriber.

Reflect on the care of a patient you have been involved with in the community setting:

- Did the nurse check what medicines the patient was taking?
- Did they ask how the patient took their medication?
- Did they check whether the patient understood what their medicines were for?
- Did they ask whether the patient had any medicines which they were not using?

Now read the report and consider how you can apply the findings to your practice.

ADMINISTERING MEDICINES

A number of 'rights' are identified to aid you to optimise the medicinal treatment received by patients. While they can really only be considered as a starting point for you as you prepare to administer medicines, they can act as a useful aide memoire for the main features of clinical practice. We will use Hall's (2002) version, which includes eight rights, as this is viewed to be comprehensive, applicable to all settings and all patients, and simple to apply.

> **THE RIGHT MEDICATION**
> is given to
> **THE RIGHT PATIENT**
> at
> **THE RIGHT TIME**
> on
> **THE RIGHT DATE**
> in
> **THE RIGHT DOSE**
> via
> **THE RIGHT ROUTE**
> in
> **THE RIGHT PREPARATION**
> and
> **THE RIGHT DOCUMENTATION**
> is completed

Figure 29.1   Eight rights of medicine administration

Source: Hall (2002)

ACTIVITY 29.2: REFLECTION

Reflect on an experience when you have assisted your practice educator to administer medication to a patient:

- Did they apply the eight rights of medication?
- If not, did they use another, similar system?
- How do the eight rights, or other systems, assist nurses to administer medication safely?

Administering medication to a patient

When administering medication, safety and accuracy are of fundamental importance. As previously identified, there are three stages of the nurse's role with respect to medication. Following the steps outlined in Clinical Skill 29.1, which relate to these stages, will enable you to safely administer medication, either orally or by topical application.

CASE STUDY 29.2: GUY, HIS MUM AND BENJI

Guy is 42 and has a moderate learning disability. He lives with his mum, who is his main carer, and requires only minimal assistance with his daily activities. Guy doesn't like to socialise, preferring to spend most of his time caring for and walking Benji, his dog, a 2-year-old Irish Wolfhound.

Over the last three months, Guy has been feeling increasingly unwell and he has recently been diagnosed with diabetes. He has been prescribed tablets to control his blood sugar, but is very confused about when he should take them and why. His mum has been searching the internet to find out information about diabetes, but she is confused about what she has found and is unclear as to how Guy's condition will be improved by the tablets.

Guy has been up all night because he is very worried about who will look after Benji if he becomes ill, as 'Benji is too big and naughty for Mum to manage'. Guy's mum has brought him to see the practice nurse at his GP surgery, to help her and Guy understand his treatment.

- What type of information is it necessary to share with Guy and his mum to help them to understand his medication?
- Who else could be involved in offering Guy and his mum the support they require?

CALCULATING THE RIGHT DOSE

When administering any medication, it is fundamentally important to calculate the right dose. It is often very much easier to calculate medicines in practice because you have non-verbal cues to help you. Some universities use computer-aided or pictorial packages to help you too. It is good practice to assist your practice educator to work out doses, so you can become experienced in pouring out and measuring the correct amounts. Numeracy for medicines does not end at simply getting the calculation correct, as the medicine still needs to be accurately measured and given to the patient.

There are many ways to work out the calculation and each person may choose a different method. Indeed, you might choose different methods of calculation depending on the complexity of the equation.

STEP-BY-STEP CLINICAL SKILL 29.1: ADMINISTERING MEDICATION (ORAL OR TOPICAL ROUTE)

☑ Essential equipment

- Drug to be administered
- Medication pots (or suitable vessel) to take the drug to the patient in
- Jug of water and clean glasses
- Medicine Administration Record (MAR)

☑ Field-specific considerations

When caring for patients, it is important to remember that many have needs which cross the boundaries of the fields of nursing, so consider all of this information as potentially relevant to the patients you may care for.

It is important at all times to empower all patients with respect to medicine administration.

Learning disability – ensure that the patient and their main carers, as appropriate, are informed about their medicine and about how it assists them. To do this you need to undertake an assessment of the individual's capability. Some people with a learning disability will be able to manage their own medications, while others may need varying amounts of support. The use of preloaded and timed pill boxes may be useful in some cases to establish a regular routine and to ensure that your patient takes the correct medicine. Medication administration records which include a photograph of the individual are frequently used in community settings as they provide a safe method of identifying an individual (as identity bands are unlikely to be worn). Another method can be the use of two identifiers (for instance, name and date of birth as well as photo or ID band).

Mental health – the use of physical and psychological supportive techniques and a good understanding of how your patient feels about their medications will assist you in appreciating the extent to which the monitoring of medications and support is required. Remember that some patients will be receiving treatment under the Mental Health Act, so may not wish to comply with this. It is also important to consider different models of health belief and self-care in establishing the best care possible for your patient. The therapeutic relationship you have with your patient will influence the information they share in respect of their drug treatment. Remember that other forms of treatment, such as psychotherapy, counselling or cognitive behavioural therapies, may be in effect simultaneously with medication. For some patients with mental health problems, including those who are severely depressed or with suicidal tendencies, when administering medicines you must ensure any medicines given to your patient have been taken. It is important to be aware that medicines may be hidden in the mouth and then secretly stockpiled.

Child – encourage, assist and educate children of all ages, as well as their parents or carers, to be involved in the administration of medicines. This will enable you to determine the capabilities the child may have, their likely behaviour and their understanding of the situation. Ensure you tailor your communication skills to reflect the needs of different age groups. An awareness of pharmacology and calculation skills to work out patient-specific drug doses is necessary in all fields, but as many drug dosages are determined by a child's weight in kilogrammes it is essential in this field of nursing. It is important that any medication administration is always undertaken away from 'safe' areas, such as the playroom or bedside, especially if the medicine administration is unpleasant. For neonates or in specialised circumstances, you may also need to learn to calculate very small doses using microgrammes.

Adult – in adult nursing, all of the above might apply, and your role involves assessing a diverse range of individuals who need your care. While most adults will be able to actively participate in their treatment, you will certainly encounter patients with dementia and those who are confused.

☑ **Care-setting considerations**

It is possible for medications to be administered orally or topically in all care settings.

☑ **What to watch out for and action to take**

Monitor the effectiveness of the treatment by pre- and post-administration observations. For example, has the patient's temperature reduced? Is the patient still in pain, or feeling nauseous, following the administration of medication?

Ensure you are aware of the therapeutic application of the medicine to be administered, its normal dosage, side-effects, precautions and contraindications before you administer it. Ensure you refer to an up-to-date version of the British National Formulary (BNF) to ascertain this information before administering any medicines with which you are unfamiliar.

Monitor for any reactions to the medication, report any concerns to your practice educator or a registered nurse and ensure they report this to the person prescribing the drug without delay. All drug reactions need to be treated appropriately as soon as they become apparent.

Contact the person prescribing the drug if an assessment of the patient indicates that the medicine is no longer suitable or the patient declines to take it.

☑ **Helpful hints**

- Gloves and aprons must be worn if contact with blood/body fluids/excreta is anticipated or the patient is in isolation.
- Gloves should be worn if contact with the medication is potentially harmful to the nurse – for example, in the case of topical steroid preparations.
- Hand hygiene must be performed before touching a patient, before clean/aseptic procedures, after body fluid exposure/risk, after touching a patient and after touching a patient's surroundings.
- Waste should be disposed of in a clinical waste bag if it is contaminated with blood/body fluids/excreta.

To aid you to administer oral medications safely, always follow the top tips below.

Top tips for administering oral medications (Hall, 2002)

- Check the prescription chart and the BNF for any special instructions relating to how to administer medications, such as:
  - administer with food, before food or after food
  - any possible interactions with other medications, substances such as herbal medicines or grapefruit juice
  - 'slow-release' tablets must be swallowed whole to allow the medication to be released gradually.
- Do not crush coated tablets as in doing this you are making their use unlicensed.
- Do not break tablets that are unscored as you are likely to be giving an inaccurate dose.
- If medication is to be administered via a **nasogastric (NG)** or percutaneous endoscopic gastrostomy (PEG) tube, ask the pharmacist to dispense a suspension which will not block the tube.
- If a medication is in liquid form, shake the bottle before you pour it out to ensure it is evenly concentrated.
- When using a medicine pot to measure a liquid, place it on a flat surface and ensure you are at eye level to it in order to read the graduations accurately.
- As well as being ingested via an oral route, tablets may be administered via the
  - sublingual route, which means they are placed under the tongue
  - buccal route, which means they are placed between the cheek and the upper gum.
- Liquids can be administered via a nasogastric (NG) or percutaneous endoscopic gastrostomy (PEG) tube.

(Continued)

MEDICINE ADMINISTRATION GUIDELINES

ENSURING SAFE AND EFFECTIVE STORAGE AND ADMINISTRATION OF MEDICATION TO PATIENTS

1 **Introduce yourself to the patient, explain the procedure and gain their consent**
Adapt communication style to meet the needs of the individual patient and their family or carers
Patients should be involved as desired in decisions relating to their medicines. Fully informed consent may be difficult if the patient is a child or has severe mental health issues or learning disabilities, but every effort should be made to explain the procedure in a way the patient can understand. This is respectful of individual human rights, supports informed participation and reduces anxiety. For patients unable to provide consent because they are unconscious, advice should be sought from your practice educator or another qualified nurse

2 **Gather required equipment**
Ensure cleanliness
Reduces risk of cross-infection and maintains patient and nurse safety

3 **Identify an appropriate place to prepare medications, away from interruptions and distractions**
Clear sufficient space within the environment where the drug is administered
Ensures patient safety, as interruption is associated with medication error
Enables clear access for the patient and the nurse to safely administer the medication

4 **Wash your hands with soap and water before you start administering medication. Ensure your use of Personal Protective Equipment (PPE) such as gloves and disposable aprons is appropriate by considering the individual patient situation and the risk presented**
Wearing an apron and gloves as part of PPE is standard infection-control procedure when dealing with body fluids or patients in isolation. When administering medications, you may need to wear gloves to protect yourself from exposure to the drug (such as when applying topical skin preparations)

5 **Follow local policy for the administration of medicines. This may mean you must observe rather than participate in administration directly yourself. As a nursing student, you must ensure you are supervised by a registered nurse when administering medication**
To ensure patient safety and support your learning
To meet local policy guidance requirements which ensure employees and students are fully insured for the care that they give

6 **Before you give any medication, you will need to complete a full assessment of your patient's medication needs. This involves:**

a. **Checking the patient's care plan for specific requirements**
b. **Checking the Medicine Administration Record (MAR) to determine the correct medicine to be given to the correct patient, taking account of all eight rights of medicine administration (see Figure 29.1)**

To ensure patient safety
You need to be aware of the patient's plan of care to ensure no changes have been made and that the medication administration remains appropriate
To ensure the drug is administered accurately and safely
Medicines must be given in a timely manner in order to ensure optimum benefits from treatments
It is dangerous to administer a medication which is not specifically **licensed** for a particular route

7 **If a number of medicines need to be given at the same time, prioritise which one to administer first**
Some medicines require specific conditions for best effect
If the medications are to be administered orally, it may be possible to take them to the patient simultaneously provided they do not interact with one another. If medication is required via different routes (e.g. injection and oral), then this will need to be managed to enable optimum treatment. Seek advice from the pharmacist

Decide if there is reason not to administer the medicine at this time and record and report accordingly
If there has been a change in the patient's condition, a medication may no longer be appropriate, or the patient may be unable to take it. If a patient is 'nil by mouth', check with the drug prescriber whether any of their oral drugs still need to be given (for example, cardiac drugs), possibly by a different route

Locate medicine to be administered, ensuring it is:

a.   in date
b.   the correct formulation for the route to be given and appropriate for your patient's preferences
c.   the correct dose strength for the prescription
d.   the correct medicine according to the prescription

a.   The quality of an out-of-date medicine may have deteriorated
b.   To prevent error and ensure the best possible outcome in terms of patient care
c.   To ensure safe practice, as medicines are available in different strengths
d.   You must check that the prescription and the label on the medicine are both clearly written and are the same to ensure patient safety

If your patient is a child or the drug dose is calculated according to the patient's weight, check that the prescribed dose is correct for the patient's current weight or BMI
To ensure patient safety, the dose must be checked using accurate patient weight. Some adult drugs are prescribed according to patient weight to ensure accuracy of treatment. Patient weights can change considerably through the illness process

Children's medicines are calculated on the basis of milligrams per kilogramme per day. Some specialised areas use BMI and surface area for drug doses. A calculator can be found on the BNF website

Calculate the amount of medicine to administer and measure the required amount accurately
An accurate amount of medication must be given to the patient

Medicine must always be measured accurately using appropriate equipment. For example, measuring a dose of 5 ml using a 50 ml medicine pot makes accuracy difficult. The difference of even a few ml can cause problems. Always use the smallest appropriate measuring device

Ensure medication is placed in an appropriate receptacle for administration to the patient
To make taking the medicine as easy as possible for the patient

Medication which is not needed must be returned to its place of secure storage or disposed of in accordance with local policy and legal requirements
Safe disposal of medicine is important to keep patients, families, carers and staff safe from unwanted effects. Controlled medicines and highly toxic materials will have specific handling and disposal guidelines

Complete final checks, which always include patient identity and allergies, but may also include specific checks for individual drugs. Provide patients with necessary information regarding their medication, using an appropriate means of communication to aid explanation
To ensure patient safety:

a.   be certain of the identity of the patient to whom the medicine is to be administered
b.   check that the patient is not allergic to the medicine before administering it
c.   before administering some drugs, cardiac ones for example, it is necessary to check that the patient's heart rate or blood pressure is within acceptable parameters

(Continued)

Patients and carers must be aware of the main features of the medicines given and how to manage them effectively and **concordantly**. They need to know what to do if the medicine is taken inappropriately and the implications of missing doses

 Ensure your patient is fully prepared for the administration of the medication and is in an appropriate position. Provide protective clothing or tissues if needed, or a drink, etc. An infant may need to be held securely
Patients should be in a position which ensures both comfort and safety

Protective clothing can maintain dignity through avoiding spills

 Ensure medication is administered in accordance with the prescription, local policy and patient preferences (see Clinical Skill 29.1). If given orally, ensure medication has been swallowed
To ensure patient safety and involvement and that the medication is received as prescribed

RECORDING ADMINISTRATION AND OUTCOME

 Record that the medicine has been administered on the Medication Administration Record to ensure a legal record of the medicine administered
You must make a clear, accurate and immediate record of all medicine administered, or any intentionally withheld or refused by the patient. You must ensure your signature is valid and is clear and legible. If local policy has allowed you to administer the medication, ensure the registered nurse supervising you countersigns your signature

EVALUATION OF THE IMPACT AND EFFECTIVENESS OF THE MEDICATION AND ASSESSMENT OF ANY UNTOWARD EVENTS

 Document relevant information on the patient's observation chart and/or in the patient's notes as necessary
Monitor the effectiveness of the medication and any reactions, reporting these to a registered nurse and the medication prescriber and instigating treatment as appropriate
Maintains patient safety and accurate records. Failing to complete documents may mean a patient could receive the medication on more than one occasion

Ensure you are fully aware of the therapeutic uses of the medicine to be administered, its normal dosage, side-effects, precautions and contraindications

Adverse reactions to medications can range from discomforting to life-threatening. By administering a medicine, you undertake to ensure that you are aware of any possible reactions and know what to do in response

Ensure you advise patients of any signs to watch out for and identify how they can inform you

 After the medication administration has been completed, ensure the patient is in a comfortable position, with drinks and call bells available as necessary
Promotes patient comfort and ensures they are well nourished and hydrated

 Discard PPE, any single-use equipment and other used materials as per policy. Clean any equipment used as per the relevant policy every time it is used and perform hand hygiene
Prevents cross-infection and maintains equipment in working condition

Source: BNF (2014); NPC (n.d.); NMC (2007); Westbrook et al. (2010); WHO (2009)

This is perfectly acceptable as long as you know how your method works and that it produces the correct answer. The following steps can be used as guidelines to assist you to administer the correct dose.

1. Identify the component parts of the calculation:

    *   What is the required dose prescribed on the prescription?
    *   What is the dose of the medicine you have available?
    *   What is the volume in ml (if a liquid)?

2. Identify an estimated amount of drug required.

This will help to ensure your calculation is accurate and may allow you to work out the required dose without resorting to a calculation. For example, if the dose prescribed is 75 mg and:

- the available dose is 100 mg
- in a volume of 10 ml

your estimate would begin by recognising that the required dose is not more than 100 mg, therefore **not more** than 10 ml.

- A little more consideration would enable you to also recognise that the required dose of 75 mg is more than half of the stock requirement – so will be **more than** 5 ml.

At this point, you have some parameters and may decide to carry on using maths facts or to use a formula for calculation, depending on the complexity of the sum.

The maths facts route

In this method, you would gather together useful knowledge about the equation and complete your calculation through reasoning:

- Some further thinking might identify two other maths facts. First, 75 is three quarters of 100. If you apply this to 10, three quarters is 7.5 ml.

OR

- If there is 100 mg in 10 ml, then every 1 ml must contain 10 mg because 10 mg × 10 mg = 100 AND 10 × 1 ml = 10 ml.

75 mg must therefore be 10 mg × 7 = 70 mg (= 1 ml × 7 = 7ml) + 0.5 ml = 5 mg = 7.5 ml

The formula route

Through this route you would use the same information, but it can be set into an equation using the formula.

What you want (dose required by prescription) x What it is in (volume)

What you have got (the available dose).

So the equation would be:

What you want = 75 mg × What it is in = 10 ml

What you have got = 100 mg

which becomes   75 × 10

and can be calculated as: 75 × 10 becomes 750 (divided by) 100

Answer is **7.5 ml**

ACTIVITY 29.3: CRITICAL THINKING

Mr Jones is prescribed 1 g of paracetamol, which comes in 500 mg tablets:

- How many tablets would you give him?

Lizzie, a 3-year-old patient, is prescribed 250 mg of ampicillin, which comes in liquid form in 50 mg per ml:

- How many ml would you give her?

You need to give Mr Singh a 50 mg dose of oral morphine. You have a bottle of morphine elixir at a concentration of 2 mg/ml:

- How much should you give him?

The dose of a drug required is 1 g and the solution available has 50 mg per ml:

- How many ml are required for the dose?

Miss MacTavish weighs 50 kg. The dose of a drug prescribed for her is 10 mg per kg and the medicine strength is 50 mg per ml:

- How many ml are required for a single dose?

An injection contains 200 mg in 10 ml and the dose required is 60 mg:

- How many ml should be injected?

WEBLINK:
DRUG CALCULATIONS
AND CONVERSION

For some further practice, the Queens University Belfast website offers a useful resource with short video clips included alongside practice tests focusing on specific aspects of arithmetic related to medicine administration:

www.qub.ac.uk/elearning/public/NumeracySkillsforDrugCalculations/Year1FinalExam/Basic DrugCalculations

www.qub.ac.uk/elearning/public/NumeracySkillsforDrugCalculations/Year1FinalExam/Conversions

For more real-life practice, you may like to try the www.nursingnumeracy.info exemplar assessment, which allows you to read a medicine prescription, make a calculation and place the right number of tablets in a pot (see www.nursingnumeracy.info/page11/page5/page5.html)

Numeracy and technical skills

As a nursing student, it is necessary to:

- have a good conceptual understanding of maths

This is a 'demonstration of competence and confidence with regard to judgements on whether to use calculations in a particular situation and, if so, what calculations to use, how to do it, what degree of accuracy is appropriate, and what the answer means in relation to the context' (NMC, 2010, Annex 3: 2). This means that you must realise why you are making a calculation and how accurate you need to be. You will use calculations every day within nursing and some will need to be more specific than others. Pouring a drink, for example, needs to be more accurate for someone with a kidney disorder than a healthy adult. In respect of medicines, this will depend on the prescription order. Some medications are prescribed in small volumes using small units, while others may be in much larger and less specific units.

It is also critical to ensure that you have a working appreciation of volume. This can help to protect against errors of magnitude (for instance, giving ten times the dose prescribed), which is a common error resulting from poor arithmetical ability combined with poor conceptual understanding of maths. Realising that 100 millilitres is about half a cup of fluid will often prevent a medication prescribed at 10 millilitres being wrongly concluded. As a new student, it is helpful to pour out different volumes of fluid and describe them – for example, 0.1 ml, 1 ml, 10 ml, 20 ml, 50 ml, 100 ml, 1 litre. Think about where you might see these different volumes and have to measure them. Examples might include maintaining a fluid balance record in a child or adult acute hospital setting, which might include measuring urine output as fluid input, drawing up a vaccination in a GP clinic, or in a mental health setting determining the volume of an injectable antipsychotic medication.

- have arithmetic ability

This means you must be able to undertake multiplication and division, addition and subtraction accurately and with confidence and be able to use formulae. You must also be competent in the conversion of decimals and fractions, be able to use Standardised International (SI) units with confidence (be able to convert milligrammes to microgrammes or grammes) and be able to input information into a calculator according to a formula and know if the answer is wrong.

- have good technical measurement skills

This means you must be able to use measuring equipment (such as syringes and medicine pots) properly. This is important because, once you have correctly calculated a dose of medication, if you are unable to accurately draw this amount up in a syringe or measure it in a medicine pot, the patient will not receive the correct amount of medication.

The key to developing your numeracy and technical skills when dispensing medications is practice. As a student I always had a notepad in my pocket; I wrote down medication names and doses that I can came across, as well as the calculations to work out doses. I asked my placement practice educators, when appropriate, if I could work out dose calculations with them whenever the opportunity arose.

Charlie Clisby, NQN

ACTIVITY 29.4: CRITICAL THINKING

Aodhan is six months into his nursing programme and has enjoyed his first placement, apart from feeling very confused as to how to calculate drug doses. He is convinced he is not able to get the correct answers and is concerned that he may give the wrong amount of a drug to a patient.

- What advice would you give Aodhan?

CONCLUSION

As individuals, patients will have personal preferences, and it is important for you to use your knowledge about their medication to empower them. To do this, you need a clear understanding of the fundamental principles of pharmacology, and to be able to understand the patient's view, assess their capability for informed consent and explore the options for those who refuse prescribed treatment with medicines.

There are three stages of the nurse's role in medicine administration, namely ensuring the safe and effective storage and administration of medications to patients (or supporting patients or their carers to self-medicate), recording the administration of the medication and the outcome, and evaluating the impact and effectiveness of the medication given and assessing any untoward effects.

Although the administration of medicines is mostly subject to professional requirements, many of the wider aspects of 'medicines management' are bound by law, which your practice must uphold. In order to assist you to ensure your practice is effective and optimises the medicinal treatment patients receive, always consider Hall's eight rights of medication (2002) during administration, as this will promote patient safety.

When administering any medication, accuracy and safety are fundamentally important. This includes calculating the right dose. There are many ways to do this, and each person may choose a different method. Indeed, you might choose different methods of calculation depending on the complexity of the equation. This is perfectly acceptable as long as you know how your method works and that it produces the correct answer.

CHAPTER SUMMARY

- Medicine administration is a holistic and integral patient-caring activity within all fields of nursing.
- The safe storage and management of medicines is an important aspect of the nurse's role.
- As a nursing student, you must always be supervised by a registered nurse when administering medications.
- Applying the eight rights of medication will aid you to optimise the medicinal treatment patients receive.
- You must never give a medicine without being certain that the dosage (relating to the patient's weight where appropriate), the method of administration, the route and the timing are all correct.
- Patient empowerment with regard to their medication is fundamentally important.
- Nurses need both the technical skills to accurately dispense medications and the mathematical skills to calculate the correct dose.

CRITICAL REFLECTION

Holistic care

This chapter has highlighted the wider importance of providing holistic care in administering medicines to patients. Review the chapter and note down some instances in which you think assessing and empowering an individual in meeting their need for medicine treatment could help to address their wider physical, emotional, social, economic and spiritual needs. Try to think of a variety of different patients across the fields, not just within your own field. You may find it helpful to make some notes to refer back to the next time you are in practice, and then write your own reflection after your practice experience.

GO FURTHER

Books

Baileff, A., Davis, J. and Davey, N. (2012) 'Managing medicines', in I. Bullock, J. Macleod-Clark and J. Ryecroft-Malone (eds), *Adult Nursing Practice: Using Evidence in Care*. Oxford: Oxford University Press. pp. 378–94. A good review of the evidence underpinning medicine administration to adults.

Hall, C. (2010) 'Medicines administration', in A. Glasper, M. Aylott and C. Battrick (eds), *Developing Practical Skills for Nursing Children and Young People*. London: Hodder Arnold. pp. 148–66. This book chapter covers the administration of medicines to children in considerable depth and provides a protocol for reading the Medication Administration Record, which applies to all fields, and a table which outlines the main routes of medicine administration.

Mutsatsa, S. (2011) *Medicines Management in Mental Health Nursing*. Exeter: Learning Matters. An excellent textbook which will develop your knowledge of medicines administration and management in mental health nursing. This book also includes a good section on administering injections.

Journal articles

Dickens, G., Doyle, C. and Calvert, J. (2006) 'Reducing medication administration errors in learning disability nursing', *Nurse Prescribing*, 4(11): 470–4. This article applies considerations around the safe administration of medicines to those caring for patients with a learning disability specifically. In this field, there are particular concerns, since these patients may be less likely than others to identify if the medications they are receiving are not correct, and in severe situations may not be able to tell you their name or provide you with other details which would help you to identify them.

Hutton, B.M., Coben, D., Weeks, K., Hall, C., Rowe, D., Sabin, M., et al. (2010) 'Numeracy for nursing, report of a pilot study to compare outcomes of two practical simulation tools: An online medication dosage assessment and practical assessment in the style of objective structured clinical examination', *Nurse Education Today*, 30(7): 608–14. This article looks in considerable detail at the component parts of medicine calculation, identifying why you may be getting wrong answers! It is important to understand this when trying to improve your numeracy skills, and you may like to share this with those who are helping you to learn too.

Westbrook, J., Woods, A., Rob, M., Dunsmuir, W. and Day, R. (2010) 'Association of interruptions with an increased risk and severity of medication administration errors', *Archives of Internal Medicine*, 170(8): 683–90. This article underlines the point that simple interruptions while in practice settings can leave patients vulnerable to medication error.

Weblinks

Go to https://study.sagepub.com/essentialnursing2e for weblinks related to this chapter. If you are using the interactive ebook, simply click on the book icon in the margin to go straight to the resource.

www.bnf.org.uk – this site offers comprehensive information about medicines licensed for use within the UK. It provides information about the pharmacology, dose of the medication, its brand and its generic name. They are very useful resources for nurses in practice and your clinical practice areas will also have access to copies of these. British National Formulary Child (BNFC) is for those caring for children and young people, while British National Formulary (BNF) is for those caring for adult patients, including those with a mental health need.

www.nice.org.uk/Search.do?searchText=medicines&newsearch=true&x=14&y=23 – NICE provides a range of guidance and evidence relating to the optimisation of medicines treatment for patients. A simple search using medicines as a keyword will produce a useful starting point for further exploration.

www.nmc-uk.org/Documents/NMC-Publications/NMC-Standards-for-medicines-management.pdf – this NMC pdf offers the professional standards for the administration and management of medicines which must be adhered to by every qualified nurse.

www.nursingnumeracy.info/page11/page5/page5.html – this website includes an example of a short, free interactive test, which allows you to calculate medicines and prepare them for the patient, including measurement. The visual cues show you how the same calculation can look different in practice, as compared to undertaking a calculation using formulae on paper.

————— ACE YOUR ASSESSMENT —————

Review what you have learned by visiting the book's online resources at: https://study.sagepub.com/essential nursing2e If using your interactive ebook, just click on the icon in the margin to go straight there.

- Test yourself with multiple-choice and short-answer questions.
- Revise key terms with the interactive flash cards.

REFERENCES

British National Formulary (BNF) (2014) *British National Formulary 68*. London: Pharmaceutical Press.

Hall, C. (2002) An Evaluation of Nurse Preparation and Practice in Administering Medicine to Children. PhD thesis, School of Education, University of Nottingham.

Medicines and Healthcare Regulatory Agency (MHRA) (2013) Policy Development and Delivery. Available at: http://webarchive.nationalarchives.gov.uk/20141205150130/htttp://www.mhra.gov.uk/Howweregulate/Howwedevelopolicy/index.htm (accessed 17 November 2014).

National Institute for Health and Care Excellence (NICE) (2015) Medicines Optimisation: The safe and effective use of medicines to enable the best possible outcomes. Available at: www.nice.org.uk/guidance/ng5live/14175/65802/65802.pdf (accessed 6 March 2018).

National Institute for Clinical Excellence (NICE) (2016) Controlled Drugs: Safe use and management. Available at: www.nice.org.uk/guidance/ng46 (accessed 3 October 2017).

National Prescribing Centre (NPC) (n.d.) A Guide to Good Practice in the Management of Controlled Drugs in Primary Care (England). Available at: www.harrogateandruraldistrictccg.nhs.uk/data/uploads/medicines-management/controlled-drugs/clinical-governance/npc-controlleddrugsthirdedition-dec2009.pdf (accessed 28 March 2018).

Nursing and Midwifery Council (NMC) (2007) *Ratified 2008 Standards and Guidance for Medicines Management*. London: NMC.

Nursing and Midwifery Council (2010) *Standards and Guidance for the Delivery of Pre-registration Nursing Education*. London: NMC.

Westbrook, J., Woods, A., Rob, M., Dunsmuir, W. and Day, R. (2010) 'Association of interruptions with an increased risk and severity of medication administration errors', *Archives of Internal Medicine*, 170(8): 683–90.

World Health Organization (WHO) (2009) WHO Guidelines on Hand Hygiene in Health Care. Available at: http://whqlibdoc.who.int/publications/2009/9789241597906_eng.pdf (accessed 7 March 2018).

ASSISTING PATIENTS WITH THEIR NUTRITIONAL NEEDS

KATE GOODHAND AND JANE EWEN

THIS CHAPTER COVERS

- Malnutrition in the UK
- Nutritional screening and assessment
- Care planning

- Providing assistance and support
- Adjuncts assisting a patient's nutritional intake

REQUIRED KNOWLEDGE

- It will be helpful to have an understanding of the anatomy and physiology of the digestive system before you start this chapter.

> Hi! I am 15 years old and was admitted to hospital to have investigations … I had to stay in overnight, which was fine, but when it came to tea time there was nothing on the menu I could eat. I am gluten-free and I think a lot of people are, so I don't know why there was no choice for me. My mum ended up buying me some chocolate from the hospital shop … she wanted to complain but I was too scared to let her!
>
> **Rebecca, patient**

> At present I am working with a patient who is struggling to eat effectively. As a team we have written care plans that monitor her food and fluid intake and provide her with the support to address her poor eating habits. Not only has lack of nourishment affected the condition of her skin, it has also exacerbated her mental health symptoms.
>
> **Alice Rowe, NQ RNMH**

> Hello! I need 24-hour care, I am 29 and have physical disabilities as well as learning difficulties. When I am at home I have a carer who visits me at meal times. When I go into hospital, which is frequently, I don't like the food and refuse to eat! The last time I went in the specialist nutrition nurse came to see me with the catering manager. They read the menus to me and I was allowed to choose things from both the child and adult menus and they found things I actually liked. They also arranged for my meal to be delivered when my carer was there so she could help me eat and drink. I won't say I am looking forward to going into hospital next time, but I feel a lot happier about it!
>
> **Colin, patient**

INTRODUCTION

This chapter provides information that will help you, as a student, assist patients with their nutritional needs. Assisting a patient to eat and drink is part of providing holistic, person-centred care, but, as you can see by reading what Rebecca has to say, we often get it wrong. Sadly, current evidence shows that once a patient is admitted to hospital, their risk of malnutrition increases. As Colin's story shows, how-ever, with a little thought, it is so easy to get right. Providing patients with food they want to eat that is good for them, is so important to promote recovery and wellbeing. It is the nurse's role to lead and coordinate patient-centred care for all of their patients' nutritional needs.

Sometimes patients being cared for in a variety of settings may not be able to take food and drink by mouth and need extra help in the form of an adjunct, such as a nasogastric or enteral tube. Therefore, you will need to be able to competently and confidently maintain a patient's nutrition and hydration using these, no matter which field of nursing you are practising in.

MALNUTRITION IN THE UK

The provision of appropriate nutrition, including hydration, is a fundamental part of patient care, whatever the context in which you are working: community, care home or hospital. Unfortunately in the UK, malnutrition in health and social care is estimated to cost £19.6 billion of public money. Older adults account for 52% of this total, younger adults for 42% and children for 6%. Individuals that were either hospital inpatients or care home residents accounted for up to £9.3 billion (BAPEN, 2015).

Around 30 per cent of patients who are admitted to hospital are at risk of malnutrition, with 6–14 per cent of that total being children (Brotherton and Simmonds, 2012). As has already been high-lighted, once a patient is admitted to hospital the risk of malnutrition increases; this is due to a number of factors, including their changing physical or psychological condition. Malnutrition can result in longer hospital stays and poorer outcomes for patients. Malnutrition was found to be a problem in care homes too, affecting 35% of residents. Most residents with 'malnutrition' were underweight and at high risk, thus requiring treatment (BAPEN, 2015).

ANSWER:
ACTIVITY 30.1

ACTIVITY 30.1: CRITICAL THINKING

Malnutrition is defined as the state in which a deficiency, excess or imbalance of energy, protein and other nutrients causes measurable adverse effects on tissue, body form, function or **clinical outcome** (Elia and Russell, 2009):

• Make a list of which patients you think will be at risk from malnutrition.

Malnourished patients visit their GP twice as frequently as those who are well nourished and have an increased risk of being admitted to hospital. The effects of malnutrition are numerous. It often goes undetected and therefore untreated, which can result in a number of adverse consequences such as:

• difficulty in keeping warm
• increased susceptibility to respiratory problems and other infections due to poor immune responses
• wounds are slow to heal
• increased recovery time from illness
• in children, growth and development can be impaired

- in women of child-bearing age, conceiving can be difficult
- psychologically, individuals can become low in mood, uninterested in eating and drinking and may lack self-esteem.

People who are overweight may also become malnourished by eating too much sugary and fatty food in preference to healthy alternatives. Generally, eating more calories than are burned off leads to obesity. An overweight person with a lot of body fat is termed obese. Obesity is a public health concern in all fields of nursing. In the UK, obesity is estimated to affect around one in every four adults and around one in every five children aged 10 to 11 (NHS Choices, 2016). Being obese can lead to lots of health issues such as diabetes, heart problems and some cancers.

ACTIVITY 30.2: RESEARCH

- What does the literature tell us about obesity in the UK?
- List all the health issues that can be caused by obesity.
- What help is available in your local community and acute hospital settings to help people eat more sensibly and be aware of the risks?

ANSWER:
ACTIVITY 30.2

ACTIVITY 30.3: REFLECTION

- How would you use the 'food plate' (Figure 30.1) to help you to explain to a patient what their diet should include?
- Thinking about what you ate yesterday, is your diet balanced?

ANSWER:
ACTIVITY 30.3

Maintaining nutritional balance requires that patients have access to the correct information and can make informed choices about what they eat. The 'food plate' (see Figure 30.1) explains what is meant by 'a balanced diet'.

> I always found when working on a busy ward that organisation was very important at lunchtime. There were usually varying numbers of patients who required assistance with eating; this can be time-consuming, so it was a group effort to ensure they all were fed in timely fashion. Protected mealtimes often help, and why not ask family members if they would like to help their loved one?
>
> Charlie Clisby, NQN

Improving nutritional care is the responsibility of all members of the healthcare team, each of whom play a key role within a patient's journey. As a nursing student, you are included within this and have a vitally important role to play in nutritional assessment and providing ongoing care.

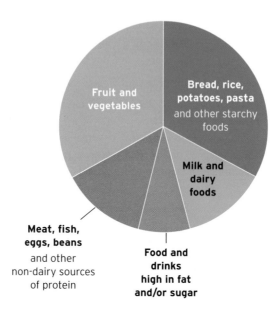

Figure 30.1   The 'food plate'

NUTRITIONAL SCREENING AND ASSESSMENT

Nutritional screening and assessment are a key priority for all patients (NICE, 2006). When a patient is admitted to hospital, screening for the risk of 'under-nutrition' should be undertaken first within 24 hours of admission, and then on a continual basis (NHS Quality Improvement Scotland, 2014).

There are over 70 screening tools available for adults and children. Some tools claim to be valid for all patient groups and settings, while others have been developed for screening specific patient groups. It has also been recognised that there is no single 'best' tool to use (van Bokhorst-de van der Schueren et al., 2014). So, it is essential that the selected screening tool is 'fit for purpose', and therefore the use of a **validated** screening tool is stipulated. In addition to this, it is important to remember that screening tools validated for adult patients, such as the Malnutrition Universal Screening Tool (MUST), the Modified Malnutrition Screening Tool (Mod-MST) and the Mini Nutritional Assessment (MNA), are inappropriate for use in children, as malnutrition presents differently within paediatrics.

For paediatrics, validated tools such as the Screening Tool for the Assessment of Malnutrition in Paediatrics (STAMP) or Paediatric Yorkhill Malnutrition Score (PYMS) are commonly used. Both of these tools were developed specifically to be used by nurses and apply a simplistic, step-by-step approach in order to assess nutritional status on admission. Other paediatric tools, such as the Paediatric Nutrition Risk Score (PNRS), aim to predict clinical outcome without nutritional intervention (Joosten and Hulst, 2014). It also has to be remembered that due to their rapid growth and potentially complex issues relating to the prematurity of children under the age of 1 year, these tools are not suitable for such young children and a specialised tool is required.

Despite these issues, however, in general, screening tools are easy to use. One important factor is that you need to be able to communicate effectively with the patient, which can prove more difficult for some patient groups and makes the tools' practicality for all patients questionable.

ACTIVITY 30.4: REFLECTION

Reflect on your experience of caring for patients:

- Are you able to identify any groups of patients with whom you would wish to undertake an assessment of nutritional status, but are likely to also have communication difficulties?

ANSWER:
ACTIVITY 30.4

Most screening tools divide nutritional risk into three groups – low, moderate and high risk – and most provide some form of nutritional advice, including dietetic assessment.

Prior to carrying out nutritional screening on a patient, you need to be competent in using the tool and be supervised by your practice educator or another registered nurse.

The outcome of the screening will determine if the patient is low, medium or high risk, and will be followed by setting out a plan to ensure the patient receives the care they require. Determining the level of risk of malnutrition will give you a clear plan of action regarding how to manage the nutritional requirements of the individual in a consistent manner and reduce the risk of future weight loss while they are in your care. This action will support any future intervention by a dietician, who will be responsible for undertaking a more detailed nutritional assessment. Always remember to follow local protocols.

The Malnutrition Universal Screening Tool (MUST) (see Figure 30.2) is the most common nutritional screening tool used in the UK (BAPEN, 2013). MUST is the first step in identifying patients who may be nutritionally at risk or potentially at risk. The rapid, simple, five-step procedure calculates the patient's risk score and therefore their level of malnutrition risk. This is done by considering weight, height, recent weight loss and current acute clinical/psychological condition.

Before nutritional support is initiated, a full nutritional assessment must take place. Much of the information relating to a patient's nutritional intake, and any unintentional weight loss, can be obtained through history-taking and health records, but in the first instance information should be obtained by talking to the patient. The use of probing questions will be required to establish all the necessary information. In some cases, this information may be sought from people other than the patient, including their family or carer, especially if the patient is a child or has communication difficulties. You would want to obtain the following information when undertaking a full nutritional assessment:

- a diet history
- information about special diets due to health reasons, such as gluten-free, low fat or diabetic
- food allergies
- the patient's particular likes and dislikes
- religious and cultural dietary requirements
- swallowing difficulties
- nausea and pain
- state of mouth, teeth or dentures
- height, weight, BMI (a measure of body fat based on height and weight that applies to adult men and women), WHO (2009) growth charts (it is vitally important to be accurate with these – see relevant clinical skills guides)
- if a baby or toddler, whether they are being breast-fed
- how much help the patient needs to eat and drink
- any equipment the patient uses for eating and drinking
- clinical examination, including biochemical blood tests.

Step 1 BMI score	+	Step 2 Weight loss score	+	Step 3 Acute disease effect score

Step 1 — BMI score

BMI kg/m^2	Score
>20(>30 Obese)	= 0
18.5-20	= 1
<18.5	= 2

Step 2 — Unplanned weight loss in past 3-6 months

%	Score
<5	= 0
5.10	= 1
>10	= 2

Step 3 — If patient is acutely ill **and** there has been or is likely to be no nutritional intake for >5 days

Score 2

Step 4 Overall risk of malnutrition

Acute disease effect is unlikely to apply outside hospital. See 'MUST' Explanatory Booklet for further information

Add scores together to calculate overall risk of malnutrition

Score 0 Low Risk   Score 1 Medium Risk   Score 2 or more High Risk

Step 5 Management guidelines

0 Low Risk Routine Clinical Care

- Repeat screening
  Hospital – weekly
  Care homes – monthly
  Community – annually
  for special groups
  e.g. those > 75 yrs

1 Medium Risk Observe

- Document dietary intake for 3 days
- If adequate – little concern and repeat screening
  Hospital – weekly
  Care home – at least monthly
  Community – at least every 2-3 months
- If inadequate – clinical concern – follow local policy, set goals, improve and increase overall nutritional intake, monitor and review care plan regularly

2 or more High Risk Treat

- Refer to dietician, Nutritional Support Team or implement local policy
- Set goals, improve and increase overall nutritional intake
- Monitor and review care plan
  Hospital – weekly
  Care home – monthly
  Community – monthly
- Unless detrimental or no benefit is expected from nutritional support e.g. imminent death

All risk categories:

- Treat underlying condition and provide help and advice on food choices, eating and drinking when necessary
- Record malnutrition risk category
- Record need for special diets and follow local policy

Obesity:

- Record presence of obesity. For those with underlying conditions, those are generally controlled before the treatment of obesity

Re-assess subjects identified at risk as they move through care settings

See the 'MUST' Explanatory Booklet for further details and the 'MUST' Report I for Reporting evidence.

Figure 30.2   Malnutrition Universal Screening Tool (MUST)

While some of the questions we need to ask may seem sensitive, without the full picture, safe, effective and person-centred nutritional care cannot be provided. Before gathering nutritional information from a patient or performing nutrition-related skills in any care setting, there are a number of issues and common steps you need to consider.

Guidelines

There are various national and local guidelines of which you must be aware. Remember never to undertake any of the following procedures unless you are, or have supervision from, a trained, experienced and competent person. The types of guidelines you need to consider will be contained in:

- infection prevention and control policy
- local organisational policies.

Once you are aware of these, you need to take a number of steps that will be common for all nutrition-related skills (see Clinical Skill 30.1).

Weighing a patient

Careful weighing and recording are vital to achieving holistic patient care for nutritional screening. In addition to this, as the dosage of many drugs is calculated depending on the weight of a child, it is especially important to weigh children accurately. Following the steps outlined in Clinical Skill 30.2 will enable you to do this.

Once a patient's weight has been obtained, effective communication between healthcare professionals, patients and carers is essential in order to meet the patient's needs and provide successful treatment and care. As was made clear by Colin at the start of the chapter, communication with the catering staff can ensure a patient is able to choose the food they like. If a patient has additional nutritional needs, a dietician or speech and language therapist (if there are swallowing problems) will need to be informed, to ensure a person-centred approach is taken to the patient's particular requirements.

Letting them collect a different toy from the play area is normally the best way to distract a child. A stethoscope can be pretty fascinating for them also. With toddlers I always ask them to stand on the special machine to see how big and grown up they are now, and also ask, if age-appropriate, if they are good at musical statues, and ask them to show how brilliant they are.

Alice Rowe, NQ RNMH

CARE PLANNING

In any care setting, all patients are required to have an appropriate multi-disciplinary care plan, which is reviewed and refined on an ongoing basis. Care plans are required to be person-centred,

STEP-BY-STEP CLINICAL SKILL 30.1: COMMON STEPS FOR ALL NUTRITION-RELATED SKILLS

☑ **Essential equipment**

Depends on skill but is likely to include one or more of the following: utensils, crockery with or without adaptations, plate guard, slip mat, napkin/disposable clothes protection.

☑ **Field-specific considerations**

When caring for a patient with a learning disability, it is important to know their level of understanding so that consent for and cooperation with the care can be gained. You will need to allow time to explain what you are doing and whether it will cause discomfort or pain.

Patients who have mental health problems may not understand why you need to undertake nutrition-related tasks. They may also be so depressed that they don't have the energy to eat, or those with cognitive impairment may have forgotten to eat. They may withhold consent to have their measurements taken and you may need to refer to the Mental Capacity Act 2005 and best interest.

Children have a different anatomy and physiology to adults, which varies from birth through to adolescence. You will need knowledge of paediatric anatomy and physiology to enable you to interpret the results. As younger children may not understand why you need to undertake the task, you will need to modify your approach. It is usually helpful to have parents or carers present to assist.

☑ **Care-setting considerations**

In hospital or a care home, seek the patient's preference for eating alone or in company. At home, individuals may need food and drink prepared and served by healthcare workers.

☑ **What to watch out for and action to take**

While undertaking any nutrition-related skill, you should also assess:

- the position of the patient
- their neurological condition – are they alert and responsive?
- any signs or complaints of pain or discomfort
- the patient's or relatives' views – these may provide you with important additional information.

The information gained from these observations will enable you to fully assess the patient's condition, institute appropriate treatment as necessary and escalate needs care to senior nurses and the medical team.

☑ **Helpful hints**

- Gloves and aprons must be worn if the patient is in isolation.
- Hand hygiene must be performed before touching a patient, after touching a patient and after touching a patient's surroundings.
- Waste should be disposed of in a clinical waste bag.

NUTRITION GUIDELINES

 The first step of any procedure is to introduce yourself to the patient, explain the procedure and gain their consent
Fully informed consent may not always be possible if the patient is a child or has mental health problems or learning disabilities, but even in these circumstances, every effort should be made to explain the procedure in terms that the patient can understand

This is not only respectful of their individual human rights, but also helps to ensure that they will be more accepting of the treatment and that their anxieties are reduced

For patients who are unable to provide consent because they are unconscious, advice should be sought from your practice educator or another qualified nurse

 Gather the equipment required (see individual skills for equipment required). Ensure these are clean and in working order
Reduces the chance of infection and maintains patient and nurse safety

 Clear sufficient space within the environment, for example around the bed space or chair
Enables clear access for the patient and the nurse to safely use the equipment required

 Wash your hands with soap and water before you start the task. Apron and gloves should only be worn if appropriate
Wearing an apron and gloves as part of personal protective equipment (PPE) is a standard infection-control procedure when a patient is in isolation

Ensure your use of PPE such as gloves and disposable aprons is appropriate by considering the individual patient situation and the risk presented

 Ask the patient if they wish to have the curtains drawn for privacy or to be in a separate room
Some patients may feel exposed
Maintain patient privacy, dignity and comfort as required

 Patients need to be in a comfortable position, either sitting in a chair, resting on a couch or in bed
Promotes patient comfort and reduces anxiety

 After performing the task, ensure the patient is in a comfortable position, with drinks and call bells available as necessary
Promotes patient comfort and ensures they are well nourished and hydrated

 Discard PPE, any single-use equipment and other used materials as per policy. Clean any equipment used as per the relevant policy every time it is used and perform hand hygiene
Prevents cross-infection and maintains equipment in working condition

 Document findings on the patient's observation chart and/or in the patient's notes
Maintains patient safety and accurate records

 If any changes are observed, escalate to senior nursing staff/your practice educator immediately
It is vital to report any changes to a registered nurse immediately so they can ensure care is escalated

Source: Dougherty and Lister (2015); WHO (2009)

STEP-BY-STEP CLINICAL SKILL 30.2: WEIGHING A PATIENT (WT)

☑ What is normal

Most adults will know their height but often get their weight wrong!

Refer to the BMI chart to determine if weight is in proportion to height.

☑ Before you start

Remember the common steps for all nutrition-related skills (Clinical Skill 30.1).

☑ Essential equipment

Appropriate weighing scales:

- 0-2 years – baby scales
- Over 2 years – sitting or standing scales
- For patients with mobility needs – hoist scales

☑ Field-specific considerations

When caring for a patient with a learning disability, it is important to know their level of understanding so that consent for and cooperation with the measurement can be gained. You will need to allow time to explain what you are doing and why.

Patients who have mental health problems may not understand why you need to undertake nutrition-related skills, or may simply require further details, full explanation and reassurance.

If you are weighing a child, prepare them using an age-appropriate explanation (you may use a play specialist to assist). If possible, involve the child's parents or carers to reassure the child. If a child becomes upset, do not weigh them, but document the reason and return later.

☑ Care-setting considerations

Patients can be weighed in any care setting, as long as the scales are in working order and accurately calibrated.

☑ What to watch out for and action to take

While undertaking any nutrition-related task, you should also assess:

- the patient's positioning and ability to mobilise
- their neurological condition – are they alert and responsive?
- any signs or complaints of pain or discomfort
- the patient's or relatives' views, as these may provide you with important additional information.

The information gained from these observations will enable you to fully assess the patient's condition, institute appropriate treatment as necessary and escalate needs care to senior nurses and the medical team.

WEIGHING GUIDELINES

 Perform steps 1-6 of the common steps (Clinical Skill 30.1)
To prepare the patient and yourself to undertake the task

 Remove clothing as appropriate:

- **0-2 – remove clothing**
- **Over 2 – remove shoes or slippers, and empty pockets**

To reduce the chance of abnormal readings

 Ensure scales are on flat surface and the dial is on zero, and apply brakes if appropriate

If the scales are the 'stand on' type, ensure the patient stands on scales centrally, with feet slightly apart, and keeps still
To ensure patient safety and promote accuracy of reading

 Perform steps 7-10 of the common steps (Clinical Skill 30.1)
To ensure that:

- the patient is safe, comfortable and receiving the appropriate care
- the results have been documented in the patient's records
- the equipment is clean and in working order

Source: Dougherty and Lister (2015); RCN (2011)

and information relating to the patient's initial and continued nutritional screening and assessment will be recorded. If the findings of the patient's nutritional screening and assessment indicate there is a need, actions to provide the care required will be planned and documented here (NHS Quality Improvement Scotland, 2014).

WHAT'S THE EVIDENCE?

Russell, C.A. and Elia, M. (2011) Nutrition Screening Survey in the UK and Republic of Ireland in 2011. Available at: www.bapen.org.uk/pdfs/nsw/nsw-2011-report.pdf.

A report by BAPEN (Russell and Elia, 2011) considers nutritional status in UK hospitals, care homes and the community, providing many issues to consider in nursing practice:

- Reflect on the care you have been involved in of a patient who needed assistance to eat and drink.
- Did the nurses offer assistance appropriate for the patient?
- Why might nurses not see assisting a patient to eat and drink as a fundamentally important aspect of their role?
- Now read the report and consider how you can apply the findings to your practice.

FURTHER READING: NUTRITION

The actions taken may be determined by local policy but, in the main, will include regular monitoring of the patient's weight, usually weekly for patients who are deemed as low risk. Patients who are

Total Intake Chart

Please record all food and drink taken by the patient. Fluids may also need to be recorded on a fluid balance chart

Patient's Name: JOHN SMITH   **Ward/ Room:** 3   **Date:** 9/5/14

Meal		Food/Drink offered Please give detailed description	Amount offered Please record actual amount offered, e.g. small, medium, large portion/bowl/slice/ spoonfuls/ volume	Amount taken (Please circle the amount)	Dietician's use	
					Energy (kcals)	Protein(g)
Breakfast	Cereal:	1 BOWL PORRIDGE	MED	none (½) all		
	Milk:	1 CUP	200 ml	none (½) all		
	Bread/toast/roll	1 SLICE	MED SL	none ½ (all)		
	Drink e.g. tea/ coffee:	1 COFFEE	200 ml	(none) ½ all		
	Supplement:			none ½ (all)		
	Other:	1 FRUIT JUICE	75ml	none (½) all		
Mid-morning	Drink:	HOT CHOC	200 ml	none ½ all		
	Biscuit:	CHOC BISCUIT	ONE	none ½ (all)		
	Supplement:	STRAWBERRY	200 ml	none ½ (all)		
	Other:			none ½ all		
Lunch	Soup:	POTATO+LEEK	MED	none (½) all		
	Fruit juice:			none ½ all		
	Potato/rice/pasta:	POTATO	1 SCOOP	none (½) all		
	Vegetable:	PEAS	MED	(none) ½ all		
	Main Course:	MINCE	MED	none (½) all		
	Pudding:	CUSTARD	1 BOWL	none ½ all		
	Drink:			none ½ all		
	Supplement:			none ½ all		
	Bread/Other:	WHITE BREAD	1 SLICE	(none) ½ all		
Mid-afternoon	Drink:	COFFEE	200 ml	none (½) all		
	Biscuit:	BISCUITS	TWO	none (½) all		
	Supplement:			none ½ all		
	Other:	CHEESE	1 PORTION	none ½ (all)		
Evening meal	Soup:			none ½ all		
	Potato/rice/pasta:	RICE	MED	none (½) all		
	Vegetable:			none ½ all		
	Main Course:	FISH	MED	none ½ (all)		
	Sandwich:			none ½ all		
	Pudding/Cake:			none ½ all		
	Fruit:	1 APPLE	ONE	none (½) all		
	Drink:	TEA	200 ml	none ½ (all)		
	Supplement:			none ½ all		
	Bread/Other:			none ½ all		
Bedtime	Drink:	HORLICKS	200 ml	none ½ (all)		
	Biscuit:			none ½ all		
	Supplement:			none ½ all		
	Other:	TOAST	1 SLICE	none (½) all		
		TOTAL FLUID INTAKE (ml)				

Reviewed 2013

Figure 30.3   Total intake chart

recorded as having a medium to high risk score will have their weight recorded on an ongoing basis, with other necessary actions identified by local protocols and a dietician. Supplementary high energy and nutrient-dense snacks are often suggested; these might include foods such as whole milk, full-fat yoghurts, cakes and biscuits.

Many patients are commenced on a total intake chart or a food diary if they are recorded as being at medium or high risk of malnutrition (see Figure 30.3).

A total intake chart (Figure 30.3) provides detailed information relating to all food and fluids consumed over a 24-hour period. This detailed breakdown of information provides a foundation for a further, more comprehensive nutritional assessment and enables a calculation of the nutrients consumed, usually undertaken by a dietician. It is therefore critical that such charts are kept up to date and food intake is recorded at the time of the meal and not retrospectively; otherwise, it can lead to inaccuracies and may have a future impact on the patient's wellbeing and clinical outcomes.

Community and hospital-based dieticians play a key role in prescribing nutritional supplements and ongoing management and review. All supplements are prescribed products (in a similar manner to medications), and, as such, adherence to the NMC (2008) *Standards for Medicine Management* and local medicines management policy is required.

ACTIVITY 30.5: REFLECTION

Make a copy of Figure 30.3 and use it to keep a record of the food you eat over a 24-hour period:

- Does the record you produce surprise you?
- Reflect on what you have eaten in light of Figure 30.1, the 'food plate', and consider the answer you gave in Activity 30.3 when you were asked whether your diet is balanced. Does the evidence from this activity support your previous answer?

Nutritional care and the mealtime experience

In a community setting, a patient's access to food may vary; some may receive 'meals on wheels' while others may have carers who assist with meal preparation, thus allowing the patient to remain as independent as possible. For those who may require additional nutritional support, attending lunch clubs and day hospitals may facilitate the provision of a balanced diet and afford the opportunity for close observation and ongoing monitoring of nutritional intake. For children, breakfast clubs and free school meals may mean they are able to access adequate nutritional requirements for growth and development.

Mealtimes in hospital and the care home setting are particularly important for any patient. They form a key part of the patient's daily routine and a time that they can look forward to. Interruptions at mealtimes can be frequent due to the unpredictable nature of healthcare: medication rounds, ward rounds or the patient having investigations off the ward, for instance. Taking steps to ensure that there is a structured and organised approach to mealtimes is paramount in ensuring patients receive their meals in a manner which suits their individual needs. Take a moment to read the 'Making meals matter' pack available from Healthcare Improvement Scotland (2011).

Inpatient experience surveys have shown that 40 per cent of patients feel they need help at mealtimes, yet 11 per cent of these do not get the help they require (Scottish Government, 2014). Such surveys highlight that staff need to prioritise their time to ensure that patients are served their meals at the correct temperature, as well as ensuring that they receive the assistance and encouragement they require. One way of achieving this is the concept of 'protected mealtimes'. This initiative was introduced in 2004 in England and makes mealtimes a period in which eating and drinking are the focus of the ward routine (NPSA, 2007). During these times, patients are able to eat and drink in a clean, quiet and safe environment because non-essential interruptions are limited to allow staff to provide assistance and encouragement.

Although activity can be unpredictable within a hospital setting and the needs of patients change on an ongoing basis, it is possible to take some simple steps to help patients be ready for their meals, have sufficient time to eat them and enjoy what they are eating. The following can help to improve the mealtime experience:

- **Take just a few extra minutes** – preparing for mealtime is crucial. This ensures that mealtimes run to plan and that patient care and comfort are the focus. Ensuring that the patient is prepared and the environment is conducive to eating and drinking, whether in a hospital, care home or home setting, is important for all in promoting oral intake.
- **Ensure that patients of all ages** are offered the opportunity to wash their hands prior to eating food. Also ensure that they have a clean mouth and teeth or dentures; if not, this may affect the patient's appetite.
- **Think about the setting** – depending on the facilities available and the patient's condition, meals can be offered either in a dedicated dining room or by the patient's bed. Where there are dining room facilities, these should be widely encouraged to be used by patients whose condition allows, as socialisation at mealtimes can promote a patient's appetite as well as improve the mealtime experience.

PROVIDING ASSISTANCE AND SUPPORT

Many hospitals and care homes implement a range of local processes to ensure that patients who are nutritionally at risk or who are unable to eat or drink independently are identified. Some areas promote the role of mealtime coordinator – a staff member who takes the lead at mealtimes to ensure all patients receive the help they require and the mealtime is structured and organised. The use of 'safety briefs', where those patients who are at high risk or require assistance with eating and drinking are identified at the start of each shift, is also a helpful and consistent approach to the provision of assistance. Another initiative is the 'red tray or mat system', in which a patient's food is served on a red tray or mat, to highlight at a glance those requiring additional assistance. Such systems, however, can be criticised as they can detract from others who could be vulnerable and impact on patients' dignity and anonymity. Boards situated either at patients' bedsides or in the ward pantry can assist in providing information in relation to any special dietary requirements patients may have, or if they require any aids for eating and drinking (see Figure 30.4 below). Required eating and drinking aids, such as cutlery or plate guards, should be easily accessible at all times. Occupational therapists may be involved in assessment as to when additional assistance is needed and may prescribe the use of plate guards, adapted cutlery or non-slip mats to promote independence.

I have ensured the food was within their reach, they were comfortable and they had food they liked to eat. I would assist my patients if they required it. I would chat and gently encourage them to eat. I would give them the time to finish their meal and enjoy it.

Julie Davis, LD nursing student

Figure 30.4   Essential equipment

Some patients may require simple assistance such as unwrapping cutlery from a napkin, opening packets and removing lids. Others may require additional assistance, including cutting up food or placing cutlery in their hands, particularly if they have poor manual dexterity or limited use of limbs. Some will require full physical assistance from a member of the nursing staff or allied health professional. Patients with dysphasia will require a swallowing assessment that can be performed by a speech and language therapist (SALT) or a suitably qualified professional. Before assisting dysphasic patients with their nutritional needs, always check your local hospital guidelines as supplementary training may be required.

Allowing patients sufficient time to eat their meal will assist with their food and fluid consumption. Within a hospital setting where mealtimes are offered at pre-set times, fixed around trolley delivery and collection times, this can be challenging. However, it is important from the patient's perspective that those who may be slower eaters are not rushed by activities such as the collection of meal trays, as this can have a negative impact on their meal consumption.

CASE STUDY 30.1: ROISIN

Roisin is 3 years old and has been admitted to hospital for an appendectomy. She will usually only eat and drink when her mother is present. Unfortunately, her mum, who is pregnant with her second baby, has had to be admitted to hospital for bed rest. Roisin's dad works on an oil platform and will be away from home for three weeks.

- How can you encourage Roisin to eat and drink?
- Who else could you involve?

ANSWER:
CASE STUDY 30.1

Assisting a patient to eat and drink

It is important that the distribution of meals in a hospital or care home is not viewed as a 'one off' task. It should not be assumed that mealtime is complete once lunch or dinner is served. Many patients require continuous support or encouragement. They may forget that their meal is in front of them and need reminding, or their appetite may be poor and they may require prompting. At this time, observation and monitoring of the patient's consumption of food and drink should be carried out.

When assisting someone to eat and drink, adoption of a comfortable seated position is not only required from a moving and handling safety perspective, but also provides patients with non-verbal cues indicating that the mealtime is not being rushed and the nurse has time to sit and chat. Standing over a patient or chatting with a colleague conveys a very different message. Using language which is degrading or belittling, or does not promote dignified care, is not accepted in caring organisations; such expressions include 'feeding patients' or 'bib' (Care Quality Commission, 2011).

Consideration should be given to family or carer involvement at mealtimes. Patients, particularly children or those who have a cognitive impairment, such as dementia or delirium, may benefit from the familiarity of having a family member involved in their care. Family members and carers may also benefit from feeling fully involved in the care of their loved one, so this should be encouraged. Some organisations use volunteers who are recruited and trained specifically to assist with such duties, and both patients and volunteers can get a lot of satisfaction from the assistance and interaction this provides. Following the steps outlined in Clinical Skill 30.3 will enable you to effectively assist a patient to eat and drink.

ACTIVITY 30.6: REFLECTION

Recruit the assistance of either a fellow nursing student, a friend or family member who agrees you may assist them with eating and drinking, and then swap roles. Carry out the steps recommended in Clinical Skill 30.3 and reflect on your experience:

- What went well when you were assisting them with eating and drinking?
- What would you do differently if you repeated the experience?
- What was important to you when you were being assisted with eating and drinking?
- How will you translate your experience to the care you deliver to patients in future?

I assisted a young boy with eating his meal who was very physically disabled and also had visual and hearing impairments. I tried to put myself in his shoes and think about how I would want to be assisted. I ensured I was aware of whether he had any prompts or cues to let him know the food was near his mouth, which he did, so he could demonstrate he was ready for the next mouthful; this also gave plenty of time for him to chew and swallow his food so he was not rushed. Also, I gave different parts of the meal separately so he could experience all the different flavours, rather than having it all mashed up together.

Siân Hunter, child nursing student

Caring for those who may be vulnerable

Patience and careful and simple explanation given to patients is vital to ensure correct meal selection and subsequent consumption. Patients may have a limited attention span; therefore, using pictorial menus can provide a more person-centred approach for patients choosing meals from a menu card. This approach can also be useful for people with learning difficulties or for whom English is not their first language.

Offering a café-style approach, where patients can see and smell what they are ordering before they choose it, is an alternative and makes a significant difference to whether the patient consumes a meal or not. The pleasure of eating, drinking and mealtimes may be lost for some patients. Patients with dementia may have a reduced or limited recognition of hunger or thirst and any patient who is disorientated with regard to time and place is unlikely to appreciate that it is mealtime, or may not recognise the meal that is put in front of them. Often, small reminders can help; for example, a favourite cup or tumbler may well aid fluid consumption.

The principle of protected mealtimes is very relevant to such groups, and other measures can also be helpful. However, getting to know a patient is fundamentally important in ascertaining what time the person normally eats, plus what food and fluids they like, dislike or choose not to intake for cultural or religious reasons.

ACTIVITY 30.7: REFLECTION

Read the Better Health fact sheet (2011), Food Culture and Religion, to investigate the diets followed by members of common religions and cultures within your local area:

- What are the particular religious or cultural dietary requirements for these groups?
- When you have been on placement, have you seen any menu options designed to meet the specific needs of these patients?

ANSWER:
ACTIVITY 30.7

Individuals with dementia can neglect their needs when it comes to remaining well nourished and hydrated. Sometimes people with dementia can believe that they have already eaten when they haven't or they won't recognise that they are hungry. It can also be the case that even though they are hungry or thirsty they become so confused by preparing a meal or drink that they will avoid doing so. Being under nourished and dehydrated can lead to other health problems that can exacerbate the symptoms of dementia; developing a UTI because of dehydration can lead to the person becoming delirious. This could be misinterpreted as a deterioration in their dementia rather than what it actually is.

Samantha Vanes, NQ RNMH

Finding out further information

A 'patient passport' can be a useful tool in finding out the normal daily needs, including diet, of a vulnerable person, and is particularly useful for those with mental health conditions or cognitive impairment. Making sure the person is comfortable and settled and then talking about the meal about

STEP-BY-STEP CLINICAL SKILL 30.3: ASSISTING A PATIENT TO EAT AND DRINK

☑ What is normal

It is normal for patients, children included, to eat and drink with only minimal assistance, so remember to enable the patient to be as independent as possible.

☑ Before you start

Remember the common steps for all clinical measurements (Clinical Skill 30.1).

Check the patient's plan of care to ascertain whether there is a known swallowing difficulty.

☑ Essential equipment

- Utensils – adapted if appropriate
- Crockery and any necessary adapted items, such as a plate guard
- Clothing protection for the patient, such as disposable covers or napkins, as required
- The meal and a suitable drink

☑ Field-specific considerations

When caring for a patient with a learning disability, ascertaining their likes and dislikes is imperative to maintaining nutritional needs.

Many mental health conditions can affect appetite and the ability to prepare food as well as to eat and drink normally, so extra support may be required.

For children, age-appropriate food and choice of utensils are important safety issues.

Elderly patients may not eat or drink adequately due to problems with dentures and oral hygiene, plus the accessibility of food, or because of the effects of medication.

☑ Care-setting considerations

It is possible to assist a patient to eat and drink in any care setting. In community settings, you may need to involve other agencies to help a patient maintain adequate nutrition throughout the whole day.

☑ What to watch out for and action to take

If the patient seems to have any difficulty swallowing at any time, stop immediately and report your concerns straight away to your practice educator or another registered nurse.

When assisting a patient to eat or drink, you should also assess:

- the patient's positioning and ability to mobilise
- their neurological condition – are they alert and responsive?
- any signs or complaints of pain or discomfort
- the patient's or relatives' views, as these may provide you with important additional information.

The information gained from these observations will enable you to fully assess the patient's condition, institute appropriate treatment as necessary and escalate needs care to senior nurses and the medical team.

EATING AND DRINKING ASSISTANCE GUIDELINES

Perform steps 1-6 of the common steps (Clinical Skill 30.1)
To prepare the patient and yourself to undertake the skill

Prepare the patient for the meal by:

- **offering toilet and hand-washing facilities before the meal arrives**
- **ascertaining where the patient wishes to eat**
- **if using a bed table, removing surplus equipment, particularly items such as sputum pots and vomit bowls**
- **cleaning the table and ensuring it is at the correct height**
- **collecting the correct diet for the patient and the utensils they require**
- **ensuring you have a supply of fresh water or appropriate fluid**

To empower the patient and reduce infection risks
    A social environment is often preferred to encourage normality, but some may wish to eat alone
    To promote an environment conducive to eating and drinking
    To ensure everything is to hand so you do not have to leave the patient

Position yourself close to the patient, at the same level as them, in a comfortable position
To promote the patient's dignity and ensure you are in a position that protects your back

Ensure the patient approves of the food choice and that food is at an appropriate temperature and consistency
To empower the patient and prevent harm from heat or swallowing difficulties

Offer as much or as little assistance as is required. While assisting the patient, ensure
pace is correct by asking for feedback. **Ensure you offer food in the order the patient wishes, following their preferences**
Communicate appropriately with the patient while they are eating, to make the experience a sociable and enjoyable one
To empower the patient while promoting autonomy and dignity

Remember to offer and encourage fluids at frequent intervals while the patient is eating
To aid swallowing and promote digestion

Ensure the patient is not rushed and has sufficient time to complete their meal
To ensure the patient eats and drinks the amount they wish

Clear away crockery and utensils; offer patient appropriate hygiene, such as hand-washing, mouth care, clean dentures and clean bed table
To promote patient comfort and a clean environment

Leave patient in a comfortable, upright position for at least 30 minutes, with their call bell to hand
To promote digestion and ensure patient safety
    For children, this will depend on their condition and stage of development, but in general aim to disturb the child as little as possible after feeding and encourage quiet activities for a while

Perform steps 7-10 of the common steps (Clinical Skill 30.1)

Source: Dougherty and Lister (2015); NICE (2006, 2012); RCN (2011) to be served is also helpful in preparing the patient. Within some settings, such as care homes, it is beneficial to involve patients in the setting of tables and general mealtime preparation. Keeping noise to a minimum and limiting distractions such as television or unnecessary activity, can also aid in ensuring the focus is solely on mealtime.

Patients who are visually impaired will have different needs. Explaining where food is situated on a plate by using a clock as a comparison can be helpful – for example, potatoes at 12 o'clock; peas at 3 o'clock. For those who are visually impaired, it is possible to offer the use of different-coloured crockery, or contrasting colours of plates, utensils and drinking vessels and crockery that has a rim.

Other patients may find it hard to chew their food and swallow solids, so will require additional assistance.

After mealtime

Ensuring that patients are left feeling comfortable after a meal is also important. Making sure hand-washing facilities are offered and food debris is removed from clothes or around their mouth, plus offering mouth care, will promote patient comfort. Patients should be left upright after their meal for at least 30 minutes, either in their chair or bed, to aid digestion. For children, this will depend on their condition and stage of development, but in general aim to disturb the child as little as possible after feeding and encourage quiet activities for a while.

There may be occasions where a patient misses a meal, perhaps where they are fasting for a procedure or an operation, or have returned later from a clinical area. In such cases, organisations will have in place a protocol to enable the patient to receive an appropriate meal at a different time to the rest of the area (DH, 2010).

CASE STUDY:
LACHLANN

Apply your understanding of supporting nutritional needs by reading Lachlann's case study, at https://study.sagepub.com/essentialnursing2e.

Assisting with nutritional needs in a community setting

It is important to remember that many patients cared for in a community setting are likely to be considered at risk of malnourishment and will therefore require effective assessment and care. The previously outlined points apply to patients in their own homes or other community-based environments, but you may need to source further health and social care support to ensure patients' nutritional needs are met throughout the entire day.

CASE STUDY 30.2: SYDNEY

Sydney Day is a 32-year-old woman who has a history of mental health problems and lives alone in a remote rural area. Sydney does not drive a car. The village shop is 2 miles away but there is no frequent public transport. Twice a week, a bus goes from the hamlet where she lives to the nearest town, 11 miles away, where there are several shops.

You accompany your practice educator on a visit to Sydney and find that she appears to have lost weight and is complaining of a lack of energy. You assess her BMI and find that it is 16. Sydney appears to be very preoccupied with a number of issues, but in particular feels acutely uncomfortable going into shops and public areas.

- What questions would you ask Sydney to assess her nutritional needs?
- How could you assist Sydney to maintain an adequate intake of food and fluid?
- What further support could be offered to Sydney?
- How would the care you offer differ if Sydney was an 86-year-old man undergoing investigations to ascertain whether he has dementia?

ADJUNCTS ASSISTING A PATIENT'S NUTRITIONAL INTAKE

The final section of this chapter considers the adjuncts that may be used within any care setting to assist with a patient's nutritional intake.

Enteral feeding

A number of conditions may affect a patient's ability to eat and drink sufficient amounts to meet the body's requirements. Sometimes a patient may have difficulty swallowing, so it becomes necessary to bypass the mouth and oesophagus. In this case, nutritional needs can be met artificially by enteral feeding, which involves the insertion of an enteral tube; nutrition, fluids and medication can then be administered safely. This is defined as complex nutritional care (Healthcare Improvement Scotland, 2011). Table 30.1 identifies the types of enteral tubes used for feeding.

Table 30.1 Types of enteral tubes used for feeding

1.	Nasoenteric tubes
	a. Nasogastric
	b. Nasojejunal
	c. Post pyloric
2.	Enteric tubes
	a. Gastrostomy
	b. Jejunostomy

The decision on how to feed a patient must be a result of multi-disciplinary team discussion and, where possible, made in conjunction with the patient and their family. As these are the adjuncts used most commonly, we will now further discuss nasogastric tubes and then gastrostomy tubes, in the form of percutaneous endoscopic gastrostomy tubes (PEGs).

Nasogastric (NG) tube feeding

The decision to commence enteral feeding will be governed by agreed local protocols that specifically address the criteria that permit enteral tube feeding.

Nasogastric (NG) tubes can be used in both children and adults, being passed through the nostril of the patient down the oesophagus and into the stomach.

A&P LINK: THE ALIMENTARY CANAL

Normal ingestion of food travels from the buccal cavity, through the oesophagus and then into the stomach before entering the intestine. When patients are unable to eat and drink, a nasogastric tube can be passed through their nasal cavity to the stomach, thus bypassing the mouth.

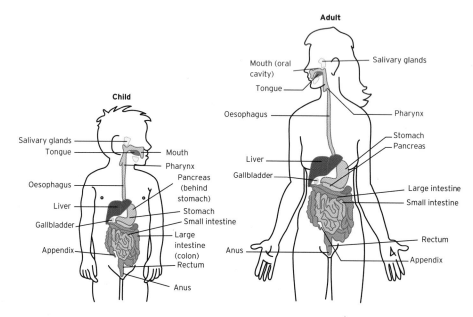

Figure 30.5   Child and adult alimentary canal

Image © Robin Lupton

Passing an NG tube can be achieved quickly and easily while the patient is conscious, although some may find it unpleasant. The technique has low procedure-related mortality (SIGN, 2001) but complications can occur, including displacement.

Unfortunately, NG tubes are less well tolerated than gastrostomy tubes and need to be replaced more frequently. Common problems when an NG tube is passed are oesophagitis and upper gastrointestinal ulceration; any gastric intolerance may mean that nutritional status is compromised. NG feed tubes usually need replacing every 10–28 days, depending on the type and material of the tube and the manufacturer's recommendations.

Ensure that the patient has been cleared of any possibility of facial fractures to have confidence when passing the NG tube. Measure twice before attempting to insert the NG tube, and check this with a colleague where possible. Once the tip of the tube is in the nose, angle it downwards. It is important to be firm to get the tube over the nasal arch. If the patient is able to assist, ask the patient to take a few sips of water to avoid the NG spooling into the patient's mouth.

Laura Grimley, adult nursing student

Insertion of an NG tube can be performed by a registered nurse or by a nursing student under direct supervision, as long as this is in accordance with local policy.

Extreme care is required as inadvertent placement into the lungs can be a problem and, if unrecognised, will have serious consequences. The position of all NG tubes should be confirmed after placement by X-ray (NICE, 2006), and before each use the position of the NG tube should be checked by aspiration and pH-graded paper, as per advice from the National Patient Safety Agency (NPSA, 2011). Local hospital criteria should also include how to proceed when the capacity to make repeated checks of the tube position is limited by an inability to aspirate the tube, or the checking of pH is invalid because of gastric acid suppression.

Patients who are receiving enteral tube feeding can be cared for in any setting. NICE guidelines set out the requirements and level of support that should be provided to patients, their families and carers, which should include:

- care provision by a wide multi-disciplinary team
- a personalised care plan
- information and training about enteral tube feeding
- for those receiving enteral tube feeding in a community setting, routine and emergency contact numbers of a healthcare professional who understands the needs and potential problems of those having community-based enteral tube feeding. (NICE, 2006)

Percutaneous endoscopic gastrostomy (PEG) tube feeding

Percutaneous endoscopic gastrostomy (PEG) tubes are suitable for both adults and children, facilitating direct access to the stomach from outside the abdomen. As an endoscope is required to insert a PEG tube, the patient must be fit for sedation and considered as someone who would benefit from such a procedure; therefore, the multi-disciplinary team needs to be involved in the decision-making process. Careful monitoring is required after the insertion as peritonitis and perforation of the colon may occur.

The National Patient Safety Agency (NPSA, 2011) has developed 'red flag' alerts for these complications, which include:

- severe pain that is not relieved by simple analgesia or that is made worse by using the tube
- fresh bleeding or gastric fluid or feed leaking from the wound site
- a sudden change in the patient's vital signs or changes in levels of responsiveness or behaviour.

Any concerns must be reported to a registered nurse and the medical team immediately.

The tube can be flushed with 50 ml of water four hours after the procedure; if no pain occurs, then the tube can be used (NICE, 2006). Feeding must be commenced slowly and follow a prescription issued by a dietician. This will be specific to each individual patient, taking into account factors such as their age and weight. Management of constipation is something that has to be considered when feeding a patient enterally.

Following successful insertion and close monitoring during the first 72 hours, the PEG tube and the site of insertion must be monitored daily or more often if required.

ACTIVITY 30.8: REFLECTION

Reflect on how you might explain the need for enteral feeding to a patient and their family or carers.

Peripheral venous cannula

As many as a third of patients cared for in hospital have a peripheral venous cannula, so it is likely that you will be involved in caring for a patient with one during a hospital-based placement. A peripheral cannula is a small hollow tube which is inserted through the skin into a peripheral vein to be used for intravenous (IV) therapy, which could include the administration of medications, blood and blood products or fluids. Peripheral cannulae are not without complications, however, including infection and phlebitis, so you need to be able to provide effective care in order to minimise this risk.

Stoma care

A stoma is any artificial opening usually leading to the surface of the body, e.g. abdominal surface. Keeping the stoma site healthy and clean is an important role.

CONCLUSION

Assisting patients with eating and drinking is a fundamental role of the nurse. Ensuring this is carried out in a safe and effective way while considering the patient's individual requirements will promote recovery, aid the healing process and help prevent deterioration in a patient's condition and general health. You, as a nursing student, can play a vital role in this aspect of care delivery.

--- **CHAPTER SUMMARY** ---

- Malnutrition, or the risk of malnutrition, affects more than three million people in the UK. Admission to hospital increases this risk.
- Undertaking nutritional screening using a validated tool and carrying out a full assessment are essential for all 'at risk' patients, especially when they are admitted to hospital.
- Communication with the patient, family, carers and multi-disciplinary team is vital to promote a good outcome for the patient. This includes good record-keeping.
- Providing a patient with adequate nutrition, including hydration, involves a person-centred, holistic approach on the part of the entire multi-disciplinary team.
- As a nursing student, you can assist a patient to choose healthy options and ensure they receive the appropriate food and drink safely.

--- **CRITICAL REFLECTION** ---

Holistic care

This chapter has highlighted the wider importance of assisting a patient with their nutritional needs in providing holistic care for a patient. Review the chapter and note down all the instances where you think caring for a patient's nutritional needs can help meet their wider physical, psychological, social, economic and spiritual needs. Think of a variety of different patients across the fields, not just within your own field. You may find it helpful to make a list and refer back to it next time you are in practice, and then write your own reflection after your practice experience.

GO FURTHER

Books

Dougherty, L. and Lister, S. (eds) (2015) *The Royal Marsden Hospital Manual of Clinical Nursing Procedures*, 9th edn. London: Blackwell Science. This text contains useful clinical nursing skills procedures and always provides rationales with up-to-date evidence.

Glasper, A., Aylott, M. and Battrick, C. (2010) *Developing Practical Skills for Nursing Children and Young People*. London: Hodder Arnold. This is an excellent book covering skills for children and young people which is very easy to read, with good references for further reading.

SAGE journal articles

Go to https://study.sagepub.com/essentialnursing2e for free online journal articles for this chapter. If you are using the interactive ebook, simply click on the book icon in the margin to go straight to the resource.

FIND OUT
MORE!

FURTHER
READING:
JOURNAL
ARTICLES

Brown, A., Forbes, M.L., Vitale, V.S., Tirodker, U.H. and Zeller, R. (2012) 'Effects of a gastric feeding protocol on efficiency of enteral nutrition in critically ill infants and children', *Infant, Child and Adolescent Nutrition*, 4(3): 175–80. This article explores enteral feeding for critically ill children.

Pratt, H.D., Phillips, E.L., Greydanus, D.E. and Patel, D.R. (2003) 'Eating disorders in the adolescent population: Future directions', *Journal of Adolescent Research*, 18(3): 297–317. An excellent article considering eating disorders that remains current.

Other journal articles

Tappenden, K.A., Quatrara, B., Parkhurst, M.L., Malone, A.M., Fanjiang, G. and Ziegler, T.R. (2013) 'Critical role of nutrition in improving quality of care: An interdisciplinary call to action to address adult hospital malnutrition', *Journal of Parenteral and Enteral Nutrition*, 37: 482–97. This article presents an interdisciplinary approach to dealing with malnutrition in hospitals.

Weblinks

Go to https://study.sagepub.com/essentialnursing2e for weblinks related to this chapter. If you are using the interactive ebook, simply click on the book icon in the margin to go straight to the resource.

FURTHER
READING:
WEBLINKS

http://guidance.nice.org.uk/CG32 – these are very useful guidelines looking at how to care for patients who require support with eating and drinking.

http://sign.ac.uk/sign-119-management-of-patients-with-stroke-identification-and-management-of-dysphagia.html – these are very useful guidelines looking at how to care for patients with dyspaghia.

www.bapen.org.uk/pdfs/nsw/nsw-2011-report.pdf – a nutrition screening survey in the UK and Republic of Ireland in 2011, considering nutritional status in UK hospitals, care homes and the community, providing many issues to think about in nursing practice.

ACE YOUR ASSESSMENT

ONLINE
QUIZZES

Review what you have learned by visiting the book's online resources at: https://study.sagepub.com/essential nursing2e If using your interactive ebook, just click on the icon in the margin to go straight there.

- Test yourself with multiple-choice and short-answer questions.
- Revise key terms with the interactive flash cards.

REFERENCES

Better Health (2011) Food Culture and Religion Fact Sheet. Available at: www.betterhealth.vic.gov. au/bhcv2/bhcpdf.nsf/ByPDF/Food_culture_and_religion/$File/Food_culture_and_religion.pdf (accessed 16 March 2015).

British Association for Parenteral and Enteral Nutrition (BAPEN) (2013) Introducing 'MUST'. Available at: www.bapen.org.uk/screening-for-malnutrition/must/introducing-must (accessed 7 March 2018).

British Association for Parenteral and Enteral Nutrition (2015) Nutrition Screening Surveys in Care Homes in the UK. Available at: www.bapen.org.uk/pdfs/nsw/care-homes/care-homes-uk.pdf (accessed 10 December 2017).

Brotherton, A. and Simmonds, N. (2012) *Malnutrition Matters: Meeting Quality Standards in Nutritional Care.* Redditch, Worcester: British Association of Parenteral and Enteral Nutrition.

Care Quality Commission (CQC) (2011) *Dignity and Nutrition for Older People: Inspection Programmes.* Newcastle upon Tyne: CQC.

Department of Health (DH) (2010) *Essence of Care: Benchmarks for Food and Drink.* London: DH.

Dougherty, L. and Lister, S. (2015) *The Royal Marsden Hospital Manual of Clinical Nursing Procedures,* 9th edn. Oxford: Wiley-Blackwell.

Elia, M. and Russell, C.R. (2009) *Combating Malnutrition: Recommendations for Action.* Output of a meeting of the Advisory Group on Malnutrition. London: BAPEN.

Healthcare Improvement Scotland (2011) *'Making Meals Matter' Pack: Improving Nutritional Care Programme.* Edinburgh: Healthcare Improvement Scotland.

Joosten, K. and Hulst, J. (2014) 'Nutritional screening tools for hospitalized children: Methodological considerations', *Clinical Nutrition,* 33(1): 1–5.

National Institute for Health and Clinical Excellence (NICE) (2006) *Nutrition Support in Adults. Oral Nutrition Support, Enteral Tube Feeding and Parenteral Nutrition.* Clinical Guideline 32. London: NICE.

National Institute for Health and Clinical Excellence (2012) *Quality Standard for Nutritional Support of Adults.* London: NICE.

National Patient Safety Agency (NPSA) (2007) Protected Mealtimes: Review Findings and Recommendations Report. Available at: www.nrls.npsa.nhs.uk/resources/patient-safety-topics/ patient-treatment-procedure/?entryid45=59806 (accessed 7 March 2018).

National Patient Safety Agency (2011) Reducing the Harm Caused by Misplaced Nasogastric Feeding Tubes in Adults, Children and Infants. Available at: www.nrls.npsa.nhs.uk/ alerts/?entryid45=129640 (accessed 7 March 2018).

NHS Choices (2016) Eatwell Guide. Available at: www.nhs.uk/Livewell/Goodfood/Documents/The-Eatwell-Guide-2016.pdf (accessed 10 December 2017).

NHS Quality Improvement Scotland (2014) Food, Fluid and Nutritional Care in Hospitals. Available at: www.healthcareimprovementscotland.org/our_work/patient_safety/improving_nutritional_ care/nutritional_care_standards.aspx (accessed 10 December 2017).

Nursing and Midwifery Council (NMC) (2008) *Standards for Medicine Management*. London: NMC. Available at: www.nmc-uk.org/Documents/NMC-Publications/NMC-Standards-for-medicines-management.pdf (accessed 7 March 2018).

Royal College of Nursing (RCN) (2011) Nutrition Now: Enhancing nutritional care. Available at: www.rcn.org.uk/__data/assets/pdf_file/0006/187989/003284.pdf (accessed 7 March 2018).

Russell, C.A. and Elia, M. (2011) Nutrition Screening Survey in the UK and Republic of Ireland in 2011. Available at: www.bapen.org.uk/pdfs/nsw/nsw-2011-report.pdf (accessed 24 February 2015).

Scottish Government (2014) Eating Well with Dementia: A carers' guide. Available at: www.gov.scot/Resource/0044/00449379.pdf (accessed 7 March 2018).

SIGN (2001) Guideline 119: Management of Patients with Stroke – Identification and management of dysphagia. Available at: www.sign.ac.uk/guidelines/fulltext/119/section6.html (accessed 24 February 2015). [Updated 2013]

van Bokhorst-de van der Schueren, M., Guaitoli, P., Jansma, E. and De Vet, H. (2014) 'Nutrition screening tools: Does one size fit all? A systematic review of screening tools for the hospital setting', *Clinical Nutrition*, 33(1): 39–58.

World Health Organization (WHO) (2009) WHO Guidelines on Hand Hygiene in Health Care. Available at: http://whqlibdoc.who.int/publications/2009/9789241597906_eng.pdf (accessed 7 March 2018).

ASSISTING PATIENTS WITH THEIR ELIMINATION NEEDS

MAIREAD COLLIE AND DAVID J. HUNTER

THIS CHAPTER COVERS

- Assisting patients with their elimination needs
- Assessing bowel function
- Bedpans, urinals and commodes

- Use of incontinence pads
- Caring for a patient with a urinary catheter
- Urinalysis

REQUIRED KNOWLEDGE

- It will be helpful to have a clear understanding of the anatomy and physiology of the digestive and urinary systems before starting this chapter.

> My name is Miss Annie Jones. I am 83 years young and live in assisted living accommodation, and you can call me Annie. I was a schoolteacher, never married because teaching was my life. I have two nephews but they live miles away, although they send me Christmas cards. I have some good friends but like me their mobility is not great and I do not see them very often now, so we keep in touch by telephone.
>
> Over the past three years I have developed osteoarthritis in both my knees, which has affected my mobility. I used to get out and about and enjoyed long walks; now I can get around my bungalow but require someone to help if I have to leave my home. The doctor has given me strong painkillers, which do help, but they give me terrible constipation which I do not like to discuss with anyone. The doctor has given me medicine for my bowels but recently it has not been working so well and my stomach is really sore. Today I had to call the GP as the stomach pain and cramps were so bad; the district nurse is coming out to see me.
>
> I am really embarrassed as I do not know what they will ask me or what they might do.
>
> **Annie, patient**

> Helping someone who needs care relating to elimination is a challenging aspect of nursing, as you are dealing with intimate and embarrassing issues. However, it is an extremely important, fundamental role and one which nurses need to take seriously. Patient education is an important aspect of elimination care as it empowers the patient and promotes independence.
>
> **Joanne, MH nursing student**

INTRODUCTION

Assisting patients with their elimination needs involves undertaking a series of procedures. The role of the nurse within these is to maintain the dignity and privacy of the patient while delivering the fundamental care required. In the patient voice, Annie outlines how difficult it can be to have to discuss elimination needs with others – if you were in her position, what would you value most in the care you received?

Patients are in a very vulnerable position when you are assisting them with their elimination needs and, as a nursing student, you may also feel embarrassed or awkward in dealing with these issues. As Joanne outlines in the student voice, however, this is an important aspect of care, which nurses need to respond to with sensitivity.

Solomon (2008) defines elimination as activity which we undertake several times a day to remove waste products from metabolism (urine and faeces) from the body. Elimination is normally undertaken in private and methods are influenced by societal and cultural norms.

This chapter will explain and discuss the fundamental skills involved in assisting patients with their elimination needs. We will discuss the practical skills involved in a range of procedures and consider the ways in which we keep comfort, dignity, respect, privacy and compassion at the heart of what we as nurses do to help patients with this aspect of their lives.

ASSISTING PATIENTS WITH THEIR ELIMINATION NEEDS

The need to assist patients with their elimination needs arises within all fields of nursing and the underlying principles are the same. The fundamental skills are:

1. Bowel assessment
2. Assisting a patient to use a bedpan or urinal
3. Assisting a patient to use a commode
4. Emptying a catheter
5. Providing catheter care
6. Urinalysis

However, your approach to the patient and the care you deliver will vary based on individual patient need and response. No matter which of the skills relating to elimination you are going to undertake or the care setting in which you will do so, there are a number of issues and common steps you need to consider first.

Guidelines

There are various national and local guidelines of which you must be aware when assisting patients with their elimination needs. Remember never to undertake any of the following procedures unless you are, or have supervision from, a trained, experienced and competent person. The types of guidelines you need to consider will be contained in:

- infection prevention and control policy
- local policies and documentation relating to the particular skill
- The Code: Professional Standards of Practice and Behaviour for Nurses and Midwives (NMC, 2015)
- Record Keeping: Guidance for Nurses and Midwives (NMC, 2009)
- local consent policy

- local health and safety policy
- disposal of clinical waste policy
- chaperone and intimate care policy.

Once you are aware of these, you need to take a number of steps that will be common for all care delivered to assist patients with their elimination needs (see Clinical Skill 31.1).

CASE STUDY 31.1: MISS JONES

You and your practice educator, a district nurse, have been asked to make a home visit to assess a patient called Miss Annie Jones, whom you met at the start of the chapter. Miss Jones contacted her GP for advice about changes in her normal bowel routine.

Miss Jones has a past medical history of osteoarthritis in both knee joints which has greatly reduced her mobility over the past three years, mainly due to pain. Annie takes co-codamol 30/500 mg and a non-steroidal anti-inflammatory drug (NSAID) as prescribed, but her pain continues to be a problem and she suffers from one of the side-effects of these analgesics – constipation. Miss Jones has discussed this with her GP, who has advised her to eat a high-fibre diet and has also prescribed laxatives when required.

Despite doing this, however, Annie continues to experience constipation. Over the past 72 hours, she has not opened her bowels and has abdominal cramps and a distended abdomen.

- What essential nursing skills do you think will be involved in taking Miss Jones' history and carrying out an examination within her home?
- What are the signs and symptoms of constipation, why do they occur and how would you describe them to a patient?

ANSWER:
CASE STUDY 31.1

When I am completing the patient's chart and need to ask whether they have been to the toilet I am aware this can be very embarrassing for some. I always ensure if in an open bay I am furthest away from the patient in the next bed and have my back to them. This allows me to shelter the patient to whom I am speaking, which I feel is more discreet. I also ask quietly, not loudly so the whole ward can hear, but also in keeping with all other questions I have asked so as not to make a big thing out of it and draw attention to the fact they may be embarrassed.

Alice Rowe, NQ RNMH

ASSESSING BOWEL FUNCTION

As is clear in the case of Annie Jones, patients can find it very difficult to discuss any issues relating to elimination, as this is an intimate and private activity. Assessment of a patient's bowel function provides us with precise information relating to their eliminatory functioning.

Although it is important for you to undertake the clinical skill accurately by following the steps outlined in Clinical Skill 31.2, it is just as important that you communicate effectively with the patient, making them feel as comfortable as possible with your presence while reducing their anxiety and embarrassment.

STEP-BY-STEP CLINICAL SKILL 31.1: COMMON STEPS FOR ALL ELIMINATION-RELATED SKILLS

☑ **Essential equipment – depends on skill but is likely to include one or more of the following:**

- Suitable personal protective equipment (PPE)
- Bedpan and paper cover, urinal, commode
- Toilet paper
- Equipment to enable the patient to wash their hands
- Manual handling equipment and possibly assistance from another member of the healthcare team
- Soap and warm water, single-use washcloths and towels

☑ **Field-specific considerations**

When caring for a patient with a learning disability, it is important to know their level of understanding so that consent for and cooperation with the care can be gained. You will need to allow time to explain why you are doing the measurements and whether they will cause discomfort or pain.

Patients who have mental health problems may not understand the relevance of the care you plan to deliver. They may therefore withhold consent and you may need to refer to the Mental Capacity Act 2005, or the Adults with Incapacity (Scotland) Act 2000, and best interest.

When assisting children with elimination needs, if possible it is usually helpful to have the parents or carers present to assist.

☑ **Care-setting considerations**

Assisting patients with elimination needs can occur within all settings, although you may not have all the equipment available to assist you. For example, in a patient's home you may not have manual handling equipment, so to ensure patient safety and your own, thorough risk assessments need to be undertaken.

☑ **What to watch out for and action to take**

While assisting a patient with their elimination needs, as appropriate, you should also observe and assess:

- the condition of their skin
- their ability to move or mobilise independently
- their neurological condition – are they alert and responsive?
- any signs or complaints of pain or discomfort
- the patient's or relatives' views – for example, saying that their needs have changed or that they are experiencing problems
- any changes reported by the patient regarding the colour, smell and consistency of their urine and any changes in their stool.

The information gained from these observations will enable you to fully assess the patient's condition and institute appropriate treatment as necessary.

☑ **Helpful hints**

- Gloves and aprons must be worn if contact with blood/body fluids/excreta is anticipated or the patient is in isolation.
- Hand hygiene must be performed before touching a patient, before clean/aseptic procedures, after body fluid exposure/risk, after touching a patient and after touching a patient's surroundings.
- Waste should be disposed of in a clinical waste bag if it is contaminated with blood/body fluids/excreta.

ELIMINATION ASSISTANCE GUIDELINES

 The first step of any procedure is to introduce yourself to the patient, explain the procedure and gain their consent
Fully informed consent may not always be possible if the patient is a child or has mental health problems or learning disabilities, but even in these circumstances, every effort should be made to explain the procedure in terms that the patient can understand. This is not only respectful of their individual human rights, but also helps to ensure that they will be more accepting of the treatment and that their anxieties are reduced

For patients who are unable to provide consent because they are unconscious, advice should be sought from your practice educator or another qualified nurse

 Gather the equipment required (see individual skills for equipment required). Ensure these are clean as appropriate and in working order
Ensures the skill is performed effectively
Reduces the chance of infection and maintains patient and nurse safety

 Clear sufficient space within the environment, for example around the bed space or chair
Enables clear access for the patient and the nurse to safely use the equipment required

 Wash your hands with soap and water before you start any care activity. Apron and gloves should only be worn if appropriate
Wearing an apron and gloves as part of personal protective equipment (PPE) is a standard infection-control procedure when dealing with body fluids or patients in isolation
Ensure your use of PPE such as gloves and disposable aprons is appropriate by considering the individual patient situation and the risk presented

 Ensure you promote patient dignity and privacy as appropriate, for example by drawing curtains or moving the patient to a bathroom if at all possible
Elimination needs are intimate and personal. At all times you need to maintain patient privacy, dignity and comfort as required

 Patients need to be in a comfortable position
Promotes patient comfort and reduces anxiety

 After performing the task, ensure the patient is in a comfortable position, with drinks and call bells available as necessary
Promotes patient comfort and ensures they are well nourished and hydrated

 Discard PPE, any single-use equipment and other used materials as per policy. Clean any equipment used as per the relevant policy every time it is used and perform hand hygiene
Prevents cross-infection and maintains equipment in working condition

 Document findings as appropriate, for example on the patient's observation chart and/or in the patient's notes
Maintains patient safety and accurate records

 If any abnormalities are observed, escalate to senior nursing staff or your practice educator immediately
It is vital to report any abnormalities to a registered nurse immediately so they can ensure the patient receives the care required

Source: NMC (2009, 2015); WHO (2009)

STEP-BY-STEP CLINICAL SKILL 31.2: ASSESSING BOWEL FUNCTION

☑ **What is normal?**

'Normal' bowel function can vary greatly: some patients open their bowels daily, others every two or three days. If possible, it is best to ask the patient what is 'normal' for them and whether they take laxatives.

☑ **Before you start**

Remember the common steps for all care delivered to assist patients with their elimination needs (Clinical Skill 31.1).

Remember to review any documentation regarding the patient and update any relevant care plans. Other factors need to be considered when assessing a patient's bowel function, as this will enable you to assess the patient's overall condition. As you approach the patient, observe them carefully to assess whether they are well nourished and hydrated. Do they look in good health or do they appear unwell, and are they able to move unaided?

☑ **Essential equipment**

Relevant documentation with regard to bowel assessment. This can vary between patients depending on the field, as well as between care settings.

Appropriate personal protective equipment (PPE).

☑ **Field-specific considerations**

If assessing a patient who has a learning disability, it is important to ascertain their level of understanding. If appropriate, involve a family member or carer in the discussion.

When assessing a patient with mental health problems, their level of capacity may need to be considered, so they may require support and assistance to enable them to recognise that they are constipated.

As appropriate depending on the age of a child, encourage and assist their parents or carers to become involved, as they will provide useful information.

☑ **Care-setting considerations**

An assessment of bowel function can be undertaken in any care setting.

☑ **What to watch out for and action to take**

Remember that the questions you are going to ask may cause anxiety and embarrassment.

If any abnormalities are found, this must be reported to a qualified nurse immediately and recorded in the patient's notes.

BOWEL FUNCTION ASSESSMENT GUIDELINES

1 Perform steps 1–6 of the common steps (Clinical Skill 31.1)
To prepare the patient and yourself to undertake the task

2 Document the history of the present bowel complaint
To gain an understanding of the patient's needs and to direct management or treatment decisions

3 Undertake a holistic assessment of the patient's condition, which includes details of their diet, fluids, mobility, dexterity, cognitive function and usual environment
To obtain a comprehensive and holistic assessment which may identify the underlying reason for the patient's altered bowel habit, whether constipation or diarrhoea

4 Document the patient's usual bowel pattern
To ascertain what is 'normal' for the patient

5 Ask the patient what medications they are currently taking
To assess if medication has affected the normal bowel routine

6 Ask the patient to identify their stool formation using the Bristol Stool Chart
To enable clear identification of the patient's needs and allow for effective management

7 As is appropriate within the care setting, ensure that future bowel actions are monitored and accurately recorded
To monitor condition and detect abnormalities

8 Develop a plan of care in partnership with the patient and their parents or carers as appropriate
To produce a clear plan of care to be delivered to the patient and ensure that the patient is aware of and happy with the ongoing management of the condition

9 Perform steps 7–10 of the common steps (Clinical Skill 31.1)
To ensure that:

- the patient is safe, comfortable and receiving the appropriate care
- the results have been documented in the patient's records

Source: NMC (2009, 2015)

The Bristol Stool Chart

The Bristol Stool Chart (Lewis and Heaton, 1997) is a simple method used to assess how a patient's digestive system is working. According to the chart, there are seven types of stool (see Figure 31.1), with each stool type being formed as a result of the time it spends in the colon.

Type 1		Separate hard lumps, like nuts (hard to pass)
Type 2		Sausage-shaped but lumpy
Type 3		Like a sausage but with cracks on its surface
Type 4		Like a sausage or snake, smooth and soft
Type 5		Soft blobs with clear-cut edges (passed easily)
Type 6		Fluffy pieces with ragged edges, a mushy stool
Type 7		Watery, no solid pieces. Entirely liquid

Figure 31.1   Bristol Stool Chart

Source: Heaton and Lewis (1997). © Informa Healthcare, 1997. Reproduced with permission of Informa Healthcare

> Many parents/carers normally change their babies' nappies and take their children to the toilet when on the ward, however this should not be an expectation. Nurses are there to provide all aspects of care. I think it should be discussed with the parents/carers and child as to what their needs are and what they would like to do, or what/how the child would like to be cared for when they need to use the bathroom, or pads need to be changed. When assisting with elimination, changing nappies or older children's pads, dignity and respect are paramount. You should empower them as much as you can, think what their abilities are, and what they can and would like to do for themselves … never assume they can't.
>
> **Siân Hunter, child nursing student**

ACTIVITY 31.1: CRITICAL THINKING

Using Clinical Skill 31.2 as a guide:

- How would you use the Bristol Stool Chart to offer further information on an adult patient's bowel functioning?
- What would be different if you were undertaking an assessment of bowel function with a patient who was 2 years old?

A&P LINK: DIGESTION

Simply put, when we are monitoring a patient's bowel function we are observing the end products of digestion. The function of the digestive system is to convert food from the diet into substances which can be used by the various cells of the body to perform everyday functions. The digestive system can be divided into four parts: the upper part, the middle portion, the lower segment and the accessory organs (see Figure 31.2).

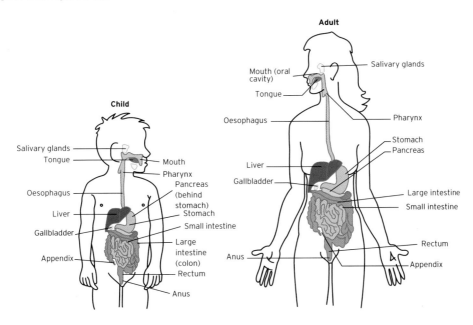

Figure 31.2   The digestive system

Image © Robin Lupton

The gastrointestinal tract is, in essence, a long hollow tube running from the mouth to the anus. The digestive process begins in the mouth, where food is broken down into smaller components through the action of the teeth, lips and cheeks in chewing (**mastication**) and saliva, which includes digestive enzymes and which provides moisture to aid swallowing (McErlean, 2011). Food boluses then travel to the stomach via the oesophagus – a muscular, collapsible tube which is approximately 25 cm long (Porth, 2007). The stomach sits in the abdominal cavity; its shape and size vary between people and in accordance with the amount of food being stored. Gastric acid and pepsin in the stomach contribute to the breakdown of food, with most meals leaving the stomach four hours after being ingested. On leaving the stomach, the partially digested foodstuffs, or 'chyme', move into the small intestine (Burch, 2013). The small intestine is approximately 6 m long and has three subdivisions: the duodenum, the jejunum and the ileum. As the chyme progresses along the small intestine, additional digestive enzymes are added, including pancreatic juice (from the pancreas) and bile (from the liver), which enter the duodenum. Chyme spends 3–6 hours in the small intestine, where nutrients and fluids are absorbed. As the process continues, the chyme enters the large intestine as fluid faeces, where it travels through the caecum, ascending colon, transverse colon, descending colon, sigmoid colon and finally reaches the rectum in preparation

(Continued)

for defecation (Burch, 2013). The primary function of the large intestine is the absorption of water to turn fluid faeces into semi-solid faeces (McErlean, 2011). **Defecation** occurs when the stretching of the rectum, as it fills with faeces, initiates the defecation reflex. It is controlled by the action of the internal and external anal sphincters and is consciously controlled in a healthy adult (Porth, 2007).

BEDPANS, URINALS AND COMMODES

You will find that assisting a patient to use a bedpan, urinal or commode is one of the most frequent elimination-related tasks you carry out. While this at first may seem a very simple process, you will find that this is not always the case.

The principles outlined in Clinical Skill 31.3 relate to assisting a patient to use either a bedpan or commode or, for male patients, a urinal. Remember that some male patients may prefer, if they are able, to stand with support from either one or two nurses to use a urinal in an upright position. If this is the case, consider safe patient handling requirements to keep both you and the patient safe.

Create a comfortable environment for that patient. Find out what they need to feel able to use the toilet, promote dignity, and give people plenty of time.

Michelle Hill, NQ RNLD

I find it easy to put patients on a bedpan and remove a full one as long as you take your time.

Hannah Boyd, adult nursing student

ACTIVITY 31.2: REFLECTION

Reflect on an experience where you have assisted a patient with their elimination needs:

- Was the patient's dignity and privacy maintained at all times?
- If you had been the patient, would you have been happy with the care you delivered?
- At the time you assisted the patient with their elimination needs, were you aware of the significance of maintaining their privacy and dignity and communicating effectively with them?
- After reflecting on your experience, would you do anything differently next time you deliver this care?

STEP-BY-STEP CLINICAL SKILL 31.3: ASSISTING A PATIENT TO USE A BEDPAN, URINAL OR COMMODE

☑ **What is normal?**

Female patients may need to use a bedpan or commode to both **micturate** and defecate; male patients may prefer to micturate in a urinal, which may be easier if they stand up (if this is appropriate).

☑ **Before you start**

Remember the common steps for all care delivered to assist patients with their elimination needs (Clinical Skill 31.1).

☑ **Essential equipment**

- Appropriate personal protective equipment (PPE)
- Appropriate bedpan and paper cover or commode or urinal and paper cover
- Toilet paper
- Facilities to allow the patient to wash their hands
- Manual handling equipment as required
- Possible assistance from a further member of the healthcare team

☑ **Field-specific considerations**

If assisting a patient who has a learning disability or cognitive impairment, it is important to ascertain their level of understanding.

As appropriate depending on the age of a child, encourage and assist parents or carers to become involved in care to maintain their normal caring role as far as is possible.

☑ **Care-setting considerations**

A patient can be assisted to use a bedpan, commode or urinal in any care setting.

☑ **What to watch out for and action to take**

Elimination is an intimate and personal activity. Ensure you promote the patient's dignity and provide privacy at all times.

(Continued)

ELIMINATION ASSISTANCE GUIDELINES

1 **Perform steps 1-6 of the common steps (Clinical Skill 31.1)**
To prepare the patient and yourself to undertake the task

2 **Bedpan or urinal**
Assess the moving and handling needs of the patient

Commode
Assess the moving and handling needs of the patient. Ensure the patient's weight does not exceed the manufacturer's recommendations

To maintain a safe environment and to determine whether or not additional assistance is required

3 **Remove the bedclothes and, if the patient is able, assist them to sit upright. Ask the patient (or use moving and handling equipment if required) to raise their hips/ buttocks to allow the bedpan or urinal to be correctly positioned. If the patient cannot raise their hips/buttocks, a rolling motion may be used with appropriate moving and handling techniques to roll the patient onto the bedpan**
Support with pillow if required

Take the equipment to the bedside, checking that the wheels on the commode are secured and that there is a bedpan receiver placed under the commode
  Remove the commode cover and assist the patient to transfer from bed/chair to the commode. Ensure the patient is comfortable
    A comfortable position may make it easier for the patient to open their bowels
    To ensure patient safety

4 **When the patient is on the bedpan or has the urinal in position, ask them to move their legs slightly apart so that you can check the position is correct**

Check the patient is positioned correctly on the commode
Checking the position will reduce the risk of spillage and associated contamination or cross-infection

5 **If safe to do so, leave the patient, ensuring that toilet paper is close at hand and giving them a nurse call button. Cover the patient's legs with a towel or sheet**
This step is not possible if you are supporting a patient to use a urinal while standing
To maintain privacy and dignity

6 **When the patient has finished using the bedpan, commode or urinal, you may need to assist them with personal hygiene. As indicated, select the appropriate PPE and clean the patient's bottom using toilet paper, wiping from front to back. Skin cleanser or warm soapy water may be required**
Assisting the patient to be clean will ensure patient comfort

Wiping from front to back will reduce the spread of infection from the bowel to the urethra (especially in women)

Pat the skin dry after assisting the patient with their personal hygiene
To prevent deterioration of the patient's skin

Help the patient to wash and dry their hands
To promote patient comfort, dignity and infection control

Perform steps 7-10 of the common steps (Clinical Skill 31.1)
To ensure that:

- the patient is safe, comfortable and receiving the appropriate care
- the results have been documented in the patient's records
- any equipment is clean and ready to be reused

Source: Ballentyne and Ness (2009); NMC (2009, 2015); Oxford University Hospitals NHS Trust (2013)

USE OF INCONTINENCE PADS

Although it is likely that you will see incontinence pads being used frequently with a wide range of patients, this practice is controversial. It is important that the use of incontinence pads meets the individual needs of the patient, so a continence assessment should always be undertaken before they are used. Incontinence pads should never be routinely applied or used instead of assisting patients to use a toilet, commode, urinal or bedpan. The main issues to consider when applying and changing incontinence pads are as follows:

- The manufacturer's instructions should be followed to ensure the pad is used to its full effectiveness.
- Only one pad should be applied to the patient at a time; if one pad is insufficient then further assessment is required, because using two pads may damage the patient's skin.
- Skincare and personal hygiene should be carried out every time a pad is changed to maintain the condition of the patient's skin.
- Always be cautious with the use of barrier creams and do not apply talcum powder under an incontinence pad.
- The patient's dignity should be maintained at all times and terms like 'nappy' should be avoided.
- Appropriate infection-control steps should be taken as you are dealing with bodily fluids.
- The need for a patient to use an incontinence pad must be frequently reassessed. (Payne, 2013)

ACTIVITY 31.3: REFLECTION

Reflect on an experience you have had when incontinence pads have been used as part of a patient's plan of care:

- Were the issues highlighted in the list above evident in the patient's care?
- Might you do anything differently in future?

A&P LINK: MICTURITION

The production of urine and micturition involves the renal system.

Urine is composed of approximately 95 per cent water and 5 per cent dissolved solids in the form of metabolic waste. It is a clear, amber-coloured liquid and around 1.5 litres are produced each day in a healthy adult.

Urine is formed in the kidneys by three processes:

- Filtration: where blood enters the glomeruli of the kidney and fluid crosses the membrane by osmosis and diffusion.
- Selective reabsorption: where around 99 per cent of the filtrate from the filtration stage is reabsorbed; this includes substances like sodium, calcium and potassium.
- Secretion: the remaining waste products are secreted by the nephron into the collecting duct, eventually leaving the kidney via the ureter.

When fully grown, the ureter is approximately 25–30 cm in length and connects the kidneys to the bladder. Although urine is formed within the kidneys, it is the bladder which stores urine and controls its elimination from the body.

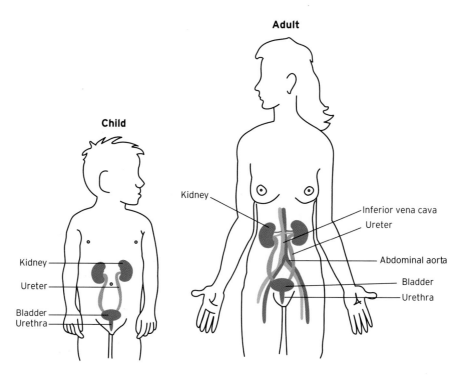

Figure 31.3   The urinary system

Image © Robin Lupton

The bladder is a hollow muscular organ which, in an adult, can hold approximately 350–750 ml of urine (Nair, 2011). The process of micturition is controlled via a complex series of neurological links between the bladder, spinal cord and brain stem, with the urge to pass urine beginning as the bladder stretches as it fills, typically at around 150–200 ml (Naish, 2008). A healthy adult is able to control the process of micturition. When urinating, the detrusor muscle of the bladder contracts, the bladder neck is widened, the resistance of the internal sphincter reduces and the external sphincter relaxes to allow the urine to leave the bladder. The urine travels from the bladder outside the body via the urethra, which is longer in men than in women (Nair, 2011).

Children's bladders are much smaller, with their size and capacity gradually increasing during the first eight years. As their bladder size increases, the frequency of micturition reduces and full control of this is usually gained by the age of 3 or 4 years, when they are dry throughout both the day and night. Children have a reduced ability to concentrate urine, so are at greater risk of dehydration.

CARING FOR A PATIENT WITH A URINARY CATHETER

A high standard of catheter care is required to reduce the complications associated with the use of an indwelling catheter, especially if this is going to be for long-term use (Pomfret, 2006). Catheters should only ever be used when absolutely necessary and those caring for patients with a catheter need to ensure they provide effective catheter care. This includes strict hand-washing principles when coming into contact with the catheter, keeping the catheter clean and encouraging the patient to drink sufficient fluids, all of which will reduce the chance of infection. Clinical Skill 31.4 outlines the steps you need to take to 'perform catheter care', which means assisting a patient to maintain their hygiene and keep the catheter clean.

ACTIVITY 31.4: CRITICAL THINKING

Maintaining dignity has been mentioned frequently throughout this chapter, as attending to our elimination needs is personal and intimate and normally something we undertake in private. The loss of dignity felt by people with continence problems can be devastating and many feel it reduces their self-worth as a competent adult.

Receiving assistance with elimination needs can be acutely embarrassing for a patient, but can also be uncomfortable for the nurse providing the care.

- What skills, in addition to accurately performing a procedure, does a nurse need to apply in order to maintain a patient's dignity when assisting a patient to meet their elimination needs?
- Does the fundamental importance of maintaining a patient's dignity when assisting with elimination needs alter if the patient is confused, disorientated or unaware of their surroundings, or is a child?

ANSWER:
ACTIVITY 31.4

Apply your understanding of caring for a patient with a catheter by watching videos on catheter care.

After providing catheter care, it may be appropriate to empty the patient's catheter bag (see Clinical Skill 31.5). It is important to recognise that performing catheter care and emptying a patient's catheter bag are two separate procedures and that you must adhere to strict infection control and prevention measures between the procedures, rather than continuing without performing the appropriate hand hygiene.

STEP-BY-STEP CLINICAL SKILL 31.4: PERFORMING CATHETER CARE

☑ What is normal?

Catheter care should be undertaken as a part of the patient's routine hygiene care.

☑ Before you start

Remember the common steps for all care delivered to assist patients with their elimination needs (Clinical Skill 31.1).

☑ Essential equipment

- Appropriate personal protective equipment (PPE)
- Soap and warm water
- Single-use washcloths
- Towel

☑ Field-specific considerations

If assisting a patient who has a learning disability, it is important to ascertain their level of understanding.

As appropriate depending on the age of a child, encourage and assist parents or carers to become involved in care to maintain their normal caring role as far as is possible.

☑ Care-setting considerations

Catheter care can be undertaken in any care setting.

☑ What to watch out for and action to take

Performing catheter care is an intimate and personal activity. Ensure you promote the patient's dignity and provide privacy at all times.

CATHETER CARE GUIDELINES

1 **Perform steps 1–6 of the common steps (Clinical Skill 31.1)**
To prepare the patient and yourself to undertake the task

2 **Assist the patient to be correctly positioned for the procedure**
To allow ease of access, maintain patient comfort and adhere to moving and handling regulations

3 **Clean the genital area using soap and water**
Soap and water are appropriate; anti-bacterial or antiseptic solutions are not required

4 **Perform meatal cleansing:**

a) **in male patients by pulling back the foreskin (if uncircumcised). Note that the foreskin should not be forcibly pulled back. It can take until the late teenage years before the foreskin can be retracted**

Clean around the glans, moving away from the meatal opening; clean the area where the catheter enters the penis and then downwards along the catheter
Rinse and dry the area
Return the foreskin to the original position
b) **in female patients by gently parting the labia**
Clean the area where the catheter enters the meatus and then downwards along the catheter
Rinse and dry the area
To reduce the risk of spreading infection
   To expose the glans penis and the urethral meatus
   To reduce contamination
   To remove any buildup of **smegma**
   To reduce the risk of irritation from soap and to maintain skin integrity
   To reduce the risk of **paraphimosis** developing
   To expose the inner genitals (labia minora) and the urethral meatus
   To reduce contamination, particularly from the anus

To reduce the risk of irritation from soap and to maintain skin integrity

Make sure that the area is completely dry
To reduce the risk of skin breakdown. Talcum powder should be avoided as irritation may be caused

Ensure that the patient is comfortable and re-dressed following the procedure
To promote patient comfort and dignity

Perform steps 7-10 of the common steps (Clinical Skill 31.1)
To ensure that:

- the patient is safe, comfortable and receiving the appropriate care
- the results have been documented in the patient's records
- any equipment is clean and ready to be reused

Source: Hunter (2012); Leaver (2007); NMC (2015)

CASE STUDY 31.2: MR PARIS

Mr Timothy Paris is a 77-year-old gentleman who lives alone in a two-bedroom, ground floor apartment. He lives in a semi-rural location, in a small town with good local amenities, and his home is well maintained. His wife, Kathryn, died three years ago. Timothy has an excellent relationship with his two daughters, who live a few miles away. They each spend part of the day with him, assisting him with all of his activities of living, and Mr Paris spends alternate weekends with them and their families at their homes.

Mr Paris worked as a civil servant and retired aged 65. He has never smoked and drinks alcohol in moderation. Until recently, he enjoyed playing golf, socialising with his friends and having meals out with his extended family. His past medical history includes arthritis and high blood pressure (hypertension). His blood pressure is monitored at his local GP surgery and is stable due to the anti-hypertensive medication he takes.

Over the past 12 months, Timothy has experienced frequent episodes of urinary incontinence, which have been managed at home. However, during this time he has been diagnosed with dementia and his physical and psychological condition has deteriorated.

Mr Paris now needs additional support to care for himself, which is provided by his daughters and extended family, the district nurse and carers. As a result of his general deterioration, Timothy, his family and the healthcare team have decided to manage his incontinence through long-term catheterisation.

- What information would you give Mr Paris and his daughters to assist them to care for the catheter?
- How would you ascertain exactly what catheter care activities Mr Paris was happy for his daughters to provide and what Mr Paris' daughters felt it was appropriate for them to undertake?

STEP-BY-STEP CLINICAL SKILL 31.5: EMPTYING A PATIENT'S CATHETER BAG

☑ What is normal?

Catheter bags should only be emptied when they are full, as each time you perform this procedure you are potentially introducing an infection risk.

☑ Before you start

Remember the common steps for all care delivered to assist patients with their elimination needs (Clinical Skill 31.1).

Do not forget that a catheter bag is attached to a patient and that you need to ask for their consent to perform this procedure.

☑ Essential equipment

- Appropriate personal protective equipment (PPE)
- Alcohol swabs
- Sterile jug or disposable container

Figure 31.4   Essential equipment

☑ Field-specific considerations

If assisting a patient who has a learning disability, it is important to ascertain their level of understanding.

As appropriate depending on the age of a child, encourage and assist parents or carers to become involved in care to maintain their normal caring role as far as is possible.

☑ Care-setting considerations

Emptying a catheter bag can be undertaken in any care setting.

☑ What to watch out for and action to take

Emptying a catheter bag can be seen by patients to be the same activity as using the toilet. Ensure you promote the patient's dignity and provide privacy at all times. If the patient's urine output is not being monitored frequently and you notice when emptying the bag that the patient has passed little or no urine, check the patient's fluid balance chart, as their catheter bag may have just been emptied. If this is not the case, you must inform your practice educator or a registered nurse, as it may indicate a problem relating to catheter drainage or an alteration in the patient's condition. Patients who are catheterised may have an overnight drainage bag attached, which will be removed when the patient mobilises and replaced with a leg bag.

CATHETER CARE GUIDELINES

 Perform steps 1–6 of the common steps (Clinical Skill 31.1)
To prepare the patient and yourself to undertake the task

 Clean the outlet port of the catheter bag with the alcohol swab and allow to fully dry

To reduce the risk of infection

 Open the port and allow the urine to drain into the jug

To empty the bag and, if required, to allow measurement of the volume of urine passed

 Close the port and clean again with an alcohol swab

To reduce the risk of infection

 Reposition the catheter bag and check that the patient is comfortable
To ensure the patient is comfortable

 Cover the jug and transfer to the sluice where the urine can be disposed of
If required, the urine should be measured
To reduce the risk of contamination
   To monitor the patient's condition and to maintain accurate documentation

 Perform steps 7–10 of the common steps (Clinical Skill 31.1)
To ensure that:

- the patient is safe, comfortable and receiving the appropriate care
- the results have been documented in the patient's records
- any equipment is clean and ready to be reused

Source: NHS Greater Glasgow and Clyde (2014); NMC (2015)

STEP-BY-STEP CLINICAL SKILL 31.6: URINALYSIS

☑ **Before you start**

Remember the common steps for all care delivered to assist patients with their elimination needs (Clinical Skill 31.1).

Assess the colour and smell of the urine.

☑ **Essential equipment**

White-top sterile specimen containers (see Figure 31.5) or bedpans are the most commonly used receptacles. To undertake accurate urinalysis, the receptacle needs to be clean but not necessarily sterile, so any clean receptacle which can hold water may be used.

☑ **Care-setting considerations**

Can be measured in any care setting.

Ensure that the patient has the mobility necessary to use the commode, urinal or bedpan. If this is not the case, offer assistance and support and apply safe patient moving techniques. Catheterisation may be considered, but the need for this would be carefully risk-assessed.

Note: Step-by-step Clinical Skill 31.6 was contributed by Valerie Foley.

Figure 31.5   Sterile specimen containers

SPECIMEN COLLECTION GUIDELINES

1 **Perform steps 1-5 of the common steps (see Clinical Skill 31.1)**
To prepare the patient and yourself to undertake the task

2 **Ensure the container you are going to use to obtain the specimen is appropriately labelled with the patient's identification details**
To ensure that you test the correct specimen

3 **First voided morning urine is best suited for urinalysis**
Its concentration provides the most reliable results

4 **It is best to test specimens immediately; if not possible, then do so within two hours**
This provides the most reliable results

5 **After shaking the sample, briefly completely immerse the whole section of the strip where the test pads are located into freshly voided urine**
Shake the sample to ensure it is mixed so the concentration will be constant throughout
Dip the strip briefly to avoid dissolving out **reagents** from the test pads which would produce incorrect results

6 **As you remove the strip from the sample, run its edge against the edge of the receptacle – apply the 'dip and drag' stages of the 'dip, drag, blot, read' technique (see Figure 31.6)**
To remove excess urine and prevent the strip from dripping

7 **Hold the strip horizontally**
To avoid potential mixing of reagents due to them running down the strip. This would cause cross-reactions that will produce unreliable results

8 **Remove excess urine by applying the 'blot' stage of the 'dip, drag, blot, read' technique (see Figure 31.6)**
Blot the edge of the strip on absorbent material such as a paper towel. Take care not to touch the test pads and maintain the strip in a horizontal position
To prevent the strip from dripping

9 **Compare all test pads with the corresponding colour chart. At the time specified, record all results**
This is the 'read' stage of the 'dip, drag, blot, read' technique (see Figure 31.6). Make sure that when you are comparing the test pads with the corresponding colour, you do not hold the strip directly against the container, as there may be urine remaining on the strip which you would transfer to the container
It is important to follow the timings specified to ensure that your results are correct. Colour changes that have occurred after two minutes are invalid and will not provide accurate results

10 **Perform steps 8-10 of the common steps (see Clinical Skill 31.1)**
To ensure that:

- the patient is safe, comfortable and receiving the appropriate care
- the results have been documented in the patient's records

Figure 31.6 Dip, drag, blot, read technique

Source: Smith and Roberts (2011)

WHAT'S THE EVIDENCE?

FURTHER
READING:
FAMILY
INVOLVEMENT

Nayeri, N.D., Gholizadeh, L., Mohammadi, E. and Yazdi, K. (2015) 'Family involvement in the care of hospitalized elderly patients', *Journal of Applied Gerontology*, 34(6): 779-96.

In case study 31.2, Mr Paris' daughters' involvement in assisting him to maintain his elimination needs highlights an important aspect of the role of the nurse, which is being able to work not only in partnership with a patient, but also with their family or carers. When caring for children, a family-centred care model is accepted practice; however, when caring for adult patients this is not always the case.

Family members' involvement in the care of adults has been investigated by Nayeri et al. (2015):

- Reflect on the care of an adult patient you have been involved in where family members or carers were also involved in delivering care.
- Did the other nurses express any views about this?
- Why might nurses not be open to involving a patient's family members or carers in the delivery of care?
- Now read the article and consider whether:

  o   there are any similarities with your experience?
  o   it is possible to translate the findings of a study undertaken in Iran to a UK setting?

URINALYSIS

The final section in this chapter considers urinalysis, an important skill in the care of all patients, whether or not they require assistance with their elimination needs. Urinalysis can reveal diseases that may go otherwise unnoticed because they do not produce clear signs or symptoms, especially not in the early stages. Examples of such diseases include diabetes mellitus, various forms of glomerulonephritis and chronic urinary tract infections. This makes urinalysis an important skill to master, but, as with all other clinical measurements, you need to ensure your results are accurate. Following the steps in Clinical Skill 31.6 will enable you to achieve this.

The 'This is me' book is great for patients who do not have capacity or have a communication impairment. Family members can get involved by writing in specific details about how their loved one likes to be cared for, their likes and dislikes – these details can really have an impact on the patient's experience while under your care.

Charlie Clisby, NQN

CONCLUSION

Although they appear straightforward or even mundane, the skills detailed in this chapter are fundamental and associated with multiple facets of nursing care. Quite correctly, in the general public's point of view, assisting patients with their elimination needs is very much associated with the role of the nurse (Dean, 2012). Throughout this chapter, frequent reference has been made to maintaining and promoting dignity, as this is both a professional and an ethical requirement for nurses (Baillie and Gallagher, 2012). In addition to this, as with all aspects of nursing practice, there are legal issues to consider, such as documentation and maintaining confidentiality.

Dewar (2013) highlights that compassion in nursing practice is at the forefront of current health-care policy, but that asking questions about how people feel about their care is not always easy. This is particularly true when dealing with the intimate issues associated with elimination. Compassion and person-centred care are closely linked, because person-centred care is about understanding people as individuals, what matters to them and how best to support them to manage their conditions or symptoms (Sanderson, 2013).

With regard to elimination needs, the nurse should provide information about the various options available to the patient to ensure their elimination needs are met in a person-centred and compassionate manner. Central to the success of undertaking the skills discussed in this chapter is good communication between the nurse, or nurses, and the patient. Communication is at the core of professional nursing practice (Jootun and McGhee, 2011). We communicate to explain the procedure and to gain consent (NMC, 2015), but it plays just as important a role in reassuring the patient during the procedure, answering any questions and acting as part of building an ongoing therapeutic relationship with a patient while they are in our care.

CHAPTER SUMMARY

- Assisting a patient with their elimination requires the nurse to be aware of the professional, legal and ethical issues associated with performing intimate care.
- Constipation has various signs and symptoms which nurses should be aware of in relation to their particular patient group.
- The Bristol Stool Chart is a widely recognised tool in relation to bowel assessment.
- A wide range of professional and local policies must be adhered to in relation to elimination needs.
- The key function of micturition and the digestive system is the removal of waste products from the body.
- As assisting a patient with their elimination needs involves dealing with bodily fluids, awareness of local infection prevention and control procedures is vital.
- Maintaining a patient's privacy and dignity is an essential component of all aspects of elimination care.

CRITICAL REFLECTION

Holistic care

Helping a patient with their elimination needs is clearly linked to providing holistic care. Elimination is a fundamental part of human existence. Review the chapter and note down all the instances where you think assisting a patient with their elimination needs can help meet their wider physical, psychological, social, economic and spiritual needs. Think of a variety of different patients across the fields, not just within your own field. You may find it helpful to make a list and refer back to it next time you are in practice, and then write your own reflection after your practice experience.

GO FURTHER

Books

Marshall, P., Gallacher, B., Jolly, J. and Rinomhota, S. (2015) *Anatomy and Physiology for Nurses*. Bloxham: Scion Publishing. An excellent anatomy and physiology textbook, written using case studies, which covers the knowledge required to ensure you understand the anatomy and physiology related to elimination.

University of Stirling (2008) *Continence and People with Dementia*. Stirling: University of Stirling Dementia Services Development Centre. A thought-provoking and person-centred book providing an insight into a range of key issues.

SAGE journal articles

FURTHER
READING:
JOURNAL
ARTICLES

Go to https://study.sagepub.com/essentialnursing2e for free online journal articles for this chapter. If you are using the interactive ebook, simply click on the book icon in the margin to go straight to the resource.

Gray, E., Blackinton, J. and White, G. (2006) 'Stoma care in the school setting', *The Journal of School Nursing*, 22: 74–80. An informative article discussing stoma creation and care of a stoma, as well as the complications and effects of living with one.

Rivers, C. (2010) 'School nurse interventions in managing functional urinary incontinence in school-age children', *The Journal of School Nursing*, 26: 115–20. A very interesting article considering functional urinary incontinence, a common problem for school-aged children.

White, J., Patterson, K., Jordan, L., Magin, P., Attia, J. and Sturm, J. (2014) 'The experience of urinary incontinence in stroke survivors: A follow-up qualitative study', *Canadian Journal of Occupational Therapy*, 81: 124–34. A study exploring the experiences of individuals living in the community who have urinary incontinence following a stroke.

Weblinks

FURTHER
READING:
WEBLINKS

Go to https://study.sagepub.com/essentialnursing2e for weblinks related to this chapter. If you are using the interactive ebook, simply click on the book icon in the margin to go straight to the resource.

www.healthcareimprovementscotland.org/previous_resources/best_practice_statement/urinary_dysfunction_in_adults.aspx – excellent advice from Healthcare Improvement Scotland focusing on the nursing contribution to continence care for adults with urinary dysfunction within a multi-disciplinary context.

http://pathways.nice.org.uk/pathways/faecal-incontinence – an excellent NICE overview of the care required by patients with faecal incontinence.

www.nice.org.uk/guidance/CG171 – specific NICE guidelines relating to continence care and female patients.

http://pathways.nice.org.uk/pathways/urinary-incontinence-in-neurological-disease – an excellent NICE resource relating to continence care in patients with neurological disease.

http://journals.rcni.com/doi/full/10.7748/ns2013.10.28.9.19.s25 – clear identification of the role of the nurse in providing effective continence-related care, from the RCN.

Video links

VIDEO
LINKS

Have a break from the text and go to https://study.sagepub.com/essentialnursing2e for useful videos related to this chapter. If you are using the interactive ebook, simply click on the lightbulb icon in the margin to go straight to the resource.

ACE YOUR ASSESSMENT

ONLINE
QUIZZES

Review what you have learned by visiting the book's online resources at: https://study.sagepub.com/essential nursing2e If using your interactive ebook, just click on the icon in the margin to go straight there.

- Test yourself with multiple-choice and short-answer questions.
- Revise key terms with the interactive flash cards.

REFERENCES

Baillie, L. and Gallagher, A. (2012) 'Raising awareness of patient dignity', *Nursing Standard*, 27(5): 44–9.

Ballentyne, M. and Ness, V. (2009) 'Eliminating', in C. Docherty and J. McCallum (eds), *Foundation Clinical Nursing Skills*. Oxford: Oxford University Press. pp. 275–307.

Burch, J. (2013) 'Care of patients with a stoma', *Nursing Standard*, 27(32): 49–56.

Dean, E. (2012) 'Dignity in toileting', *Nursing Standard*, 26(24): 18–20.

Dewar, B. (2013) 'Cultivating compassionate care', *Nursing Standard*, 27(34): 48–55.

Hunter, D. (2012) 'Conditions affecting the foreskin', *Nursing Standard*, 26(37): 35–9.

Jootun, D. and McGhee, G. (2011) 'Effective communication with people who have dementia', *Nursing Standard*, 25(25): 40–6.

Leaver, R.B. (2007) 'The evidence for urethral meatal cleansing', *Nursing Standard*, 21(41): 39–42.

Lewis, S.J. and Heaton, K.W. (1997) 'Stool form scale as a useful guide to intenstinal transit time', *Scandinavian Journal of Gastroenterology*, 32: 920–4.

McErlean, L. (2011) 'The digestive system and nutrition', in I. Peate and M. Nair (eds), *Fundamentals of Anatomy and Physiology for Student Nurses*. Chichester: Wiley-Blackwell. pp. 406–45.

Nair, M. (2011) 'The renal system', in I. Peate and M. Nair (eds), *Fundamentals of Anatomy and Physiology for Student Nurses*. Chichester: Wiley-Blackwell. pp. 446–75.

Naish, W. (2008) 'An overview of female voiding dysfunction', *Nursing Standard*, 22(30): 49–57.

Nayeri, N.D., Gholizadeh, L., Mohammadi, E. and Yazdi, K. (2015) 'Family involvement in the care of hospitalized elderly patients', *Journal of Applied Gerontology*, 34(6): 779–96.

NHS Greater Glasgow and Clyde (2014) Standard Operating Procedure (OP): Insertion and maintenance of adult indwelling urethral urinary catheters. Available at: http://library.nhsggc.org.uk/mediaAssets/Infection%20Control/SOP%20Urinary%20Catheters%20V4%20-%20BICC%2006.10.14.pdf (accessed 4 December 2017).

Nursing and Midwifery Council (NMC) (2009) *Record Keeping: Guidance for Nurses and Midwives*. London: NMC.

Nursing and Midwifery Council (2015) *The Code: Professional Standards of Practice and Behaviour for Nurses and Midwives*. London: NMC.

Oxford University Hospitals NHS Trust (2013) Oxford Pelvic Floor Service: Obstructive defaecation. Patient advice and information leaflet on the management of obstructive defaecation. Available at: www.ouh.nhs.uk/patient-guide/leaflets/files%5C130124obstructivedefaecation.pdf (accessed 24 February 2015).

Payne, D. (2013) 'How to ... apply and change incontinence pads', *Nursing & Residential Care*, 15(12): 803.

Pomfret, I. (2006) 'Urinary catheter care', *Nursing & Residential Care*, 8(10): 446–8.

Porth, C.M. (2007) *Essentials of Pathophysiology: Concepts of Altered Health States*. Philadelphia, PA: Lippincott Williams & Wilkins.

Sanderson, H. (2013) 'Personalisation: Three steps to transform practice', *Learning Disability Practice*, 16(5): 34–7.

Smith, J. and Roberts, R. (2011) *Vital Signs for Nurses: An Introduction to Clinical Observations*. Oxford: Wiley-Blackwell.

Solomon, J. (2008) 'Eliminating', in K. Holland (ed.), *Applying the Roper, Logan, Tierney Model in Practice*. Edinburgh: Churchill Livingstone Elsevier. pp. 229–64.

World Health Organization (WHO) (2009) WHO Guidelines on Hand Hygiene in Health Care. Available at: http://whqlibdoc.who.int/publications/2009/9789241597906_eng.pdf (accessed 7 March 2018).

ASSISTING PATIENTS WITH THEIR HYGIENE NEEDS

32

CATHERINE DELVES-YATES

THIS CHAPTER COVERS

- Hygiene and person-centred care
- Your role as a nurse in assisting a patient with their hygiene needs
- Bed-bathing
- Shaving
- Oral care
- Washing and trimming nails

REQUIRED KNOWLEDGE

- It will be helpful to understand the anatomy and physiology of the skin, mouth, nails and hair before you start to read this chapter.

> " I am 13 and every three months I go to respite care, so my mum can have time to herself. The first time I went, to be honest, I felt really vulnerable and worried that it wouldn't be possible for me to have a bath, as I need to use a hoist. Fortunately I had a great nurse who asked me how I wanted to be washed, used the hoist, saw my arms were weak – but most importantly, realised I liked lots of bubbles!
>
> **Flo, patient** "

> " Washing a patient who is incapable of washing themselves is an extremely personal and intimate activity, requiring the highest level of skill in terms of communication and making the patient feel relaxed enough to fully trust you. This is fundamental to establishing a therapeutic relationship.
>
> **Alexander MacFarlane, adult nursing student** "

Visit https://study.sagepub.com/essentialnursing2e to access a wealth of online resources for this chapter – watch out for the margin icons throughout the chapter. If you are using the interactive eBook, simply click on the margin icon to go straight to the resource.

INTRODUCTION

How would you feel if you couldn't perform your own personal hygiene care? What would be the important things you would like your nurse to do? Flo's story above outlines how important it is that a nurse aids a patient to look after their personal hygiene in a way the patient finds acceptable. It can also be intimidating for you, as a nursing student, to wash someone, as Alexander's comment shows.

The World Health Organization (WHO) defines hygiene as 'practices that help to maintain health and prevent the spread of diseases' (WHO, 2014). However, assisting a patient to maintain their hygiene is more than this. These procedures are the core of nursing care, ensuring a patient's individual needs and preferences are met. While maintaining hygiene describes the physical act of cleansing the body, this activity is closely linked with the provision of compassionate care which maintains comfort, dignity, self-esteem and a positive body image, all of which are integral aspects of nursing practice.

This chapter outlines the fundamental role of the nurse in maintaining a patient's hygiene. We will first consider what hygiene means to your patient within your nursing role, and why it is so important. We will then describe how to perform a bed bath, assist a patient with washing and shaving and undertake mouth, nail and hair care in a variety of settings, while – most importantly – promoting the patient's independence and dignity.

HYGIENE AND PERSON-CENTRED CARE

ACTIVITY 32.1: REFLECTION

- Compile a list of all of the measures you have undertaken to maintain your hygiene over the past week.
- Why do you follow the routines you have included in your list?
- Besides 'clean', how else do your preferred hygiene routines make you feel?

We all have personal hygiene practices, formed by our culture, the practices of our family and our own choices. These choices will involve whether we prefer to bathe or shower and if we do this before going to bed, when we wake up or once a week. Further choices are made as to whether we shampoo our hair daily, weekly or whenever we feel it is necessary. Within these personal preferences, illness may be a limiting factor, but encouraging the patient to maintain their usual routine, enabling them to be as independent and feel as in control as possible while offering assistance, is an important aspect of a nurse's role. It may also be that you could be caring for patient – a child, for example – who already has a carer, so your role may be to assist the carer to adapt their routine to accommodate the patient's additional needs.

For personal, social, health and psychological reasons, most people are conscious of their hygiene needs. As children, we are taught the importance of good hygiene; it is part of feeling accepted and prepared for whatever is ahead – just think about how cleaning your teeth or styling your hair in the way you prefer makes you feel. While the focus in maintaining a patient's hygiene is frequently on cleansing, it is also important to remember that most individuals' daily routines do not end when they are clean. We all rely on the toiletries we are used to, such as deodorant, hair products and cosmetics, to keep us looking how we wish throughout the day. This is the patient's choice and there is no reason why we cannot assist them to continue to present themselves as they desire.

Although we may think of activities of assisting patients to maintain their hygiene occurring at the start or end of the day, the importance of offering the opportunity to undertake such activities throughout the entire day must not be forgotten. Patients should not only be assisted with washing their hands before meals and after they have used the bedpan or commode; they may well also wish to clean and floss their teeth or dentures after a meal, or wash their hands and face, brush their hair and reapply make-up before visitors arrive.

In considering the different settings within which you will be caring for patients, there is a priority to ensure cleanliness to reduce a patient's risk of contracting infections such as MRSA. Due to this, hygiene interventions in hospital settings may include the use of antiseptic washes and wipes. This requires explanation, as it may be different from the patient's usual routine. When caring for patients in their own home, you may be supporting them and their carers to acquire the skills necessary to maintain their own hygiene, or promoting personal hygiene because they may have lost interest in their appearance due to illness.

When assisting patients with hygiene needs like washing by the side of or in the bed, I always promote the patient doing as much as they can, especially when it comes to washing intimate areas. It may take longer but it can be a lot more dignified for a patient to be involved in these aspects of their care.

Charlie Clisby, NQN

YOUR ROLE AS A NURSE IN ASSISTING A PATIENT WITH THEIR HYGIENE NEEDS

There are five components of care to consider when working in partnership with a patient and supporting them to maintain their hygiene. Remembering **CLEAN**, as shown in Figure 32.1, will help!

Consider and assess the patient's needs:

- What are their exact personal hygiene needs?
- Are they able to maintain their own hygiene with minimal support, or do they need full assistance?

Listen to the patient's preferences and devise a plan:

- How is it appropriate to meet the patient's needs?
- Are there any religious/cultural issues you need to consider?
- Is a bed bath needed or can they go to the bathroom for a wash, bath or shower?
- Always remember to obtain consent and maintain patient safety. If uncertain what is appropriate, *ask*.

Environmental and equipment factors:

- Can the patient's needs be safely met in their environment?
- If the patient has a carer, can they meet the patient's needs without putting the patient or themselves at risk?
- Don't forget other equipment - are the patient's preferred toiletries available?

Assistance:

- Provide the patient with the care they require.

'**N**owledge and skills:

- Ensure that the patient and/or their carer have sufficient knowledge and skills to continue maintaining their hygiene and that they are satisfied with how their needs have been met.

Figure 32.1 CLEAN

Source: Adapted from DH (2010)

Working in this manner ensures you promote patient independence, take account of patient preferences, treat them as individuals and maintain their dignity. Remember that, as a nurse, it is your role to assist a patient to maintain their hygiene, not only to keep them physically clean but, just as importantly, for personal, social and psychological reasons.

The intimate nature of personal hygiene care can trigger inappropriate or challenging behaviour from some patients. Challenging behaviour is deliberate or non-deliberate non-verbal, verbal or physical behaviour which makes it difficult to deliver good care. Individualised, carefully planned and risk-assessed care is an important strategy to reduce the potential for this. Remember the importance of talking to a patient and understanding their psychological, emotional and physical needs, and involve them in care. Ensure you are aware of their behaviour patterns and any triggers that may act as a precursor to challenging behaviour. If a patient behaves in a challenging or an inappropriate way:

- De-escalate the situation by using effective communication skills. Be empathetic and non-confrontational; minimise any threat; negotiate, compromise, agree to reasonable requests, distract them and, if appropriate, offer a change of nurse.
- Consider leaving and returning, as long as patient safety is not compromised. This will give the patient 'time out', which may be all that is necessary.
- Be understanding and tolerant. Intimate hygiene care can be misinterpreted, so view the situation from the patient's perspective and be reassuring and non-judgemental. Disapprove of the behaviour, not the individual. (Adapted from NHS, 2013)

Guidelines

There are various national and local guidelines of which you must be aware when performing hygiene activities. Remember never to undertake any of the following procedures unless you are, or have supervision from, a trained, experienced and competent person. The types of guidelines you need to consider will be contained in:

- infection control policy
- local organisational policies.

To effectively assess and care for a patient's skin, lips, nail beds and mouth, you need to understand how they should look and what their normal functions are.

BED-BATHING

Washing removes perspiration, dirt and odours, stimulates circulation, exercises body parts, refreshes, relaxes, promotes comfort and enables evaluation of a patient's skin. Just as importantly, it is also a time at which the patient has your complete attention, when you can develop your therapeutic relationship with the patient and also assess their mood, whether they are in pain and how they are feeling in general. You may find that they will express their concerns or tell you things that are important to them at this time, so maximise the opportunities for them to do so. As this time is devoted to personal and intimate matters, it can be a good opportunity to find out about the patient's bowel function. However, if they do not wish to talk, you must respect this. If your patient is unable to speak or understand you, do not forget to talk to them and explain what you are doing, to reassure them and involve them in their care.

Always make sure that before you start you have all the equipment you need. I always look at how I would like to be treated and I know I would not be happy if someone kept stopping and saying I just need to go and get this and that, knowing that the patient could be left feeling vulnerable.

Sarah Parkes, LD nursing student

It is important to get everything you might need ready in advance so that you aren't running in and out of the room/curtains when helping a patient with their hygiene. I always make sure that I have plenty of towels so that I don't have to run out.

Hannah Boyd, adult nursing student

After reading about Clinical Skill 32.2, apply what you have learned in this chapter by reading Daisy's case study, at https://study.sagepub.com/essentialnursing2e.

CASE STUDY:
DAISY

SHAVING

For many men, shaving is an important part of their daily routine and they may feel unkempt if they have not shaved, although some men may choose not to shave for religious or cultural reasons. If the patient does shave, they should be offered the opportunity to do so daily. They may need you to shave them, or just need support and assistance. If you are going to shave them, an electric razor will provide the greatest safety. If the patient has their own electric razor, you can use this, but, if not, a disposable safety razor is perfectly acceptable as long as the patient is not suffering from a coagulation disorder or on anticoagulation therapy. For these patients, you must use an electric razor. If a patient is cut during a shave, use clean gauze and apply firm pressure until the bleeding stops. Due to the risk of cross-contamination, razors of any type are never shared, so encourage relatives to bring in the patient's equipment from home. Remember the importance of ensuring safety razors are stored safely, especially in settings caring for vulnerable patients or those who may self-harm.

ACTIVITY 32.2: REFLECTION

Either reflect on an experience where you have needed a nurse to assist you to maintain your hygiene, or imagine this situation:

• What behaviours do you think are important for the nurse to demonstrate as they assist you?

STEP-BY-STEP CLINICAL SKILL 32.1: COMMON STEPS FOR ALL HYGIENE PROCEDURES

☑ **Essential equipment – depends on skill but is likely to include one or more of the following:**

Single-use bowls, warm water, towels, soap, incontinence pads, disposable washcloths, skin moisturiser or talc (if the patient wishes), clean clothes, nightwear or gown for the patient, clean bedlinen.

☑ **Field-specific considerations**

When assisting a patient with a learning disability, it may be important to ascertain what a patient's usual hygiene routine is, as they may not be able to tell you. Assisting a patient to develop their ability to maintain their hygiene needs can be an important step towards independence.

Patients with mental health problems – who are severely depressed, for example – may not view their personal hygiene as important, so both physical and psychological support could be required. Those with a cognitive impairment such as dementia or psychosis may not realise or even understand what is needed.

When caring for a child, encourage and assist parents or carers to be involved in hygiene care to maintain the usual routine. Supporting, educating and enabling parents or carers to continue their care within any environment is an important nursing role.

☑ **Care-setting considerations**

It is not always possible to have all the equipment available to assist a patient to safely meet their hygiene needs in the exact manner they wish. For example, in a patient's home you may not have a hoist, so it may not be safe for them to use their bath; however, you can still assist them to meet their hygiene needs in a different way.

Always ensure you have the equipment required to safely meet the patient's needs in your current setting.

☑ **What to watch out for and action to take**

While maintaining a patient's hygiene, you should assess:

- the colour of the skin, lips, nail beds and **sclera** of their eyes
- the location and appearance of any rashes
- whether the skin is dry and/or flaky
- the condition of pressure areas, for any bruises, open areas, pale or reddened areas; the appearance of any wounds and whether or not they are draining (see Chapter 26, Skin Integrity, and Chapter 20, Safeguarding)
- any complaints of pain or discomfort
- the temperature of the patient's skin.

The information gained from these observations will enable you to fully assess the condition of the patient's skin and, if necessary, plan any changes in treatment, plus evaluate whether the current treatment is effective.

☑ **Helpful hints**

- Gloves and aprons must be worn if contact with blood/body fluids/excreta is anticipated or the patient is in isolation.
- Hand hygiene must be performed before touching a patient, before clean/aseptic procedures, after body fluid exposure/risk, after touching a patient and after touching a patient's surroundings.
- Waste should be disposed of in a clinical waste bag if it is contaminated with blood/body fluids/excreta.
- Equipment must be cleaned as identified by the relevant policy every time it is used.

HYGIENE ASSISTANCE GUIDELINES

 The first step of any procedure is to introduce yourself to the patient, explain the procedure and gain their consent
Fully informed consent may not always be possible if the patient is a child or has mental health problems or learning disabilities, but even in these circumstances, every effort should be made to explain the procedure in terms that the patient can understand. This is not only respectful of their individual human rights, but also helps to ensure they will be more accepting of the treatment and that their anxieties are reduced

For patients who are unable to provide consent because they are unconscious, advice should be sought from your practice educator or another qualified nurse

It could be that the procedure is one normally undertaken by the patient's family or carer, or they may express the wish to be involved in the care you are about to deliver. If this is so, and if it is appropriate, it is an opportunity to maintain the patient's usual routine, or you could support the patient's family or carer in adapting their usual routine to meet the patient's changed care needs

 Gather the equipment required (see relevant skill for details)
Ensure these are clean as appropriate
Reduces the chance of infection and maintains patient and nurse safety

 Clear sufficient space within the environment, for example in the bathroom or around the bed space
Enables clear access for the patient and the nurse to safely use the equipment required

 Wash your hands and put on an apron. Gloves should only be worn if absolutely necessary, never 'just in case'
Wearing gloves creates a barrier between the nurse and the patient as it sends signals that the nurse is undertaking 'dirty tasks'

Wearing an apron and gloves as part of personal protective equipment (PPE) is a standard infection-control procedure when dealing with body fluids or patients in isolation

Ensure your use of PPE such as gloves and disposable aprons is appropriate by considering the individual patient situation and the risk presented

 Ensure privacy, so close doors and curtains/ blinds as necessary. If you are at a patient's bed space, ensure you draw the curtains fully. Assist the patient to find a comfortable position and ensure they will not get cold
Do not hurry and be gentle
Only expose the area of the body you need to attend to at that particular moment
Patients will need to feel able to remove their clothing without being seen by others. Maintain patient privacy, dignity and comfort as required

Caring for a patient's hygiene is a personal and intimate procedure which takes time to perform with dignity

Washing areas of the body can result in cooling

Areas of the skin can be very delicate

 As appropriate, encourage the patient to undertake as much of the process as possible
Promotes independence

 Equipment used for hygiene needs, such as electric shavers, must not be shared between patients
Reduces the risk of infection

 After you have completed the hygiene procedure, remove any towels that have been used to protect the patient and assist them to get into a comfortable position
Promotes patient comfort

 Remove your apron and perform hand hygiene. Document in the patient's notes the care you have given and any relevant observations of pressure areas, etc.
Reduces the risk of infection

Maintains patient safety and accurate records

 Offer or support the patient to have a drink (so long as this is not contraindicated)
Promotes patient comfort and ensures they are well nourished and hydrated

Source: Baillie (2009); DH (2010); Dougherty and Lister (2015); Glasper et al. (2010); NICE (2012); NMC (2015); Sargeant and Chamley (2013); Sharples (2011); WHO (2009)

STEP-BY-STEP CLINICAL SKILL 32.2: BATHING A PATIENT IN BED

☑ What is normal

Most patients have their own hygiene practices, which may be very different from yours, so remember the stages of CLEAN (Figure 31.1) to ensure you are working in partnership with your patient.

Remember to constantly observe and assess the patient's skin.

☑ Before you start

Remember to perform the common steps (see Clinical Skill 32.1).

☑ Essential equipment

Single-use bowl x2, warm water, towel x3, soap, incontinence pads, disposable washcloths, skin moisturiser or talc (if the patient wishes), clean clothes, nightwear or gown for the patient, clean bedlinen.

☑ Care-setting considerations

It is possible to bed-bath a patient in a variety of settings as long as the necessary equipment is available.

☑ What to watch out for and action to take

If, while bed-bathing a patient, any areas of skin have been observed which are abnormal, this must be reported to a relevant individual and recorded in the patient's notes.

BED-BATHING GUIDELINES

 1 **Perform steps 1–7 of the common steps (Clinical Skill 32.1)**
To prepare the patient and you to undertake the task

 2 **Offer assistance as required to undress the patient. Only uncover the area you are washing; the rest of the patient should remain covered by either the bed sheets or a dry towel**
Maintains patient dignity and keeps them warm

 3 **Fill a bowl with fresh warm water, check the temperature carefully and, if possible, check that the patient is happy with the** temperature. **Change this water at any time if it becomes too cool or dirty. Always change the water after washing the perineal area and buttocks**
Aids patient safety
Reduces risk of contamination

4 Disposable washcloths are much better than a flannel for washing patients as you can dispense with them when they have been used
Always use new washcloths for the patient's face, torso, back and perineal area. To keep the water as clean as possible, do not put a soapy washcloth back into the water - dispose of it and use a new one
Bacteria rapidly multiply in wet, warm environments such as a flannel
Reduces risk of contamination

5 Ensure the bed is at a height at which it is comfortable for you to work, changing this throughout the procedure as necessary
Cares for your back

6 Start by washing the patient's face. If possible, check with the patient whether they prefer to use soap for areas of their body such as their face. If you use soap, rinse it off well. Avoid getting soap in eyes
Reduces risk of contamination
Prevents soap left on the skin from making it dry and itchy

7 Use a clean washcloth for each part of the body
Avoids transferring contaminants

8 Wash each area of the patient's body by wetting the washcloth and then wringing it out to prevent dripping water all over the patient. Always pat the skin thoroughly dry with a towel. If possible, ask the patient whether they feel dry
If patients are not thoroughly dried, they will become cold

9 Once you have washed the patient's face, move to the arm furthest away from you. Place a towel underneath and wash the hand, then arm, then armpit using soap. Take special care to avoid any dressings or cannulae. Rinse the soap off well and dry with the towel. Repeat the process for the other arm
Prevents dripping on areas previously washed
Reduces risk of infection

10 Next, wash the torso using soap. For female patients or men with gynecomastia, gently lift the breasts and wash underneath. Repeat this procedure with any other skin folds that may be present. Once again, be very careful not to get any dressings, drains or other lines wet
Rinse the soap off and dry the area thoroughly
Skin under the breasts or skin folds need to be cleaned and dried to avoid fungal infections

11 If the patient wishes, apply deodorant, moisturiser or talc. When finished, cover the torso with a dry towel
Continues the patient's normal routine
Maintains patient dignity and keeps them warm

12 Lift the bedsheet back to expose the patient's feet and legs, but ensure you keep the genitals covered. Place a towel under the leg furthest away and wash the foot and leg with soap. Ensure you clean very gently

(Continued)

between the toes. Rinse well. Dry thoroughly and repeat with the other foot and leg
Prevents dripping on areas previously washed
   Maintains patient dignity and keeps them warm

 13 Change the water and put on gloves if you are not already wearing them
Potential contact with body fluids/excreta

14 Ask the patient if you can wash their genitals now and obtain their consent. Some patients may wish to wash this area themselves, so offer them this opportunity
Promotes independence and maintains dignity

15 The genital/perineal area is very delicate and needs special care. Wash very gently with warm water alone, rinse well and pat dry. Work from the cleanest to the dirtiest area, so from the front to back (urethral to anal area)
To wash an uncircumcised adult male patient, you will need to gently retract the foreskin to wash the urethral meatus
Remember to gently return the foreskin after washing to prevent swelling and discomfort. If the patient is unable to do this, you will need to obtain their consent and explain exactly what you are doing while you do it
Reduces potential of contamination
   This would not be done with a child

16 If the patient has a catheter, carry out the appropriate catheter care in line with local policy
Reduces risk of infection

 17 When clean and dry, re-cover the patient and dispose of the water and the single-use bowl. Remove your gloves and wash your hands. Reapply gloves if necessary and refill a new single-use bowl with warm water
Maintains patient dignity and keeps them warm
   Reduces risk of infection

18 Even if the bedlinen is not wet or soiled, this is a good time to change it. If the patient is unable to move easily in the bed, you will need another carer to assist you to change the sheets while the patient is still in the bed
Ensure you abide by manual handling policies and that the bed is at the correct height, and use a slide sheet if required to reposition the patient
Promotes patient comfort
   Cares for your back

19 Assist the patient to roll onto their side, facing away from you and towards the other carer. Ensure the other carer is able to support the patient and the patient feels safe. Cover the patient's front with the bed sheet
Ensures patient safety
   Maintains patient dignity

 20 Roll the old sheet into the middle of the bed and place a towel behind the patient

 21 Use soap to wash the patient's back, then rinse and dry thoroughly
Keeps the patient warm

Ask the patient's consent to wash their sacral area/buttocks
If the patient is soiled, put on gloves if you are not wearing them already. Wash, rinse and dry thoroughly. If appropriate, remove gloves, dispose of them and wash your hands
Reduces risk of contamination

 Remove towel from behind patient. If sheet rolled up behind/under patient is damp or soiled, cover with an incontinence pad
Reduces risk of contamination

 Tuck a clean sheet under mattress edge closest to you; smooth it over the mattress behind the patient and roll up the part which will go under the patient

 Assist the patient to roll onto their other side; remember to tell them they will roll over a bump due to the rolled sheets
Remove old sheet and incontinence pad if appropriate. Dispose of them as per policy
Reduces risk of infection

 Unroll clean sheet and tuck tightly under the mattress
Wrinkle-free sheets promote patient comfort

 Assist the patient to re-dress as appropriate and move into a comfortable position
Promotes patient comfort and dignity

 Finish changing the bedlinen by putting clean pillowcases on the pillows, with a clean top sheet and blankets if required

 Dispose of bowl or clean with detergent and water if reusable. Store inverted to avoid dregs of water collecting in it. Dispose of/ clean any other equipment as per local policy and return any of the patient's equipment to their locker. Clean the bedside table and put any belongings you moved back in their original position. If appropriate, ensure the patient can reach the nurse call bell
Reduces risk of infection
　　Maintains patient safety

 Perform steps 8–10 of the common steps (Clinical Skill 32.1)
To ensure that:

- the patient is safe, comfortable and receiving the appropriate care
- the results have been documented in the patient's records
- the equipment is clean and in working order

Source: Baillie (2009); DH (2010); Dougherty and Lister (2015); Glasper et al. (2010); NICE (2012); NMC (2015); Sargeant and Chamley (2013)

STEP-BY-STEP CLINICAL SKILL 32.3: SHAVING

☑ **What is normal**

Most patients have their own hygiene practices, which may be very different from yours, so remember the stages of CLEAN (Figure 31.1) to ensure you are working in partnership with your patient.

☑ **Before you start**

Remember to perform the common steps (Clinical Skill 32.1).

☑ **Essential equipment**

Using an electric shaver - electric shaver, bowl, warm water, towel, mirror and moisturiser or aftershave (if the patient wishes).

Using a safety razor - safety razor, shaving foam, bowl, warm water, dry towel, mirror and moisturiser or aftershave (if the patient wishes).

☑ **Field-specific considerations**

When assisting a patient with a learning disability, it may be important to ascertain what a patient's usual shaving routine is, as they may not be able to tell you.

Patients with mental health problems - who are severely depressed, for example - may not view their personal hygiene as important, so both physical and psychological support could be required.

☑ **Care-setting considerations**

Ensure patient dignity is maintained as most individuals carry out all of their hygiene practices in private.

Shaving can be undertaken in any care setting.

☑ **What to watch out for and action to take**

If you observe any skin areas that are abnormal, you need to report this to a relevant individual, record it in the patient's notes and omit step 5, as this may potentially aggravate the areas.

SHAVING ASSISTANCE GUIDELINES

 Perform steps 1-7 of the common steps (Clinical Skill 32.1)
Prepares the patient and you to undertake the task

 Drape a towel around the patient's front
Protects clothes

 Wash the patient's face and dry it thoroughly
Cleans the area, enables observation of the skin plus any shaving preferences, such as sideburns, etc.

 If any of the stubble is more than 1 cm or so long, use a beard trimmer to cut this first
Long hairs will be pulled out rather than cut by an electric shaver or safety razor

5 **Electric shaver**

a. Shave in the opposite direction to hair growth, making small circular motions if the patient has short stubble. For longer stubble, create larger circular motions

b. Avoid repeatedly shaving the same area

Safety razor

a. Apply shaving foam to the patient's face and neck

b. Pull the area you are about to shave taut – where you start is a matter of preference

c. Angle the razor to approx. 45 degrees away from the face. Using as little pressure as possible, move the razor across the skin in the direction of hair growth

d. Repeat this process once more on the same area of skin and then move to another area

e. Frequently dip the razor into the warm water

f. If there is a large amount of stubble, you may need to use more than one safety razor

g. Rinse the patient's face with cool water when you have finished shaving all areas

Results in the closest, most comfortable shave and prevents skin from becoming sore

Removes the hair and any excess shaving foam

6 **If the patient desires apply moisturiser or aftershave, but remember if you use aftershave to apply it sparingly, as it can sting**
Enables patient to continue their usual hygiene practices

Do not apply moisturiser or aftershave to areas of sore or broken skin

7 **Assist the patient to look at his face in the mirror to ensure they approve of the result**
Helps the patient present themselves in the manner they desire

8 **Perform steps 8–10 of the common steps (Clinical Skill 32.1)**
To ensure that:

- the patient is safe, comfortable and receiving the appropriate care
- the results have been documented in the patient's records
- equipment is clean and in working order

Source: Baillie (2009); DH (2010); Dougherty and Lister (2015); NICE (2012); NMC (2015)

CASE STUDY 32.1: ADAM

Adam is 25, has a moderate learning disability and lives in a supported-living home. While returning from shopping four days ago, he was hit by a car and sustained fractures of both wrists, which have been immobilised in a plaster cast. He also has a severely sprained left ankle, on which he is unable to bear weight, which is being treated with analgesia, rest, elevation and ice packs. Adam has numerous **contusions** and a cut over his right eye, which was sutured. He came home from hospital yesterday and is in bed because he says he 'feels wobbly'. Adam is desperate to have a bath and shave because he says he 'pongs like the hospital'. Normally, he needs minimal assistance with hygiene, but he now needs full assistance.

- How are you going to assist Adam to maintain his hygiene in a manner he finds acceptable?
- Which of the step-by-step clinical skills guides in this chapter would be relevant for Adam's care, and would you need to make any modifications to these?
- What will be your priority and what additional assessments will you undertake?

ANSWER:
CASE STUDY 32.1

STEP-BY-STEP CLINICAL SKILL 32.4: TEETH-CLEANING

☑ What is normal

Most patients have their own hygiene practices, which may be very different from yours, so remember the stages of CLEAN (Figure 32.1) to ensure you are working in partnership with your patient.

☑ Before you start

Remember the common steps (Clinical Skill 32.1).

☑ Essential equipment

Toothbrush, toothpaste, disposable cup, bowl, towel, mouthwash (if the patient wishes) and mirror.

☑ Field-specific considerations

When assisting a patient with a learning disability, it may be important to ascertain what a patient's usual teeth-cleaning routine is, as they may not be able to tell you.

Patients with mental health problems – who are severely depressed, for example – may not view their personal hygiene as important, so both physical and psychological support could be required.

When caring for a child, encourage and assist parents or carers to be involved in hygiene care to maintain the usual routine. Supporting, educating and enabling parents or carers to continue their care within any environment is an important nursing role.

☑ Care-setting considerations

Ensure patient dignity is maintained, as most individuals carry out all of their hygiene practices in private.

Teeth-cleaning can be undertaken in any care setting.

☑ What to watch out for and action to take

Remember to constantly observe and assess the patient's tongue and oral structures. If you observe any areas that are abnormal, you need to report this to a relevant individual and record it in the patient's notes.

TEETH-CLEANING ASSISTANCE GUIDELINES

1 **Perform steps 1-7 of the common steps (Clinical Skill 32.1)**
Prepares the patient and you to undertake the task

2 **Drape a towel around the patient's front**
Protects clothes

3 **Apply a pea-sized blob of toothpaste to the toothbrush. Ask the patient to open their mouth and, holding the brush at 45 degrees, use small circular motions to brush the teeth**
Effectively cleans teeth

4 **Brush the upper teeth first, brushing all surfaces, paying extra attention to the area where the teeth and gums meet**
Particles gather between the teeth and gums

5 **When you have brushed all areas, offer the patient diluted mouthwash or water to rinse**
Removes toothpaste and particles

6 **Assist the patient to look at their teeth in the mirror to ensure they approve of the result**

Enables the patient to present themselves in the manner they desire

7 **Perform steps 8–10 of the common steps (Clinical Skill 32.1)**
To ensure that:

- the patient is safe, comfortable and receiving the appropriate care
- the results have been documented in the patient's records
- the equipment is clean and in working order

Source: Baillie (2009); DH (2010); Dougherty and Lister (2015); Glasper et al. (2010); NICE (2012); NMC (2015); Sargeant and Chamley (2013)

ORAL CARE

Oral care is important in maintaining patient comfort, preventing odours, infections, tooth decay and gum disease and enhancing the taste of food. Patients should be offered oral care before breakfast, after meals, at bedtime and whenever else they request it.

For babies and young children, a clean mouth is important even before the eruption of teeth, and children need to be supported to clean their teeth effectively. Good dental habits from a young age are important, as is educating parents or carers about the prevention of dental decay. Teeth-cleaning should start at around six months of age and will need to be performed for the child. As children get older, they should be supervised according to their developmental stage.

Remember that oral care does not just involve brushing a patient's teeth; patients with dentures may like to rinse their mouth with water or diluted mouthwash and some may even brush their gums with a very soft toothbrush. Use the time spent providing oral care to assess the condition of the tongue, mucosa, lips and other structures. Many patients, especially those who are dehydrated, have noticeably dry, coated tongues and cracked lips. Encourage patients to drink sufficiently and remember that petroleum jelly is soothing for cracked lips. Handle dentures with care, cleaning them in the same way as natural teeth, and store them in a labelled container whenever they are out of the patient's mouth.

ACTIVITY 32.3: REFLECTION

For this activity, either another student, or a friend or family member is needed to assist.

Using Clinical Skill 32.4 as a guide, ask your assistant if you can clean their teeth and then if they will clean your teeth:

- How did it feel when you were cleaning your assistant's teeth?
- What did it feel like having someone else clean your teeth?
- How will you apply what you have learned from this experience to your practice?

CASE STUDY 32.2: MOHAMMED

Mohammed is 3 and attends a local nursery four days a week. After lunch, he asks to clean his teeth, as he recently went for his first dental appointment and was told this is important.

- Using the relevant clinical skill guide as a resource, what are the important health education points to stress to Mohammed?
- How could you do this in a way he understands?

ANSWER:
CASE STUDY
32.2

WASHING AND TRIMMING NAILS

CASE STUDY 32.3: JOSETTE

Josette is 52 and has a long history of severe depression. The community mental health nurse has visited Josette at home today and finds her looking dishevelled. Her clothes are stained and smell of sweat, her hair is greasy and matted and her fingernails are long and dirty.

- What would your priorities be in assisting Josette to maintain her hygiene?
- How will you assist Josette to maintain her hygiene in a manner she finds acceptable?
- What additional issues do you need to consider due to the setting of her care?

ANSWER:
CASE STUDY
32.3

WHAT'S THE EVIDENCE?

Malkin, B. and Berridge, P. (2009) 'Guidance on maintaining personal hygiene in nail care', *Nursing Standard*, 23(41): 35-8.

In this literature review, Malkin and Berridge found that there is confusion amongst qualified nurses about who should perform nail-cutting, which has resulted in poor care for patients:

- Reflect on the care of a patient you have been involved with who needed assistance to cut their toenails.
- Did the nurses offer to assist the patient?
- Why might nurses not want to cut a patient's toenails and feel that this is not part of their role?
- Now read the article and consider how you can apply the findings to your practice.

FURTHER
READING:
NAIL CARE

CONCLUSION

The key to maintaining a patient's hygiene is to carry out very personal and intimate activities in a dignified and compassionate manner. To do this you must work in partnership with the patient, ascertaining their normal routines and replicating them as far as is possible. You must always have either the patient's consent or assent to your care, and if appropriate you should involve the patient's family or carers in activities. Providing hygiene-related care often gives you an opportunity to discuss any specific concerns the patient has, provide psychological support with these and undertake a thorough assessment of the physical condition of the patient's body.

CHAPTER SUMMARY

- Assisting a patient to maintain their personal hygiene is at the heart of nursing care.
- Performing the range of personal and intimate activities involved requires nursing knowledge and skill, but more than this, effective communication.
- Maintaining hygiene involves activity throughout the whole of the patient's day, not just at the start and end, promoting patient dignity, self-esteem and a positive body image.
- The key clinical skill procedures you should be familiar with in terms of patient hygiene include how to perform a bed bath, assist a patient with a wash and undertake mouth, nail and hair care.
- You will need to adapt hygiene practices to a variety of settings, while being mindful of the need to maintain patient dignity and independence and ensure patients' safety.

CRITICAL REFLECTION

Holistic care

This chapter has highlighted the wider importance of providing holistic care for your patient when assisting with hygiene needs. Review the chapter and note down all the instances where you think caring for a patient's hygiene can help meet their wider physical, psychological, social, economic and spiritual needs. Think of a variety of different patients across the fields, not just within your own field. You may find it helpful to make a list and refer back to it next time you are in practice, and then write your own reflection after your practice experience.

GO FURTHER

Books

Dougherty, L. and Lister, S. (eds) (2015) *The Royal Marsden Hospital Manual of Clinical Nursing Procedures*, 9th edn. Oxford: Wiley-Blackwell. An outstanding guide to a wide range of nursing procedures.

Glasper, A., Aylott, M. and Battrick, C. (2010) *Developing Practical Skills for Nursing Children and Young People*. London: Hodder Arnold. An excellent resource outlining how to care for children and young people.

SAGE journal articles

FURTHER
READING:
JOURNAL
ARTICLES

Go to https://study.sagepub.com/essentialnursing2e for free online journal articles for this chapter. If you are using the interactive ebook, simply click on the book icon in the margin to go straight to the resource.

Blinkhorn, F., Weingarten, L., Boivin, L., Plain, J. and Kay, M. (2012) 'An intervention to improve the oral health of residents in an aged care facility by nurses', *Health Education Journal*, 71: 527–35. How a simple oral health intervention improved patients' oral health.

Tanner, J., Gould, D., Jenkins, P., Hilliam, R., Mistry, N. and Walsh, S. (2012) 'A fresh look at preoperative body washing', *Journal of Infection Prevention*, 13: 11–15. A critique of pre-operative washing practices.

Other journal articles

de Oliveira, C., Hamer, M. and Watts, R. (2010) 'Toothbrushing, inflammation and risk of cardiovascular disease', *BMJ*, 340: c2451. Available at: http://dx.doi.org/10.1136/bmj.c2451. A look at the connections between oral hygiene and heart disease.

Kitson, A.L., Dowd, C., Calabrese, O.D., Locock, L. and Athlin, Å.M. (2013) 'Stroke survivors' experiences of the fundamentals of care: A qualitative analysis', *International Journal Of Nursing Studies*, 50(3): 392–403. An interesting article focusing upon the importance of personal care in ensuring patient dignity.

McAulife, C. (2007) 'Nursing students practice in providing oral hygiene for patients', *Nursing Standard*, 21(33): 35–9. The factors influencing nursing students' oral hygiene practices for hospitalised patients.

Weblinks

FURTHER
READING:
WEBLINKS

Go to https://study.sagepub.com/essentialnursing2e for weblinks related to this chapter. If you are using the interactive ebook, simply click on the book icon in the margin to go straight to the resource.

www.nursingtimes.net/student-nurses-should-not-underestimate-the-value-of-delivering-hands-on-personal-care/5008022.article – the importance of developing skills in essential care, from the *Nursing Times*.

www.who.int/entity/gpsc/5may/Hand_Hygiene_Why_How_and_When_Brochure.pdf – when to practise hand hygiene, from the WHO.

www.gov.uk/government/publications/essence-of-care-2010 – the benchmarks for personal hygiene.

www.deltadentalins.com/oral_health/heart.html – the link between oral hygiene and cardiovascular disease.

Video links

VIDEO
LINKS

Have a break from the text and go to https://study.sagepub.com/essentialnursing2e for useful videos related to this chapter. If you are using the interactive ebook, simply click on the lightbulb icon in the margin to go straight to the resource.

ACE YOUR ASSESSMENT

ONLINE
QUIZZES

Review what you have learned by visiting the book's online resources at: https://study.sagepub.com/essentialnursing2e If using your interactive ebook, just click on the icon in the margin to go straight there.

- Test yourself with multiple-choice and short-answer questions.
- Revise key terms with the interactive flash cards.

REFERENCES

Baillie, L. (2009) *Developing Practical Adult Nursing Skills*, 3rd edn. London: Hodder Arnold.

Department of Health (DH) (2010) *Essence of Care Benchmarks for Personal Hygiene*. London: DH.

Dougherty, L. and Lister, S. (eds) (2015) *The Royal Marsden Hospital Manual of Clinical Nursing Procedures*, 9th edn. Oxford: Wiley-Blackwell.

Glasper, A., Aylott, M. and Battrick, C. (2010) *Developing Practical Skills for Nursing Children and Young People*. London: Hodder Arnold.

Malkin, B. and Berridge, P. (2009) 'Guidance on maintaining personal hygiene in nail care', *Nursing Standard*, 23(41): 35–8.

National Health Service (NHS) (2013) Guidance: Clinically Related Challenging Behaviour – Prevention and Measurement. Consultation draft. London: NHS.

National Institute for Health and Clinical Excellence (NICE) (2012) *Prevention and Control of Healthcare-Associated Infections in Primary and Community Care*. Clinical Guideline 139. London: NICE.

Nursing and Midwifery Council (NMC) (2015) *The Code: Professional Standards of Practice and Behaviour for Nurses and Midwives*. London: NMC.

Sargeant, S. and Chamley, C. (2013) 'Oral health assessment and mouthcare for children and young people receiving palliative care', *Nursing Children and Young People*, 25(3): 30–3.

Sharples, K. (2011) *Successful Practice Learning for Nursing Students*, 2nd edn. London: SAGE.

World Health Organization (WHO) (2009) WHO Guidelines on Hand Hygiene in Health Care. Available at: http://whqlibdoc.who.int/publications/2009/9789241597906_eng.pdf (accessed 7 March 2018).

World Health Organization (2014) Health Topics: Hygiene. Available at: www.who.int/topics/hygiene/en/ (accessed 7 March 2018).

LAST OFFICES

JEAN SHAPCOTT

REQUIRED KNOWLEDGE

- It will be helpful to read Chapters 8, 12, 15 and 16 before reading this chapter.

> " My mother had dementia and somehow broke her hip without even falling. She was admitted to hospital and had an operation to replace her hip, but she never recovered and died a week later. The night before she died I asked if I could stay with her as it was obvious she was dying, but the nurses made it really hard for me to do so, and I went home. Mum died as I arrived early the next morning – I did not get to say goodbye, but this time the nurses were amazing. They let me stay with Mum as long as I wanted, but made sure I knew where to find them if I needed to. When it came time to carry out the Last Offices, the nurse asked whether I wanted to stay and I said I did, but I did not want to be involved. They said that was fine and proceeded to wash Mum gently and in a very dignified way. They talked to her as they did this, using her name throughout. When they had finished the nurse suggested that this would be a good time to leave as they were going to 'wrap her up', so I quietly said my last goodbye and left. I will never forget the way those two nurses looked after my mum – they really cared, right to the end. "
>
> **Charlotte, patient's daughter**

> " I will never forget my first Last Offices or the third-year student who guided me through it. The patient had been on the ward where I had my first placement for a while, so we all knew him. I was looking after him with my practice educator on the day he died. I had never seen anyone die before and I really didn't want to do Last Offices so early in my course. The third-year offered to do them with my practice educator, but insisted I stood by his side while he did it. He talked me through what he was doing and just made the whole experience somehow good, which I did not think it could ever be. His guidance and support helped me realise the importance of the procedure and how much of a privilege it is to do it. "
>
> **Mary-Louise, adult nursing student**

INTRODUCTION

Caring for a patient does not end at the point of death. Last Offices is the term used for care given after a patient has died and is the final act that you will perform for any patient. They should always be performed in a way that demonstrates continued respect for the individuality of the patient (NMC, 2015). Although Last Offices are based on relatively simple procedures, skilled, sensitive communication is required when addressing the needs of the bereaved and respecting the integrity of the person who has died, as was clearly evident in the relative's voice at the start of the chapter.

CULTURAL AND SPIRITUAL CONSIDERATIONS

It is essential that nurses respect cultural requirements when performing Last Offices, while ensuring legal obligations are met. Wherever possible, nurses should have discussed this with the patient and their family to ensure their wishes are fully known. Unless there are legal reasons why these wishes cannot be respected (for example, a post-mortem ordered by the coroner to determine the cause of death), they must take precedence. It is important to remember that it is possible that the religion stated by a patient may be more related to their cultural and national roots than to any significant level of adherence to that faith. If there is any doubt about the cultural requirements for undertaking Last Offices, you should seek guidance from the patient's family or community leaders.

It lies outside the scope of this chapter to provide detailed information regarding Last Offices for each culture represented in an increasingly multicultural society, but some of the considerations required for the major cultures are as follows:

- Ideally, the body of a deceased Buddhist should be moved as little as possible before a community leader arrives and Last Offices should be delayed as long as possible, since Buddhists believe that consciousness remains in the body for a while after death.
- Christians believe that the bodies of the dead should be treated with the same respect as if they were alive.
- In Hindu culture, the wishes of the dead are always honoured. The family should be consulted before the body is touched or moved by a non-Hindu and, if the body has to be moved, nurses should wear gloves. The family should also be asked if they wish to perform the Last Offices, whether the patient dies in hospital or at home. Hindus may oppose post-mortems, but there is no objection if this is required by law. All organs must be returned to the body before the funeral.
- The Jewish community has its own funeral service – the *chevra kadisha* – which ensures that the bodies of Jews are prepared for burial according to tradition and are protected from desecration. While not all Jewish patients will request the services of the *chevra kadisha*, you must remember that the body should not be touched by the ungloved hand of a non-Jew and that family or community members may prefer to perform Last Offices themselves.
- Similarly, in the Muslim community, the body should not be handled by a non-Muslim unless they are wearing gloves and should not be uncovered, except for washing. Whenever possible, the body should be washed by nurses of the same gender as the deceased – if this is not possible, the family must be informed, as they may wish to undertake this themselves. Unless required by law, post-mortem is prohibited and the body should be released to the family as soon as possible.
- In the Sikh community, family members often perform Last Offices, whether at home or in hospital. Sons and other male members of the family attend to the body of a deceased man, while daughters and other females prepare the body of a woman. The five 'Ks' (Kesh – hair; Kangha – comb; Karah – steel bracelet; Kachhera – special unisex shorts/underwear; and Kirpaan – sword (ornamental and usually very small)) should not be removed. (Adapted from Suffolk Mental Health Partnership Trust, 2009)

These are guidelines only and you should remember that individual requirements may vary, even amongst people from the same cultural background.

Spirituality

Death can be an intensely spiritual time both for the person who is dying and for their family and friends. Nurses are amongst those professionals most closely associated with the expression of individual belief, as well as the spiritual enquiry and engagement which may surface as patients and their families and friends encounter death (Holloway, 2006). In current practice, the nurse needs to be able to translate what we know and understand from contemporary experience, as well as ancient tradition, into approaches which are relevant for a particular family. Long-standing rituals and practices may be helpful for some, but for others there may be a need for customisation or adaptation in order to facilitate a spiritual understanding of death and all its meanings.

While nurses must be able to recognise the specific beliefs and values which operate within the major faiths of the world, they must equally be able to recognise spiritual needs expressed by individuals who have only very loose ties with a recognised faith system or do not express any faith. Holloway (2006) identifies four beliefs that overwhelmingly give comfort to people who report no religious affiliation at all:

1. Death is part of the cycle of life.
2. Your loved one did their best for their family and friends.
3. Forgiving allows individuals to die peacefully.
4. Death is our fate.

While these may appear somewhat stark, they represent the challenge to nursing and nurses of addressing the spirituality of death in an increasingly secular society. Many nurses would agree that performing Last Offices is not only the final act of caring for a patient, but also a privilege afforded to very few people.

ACTIVITY 33.1: CRITICAL THINKING

A strict Orthodox Jewish patient has died on the operating table. He was only the second on the list; there are still a number of patients awaiting surgery and all the other theatres are busy. It is clear that this patient will have to be moved from the table onto a bed.

- How would you manage this task while respecting the cultural needs of this patient?

ANSWER:
ACTIVITY 33.1

PERFORMING LAST OFFICES

Before Last Offices are undertaken, you must ensure that certain other important things have been done – most notably, that the death of the patient has been confirmed. In the case of an unexpected death, this is always done by a doctor, usually a senior member of the team. When the death of a patient is expected, confirmation is still usually carried out by a doctor, although, if local policy permits, senior nurses may do this in some clinical settings (Dougherty and Lister, 2015).

Caring for dying patients can be a very difficult and challenging experience, especially when you start out in nursing. You have to keep your emotions in check and act professionally – I think this is something you can't learn in a classroom: you have to experience it and learn from the more experienced staff members around you.

Charlie Clisby, NQN

Performance of Last Offices will be affected if a patient's death is to be referred to a coroner. This may occur if:

- the cause of death is unknown
- the death was violent or unnatural
- the death was sudden or unexplained
- the person who died was not seen by a medical practitioner during their final illness
- the person who died was not seen by the medical practitioner who signed the death certificate within 14 days before death or after they died
- the death occurred during an anaesthetic or before the person came out of anaesthetic. (Gov.UK, 2013)

Post-mortems can also affect Last Offices, whether this is a legal requirement or has been requested by a consultant in order to answer a specific query on the cause of death.

Infection-control measures are required for the safe performance of Last Offices for every patient, whether they die in hospital or a community setting. If a patient had a known infection, it is important that you know the nature of that infection and the causative agent. There are additional infection-control requirements for undertaking Last Offices on patients with blood-borne infections and you should seek advice from the senior nurse on duty and infection-control nurses.

Whatever the circumstances of the patient's death, they were once a living person and must be cared for with dignity. Whether in hospital or the community, the family should be allowed to sit with their relative in the period immediately after death, unless the death is suspicious. Many hospices have cold rooms which offer the family opportunities to view the body beyond the time possible in other environments. Nurses should offer age-appropriate support as it is vital that, with parental consent, children are not excluded from this experience.

While much of what constitutes Last Offices is the same whether the patient dies in hospital or at home, the latter is generally a less 'clinical' environment in which some of the requirements vary slightly, and much of the equipment used in hospital may not be available.

ACTIVITY 33.2: LEADERSHIP AND MANAGEMENT

You were present when the family of a young woman who has died unexpectedly in the emergency department were told that her death would be referred to the coroner and that a post-mortem would be required. Although clearly devastated, the family understood the need for this course of action.

While you are helping a newly qualified nurse undertake Last Offices, she insists that you remove all the cannulae, drains, etc. from the body of the deceased. You remind her that this is to be a coroner's case but she continues to insist. What should you do?

ANSWER:
ACTIVITY 33.2

> I have looked after a child who is dying and felt very privileged that they themselves and their family have allowed me to care for them at such a difficult time.
>
> Alice Rowe, NQ RNMH

FOLLOWING LAST OFFICES

Once Last Offices have been completed, the body can be transferred to the mortuary. In hospital settings, this is normally done by portering staff, while in the community the funeral directors will make all necessary arrangements, including those required for cultural reasons.

All aspects of the care given must be accurately documented in the nursing notes, identifying the professional involved. Once this has been done, the documents are made available to the bereavement team and others who require access to them – pathologists, for example.

CASE STUDY 33.1: JAKE AND ZOE (HOSPITAL)

Jake was 6 years old and had been in and out of the children's ward for the past two and a half years, having been diagnosed with a brain tumour at the age of 4. Initially it was thought that the tumour was benign and surgeons believed they had successfully removed it, but it came back in a malignant form. Despite further surgery, the tumour could not be removed and Jake had been receiving palliative care for the past six months.

Jake's mother, Terri, and his father, Max, had cared for Jake at home for much of the time he was sick, but he had wanted to die in hospital 'with his favourite nurses around him' so, when it became apparent that the end was near, the family came into hospital for the final time. They took over Jake's usual cubicle and Terri, Max and Jake's 12-year-old brother James all stayed there with him. There were pictures of other family members, the family's dog and cat and cards all around the room and it didn't really feel like a hospital cubicle.

After a bad night, Jake deteriorated and died in his mother's arms around 10 am; he did indeed have his favourite nurses around him. Terri, Max and James sat with Jake for over an hour after he died until it was time to perform Last Offices. Zoe, the nurse, tried gently but firmly to ask the family to leave, but they were insistent that, having cared for Jake in life, they wanted to perform the final caring acts for him. Although she felt very uncomfortable, the nurse reluctantly allowed Terri and Max to stay, but felt strongly that James was too young and should leave.

James' response was to take Jake's towel and gently dry the areas that his parents had just washed – talking to Jake all the time, telling him what a special brother he had been and that he (James) would look after their mum and dad. He helped Terri and Max to dress Jake in his Manchester United kit and when the time came to put identity labels on Jake's body, James took them out of the nurse's hand and carefully placed them around his brother's wrist and ankle. He then went to the pile of toys that Jake had accumulated while in hospital and picked out his favourite cuddly bunny, which he placed in Jake's hands before the body was prepared for transfer to the mortuary.

As the family left the cubicle, Terri simply said 'Thank you', but James turned and ran back to Zoe to give her a big hug.

ANSWER:
CASE STUDY 33.1

(Continued)

- Why might Zoe have been reluctant to allow Jake's family, and particularly his brother James, to participate in performing Last Offices?
- How could being involved in this procedure have assisted family members in managing their grief, both in the period immediately after Jake's death and in the following months?

STEP-BY-STEP CLINICAL SKILL 33.1: PERFORMING LAST OFFICES

☑ Before you start

Remember to ensure that the death of the patient has been confirmed, that you know whether there is going to be a post-mortem and that, if relevant/appropriate, the family has been offered the opportunity to assist in performing Last Offices. Ensure all cultural requirements can be met when undertaking Last Offices.

☑ Essential equipment

All settings

- Disposable aprons and gloves; bowl of warm water; patient's own toilet articles; disposable washcloths; towels x 2; patient's own razor/disposable razor (if male); comb and equipment for nail care; equipment for mouth care, including care of patient's dentures; plastic bags for clinical and domestic waste; container for expressed urine; clean linen; any documentation required by law or local policy; shroud or culturally appropriate clothing or patient's own clothes if requested by family.

Community setting

- Toe tag (for identification).

Hospital setting

- Linen skip for soiled linen, identification bands x 2, valuables/property book, bag(s) for patient's own property.

If required

- Gauze, dressings and tape to cover wounds, IV sites, etc.; caps/spigots for urinary catheters, drains, etc. if they are to be left in situ.

For children

- Card/envelope to keep a lock of hair, washable paint and card for hand/footprints, toy, etc. that family may wish to leave with the child after the procedure is completed.

☑ Care-setting considerations

Last Offices can be performed in both hospital and community care settings.

LAST OFFICES GUIDELINES

 Gather the equipment required. Ensure these are clean as appropriate
To be fully prepared and organised
    Reduces the chance of infection and maintains patient and nurse safety

 Ensure privacy, so close doors and curtains/blinds as necessary. If in a hospital setting, ensure you draw the curtains fully or close all doors
Maintains patient privacy and dignity as required

 Tidy the bed space; turn off monitoring equipment. If possible, remove equipment from the bedside
To normalise the environment for relatives or carers and provide access to safely perform the procedure

 Wash your hands and put on an apron. Wear apron throughout procedure and gloves whenever appropriate or required to maintain cultural sensitivity
Personal protective equipment (PPE) must be worn when performing Last Offices to protect yourself and other patients from the risk of infection. However, this needs to be done in a way that maintains dignity and respect
    If family members are present, be especially sensitive to their views relating to this; consider how they might feel if gloves are worn when, for example, washing the face of their loved one

 If the patient was being nursed on a pressure-relieving mattress or device, consult manufacturer's guidance before turning it off
If the mattress is allowed to deflate too quickly, it may pose a moving and handling challenge when performing Last Offices

 Lay the patient on their back with their limbs as straight as possible while adhering to local moving and handling policy

It will not be possible to do this at a later stage. Stiff, flexed limbs can be difficult for mortuary staff to manage and can cause additional distress to family members or carers who wish to view the body
    However, if it is not possible to straighten the patient's body or limbs, do not use force; it can be corrected later by the undertaker

 Close the patient's eyes by applying light pressure to the eyelids for approximately 30 seconds. If this is unsuccessful, moistened cotton wool can be used to maintain the position of the eyelids until they remain closed. Some policies suggest the use of tape to keep eyelids closed
To maintain the patient's dignity, for aesthetic reasons and to minimise the distress of relatives who may wish to view the body
    Only tape that does not mark the skin on removal should be used, and this should not be done to the eyelids of a child

 If it is certain that there is not to be a post-mortem, all drains, cannulae, catheters, etc. can be removed and disposed of appropriately. Gauze dressings may be applied over entry sites
If there is to be a post-mortem, leave all drains, cannulae, catheters, etc. in situ, disconnect as close to the body as possible and spigot as necessary
To leave the deceased in as natural a state as possible for family members who may wish to view the body
    To prepare the body for burial or cremation
    To comply with legal requirements and facilitate investigation into the cause of death

 Any wounds should be covered with a clean absorbent dressing and secured with an occlusive dressing or waterproof tape. Stitches and clips should be left intact

(Continued)

The dressing will absorb leakage from the wound site and prevent oozing of blood or serous fluid

 Drain the patient's bladder by applying gentle pressure over the lower abdomen
To ensure the bladder contains a minimal volume of urine, and prevent leakage of body fluids

 Leakage of body fluids from the oral cavity can be contained by the use of suction
Incontinence pads should be used to contain leakage from the vagina and bowel. Stomas should be covered with a new bag
The packing of orifices can cause damage to the body and should not be done
Leaking orifices pose a health hazard to staff coming into contact with the patient's body
Ensuring that the body is clean demonstrates continuing respect for the patient's dignity

 Wash the patient in the same way you would when undertaking a bed bath, unless requested not to do so for cultural or religious reasons or the family or carer's preference
If family members wish to assist, facilitate their participation
Male patients should be shaved unless they chose to wear a beard or moustache in life
For aesthetic and hygiene purposes. This is also both a mark of respect and a point of closure in the relationship between nurse and patient
The involvement of family members in washing the body is an expression of respect and affection as well as part of the process of adjusting to their loss and expressing their grief

 Mouth and teeth should be cleaned using foam sticks or a toothbrush. If the patient normally wore dentures, clean them and place them in their mouth. Apply petroleum jelly or equivalent to dry lips

The patient's teeth and mouth are cleaned to remove debris for aesthetic and hygiene purposes. If dentures are not re-inserted into the mouth, the patient may appear very different to the way they appeared in life

 Death in hospital
Ensure all the patient's property is gathered together and placed in a clearly labelled bag
In the presence of another nurse, remove all jewellery from the body unless the family requests otherwise. Record the jewellery and other valuables, storing them in accordance with local policy. Avoid using the names of precious metals or gems when recording jewellery – instead, use terms such as 'white metal' and 'green stone'

Death at home
Work closely with the patient's family to ensure their wishes and those of the deceased are followed
To respect relatives' wishes and comply with both legal requirements and cultural practices
Sensitivity is required when clothing is soiled and you should not assume that the family wish to keep it – always ask
To ensure items are accurately described, as it can be very difficult to tell precious metals or stones from imitation ones
To ensure it remains with the patient
To provide a formal record of what has been left on the patient
Any jewellery left on the body should be secured with tape
All jewellery remaining on the body should be documented on the Notification of Death form

 Dress the patient in a shroud or other clothing as required by cultural tradition or requested by family members. Children are not normally dressed in a shroud and parents often have specific requests as to what they should wear
Remember that at this point there may still be some leakage from body orifices, so it is not appropriate to dress the body in clothing that the family may wish them to wear for burial or cremation

For aesthetic reasons, for family members or others who may wish to view the body, to comply with religious or cultural requirements and to meet the needs of the family members or carers

 Death in hospital
Ensure two fully completed patient identification bands are attached to the patient – one on the wrist and one on the ankle Complete all necessary documentation, such as Notification of Death cards, and tape such card to the shroud or clothing

Death at home
Ensure that a toe tag (or equivalent) is attached to the patient and that all necessary documentation is completed and ready to accompany the body
To ensure accurate and easy identification of the patient's body in the mortuary

 Following local policy, prepare the body for removal to the mortuary. This may involve wrapping the body in a sheet, ensuring that all the limbs are held securely in position and the face and feet are covered. For a child, ensure any toy that the parents have requested should accompany the body is secured within the sheet. If used, secure the sheet with tape

To avoid possible damage to the patient's body during transfer and prevent distress to colleagues (such as porters in the hospital setting)
Pins should not be used as they present a health and safety hazard

 If required by local policy or for infection-control purposes, place the body in a body bag and ensure that information regarding any known infectious disease is clearly documented and visible
Placing the body in a body bag is advised for all notifiable diseases and some other infectious diseases (such as HIV), and a label clearly identifying the infection must be attached to the patient's body. While it is true that certain additional precautions are required when performing Last Offices on a patient with a disease known to be infectious who has died, the body poses no greater infection risk than it did when that patient was alive. The application of standard infection-control practices must therefore be continued when handling the body of the deceased

 Tidy up the area, complete any further documentation and clean any reusable equipment
To ensure that:

- the patient's records are updated
- equipment is clean and in working order

Source: Dougherty and Lister (2015); Green and Green (2006); HSAC (2003); NMC (2015)

PSYCHOLOGICAL CARE

It is hard for any nurse to fully understand the feelings of family members or those close to a patient when they die. The way in which a person dies will have a major impact on the way in which people behave when they are bereaved. Following a sudden, unexpected death, family and close friends may be extremely distressed and shocked. They may feel numb and express denial that the person has died. While nurses might think that relatives are prepared for the anticipated death of a loved one, the actual death can still come as a shock and the bereaved will still display the signs of grief.

When a loved one dies, a range of emotions are released, which may be difficult to control. People want to remember the person who has died and it is believed that grief and mourning enable people to integrate the character and life of the person who has died into the ongoing life of the bereaved, somehow re-establishing a relationship that others might believe had ended (Hills and Albarran, 2010). There are a number of tasks involved in doing this. Worden (1991) suggests that these include:

- coming to terms with the fact that the death has occurred
- feeling the pain both emotionally and physically
- adjusting to life without the deceased
- relocating and reinvesting in their own lives.

There are many theories that attempt to explain the ways in which people express grief and bereavement, but no single theory can explain the complexity of emotions felt by an individual (Hills and Albarran, 2010). Cultural factors will have an impact on grief behaviours. In some cultures, grief behaviours involve displaying inconsolable weeping or tearing of their own clothing; such behaviours can be difficult to manage in a hospital environment, particularly where there are many other very sick patients. The way in which nurses convey emotional concern, empathy and compassion can be critical in facilitating both acute and long-term responses and adjustment to grief. Whatever the setting or situation, there is a consensus that emotional support in the early stages of bereavement can prevent long-term ill health associated with extended grief.

The relatives of the deceased will require support from the nurses and this can facilitate the incorporation of any specific care or practices which may be required. As identified previously, in some cultures it may be unacceptable for anyone except a family member or religious/community leader to wash the body, but even where this is not the case, family members may wish to assist with Last Offices. This is particularly true when a child has died since many parents wish to be involved in this final caring act for their son or daughter (see case study 33.1). Such families and carers should be supported and encouraged to participate as this may help the grieving process.

Once the family has been informed of the death of their loved one, it is important to allow them time to understand the news and express how they are feeling. Nurses need to be supportive and provide compassionate, honest and individualised information (Hills and Albarran, 2010). The provision of appropriate care for the bereaved following the death of their loved one can be achieved through:

- finding a comfortable, non-denominational venue to ensure privacy. It may not be appropriate to suggest that a family go to the chapel, but a suggestion that they might want to sit in a quiet garden or room may well be more acceptable
- providing the family with opportunities to verbalise emotions and have their questions answered simply, clearly, sensitively and informatively
- offering relatives the opportunity to view the deceased (when appropriate).

It is clear that many of the nursing interventions and behaviours identified above are simple and basic caring acts. Relatives find comfort in the actions of nurses who respect the dignity of the patient and demonstrate insight into the needs of the family by caring for the deceased's body in a thoughtful and caring way.

It is important that nurses appreciate the significance that bereaved family members place on their presence at such a difficult time. Relatives often describe the kindness, comfort and emotional support provided by nurses, which in some way counteract the harsh reality of death. They are touched by nurses' non-intrusive presence, their expressions of emotional solidarity and the empathy they show by sharing their own emotional responses to the patient's death (Williams et al., 2012).

When there are no relatives

It is important to remember that some patients who die may not have any relatives around. These patients deserve the same dignified care as any other, and you, as the nurse, may be one of the only people who will remember them as a person. In addition, in some fields of nursing, notably learning disability, the nurses and other care staff may have acted in the role of a family member for many years and will therefore experience grief similar to that of a family member. Nurses are only human and they too can be affected by the death of a patient. How a nursing student responds to a first death and whether or not they are supported by peers and practice educators can affect how they react to future losses (Domrose, 2011).

WHAT'S THE EVIDENCE?

WEBLINK:
JORDAN
(2008)

Jordan, J.R. (2008) 'Bereavement after suicide', *Psychiatric Annals*, 38(10): 679-85.

In this literature review, Jordan investigated the impact of suicide on those left behind - suicide survivors - and the interventions that may be appropriate when providing compassionate bereavement care following a suicide.

It is estimated that there are six suicide survivors (those who are negatively affected by the suicide of a loved one) for every suicide. Suicide survivors often show high levels of distress in several aspects of their lives. The first of these is the increased risk that they too will take their own life, especially when the suicide was a family member's. Adolescents were identified as a group more likely to contemplate suicide when exposed to the suicide of either a member of their family or a peer. Survivors often display problematic grief experiences, including intense guilt, a strong desire to make sense of the death, strong feelings of rejection, abandonment and anger at the deceased, trauma symptoms and shame about the manner of the death.

A number of interventions aimed at helping suicide survivors were identified. Research into the perceived needs of the survivors themselves has identified the need to reduce the impact of the suicide on children in the family, dealing with trauma symptoms (re-living experiences, constant reflection on the frame of mind of the deceased), difficulties in finding suicide-specific support services and problems in family communication after the suicide. Interventions identified as being useful include either individual bereavement therapy with a mental health professional or bereavement support groups, whether peer or professionally led. Family therapy may be useful alongside such interventions as it can provide insight into the cause of the suicide and help to promote open communication and good bereavement self-care for all involved. Contact with other survivors has proved invaluable for many since it provides a safe space to compare and normalise experiences, reduce the sense of social isolation and stigma and receive non-judgemental support for grief.

- Reflect on what you feel are the important elements within the bereavement care delivered to all patients' friends and relatives, including those whose loved one has committed suicide.
- Now read the article and consider how you can apply the findings to your practice.

CARING FOR YOURSELF

Nurses who allow themselves to go through a grieving process seem to be healthier than those who hold in their grief, as those who hold in their grief often pay the price through not being able to deal with their feelings at the time or in an appropriate place. They may experience disenfranchised grief, feeling it is not acceptable to express their emotional response to a patient's death in the workplace environment, which may lead to them becoming reluctant to develop relationships with other patients or having physical problems such as difficulty sleeping or eating properly.

Nurses may resent being asked to support others (bereaved family members, colleagues, students) in their loss without any acknowledgement that the death is a loss for them as well (Wilson and Kirshbaum, 2011). It is therefore important that psychological support is available to nurses as well as family members. This can be provided both by the placement and the university as well as within social networks.

Creating a forum within a placement area in which staff can articulate their feelings in a safe and supportive environment benefits not only individual nurses but also the healthcare team as a whole. Less formal strategies can be seen in nurses going for a break following the death of a patient or deciding to call a ward or team meeting to debrief when a death has been particularly difficult or unexpected.

When nursing a dying patient I ensured I gave them the care they needed with empathy and compassion. To ensure I was able to do this I would talk to and gain support from my colleagues when I needed it. If I needed support I spoke to my practice educator and other students on my course as we are all learning together.

I would ensure I relaxed during my time off and if I needed to become upset I would do this in the privacy of my own home. It is important to ensure we eat and sleep well and recognise when our patients have an emotional impact on us and look for support when this happens.

Julie Davis, LD nursing student

Outside the workplace, most nurses have an extensive network of friends and family (Wilson and Kirshbaum, 2011). For many children's nurses, the first act after undertaking Last Offices on a child is to call their own child's school or their partner or parents, just to check on the welfare of their own family. Some nurses prefer to rely on these informal networks since they feel that these individuals know them best and may be able to provide support tailored to their needs.

CASE STUDY 33.2: BILL, ELLA AND HARRIET [HOSPITAL]

Ella is a final-year nursing student who has always felt it a privilege to perform Last Offices for those who die in her care.

Bill, an elderly gentleman, has died and Ella is aware that Harriet, a student on her first placement, has been involved in caring for him. She watches Harriet and her practice educator go into Bill's room to undertake Last Offices. Shortly after, she sees the practice educator leave the room, leaving Harriet alone with Bill. Ella becomes aware that the practice educator has got caught up with another patient while Harriet is still alone and goes in to check that she is OK.

Harriet is sitting by the bed of the patient looking very pale and close to tears. She tells Ella that the only other dead body she had seen was that of her grandfather, who died when she was 12 years old.

Ella suggests that they both take some time out and takes Harriet to the ward office, informing the practice educator and the HCA with whom she is working (to ensure her own patients are cared for) that they are there. She then allows Harriet to talk about how she is feeling about caring for a patient who has died and what she is worried about with regard to Last Offices. The practice educator, seeing the rapport between the two students and knowing that Ella has done Last Offices on a number of occasions, suggests that they might undertake the procedure together.

- How might this opportunity to do Last Offices together be beneficial for both Ella and Harriet?
- Often, one of the best sources of support for nursing students is other students. How might you either support another student or seek support from another student if you were in a similar situation?

CONCLUSION

Last Offices is the final act you will perform for any patient. It should always be performed in a way that demonstrates continued respect for the individuality of the patient.

It is essential that nurses respect cultural requirements when performing Last Offices, while ensuring legal obligations are met. Unless there are legal reasons why these wishes cannot be respected (for example, a post-mortem ordered by the coroner to determine the cause of death), they must take precedence.

Death can be an intensely spiritual time both for the person who is dying and for their family and friends. Nurses are amongst those professionals most closely associated with the expression of individual belief as well as the spiritual enquiry and engagement which may surface as patients and their families and friends encounter death.

The way in which nurses convey emotional concern, empathy and compassion can be critical in facilitating both acute and long-term responses and adjustment to grief. Nurses need to be supportive and provide compassionate, honest and individualised information. Relatives often describe the kindness, comfort and emotional support provided by nurses which in some way counteract the harsh reality of death. They are touched by nurses' non-intrusive presence, their expressions of emotional solidarity and the empathy they show by sharing their own emotional responses to the patient's death.

Nurses who allow themselves to go through a grieving process seem to be healthier than those who hold in their grief. Those who hold in their grief often pay the price through not being able to deal with their feelings at the time or in an appropriate place. You will find support can be offered by your placement area, university and friends and family; however, many nursing students feel that the best support is offered by other nursing students, as they have often experienced similar feelings.

ACTIVITY 33.3: REFLECTION

- How might your own personal, cultural and spiritual attitudes, values and beliefs impact on your involvement in performing Last Offices?
- How can you manage the emotions that you might experience when performing Last Offices?
- In what way has reading this chapter enhanced your understanding of the cultural and spiritual considerations inherent in performing Last Offices and caring for the bereaved?

CHAPTER SUMMARY

- Care does not end at the point of death. Last Offices involves all the care that is given to a patient after death.
- There are a range of cultural and spiritual considerations to be taken into account when performing Last Offices and caring for those who are recently bereaved. Ideally, nurses will be aware of these before death and therefore prepared, but, unless there are legal reasons for not respecting such wishes, nurses must seek to meet the cultural needs of the patient and family.
- Some deaths are referred to the coroner, which will affect the way in which Last Offices are carried out.
- The role of the family in Last Offices is particularly important, particularly in relation to culture and the needs of bereaved parents.
- When providing psychological care for bereaved family and friends, remember that simple, caring nursing interventions and behaviours are appreciated by those whose loved one has died.
- It is just as important to care for yourself as it is to care for patients and their loved ones.

CRITICAL REFLECTION

Holistic care

This chapter has highlighted the wider importance of providing holistic care for your patient's friends and family. Review the chapter and note down all the instances where you think the bereavement care you would deliver as part of Last Offices can help meet their wider physical, psychological, social, economic and spiritual needs. Think of a variety of different patients across the fields, not just within your own field. You may find it helpful to make a list and refer back to it next time you are in practice, and then write your own reflection after your practice experience.

GO FURTHER

Books

Corr, C. and Balk, D. (2010) *Children's Encounters with Death, Bereavement and Coping*. New York: Springer. An excellent resource outlining how bereaved children can be helped to cope with their experiences.

Green, J. (2006) *Dealing with Death: A Handbook of Practices, Procedures and Law*, 2nd edn. London: Jessica Kingsley Publishers. A comprehensive source of information for professionals on the procedures, laws and cultural customs that should be observed when someone dies.

McNeilly, P. and Price, J. (2008) 'Care of the child after death', in J. Kelsey and G. McEwing (eds), *Clinical Skills in Child Health Practice*. Edinburgh: Churchill Livingstone.

Journal articles

Cooper, J. and Barnett, M. (2005) 'Aspects of caring for dying patients which cause anxiety to first year student nurses', *International Journal of Palliative Nursing*, 11(8): 423-30. A very well written and informative article considering the aspects of caring for dying patients that are most difficult for nursing students at the start of their programme.

Heise, B. A. and Gilpin, L.C. (2016) 'Nursing students' clinical experience with death: a pilot study', *Nursing Education Perspectives* (National League For Nursing), 37(2): 104-106. An interesting research paper which reviews nursing students' experiences of death whilst in placement.

Higgins, D. (2008) 'Carrying out last offices: Part 1 – Preparing for the procedure', *Nursing Times*, 104(37): 20-1. A practical source of information outlining how to prepare for Last Offices.

Higgins, D. (2008) 'Carrying out last offices: Part 2 – Preparing the body', *Nursing Times*, 104(38): 24-5. A practical source of information outlining how to undertake Last Offices.

Hyoung Sook, P., Youngju, J., Soon Hee, K. andf Yoon-ji, K. (2014) 'Nursing students' first clinical experiences of death', *Korean Journal Of Hospice & Palliative Care*, 17(3): 161-169. A thought-provoking paper considering nursing students first experiences of death.

Keating, J. (2009) 'Care after death', *Nursing Standard*, 23(26): 56-9. An interesting and helpful article considering the care you should deliver to patients once they have died.

Weblinks

Go to https://study.sagepub.com/essentialnursing2e for weblinks related to this chapter. If you are using the interactive ebook, simply click on the book icon in the margin to go straight to the resource.

FURTHER
READING:
WEBLINKS

www.childbereavementuk.org – Child Bereavement UK provides information for anyone whose child has died and information for professionals about how to support them.

www.childdeathhelpline.org.uk – Child Death Helpline provides support for anyone (including healthcare professionals) affected by the death of a child from before birth to adulthood.

www.cruse.org.uk – Cruse Bereavement Care provides information for bereaved people following the death of a loved one.

www.mariecurie.org.uk/help/support/bereaved-family-friends/practical-legal/when-death-occurs – information for carers from Marie Curie about what happens around the time of death of a loved one.

Video links

Have a break from the text and go to https://study.sagepub.com/essentialnursing2e for useful videos related to this chapter. If you are using the interactive ebook, simply click on the lightbulb icon in the margin to go straight to the resource.

VIDEO
LINKS

ACE YOUR ASSESSMENT

Review what you have learned by visiting the book's online resources at: https://study.sagepub.com/essential nursing2e If using your interactive ebook, just click on the icon in the margin to go straight there.

GREAT FOR
REVISION

- Test yourself with multiple-choice and short-answer questions.
- Revise key terms with the interactive flash cards.

ONLINE
QUIZZES

REFERENCES

Domrose, C. (2011) Good Grief: Nurses cope with patient deaths. Available at: www.nurse.com/blog/2011/02/21/good-grief-nurses-cope-with-patient-deaths (accessed 24 February 2015).

Dougherty, L. and Lister, S. (2015) *The Royal Marsden Hospital Manual of Clinical Nursing Procedures*, 9th edn. Oxford: Wiley-Blackwell.

Gov.UK (2013) What to Do after Someone Dies. Available at: www.gov.uk/after-a-death/when-a-death-is-reported-to-a-coroner (accessed 7 March 2018).

Green, J. and Green, M. (2006) *Dealing with Death: A Handbook of Practices, Procedures and Law*. London: Jessica Kingsley Publishers.

Health and Safety Advisory Committee (HSAC) (2003) *Safe Working and the Prevention of Infection in the Mortuary and Post-Mortem Room.* London: Health and Safety Advisory Committee/HSE.

Hills, M. and Albarran, J.W. (2010) 'After death 1: Caring for bereaved relatives and being aware of cultural differences', *Nursing Times*, 106(7): 19–20.

Holloway, M. (2006) 'Death the great leveller? Towards a transcultural spirituality of dying and bereavement', *Journal of Clinical Nursing*, 15(7): 833–9.

Jordan, J.R. (2008) 'Bereavement after suicide', *Psychiatric Annals*, 38(10): 679–85.

Nursing and Midwifery Council (NMC) (2015) *The Code: Professional Standards of Practice and Behaviour for Nurses and Midwives.* London: NMC.

Suffolk Mental Health Partnership Trust (2009) Action in the Event of an Expected or Unexpected Death (Incorporating Last Offices): Policy and Procedure. Available at: www.smhp.nhs.uk/smhp/LinkClick.aspx?fileticket=JCEJCWUZRpo%3D&tabid=165&mid=746 (accessed 24 February 2015).

Williams, B.R., Lewis, D.R., Burgio, K.L. and Goode, P.S. (2012) 'Next-of-kin's perceptions of how hospital nursing staff support family presence before, during and after the death of a loved one', *Journal of Hospice and Palliative Nursing*, 14(8): 541–50.

Wilson, J. and Kirshbaum, M. (2011) 'Effects of patient death on nursing staff: A literature review', *British Journal of Nursing*, 20(9): 559–63.

Worden, W. (1991) *Grief Counselling and Grief Therapy: A Handbook for the Mental Health Wellbeing Practitioner.* New York: Springer.

The aim of this part of the book is to introduce you to the wider aspects of nursing, all of which are important in providing nurses with further sources of knowledge that they can apply to patient care. In nursing, a clear understanding of the rationale behind a patient's action, their beliefs or the complexities of the UK healthcare system are factors that enable us to work effectively in partnership to ensure the best possible outcomes.

Working as a nurse frequently involves combining your skills with those of other healthcare professionals, in order to offer the patient care that addresses all aspects of patients' needs. This means that you need to be able to function effectively not just individually but also as part of a much wider healthcare team, and understand the benefits this can bring to patient care when you do so.

While health policy may seem far removed from a nurse's daily role of providing care, a sound knowledge of policy-related issues is an excellent way to ensure patients receive the most up-to-date and effective care. In addition to this, being politically aware and active will enable you to do your utmost in advocating for the needs of your patients.

This part of the book covers the organisation and settings of care, interprofessional working and health policy, and introduces you to the global perspective of nursing. It highlights why an understanding of psychological and sociological issues is fundamental to all aspects of nursing care.

As Pamela reminds us, nurses frequently care for patients who are experiencing a wide range of challenging circumstances, not just those related to their health. In order to assist them, it is necessary to be able to view their situation from *their* perspective, with a sound knowledge of the wider aspects of nursing care, to ensure unfounded assumptions are not made. The voices in this part opener highlight the importance of these issues – read them and keep them in mind as you read through the chapters in this final part of the book.

INTRODUCTION TO THE ORGANISATION AND SETTINGS OF CARE

SIOBHAN MCCULLOUGH

THIS CHAPTER COVERS

- A brief overview of the development of the NHS
- Primary, secondary and tertiary care
- Organisation and delivery of healthcare in the UK
- Challenges facing the UK healthcare system
- A patient's journey through an experience of care

> My name is Jade and I am a second-year university student. I have a mental health problem and am finding it very difficult to access the mental health services I need. My GP has explained that there may be a wait to see the mental health 'crisis team' although new government policies mean mental health problems must be treated the same as physical health problems. However I am very worried because I know that in the past, early access to services in primary care helped me stay out of hospital and recover, and if I cannot access them soon, my illness will get worse.
>
> Jade, mental health service user

INTRODUCTION

Have you, a relative or a patient for whom you have cared, ever had an experience similar to Jade's? Do you find it difficult to understand the complex system of healthcare in the UK? How easy do patients find navigating this complicated system?

Jade's story demonstrates the increasingly complex and specialised nature of healthcare, with the delivery of ever more complex care outside hospitals and the increasing parity of esteem between mental and physical health. The aim of this chapter is to assist you to understand the development and organisation of the UK healthcare system, enabling you to appreciate the differences between the various settings. This will allow you to understand the experiences of the patients you care for, in a more critical and informed manner.

In order to achieve this, the chapter will introduce you to the concepts of primary, secondary and tertiary care by following a patient as they journey through these three levels of care. Within this, specific aspects of the care offered at each level will be identified and the reasons why a patient is referred on to the next level outlined. The chapter begins by briefly outlining the development of healthcare provision within the UK, which will help you to understand the current organisation and settings of NHS care.

A BRIEF OVERVIEW OF THE DEVELOPMENT OF THE NHS

Following recommendations in the 1942 Beveridge Report, the welfare state was established in 1948 with the purpose of providing a comprehensive range of services for UK citizens, including health and social care. The welfare state continues to change and evolve and has diversified into a complex set of organisations. In 1948, the National Health Service (NHS) was underpinned by key principles so that it was designed to be a comprehensive system to meet people's needs from cradle to grave, it was universal, free at the point of delivery and based on clinical need, and these principles hopefully still sound familiar to you today. Social care had a distinctly different development in 1948 and afterwards, and importantly it was not free at the point of delivery. Thus, it remains a much more complex system for patients to navigate. In order to understand how the organisation and settings of the UK health and social care system relate to patient care, we will discuss the journey of a patient, Aaeesha, through the primary, secondary and tertiary levels of care. As we will see in the case study (34.1), although we make distinctions between these settings, the boundaries between them are blurred and continuously shifting. Before we meet Aaeesha, however, in order to put her journey into context, it is necessary to clarify what is meant by the terms primary, secondary and tertiary care, to note the role of community care and to briefly discuss the development of the NHS.

PRIMARY, SECONDARY AND TERTIARY CARE

Primary care describes what, for most patients, is the first point of contact with the health system, and the level at which people receive the majority of their healthcare. It is usually based in the local community and can be provided in a variety of settings, but the most familiar one to you is probably the general practitioner's surgery (GP). Primary care can be provided by GPs, nurses, dentists, pharmacists, occupational therapists, physiotherapists, mental health practitioners, learning disability practitioners, children's community nurses and others. It is part curative and part preventative, as it includes many elements of health promotion, vaccination and screening programmes. The World Health Organization Alma-Ata Declaration (WHO, 1978) views primary care as the most effective way of addressing the main health problems in local communities, as it includes diagnosis, treatment, health conditions follow-up, diagnostic laboratory tests and prevention. Primary care involves the widest scope of healthcare, as it is directly accessible to every citizen and is often provided on an ongoing basis. Thus, primary care practitioners must possess a broad range of knowledge and when care at this level is exhausted, the patient is referred (often by their GP) on to secondary care.

Secondary care is accessed when you are referred from primary care to a more specialist service, which may be hospital-based, but can be delivered on an outpatient basis. It is care provided by a practitioner with specialist expertise, and this specialism may focus on a specific body system or disease. Thus, a cardiologist will focus on the heart, a nephrologist on the kidneys and an oncologist on treating cancer. The professionals working within secondary care include medical and surgical specialists, nurses, physiotherapists, occupational therapists, speech therapists, dieticians, podiatrists, children's specialist nurses, learning disability specialist nurses and specialist mental health nurses.

Tertiary care is the highest level of specialist care and referral is normally from a primary or secondary care professional. It is usually provided in hospital, where highly specialised facilities, equipment and expertise are available. Frequently, this will be in a specialist hospital or a large acute teaching hospital. Tertiary care includes neurosurgery, intensive care, cardiology, nephrology, neonatology services or forensic mental health services.

> Primary care is a person's first point of contact with healthcare – this could be either a GP's surgery, optician or dentist.
>
> Secondary care is provided by hospitals – contact with a hospital is often following a referral from a primary care setting.
>
> Tertiary care is provided by specialists within the hospital environment, following referrals from professionals in primary and secondary care teams. Tertiary care is provided by professionals who have a higher level of expertise than those in other care settings. This often involves complex treatments and procedures such as plastic surgery and heart surgery.
>
> **Sophie Lahe, LD nursing student**

Community care

Community care works in combination with primary, secondary and tertiary care and care is provided to people in their own homes or in non-institutional settings (Baggott, 2011). Community care services are designed to meet the needs of older people, children, people with physical or mental health problems or learning disabilities and those with long-term conditions. These services can vary, from being highly acute and specialised – such as the physical or psychological care delivered in a time of crisis in order to prevent hospital admission – to preventative care such as immunisation and health promotion. UK community care policy developed in part in response to evidence identifying the negative effects of institutional care. UK community care policy remained rather unclear and vague, and the National Health Service and Community Care Act 1990 was an attempt to address this lack of policy clarity. However, despite this Act and a consensus that care in the community is better than the provision of support in institutions, community care policy arguably continues to remain poorly defined and resourced.

Advances in mental healthcare, including the development of drugs, a greater emphasis on human rights and deinstitutionalisation, led to a decrease in the number of mental health beds, but progress to replace these with community alternatives has not kept pace. Thus, the number of adult inpatient psychiatric beds decreased by 39 per cent between 1998 and 2012, and bed occupancy is very high (NHS England, 2016). Almost two million people were in contact with specialist mental health and learning disability services in 2014/15 and of the adults with severe mental health problems 90 per cent are supported by community services (NHS England, 2016). However, there are frequently very long waits for those with common mental health problems, for some of the key interventions recommended by NICE (2011).

The importance of the provision of mental health is demonstrated by the fact that it is the second most common reason for primary care consultations, counting for 25 per cent of GP consultations and almost 11 per cent of the secondary care budget (Glasby, 2012). Mental health problems are the largest single cause of disability in the UK and cost the economy approximately £105 billion a year (NHS England, 2016). In policy terms, the National Service Framework for Mental Health (DH, 1999) led to the development of new forms of community mental health teams, with the NHS Plan (DH, 2000) providing funding. These teams included assertive outreach teams, crisis intervention teams and early intervention teams. In 2011 the coalition government published a mental health strategy, which recognised the significant challenges those with mental health problems still face, often with inadequate provision and worsening outcomes (DH, 2011). This was followed by the Independent Mental Health Taskforce in England (NHS England, 2016) which outlined a 10-year journey to transform mental health services to achieve a parity of esteem between mental and physical health, for all those who require it. This is to be achieved by improving seven-day crisis response services across the NHS and developing integrated mental and physical health services (NHS England, 2016). This includes a focus on prevention and promoting good mental health and creating mentally healthy communities, investing an additional £1 billion, developing and supporting the mental health workforce and improving data collection. The development of psychological therapies to address mental health has been a key feature of UK policy more recently, however current services are only meeting 15 per cent of the need of adults, so the aim is for this to increase to 25 per cent of need by 2020/21 (NHS England, 2016). This puts Jade's situation in the patient voice at the start of this chapter into context. Mental health nurses are also experiencing challenges, as highlighted in What's the Evidence?

WHAT'S THE EVIDENCE?

FURTHER
READING:
PRIMARY CARE

Richards, C., Rafferty, L. and Gibb, A. (2013) 'The value of mental health nurses working in primary care mental health teams', *Mental Health Practice*, 16(10): 19–23.

Richards et al. (2013) investigated the changes in mental health services and the benefits of including mental health nurses in primary care mental health teams in Greater Glasgow and Clyde. The introduction of the Increasing Access to Psychological Therapies (IAPT) service in England means interventions may be delivered by practitioners without a mental health qualification. Although IAPT had not been implemented in Scotland at the time of this study, there had been an increase in low-intensity psychological interventions by practitioners who did not necessarily have a mental health qualification. The study suggests that since the closure of large psychiatric institutions, mental health nurses have struggled to prove their therapeutic worth and cost-effectiveness.

- How important do you think it is for patients to be cared for by nurses with specialist qualifications?
- Is cost-effectiveness a crucial measure when evaluating the care delivered to patients?
- Now read the article and consider whether you would draw the same conclusions as the authors.

ORGANISATION AND DELIVERY OF HEALTHCARE IN THE UK

The organisation and delivery of UK healthcare is constantly evolving in response to demographic changes, such as the increase in the older population, as well as other changes such as developments in pharmacology, improved technology so healthcare can be delivered in and out of hospital safely, increasing patient expectations and the political context of care.

Although the organisation and delivery of healthcare is complex, a number of key themes are evident, including a focus on the quality of care, shifting care delivery from hospital to community settings, increasing patient choice and partnership, and involving the public in healthcare decisions. To enable you to understand how the NHS is currently organised, we will now consider a brief overview of how it developed. Interestingly, by examining the evolution of the UK NHS, some of the reasons why nurses are struggling to effectively define their professional roles, identity and value in the contemporary healthcare system, become clear.

Evolution of the NHS

The welfare state and state control and responsibility for healthcare in the UK only date back to 1948, following two world wars, political and economic unrest and many promises to 'improve the lot' of the UK population. Until then, the state was haphazardly involved in health and welfare – for example, with the 1848 Public Health Act, which gave local government the power to construct a clean water supply and sewerage system, and the 1875 Public Health Act, which established a framework for the subsequent development of public health. State involvement in healthcare was given even greater impetus when the 1899 Boer War recruitment drive revealed the dire standards of potential recruits' health. This led to improvements in child health through, for example, the 1906 and 1907 Education Acts, which provided the basis for school meals and medical services. The 1911 National Insurance Act established access to general practitioners and income during sickness and unemployment for some workers. However, by 1939 only 43 per cent of the population was covered by this type of insurance, although it marked the beginnings of primary care (Ham, 2009).

The hospital-based sector developed from the legacy of public hospitals, which began life attached to workhouses and were then developed to become separate infirmaries; and voluntary hospitals which were mainly established by religious and charitable organisations. By the 1940s, these hospitals provided a national but patchy hospital system, with general agreement that they were inadequate in coverage and quality (Klein, 2013). At the outbreak of the Second World War in 1939, this patchy hospital system was amalgamated into the Emergency Medical Service in order to provide hospital care during the war, thus providing a template for the NHS. The war served to galvanise political commitment to nationalised welfare services and the Beveridge Report of 1942 recommended reform of the social security system and creation of a National Health Service, amongst other reforms.

On 5 July 1948, the NHS was 'born' and 'The transformation of an inadequate, partial and muddled patchwork of healthcare provision into a neat administrative structure was dramatic' (Klein, 2013: 1). This also marked the beginning of the comprehensive primary, secondary and tertiary care sectors.

Founding principles

A number of founding principles underpin the NHS and they continue to be influential. The first is universalism, with health services being made freely available to the entire UK population. These were to be delivered in an equitable manner, available to the entire population equally on the basis of clinical need, not the ability to pay. Thus, they were 'free at the point of delivery' or use. They were to be comprehensive and cover the entire range of healthcare needs from 'cradle to grave', with high-quality care. The NHS was to be centrally funded, mainly from state taxation (with some direct charges), and staff would exercise professional autonomy.

Power and the NHS

Power differentials between the professions were soon established in 1948, when a wide range of health professionals joined the NHS as salaried employees. The medical profession achieved political representation at every influential level in the NHS and negotiated favourable terms, with GPs maintaining their independent contractor status (Ham, 2009). Hospital doctors regarded the NHS more favourably and agreed to become salaried employees, but, to ensure he gained hospital consultants' support, the then health minister Nye Bevan awarded them high salaries, merit awards and the option to combine NHS and private work. It is important to note that nurses were largely absent here and their voices went unheard (Rafferty, 1992).

ACTIVITY 34.1: LEADERSHIP

How effective is nurse leadership?

- Why were nurses' voices largely absent in the late 1940s?
- How influential are nurses as leaders in the NHS today?
- Which professional organisations exercise leadership on your behalf?

ANSWER:
ACTIVITY 34.1

CHALLENGES FACING THE UK HEALTHCARE SYSTEM

The NHS developed as a tripartite organisation, reflecting what had gone before, with a hospital system, a system of family health services, and community and public health services run by local authorities. However, problems soon emerged, such as difficulty with coordination between the three parts. This has resulted in ongoing structural reorganisations, which arguably have still not effectively addressed the problems. Undoubtedly, you will witness this in clinical practice, in the difficulties you may experience when you are involved in coordinating health and social care.

From the outset, the hospital sector was funded more generously and was considered the most powerful of the three systems. This led to claims that the NHS appeared to be a national *hospital*, not a national *health* service, and one that concentrated on sickness rather than illness prevention, at the expense of primary and community services (Klein, 2013). It was also evident that there were power differentials between professions such as nursing and medicine and within the medical profession, whereby hospital consultants were considered more powerful than GPs.

Ensuring universal standards and policy was difficult and the professional autonomy of those delivering care often guided practice instead. Inequalities in services were inherited from the previous 'patchy hospital system' in the uneven geographical distribution of beds, resources, specialist services and the distribution of healthcare professionals, despite Bevan's vision of 'as nearly as possible a uniform standard of service for all' (Klein, 2013: 35). Improving the distribution of NHS resources has proved persistently problematic, with a number of reports (Acheson, 1998; Black, 1980; Marmot, 2010) all identifying startling social class-related inequalities in health. There was great fragmentation in the delivery of some services, particularly those related to mental health and disability, children and older people, leading to the claim that these were 'Cinderella services' (Ham, 2009). The quality of care (especially for some patient groups) became an issue in the 1960s, with evidence of low standards of service provision and ill treatment of elderly patients. Evidence of the abuse and neglect of 'mentally handicapped' patients at Ely Hospital, Cardiff also emerged (Ham, 2009). Sadly, these problems and other concerns emerge periodically, and are shamefully reflected in reports relating to the Mid Staffordshire Hospital Trust and services for learning disability patients at Winterbourne View, Bristol.

Expectations of the NHS

The expectation in 1948 was that the NHS would produce a healthier population, and thus health expenditure would decrease. Today, this sounds a rather naïve view, which has never been fulfilled – in fact, demand for healthcare has constantly increased. In 1952, this led to the decision to introduce charges for prescriptions, followed by other charges, such as for eye tests and dental treatment. Thus, the NHS has had to manage the supply of care against increasing demand by a form of 'rationing' – for example, with a system of waiting lists, targets and GPs acting as 'gatekeepers' to more specialised secondary care, which helps control expenditure.

Politics and the NHS – the story from 1950 to today

The 1950s and 1960s were a time of 'consensus politics', with broad political agreement about how to run the welfare state. However, this diverged during the economic crisis of the 1970s, and the 'New Right' politics of the incoming Conservative government (1979–97) signalled a distinct ideological shift in the approach to the welfare state and the NHS. This led to the introduction of free market ideas, with privatisation of public bodies and an internal market in healthcare. This separated purchasers from providers in an attempt to introduce the concept of competition, with hospitals, for example, as semi-autonomous bodies and GPs as budget fund-holders. The assumption was that this would make services more responsive to local need and improve efficiency, with a focus on the quality of healthcare. The key legislation related to this was the National Health Service and Community Care Act 1990, which also served to highlight evidence-based healthcare, public health and primary care, as the spotlight was thrown on to what was happening in the community (Ham, 2009). This separation of purchasers and providers was retained by successive governments.

The Labour government (1997–2010) which replaced the Conservative government had a more eclectic and pragmatic approach to improving NHS performance. This involved a ten-year plan of sustained investment, increased central involvement and the development of a 'one nation NHS' (DH, 2000). The aim was to reduce variation in performance through the establishment of a variety of frameworks and organisations such as National Service Frameworks and the National Institute for Clinical Excellence (NICE). In this system, improvement in performance would be judged not just on efficiency but also on health improvement, effective delivery, fair access, and patient experience and health outcomes. Another notable shift was the replacement of the idea of the patient as a passive recipient of care, with a new philosophy of developing partnerships with patients, so they were more autonomous and in control of their own decision-making. There was also a determined political focus on quality, with the national standards set by the new frameworks and bodies to be delivered via the introduction of clinical governance. The Commission for Health Improvement, now the Care Quality Commission, would monitor this. Since 2004, healthcare trusts have evolved into foundation trusts, with increasing degrees of autonomy and accountability for the health needs of their local population. Similarly, GP fund-holding evolved into primary care groups/trusts, which purchase health services for their local population, controlling 80 per cent of the total NHS budget – a move which signalled the continuation of a primary-care-led NHS (Ham, 2009).

The Liberal Democrat/Conservative coalition government (2010–15) was elected two years after the onset of a global economic crisis, which has influenced the direction of subsequent English health and welfare policy. The key policies emanated from the 2012 Health and Social Care Act, which aimed to take account of future trends, including an ageing population and the shift in care from hospital to community. This Act was so controversial that it was temporarily paused in 2011 for a listening exercise in the NHS Future Forum. What emerged was a series of changes of considerable complexity, with the replacement of primary care trusts (PCTs) with clinical commissioning groups (CCGs), with GPs taking the lead role. Thus, clinical commissioning groups have taken responsibility for commissioning most of the NHS's services in England, supported by NHS England. A health-specific economic regulator, called 'Monitor', was created with a mandate to guard against 'anti-competitive' practices. All NHS trusts were to become foundation trusts or to be merged with more independent trusts, with many of the Department of Health's responsibilities shifted to NHS England. Patients had a greater voice via a body called 'Health Watch'. Public health had a new focus as a result of the creation of Public Health England and Health and Well-being boards, to facilitate a more integrated approach to health and social care. In the local authorities, Health and Well-being boards brought together the NHS, public health, adult social care and children's services, local Health Watch and elected representatives, to plan how to meet the needs of their local population and address local health inequalities. The National Institute for Clinical Excellence (NICE) has evolved into the National Institute for Health and Care Excellence (still NICE), with its new name identifying that its remit now extends to social care.

In terms of how this has impacted on the NHS, it appears that despite some improvement in outlook, 43 per cent of trusts expect to overspend their budgets this financial year (2017) and 50 per cent of CCGs claim that achieving this year's financial forecast is likely to depend on delaying or cancelling spending (Murray et al., 2017). NHS funding has not kept pace with the 4 per cent increase required each year, and with the year-on-year growth in demand there are increases in patients spending longer than four hours in A and E, increases in people waiting longer than 18 weeks for hospital treatment and increases in bed days lost, due to delayed transfers of care (The King's Fund, 2017). However, NHS England's Next Steps (2017) reconfirms plans to improve cancer and urgent care, primary care and mental health and this has given rise to a more optimistic perspective.

The NHS is currently undergoing massive changes but it is important to remember the essence of what the NHS is and how it began. The NHS is to provide a free health service at the point of contact which is based on need and not on the ability to pay. By having an understanding of how the NHS has grown and developed since its introduction it can give an insight into some of the current issues that are now being faced in the health service and how this is impacting on those accessing the NHS and how sustainable it really is in its current state. The NHS is under constant scrutiny and can receive a lot of negative coverage but it is often forgotten just how far the service has developed since its creation. The NHS is a 'health' service and I think it is important to understand that those working in the NHS are also responsible for keeping people well and promoting healthy living as well as treating people.

Samantha Vanes, NQ RNMH

Your placement and ongoing change

As a nursing student, you will have a range of practice placements – in hospitals, the community, primary care and other settings – and the changes identified may impact on your practice. Whilst the Health and Social Care Act 2012 only applies to England, students in the other UK countries may also directly experience how the evolution of the NHS and social care affects practice. But it will be helpful to consider if and how these types of changes foster effective communication and the coordination of care between health and social care professionals.

Telemedicine

It is not possible to fully consider all of the issues relevant to the organisation and settings of care without considering the evolving development of information and communication technology for healthcare delivery.

ACTIVITY 34.2: REFLECTION

- During your next placement, discuss with your practice educator and other members of the healthcare team if and how their role and their organisation have altered, in response to the changes in the NHS and social care.
- Reflect on your discussion, identifying the strategies which your practice educator and other members of the healthcare team use to enable them to cope with ongoing change.
- Which of these strategies could you apply to enhance your ability to function within an environment of constant change?

ANSWER:
ACTIVITY 34.2

Telemedicine has been defined as using telecommunications technology as part of medical diagnosis and patient care (Currell et al., 2010). You are likely to be familiar with this in a social context, with the use of social media, email, text, telephone and the wide variety of online forums available. Telehealth allows healthcare professionals to provide patient care from a remote location. Telehealth is a generic term, which includes tele-monitoring, which, for example, remotely captures physiological measurements such as blood pressure and sends it to the healthcare professional for review. Telehealth also includes tele-coaching which is one-to-one audio, visual and/or interactive communications to support health and social care in the community and to encourage self-care and improve management of the patient's condition. Telecare involves the use of a variety of equipment such as alarms and sensors, usually in the home, to help people live more independently by monitoring for changes and, when these are found, alerting either the person being monitored or a remote control centre. The devices used here include personal alarms, movement detectors, fall detectors and temperature-extremity sensors.

Telemedicine research is relatively youthful and thus not conclusive; although telemedicine has been found to be reliable and well tolerated, there is limited evidence of its benefits or cost-effectiveness (Currell et al., 2010). More recent studies have concluded that, although mortality is reduced (Steventon et al., 2012), telemedicine does not seem to be a cost-effective addition to standard support and treatment (Henderson et al., 2013), but telemedicine is in its infancy and this debate will continue.

ACTIVITY 34.3: REFLECTION

Reflect on a patient whose care you have been involved in providing:

• How could telemedicine be of benefit to them?

Relating to their discharge plan, consider:

• How could telehealth be of benefit?
• How could telecare be of benefit?

ANSWER:
ACTIVITY 34.3

A PATIENT'S JOURNEY THROUGH AN EXPERIENCE OF CARE

In order to consider the relevance of the organisation and settings of care for a patient, we will now meet Aaeesha and her family, following their journey through primary, secondary and tertiary care (case study 34.1).

CASE STUDY 34.1: AAEESHA

Aaeesha Hussain is a 50-year-old woman who lives with her husband, 51-year-old Aasim, and their only child, 13-year-old Munir, who is autistic. Aaeesha and Aasim emigrated from Pakistan 30 years ago and they run a small shop together. Their first language is Punjabi, but both they and Munir speak fluent English.

Aaeesha has been feeling unwell recently, with vague symptoms of lethargy, fatigue and weight loss, and more recently has felt thirsty all the time. She works in the shop until 4 pm every day and then returns home to be there for Munir when he gets back from school. Once Aaeesha is home, meeting the needs of her family takes up all her time.

Owing to his autism, Munir requires additional support to attend mainstream education; this additional support is mainly provided by Aaeesha, with regular visits from the community learning disability nurse. Every evening, Aaeesha assists Munir with his schoolwork and cooks supper for the family, then assists Munir with bathing and getting ready for bed and reads him a bedtime story before he goes to sleep. However, Aaeesha has been finding this increasingly difficult, because she is totally exhausted. Aasim is very worried and for the last six weeks he has been urging her to go to the GP.

• Why do you think Aaeesha is reluctant to visit her GP?
• If during placement with the community learning disability nurse, you were to visit the Hussains at home, how would you take a person-centred, personalised approach to the care provided for both Munir and Aaeesha?

The World Health Organization's (1946) definition of health as 'a state of complete physical, mental and social wellbeing and not merely the absence of disease or infirmity' illustrates the holistic nature of health and illness, which is not solely related to physical symptoms. However, when symptoms are insidious, as Aaeesha's are, people may tend to disregard them. So, while illness has biological aspects, it also has psychological and social aspects, with the potential to affect Aaeesha's identity as a mother and wife and alter how she views herself in terms of being in control of her life. Aaeesha, however, now feels so unwell that she allows Aasim to make an appointment with the GP.

Aaeesha is about to enter the first level of care, primary care, which is the first point of contact for healthcare and one to which you refer yourself. The GP's broad knowledge of medical conditions will contribute to Aaeesha's assessment, treatment and diagnosis, and ongoing care.

CASE STUDY 34.1: AAEESHA (CONTINUED)

When Aaeesha and Aasim arrive at Riverdale Surgery, they are feeling very anxious, but the receptionist greets them cheerfully and they are soon in the GP's room. Dr Jenny Martin listens carefully to Aaeesha and asks her lots of questions about her symptoms. She then physically examines her, tells her she wants to take some tests and sends her to see Sister Fiona Glackin, the practice nurse.

Sister Fiona is very reassuring as she asks more questions and checks Aaeesha's blood pressure and weight. Despite having lost weight recently, Aaeesha is overweight and has a BMI of 32. Sister Fiona also takes a sample of urine and a blood glucose sample, which reveals that Aaeesha's glucose levels are high. Aaeesha is unsure what this means so Sister Fiona explains that she may have type 2 diabetes and arranges for her to come back to the surgery the next morning, to have another blood test taken after fasting overnight.

- What information would you have shared with Aaeesha and Aasim to prepare them for Aaeesha potentially being diagnosed as having type 2 diabetes?

At this stage, Aaeesha's GP could also refer her to the secondary level of care in hospital, to see a specialist consultant, Dr Tara McCabe, a diabetologist and endocrinologist, who treats conditions related to diabetes and the endocrine system. However, political commitments to public health from the 1980s onwards moved the focus of this type of care from secondary to primary care, enabling the development of a range of services within primary care, which were previously only available in hospital. Thus, if Aaeesha is diagnosed with type 2 diabetes, she could be cared for exclusively by her GP in primary care, only needing to be referred to Dr McCabe at the hospital (secondary care) if she experiences significant problems.

CASE STUDY 34.1: AAEESHA (CONTINUED)

A week later, Aaeesha and Aasim return to Riverdale Surgery for the results of the blood tests and Dr Martin tells Aaeesha that the tests confirm she has type 2 diabetes, a long-term condition requiring regular self-monitoring of her blood glucose, medication, diet and exercise. Dr Martin spends a long time talking to Aaeesha and Aasim, explaining how the medication works and how Aaeesha will need to monitor her blood glucose, making sure they both understand that high blood glucose could cause damage to Aaeesha's eyesight, heart, kidneys or lower limbs.

(Continued)

Dr Martin makes an appointment for Aaeesha to see the diabetes specialist nurse and community dietician, who are attached to the surgery and part of the primary healthcare team (PHCT). At this stage, Aaeesha feels overwhelmed by the number of healthcare professionals who are now part of her life, and very concerned about the risk of complications.

Aaeesha meets the diabetes specialist nurse (DSN), Catherine O'Hare, who shows her how to use the blood glucose self-monitoring kit and how to check her blood glucose every day. DSN Catherine talks to Aaeesha about diet, medication and exercise, and introduces her to Alan Hunt, the community dietician, who discusses the dietary changes she needs to make and how these could be adapted to fit with Aaeesha's culture. Aaeesha leaves the surgery still overwhelmed and tries to follow all the advice given; however, this is difficult, because she needs to cook for the whole family and Munir refuses to eat the food she is now preparing.

When Aaeesha returns to Riverdale Surgery a few weeks later, DSN Catherine is concerned because Aaeesha is not following the recommended diet, is not losing any weight and still has high glucose levels. Aaeesha explains that food is an important part of her culture and the diet she has been given does not easily translate to include any of the foods she would normally eat. Aaeesha is also finding it difficult to exercise, because all her time is devoted to working in the family shop and then looking after her family.

- What steps could be taken to support Aaeesha to make the necessary changes required to maintain her health but still respect her cultural identity?
- Munir is being presented with significant changes to his routine at home – what support could you provide to make this transition easier?

CASE STUDY 34.1: AAEESHA [CONTINUED]

In order to develop a package of care to support Aaeesha, the PHCT meet and decide to implement a structured programme of weekly meetings with DSN Catherine, the dietician and Dr Martin. They also refer Aaeesha to Dr McCabe, at the local hospital, who has liaised closely with Dr Martin, Aaeesha's GP. Thus, Aaeesha entered the secondary care level, but continued to be mainly supported by the primary care team.

Despite this, Aaeesha's condition continued to deteriorate and, a few months later, Dr McCabe, the diabetologist, decided to commence insulin injections. With the support of DSN Catherine, Aaeesha coped with this very well. For the next few months, her glucose levels were fairly well controlled and she began to feel a little better, but this did not last. At one of her frequent visits to see Dr McCabe, Aaeesha's blood results indicated significant renal problems, so she was referred to a specialist hospital to see Dr Alex Cameron, a nephrologist. Thus, Aaeesha entered the tertiary level of care, where there are increased levels of expertise and facilities available to support her.

- Review Aaeesha's journey and identify the positive and negative aspects of her care.
- Reflect on a patient whom you were involved in caring for on a recent placement. Consider how the patient experienced their journey from primary to secondary care. How had the patient been referred to secondary care? Were there any delays in their referrals and, if so, why?

The National Service Framework (NSF) for Diabetes (DH, 2001) provided guidance for the care of patients with diabetes, to try to ensure all patients receive the best possible access to uniformly high-quality care. However, in an evaluation of this NSF, Diabetes UK (2008) found that although much good practice existed, high-quality services were not universally available across England. This had resulted in a 'postcode lottery', with variations in care, so that some people found themselves at greater risk of diabetic complications. Diabetes UK (2008) thus concluded that greater investment, prioritisation and integrated working were required to address this. In terms of improving the clinical practice of staff in the area of diabetes, local diabetes networks were set up and education and training programmes were developed. In 2011, when primary care trusts were replaced by clinical commissioning groups, there were concerns about how CCGs could adequately understand the complexity of caring for a person with diabetes. NICE (2017) guidelines emphasise the importance of continuity of care of the person with diabetes, especially if the person is using a number of different services in primary and secondary care or attending different clinics in hospital, to ensure the effective coordination and prioritisation of care. NICE (2017) guidelines require that patients are enabled to actively participate in their care and that decision-making is shared and cultural needs are fully met.

Aaeesha's experience of healthcare is not unusual. Many patients receive care in a variety of settings concurrently, and it may be difficult to tailor care to meet their individual needs in the best way possible. As with all patients, Aaeesha's case demonstrates the importance of holistic assessment and care, whilst fully understanding and taking into account the cultural and other complexities of the patient's lifestyle, to enable the healthcare professional to help the patient manage their care as effectively as possible.

CONCLUSION

This chapter has illustrated the importance of understanding the structure and organisation of the NHS and the different levels of care available.

The welfare state was established in 1948, following the recommendations in the Beveridge Report of 1942, with the purpose of providing a comprehensive range of services for UK citizens, which included health and social care.

The UK welfare state continues to evolve, in response to changing health policy, advances in technology and evidence supporting best practice. Care is currently organised within a number of settings, each offering a different level of support.

For most patients, primary care describes their first point of contact with the health system and is the level at which most patients will receive the majority of their healthcare. Secondary care is normally accessed by referral from primary care to a more specialist service, which is usually hospital-based. Tertiary care is the highest level of specialist care, again usually delivered within a hospital setting, with referral normally being from a primary or secondary care professional.

In addition to these three levels of care, a system of community care also exists throughout the UK which, through close integration of health and social care, aims to look after people in their own homes or non-institutional settings.

In an ongoing quest to deliver high-quality care, the NHS has experienced constant change since its inception in 1948. While this can bring challenges, both to those receiving and those delivering services, the organisation and settings of care in the UK provide healthcare which is universally free at the point of use, is internationally respected and where the NHS maintains very high levels of public support in the UK.

CHAPTER SUMMARY

This chapter has:

- discussed primary, secondary and tertiary levels of care
- considered the role of community care
- briefly outlined the development of the NHS
- highlighted the shift from hospital care to primary care
- identified the need for different parts of health and social care to effectively communicate and work together, in order to benefit patient care
- focused on one patient's journey, highlighting her experiences through the three levels of care
- identified a link between healthcare policy and the organisation and settings of care.

CRITICAL REFLECTION

Holistic care

This chapter has highlighted how important the provision of holistic care is to all patients in all settings of care. Read *Strengthening the Commitment: The Report of the UK Modernising Learning Disabilities Nursing Review* (DH, 2012):

ANSWER:
CRITICAL
REFLECTION

- Why are people with a learning disability still not being offered person-centred, comprehensive, integrated, well-coordinated and responsive healthcare, across all levels of primary, secondary and tertiary care?

GO FURTHER

Books

Baggott, R. (2015) *Understanding Health Policy*, 2nd edn. Bristol: Policy Press. This book comprehensively discusses health policy in the UK and internationally, party politics, the media and pressure groups.

Traynor, M. (2013) *Nursing in Context: Policy, Politics, Profession*. Houndmills: Palgrave Macmillan. This book provides a comprehensive insight into the development of nursing professionally and educationally and examines health policy related to nursing.

McCormack, B. and McCanne, T. (2010) *Person-Centred Nursing, Theory and Practice*. Oxford: Wiley-Blackwell.

SAGE journal articles

FURTHER
READING:
JOURNAL
ARTICLES

Go to https://study.sagepub.com/essentialnursing2e for free online journal articles for this chapter. If you are using the interactive ebook, simply click on the book icon in the margin to go straight to the resource.

Ellenbecker, C.H., Fawcett, J., Jones, E.J., Mahoney, D., Rowlands, B. and Waddell, A. (2017) 'A staged approach to educating nurses in health policy', *Policy, Politics and Nursing Practice*, 18(1): 44-56. Nurses have a responsibility to address health problems by participating in health policy development. This article discusses a proposal for a staged approach to educating nurses about health policy.

Lathrop, B. (2013) 'Nursing leadership in addressing the social determinants of health', *Policy, Politics and Nursing Practice*, 14(1): 41-7. This US article argues that nurses are well placed to address the social determinants of health through interdisciplinary collaboration, political involvement and community partnerships.

Other journal articles

Hope Koltveit, B.C., Gjengedal, E., Graue, M., Iversen, M.M., Thorne, S. and Kirkevoid, M. (2016) 'Telemedicine in diabetes foot care delivery: Health care professionals' experience', *BMC Health Services Research*, 16(134): 1–8. Available at: www.ncbi.nlm.nih.gov/pmc/articles/PMC4836108/pdf/12913_2016_Article_1377. pdf (accessed 16 August 2017). This study explores healthcare professionals' (mainly nurses') experiences of introducing telemedicine technology within caring for people with diabetic leg ulcers, in a variety of settings. Findings include improved wound assessment knowledge and skills and more streamlined communication between primary and secondary specialist healthcare.

Koivunen, M., Niemi, A. and Hupli, M. (2015) 'The use of electronic devices for communication with colleagues and other healthcare professionals – nursing professionals' perspectives', *Journal of Advanced Nursing*, 71(3): 620–31. This study describes nurses' experience of using electronic devices for communication with nurses and other healthcare professionals. Findings included the following: email was the favoured method and it was used for practical nursing and administrative tasks; it improved management of patient data and staff cooperation, and used working time more effectively.

Parveen, A., Watson, R. and Albutt, G. (2011) 'Are English novice nurses prepared to work in primary care settings?', *Nurse Education in Practice*, 11(5): 304–8. This study examined how prepared nurses feel for work in the primary care sector and concluded that the nursing curriculum was generally focused on acute care.

Weblinks

Go to https://study.sagepub.com/essentialnursing2e for weblinks related to this chapter. If you are using the interactive ebook, simply click on the book icon in the margin to go straight to the resource.

FURTHER READING: WEBLINKS

The following websites reflect the delivery and organisation of health within the four nations of the UK:

www.health-ni.gov.uk – Department of Health (Northern Ireland)
http://wales.gov.uk/topics/health/?lang=en – Department of Health (Wales)
www.scotland.gov.uk/Topics/Health – Department of Health (Scotland)
www.dh.gov.uk – Department of Health (England)

Access each country's health department website and identify the policies relating to health inequalities.

http://3millionlives.co.uk – this website demonstrates the UK government's focus on telemedicine and the aim that three million people in England will benefit from it over the next five years.

www.rcn.org.uk/professional-development/learning-zone – a useful RCN site which contains a range of learning resources.

www.diabetes.org.uk – the website of a leading UK diabetes charity which offers education, support, resources and research development information. It aims to influence government and healthcare professionals.

www.kingsfund.org.uk – the King's Fund is a charity which focuses on understanding how the health system in England can be improved.

www.nuffieldtrust.org.uk – the Nuffield Trust is a charity which focuses on producing independent evidence-based research and healthcare policy analysis to improve healthcare.

www.youtube.com/watch?v=Fj_9HG_TWEM – from the HSJ, the story of Mrs Andrews, who was admitted to hospital following a fall at home. It recounts her failed care pathway and illustrates why people like her need more support and care outside of hospital.

www.kingsfund.org.uk/audio-video/joined-care-sams-story – this story, from the King's Fund, demonstrates how health and social care can be successfully coordinated by a district nurse, to enable an 87-year-old widowed man, Sam, to live at home.

ACE YOUR ASSESSMENT

ONLINE
QUIZZES

Review what you have learned by visiting the book's online resources at: https://study.sagepub.com/essential nursing2e If using your interactive ebook, just click on the icon in the margin to go straight there.

- Test yourself with multiple-choice and short-answer questions.
- Revise key terms with the interactive flash cards.

REFERENCES

Acheson, D. (1998) Independent Inquiry into Inequalities in Health. Available at: www.archive. official-documents.co.uk/document/doh/ih/part1b.htm (accessed 25 July 2017).

Baggott, R. (2011) *Public Health: Policy and Politics*, 2nd edn. Houndmills: Palgrave Macmillan.

Beveridge, W. (1942) *Beveridge Report: Social Insurance and Allied Services*. London: HMSO.

Black, D. (1980) *Black Report: Inequalities in Health*. London: DHSS.

Currell, R., Urquhart, C., Wainwright, P. and Lewis, R. (2010) 'Telemedicine versus face to patient care: Effects on professional practice and health care outcomes', *Cochrane Database of Systematic Reviews*, 1: 1–34.

Department of Health (DH) (1999) A National Service Framework for Mental Health. Available at: www.gov.uk/government/publications/quality-standards-for-mental-health-services (accessed 23 July 2017).

Department of Health (DH) (2000) *The NHS Plan: A Plan for Investment, A Plan for Reform*. London: HMSO. Available at: http://pns.dgs.pt/files/2010/03/pnsuk1.pdf (accessed 12 August 2017).

Department of Health (DH) (2001) National Service Framework for Diabetes. Available at: www. gov.uk/government/uploads/system/uploads/attachment_data/file/198836/National_Service_ Framework_for_Diabetes.pdf (accessed 16 August 2017).

Department of Health (DH) (2011) *No Health without Mental Health: A Cross-Government Mental Health Outcomes Strategy for People of all Ages*. London: HMSO. Available at: www.gov.uk/government/ publications/the-mental-health-strategy-for-england (accessed 16 August 2017).

Department of Health (DH) (2012) *Strengthening the Commitment: Report of the UK Modernising Learning Disabilities Nursing Review*. London: HMSO. Available at: www.health-ni.gov.uk/publications/ strengthening-commitment-report-uk-modernising-learning-disabilities-nursing-review (accessed 16 August 2017).

Diabetes UK (2008) *The National Service Framework for Diabetes: Five Years On … Are We Halfway There?* London: Diabetes UK.

Glasby, J. (2012) *Understanding Health and Social Care*, 2nd edn. Bristol: The Policy Press and the Social Policy Association.

Ham, C. (2009) *Health Policy in Britain*, 5th edn. Houndmills: Palgrave Macmillan.

Henderson, C., Knapp, M., Fernández, J., Beecham, J., Hirani, S., Cartwright, M., et al. (2013) 'Cost effectiveness of telehealth for patients with long term conditions (Whole Systems Demonstrator telehealth questionnaire study): Nested economic evaluation in a pragmatic, cluster randomised controlled trial', *BMJ*, 346: f1035.

King's Fund, The (2017) The NHS Budget and how it has Changed. Available at: www.kingsfund.org. uk/projects/nhs-in-a-nutshell/nhs-budget (accessed 27 July 2017).

Klein, R. (2013) *The New Politics of the NHS: From Creation to Reinvention*, 7th edn. Oxford: Radcliffe Publishing.

Marmot, M. (2010) Fair Society, Healthy Lives (Marmot Review). Available at: www. instituteofhealthequity.org/resources-reports/fair-society-healthy-lives-the-marmot-review (accessed 1 July 2014).

Murray, R., Jabbal, J., Thompson, J., Baird, B. and Maguire, D. (2017) Quarterly Monitoring Report (QMR): How is the NHS performing? Available at: www.kingsfund.org.uk/publications/articles/ how-nhs-performing-june-2017 (accessed 16 August 2017).

NHS England (2016) The Five Year Forward View for Mental Health. Available at: www.england.nhs.uk/ wp-content/uploads/2016/02/Mental-Health-Taskforce-FYFV-final.pdf (accessed 12 August 2017).

NHS England (2017) Next Steps on the NHS Five Year Forward View. Available at: www.england.nhs. uk/publication/next-steps-on-the-nhs-five-year-forward-view (accessed 16 August 2017).

National Institute for Health and Care Excellence (NICE) (2011) *Common Mental Health Problems: Identification and Pathways to Care*. London: NICE. Available at: www.nice.org.uk/guidance/cg123 (accessed 16 August 2017).

National Institute for Health and Care Excellence (NICE) (2017) *Diabetes*. London: NICE. Available at: www.nice.org.uk/guidance/conditions-and-diseases/diabetes-and-other-endocrinal--nutritional-and-metabolic-conditions/diabetes (accessed 12 August 2017).

Rafferty, A.M. (1992) 'Nursing policy and the nationalization of nursing: The representation of "crisis" and the "crisis" of representation', in J. Robinson, A. Gray and R. Elkan (eds), *Policy Issues in Nursing*. Milton Keynes: Open University Press. pp. 68–83.

Richards, C., Rafferty, L. and Gibb, A. (2013) 'The value of mental health nurses working in primary care mental health teams', *Mental Health Practice*, 16(10): 19–23.

Steventon, A., Bardsley, M., Billings, J., Dixon, J., Doll, H., Hirani, S., et al. (2012) 'Effect of telehealth on use of secondary care and mortality: Findings from the Whole System Demonstrator cluster randomised trial', *BMJ*, 344: e3874.

World Health Organization (WHO) (1946) Constitution of the World Health Organization. Available at: www.who.int/governance/eb/who_constitution_en.pdf (accessed 16 August 2017).

World Health Organization (WHO) (1978) Primary Health Care. Available at: www.who.int/topics/ primary_health_care/en/ (accessed 20 July 2017).

INTRODUCTION TO INTERPROFESSIONAL WORKING

ADELE ATKINSON

THIS CHAPTER COVERS

- Understanding the importance of inter-professional and multi-professional working
- Multi-disciplinary collaboration

- Working as an individual and working in partnership with others
- Benefits and challenges of interprofessional working

"

My name is Joe. I am 16 and live in a village in Sussex. When I was 6, I got food poisoning and became very unwell with problems with my kidneys (acute renal failure). I had to go to a specialist hospital in London and was taken there by a paramedic in an ambulance.

When I was there I was in intensive care. This was very scary. I had tubes put into my stomach to give me food as I couldn't eat. A dietician came and talked to me and my mum about what was happening. After two weeks I went onto the children's ward, which was nicer. The nurses and play specialist used to play games with me. I also met the hospital teacher.

Over the next six years my kidneys were stopping working again and I needed a new kidney (a transplant). My dad said he would give me one of his kidneys. I went back to the children's ward at the hospital and my dad went onto another ward. I think there must have been a lot of coordination between the doctors and nurses in the different wards. I had surgery and was given one of my dad's kidneys. I still have to go to the hospital for check-ups every year but am quite well now.

I am so thankful to all the nurses, specialist nurses, dieticians, doctors, social worker, teacher and everyone else involved in making me better.

Joe, patient

"

"

While at university, I had been participating in an interprofessional case-based learning session with physiotherapists, radiographers, medical students and midwives. The case involved a patient with arthritis. It really helped me not only to understand my own profession's role but those of other professionals, what the differences were and how working together helped patient care. When I was on placement, I nursed a patient with severe arthritis and I had the confidence to suggest to my practice educator that it might be useful to discuss key issues regarding the patient with colleagues from other professions. I think this really helped the patient receive appropriate care quickly.

Hilary, LD nursing student

"

Visit https://study.sagepub.com/essentialnursing2e to access a wealth of online resources for this chapter – watch out for the margin icons throughout the chapter. If you are using the interactive eBook, simply click on the margin icon to go straight to the resource.

INTRODUCTION

As you can see from both Joe and Hilary's views above, it takes more than one member of the multi-disciplinary team to look after patients. So it makes sense for the multi-disciplinary team to work together interprofessionally, and this is how you will work from the very start of your nursing programme. You may have already experienced interprofessional 'days' or activities. In fact, the NMC expects pre-registration nursing programmes to prepare students so that they play an active and equal role in the multidisciplinary team, collaborating and communicating effectively with a range of colleagues.

Interprofessional education occurs when two or more healthcare professions learn with, from and about each other to improve collaboration and the quality of care.

This chapter explores the reasons behind interprofessional working and explains some of the terminology used. It also considers working in partnership with others and some of the issues this raises, such as professional role and identity, power and status, professional knowledge and skills and team structure.

UNDERSTANDING THE IMPORTANCE OF INTERPROFESSIONAL AND MULTI-PROFESSIONAL WORKING

There have been many reports on the failings of the health service (see below), which indicates that a more collaborative working culture may prevent similar tragedies from occurring. British society is ageing, as people live longer than ever before. This, and the increase in the number of people with long-term health conditions, mean that there is not just one 'specialist' who will treat and care for a patient.

MULTI-DISCIPLINARY COLLABORATION

Victoria Climbié

In 2000, an 8-year-old girl, Victoria Climbié, was tortured and murdered by her guardians. Her death led to a public inquiry headed by Lord Laming. It discovered numerous instances where Victoria Climbié could have been saved and, as a result, numerous changes were made to child protection laws. The recommendations made it clear that if support is to be effective for children and families it cannot be achieved by just one agency acting alone. Effective support depends upon a number of agencies working well together and is a multi-disciplinary task (DH and Home Office, 2003).

The Francis Report

In 2010, following complaints, a public enquiry headed by Robert Francis was set up to look at the care provided to patients at Mid Staffordshire NHS Foundation Trust.

The Laming and Francis reports, coupled with changing healthcare needs, mean it is time to re-look at how professionals work within the NHS. What is needed is effective team working, where collaborative working is central to the practice of all healthcare professionals.

Terminology

Before further discussion, it is necessary to consider the terms interprofessional, multi-professional and multi-disciplinary team. The prefix 'multi' refers to the involvement of individuals from different professions, whereas 'inter' refers to the collaboration between professions.

Rather than, for example, nurses being concerned only with their own discipline (uni-professional) or recognising that other professionals have a role to play (multi-professional), an interprofessional approach means working across professional boundaries for the benefit of the patient. Collaborative teamwork is at the heart of interprofessional working.

In order to start to think about working interprofessionally, it is helpful to consider what it is to be part of a profession and how your own code of professional conduct compares with that of others (Activity 35.1).

ACTIVITY 35.1: REFLECTION

- Reflect on what you understand by the term 'a profession'.
- Do an online search for the documents detailed in Table 35.1 and compare the NMC Code with one of the other professional codes.
- Can you identify similarities and differences between the nursing code and those for other professions?
- What do they say about interprofessional learning or working?
- How does a code help you to understand another profession?

Table 35.1 Codes

WEBLINKS:
TABLE 35.1

Professional role	Search for:
Nurse	NMC (2015): *The Code: Professional Standards of Practice and Behaviour for Nurses and Midwives*
Dietician	HCPC (2013a): *Standards of Proficiency: Dieticians*
Doctor	General Medical Council (2013): Good Medical Practice
Paramedic	HCPC (2014a): *Standards of Proficiency: Paramedics*
Physiotherapist	HCPC (2013b): *Standards of Proficiency: Physiotherapists* Chartered Society of Physiotherapy (2011): Code of Professional Values and Behaviour
Social worker	British Association of Social Workers (2012): The Code of Ethics for Social Work HCPC (2017): *Standards of Proficiency - Social Workers in England*
Occupational therapist	HCPC (2013c): *Standards of Proficiency - Occupational Therapists* College of Occupational Therapists (2015): *Code of Ethics and Professional Conduct*
Radiographer	HCPC (2013d): Standards of Proficiency - Radiographers Society of Radiographers (2013): *Code of Professional Conduct*
Pharmacist	General Pharmaceutical Council (2012): Standards of Conduct, Ethics and Performance
Psychologist (practitioner)	HCPC (2015): *Standards of Proficiency - Practitioner Psychologists*
Speech and language therapist	HCPC (2014b): *Standards of Proficiency - Speech and Language Therapists*

WORKING AS AN INDIVIDUAL AND WORKING IN PARTNERSHIP WITH OTHERS

Working in partnership, or collaborative working, means engaging with other professionals. This means that a group of individuals work together as a team to identify problems and goals, assuming joint responsibility for dealing with these, but retaining their own professional role in doing so. This can sometimes be difficult, because the individuals are both part of a team and they belong to different professions, which can cause tension (Kvarnstrom, 2008). But, if it is done effectively, interprofessional working through collaboration can produce many benefits – for example, better communication between professions and an improved understanding of each other's roles.

Individuals tend to work within their professional boundaries because each profession contributes different knowledge, competencies and experience, and if the boundaries become blurred – if team members have not been clear about what they will each contribute – there may be confusion, a lack of preparedness and duplication (Rushmer, 2005). This is similar to sharing a house and finding that no one buys the washing-up liquid because you all think someone else is going to buy it!

If everyone only focuses on their own professional agenda, they will stop interacting with other professions. Good communication within the team is key, as it can lead to an understanding of how each other's work contributes to overall patient care, can help when negotiating with other professionals and can also lead to building a trusting and respectful relationship (San Martín-Rodríguez et al., 2005).

Healthcare professionals who work effectively in an interprofessional way appear to have increased job satisfaction and improved communication skills (Maslin-Prothero and Bennion, 2010). They are also quicker to refer patient issues to other professionals within the team (Brown et al., 2003), ensuring that problems can be dealt with faster.

It is important for nurses to keep in mind the wide range of other professions that they will have to work with. These include other clinicians, such as doctors, midwives, paramedics and physiotherapists, who will share many of the same experiences as nurses in working to provide healthcare, and may have similarities of professional culture. But nurses also need to be able to work with other, less similar occupational groups including social workers and the police. This can bring different challenges. For example, consider working with the police. The police are from a separate non-NHS organisation with different priorities, and a different culture, and therefore their values may be very different to those of a profession working within the NHS.

I have really enjoyed working with other professions as it enables you to understand how closely they all work together, and how everyone's input enables professionals to deliver a complete package of care. It also highlights the fact that as a nurse is the one that can often have the most interaction with a patient therefore you also have the knowledge and understanding of the patient/family situation that need to be passed on to enable another professional to carry out their role. For example, a young girl that had anorexia was really upset that something had been put on her diet regime that she really did not like and did not understand why it had been put on, and she disclosed this information to me and my practice educator as we had a good therapeutic relationship. We were able to contact the dietician and explain what had happened and discussed how it could be resolved. The dietician then reviewed the diet and visited this young girl, aware that she was upset, and did her best to resolve it and explain the reasons why it had been done and changed it to something she liked, which made her much happier. I realise that the nurses' role in interprofessional working is important not only for the patient but also for other professionals.

Siân Hunter, child nursing student

Underlying all this, however, is the issue of accountability. Nurses and other groups are accountable for their actions within the context of their unique professional codes, and it is possible that these may not coincide. In this instance, compliance with the professional code takes priority over collaboration.

BENEFITS AND CHALLENGES OF INTERPROFESSIONAL WORKING

Interprofessional working comes with its own set of unique opportunities, such as effective knowledge sharing, which ensure the best outcomes for patients. When working interprofessionally, you may also encounter some obstacles, such as dealing with the hierarchical nature of the health profession or working within a team consisting of members across a large geographic area. The next section introduces how to make the most of the opportunities offered by interprofessional working while overcoming some of the challenges.

Power and status

Each profession has its own views on what collaborative team working is. For example, doctors may see collaborative working as meaning that other professionals should report the impact of medical decisions. Nurses may see it as doctors having an appreciation of their role as well as discussing medical issues (Collin et al., 2011). Power, status and gender have also been shown to be problems in interprofessional working, which links to the hierarchical nature of the health professions (Arslanian-Engoren, 1995), to the extent that sometimes interprofessional collaboration only happens if doctors lead this process. Although the issue of doctors' status may be difficult to overcome, the advent, in the UK, of nursing as an all-graduate profession means that nurses will have an increased knowledge base, and with it the authority and professional standing to challenge the views of their medical colleagues. There is evidence that this is happening within learning disability nursing, where nurses are seen more as a facilitator and regularly lead changes made to care (McCray, 2003).

Interprofessional working should also include the patient, who has the least power in this situation. The use of the internet though means that patients may have an increasing amount of knowledge about their condition and, at times, more than the nurses or doctors caring for them. This should be acknowledged in informed consent and the use of advanced directives. In both instances, it is important to use language that the patient will understand rather than relying on the professional terminology appropriate to communicating with colleagues.

San Martín-Rodríguez et al. (2005) found that it was important to create a collegiate atmosphere wherein all professionals were seen as partners. Ethical codes can sometimes hinder collaborative team working. For example, nurses may come into conflict with other members of the team when they are acting as a patient advocate. One way of preventing this from happening is to discuss and agree patient care within the team, for example through interprofessional case conferences.

Apply your knowledge of caring for a patient within a team by reading Kevin's case study, at https://study.sagepub.com/essentialnursing2e.

CASE STUDY:
KEVIN

Professional knowledge and skills

The differing educational backgrounds of health professions and the socialisation processes which lead to their identity have been identified as a barrier to effective interprofessional working.

Management structures within the NHS may also be seen as a hindrance (Lewy, 2010) and it has been argued that these hierarchical structures need to be flattened and those within the hierarchy made more equal for good interprofessional collaboration to be achieved. It is certainly true that, in order to work collaboratively, professionals need to know how other professions work, with this knowledge fostering mutual respect. However, this can be especially difficult when staff may not work on the same site or to the same shift pattern.

Team structure and processes

Some features tend to make team working less effective. Geographical separation leads to a lack of integration and to problems with communication. This is the case, for example, in a community setting or when paramedics hand over patients to nurses or doctors at A&E. These problems may be exacerbated where the two professional groups are part of different organisations which may have entirely different priorities and goals. For example, paramedics may be required by their managers to meet time targets getting to patients, which may run counter to A&E staff requirements to do a thorough and detailed handover. Larger teams are less effective at interprofessional work than smaller ones. However, the issue related to team size is balanced by research showing that the more professions are represented within a team, the more innovative it can be (Xyrichis and Lowton, 2008).

On a practical level, it is important that a team has somewhere to meet regularly and that time is set aside for this and other means of communication. This can be as simple as having a coffee room where staff can 'debrief' or catch up. Such meetings can provide a time for the team to explore reflective practice. Reflective practice fosters interprofessional collaboration and may lead to interprofessional policies being made and implemented. Interprofessional away-days and team-building exercises also foster collegiate working.

CASE STUDY:
MRS BIGGS

Within the hospital setting, teams often develop around the needs of individual patients, but this means that professionals are typically members of a number of such ad hoc teams, creating a great deal of complexity. The additional case study at https://study.sagepub.com/essentialnursing2e identifies how many different healthcare professionals can be involved in the elective care of just one patient during and after an uncomplicated surgical procedure.

Longer-term teams can evolve around teams of doctors treating patients with cardiac, surgical or haematological conditions, for example. Although these can provide a more stable model, there is also a danger of a reliance on traditional professional boundaries, and there needs to be mutual respect for all members of the professional team.

The increased use of IT may help to reduce some of these problems. Social media can help to create a sense of team identity, but will not be appropriate if any confidential information is to be shared. This may be addressed by the encryption offered in, for example, WhatsApp. In other instances, social media could be used for educational discussion. However, it would be appropriate to ensure that any use of social media was in line with trust policies and that advice was sought from the organisation's IT team.

Reeves et al. (2007) identified that both formal and informal communication strategies take place within interprofessional teams. Informally, there were unplanned discussions so that when one professional needed information, they would ask another for help. Formally, there were weekly multidisciplinary team meetings, although individual attendance was not consistent due to shifts and workload pressures, leading to fragmentation.

FURTHER
READING:
QUALITATIVE
STUDY

WHAT'S THE EVIDENCE?

Miller, K., Reeves, S., Zwarenstein, M., Beales, J.D., Kenaszchuk, C. and Conn, L.G. (2008) 'Nursing emotion work and interprofessional collaboration in general internal medicine wards: A qualitative study', *Journal of Advanced Nursing*, 64(4): 332-43.

This study by Miller et al. (2008) explored whether the emotional aspect of nursing facilitates or impedes interprofessional collaboration.

The study concluded that the emotional aspect of nursing causes problems for interprofessional collaboration. Although it was acknowledged that nurses' continuous care of patients gave them a unique position, this was suppressed or ignored during formal meetings. This resulted in nurses not being involved in interprofessional collaboration during formal meetings.

- Reflect on your experiences of interprofessional working. Do they support the experiences described in this study?
- Now read the article and consider how you can use the findings to improve your nursing practice.

Clear leadership within teams is also necessary to help teams work effectively. It is often suggested that in most interprofessional teams, the doctor assumes leadership, which can result in nurses not being confident enough to voice their views. This presents a problem if nurses are to act as patients' advocates. However, if nurses become more assertive, tension can be created – with, for example, GPs feeling that their power is undermined by the expanding role of nurses (Elston and Holloway, 2001).

Interprofessional learning

One way of overcoming these potential barriers to effective interprofessional working can be by introducing it into pre-registration education, in which students start to learn together and understand each other's professional beliefs and values. If students are only immersed within their own profession throughout pre-registration education, then the concepts of interprofessional practice will not be embodied. Learning with other healthcare professionals should allow for better interprofessional working once qualified.

Your nursing programme may involve interprofessional learning opportunities within the classroom, but actually most of your interprofessional learning will happen in practice.

Good communication skills are essential to interprofessional working and it may be helpful if, as well as learning to communicate with patients, you consider how to communicate with other professions. This will help improve your collaborative skills.

Interprofessional learning in placements

From your perspective, learning experiences will initially be guided by your practice educator when you are in placement. Your time in placement may be the time to explore how you become socialised into the nursing profession, but, more importantly, it also can form the basis of how you interact with other professionals and start to learn more about those professions. Exploring the nurse's role within both the professional team and the wider interprofessional team can also start in the classroom. As you progress, you can start to actively influence collaboration with other professions by suggesting this to your practice educator.

> Working and learning in a multi-disciplinary team, both in a clinical and community setting has given me the opportunity to learn the roles of others and to discover what is expected of me as a nurse. I have learnt how to put the theory into practice and to understand the importance of sharing my knowledge and skills and learning as much as I can from other professionals. Each professional has their own unique role and it is essential to appreciate this and to work together to give the patient the best care we can.
>
> Julie Davis, LD nursing student

ACTIVITY 35.2: REFLECTION

- Reflect on the experiences you have had so far when caring for patients as part of an interprofessional team in placement.
- What opportunities for interprofessional learning have you had?
- Can you identify any of the personal challenges you may face when working as part of an interprofessional team?

CONCLUSION

The concept of interprofessional working is clearly embedded in UK health policy and educational practice. The evidence suggests that there are many benefits to this approach, including an improved understanding of other professions' roles, better working relationships and improved delivery of care. However, there are barriers still to be overcome, such as the question of who should lead the interprofessional team, how to acknowledge the different input that each profession provides while continuing to work collaboratively, and team cohesiveness. It is widely agreed, however, that learning together at undergraduate, pre-registration level is crucial to improving the effectiveness of future interprofessional working.

CHAPTER SUMMARY

- Despite various reports stating that interprofessional communication/collaboration would prevent tragedies from occurring, this has not yet been fully achieved.
- All professions' standards make mention of interprofessional collaboration in some form.
- Interprofessional working is complex and multi-faceted.
- Understanding your own professional role as well as those of others is crucial to interprofessional collaboration.
- Interprofessional dynamics mean that leadership of the team may create problems.

- Team-building is crucial and time must be set aside for this.
- Working interprofessionally must begin within undergraduate pre-registration programmes.

CRITICAL REFLECTION

Holistic care

This chapter has highlighted the importance of working in teams interprofessionally in order to provide holistic care for your patient:

- Reflect on the patient care you have recently been involved in and make a list of the different professionals involved in their care and what their roles were.
- Would there be any difference if you were caring for a patient from another field, or within a different healthcare setting?
- Make a note of your thoughts and refer back to these the next time you care for a patient, and then reflect on and write about your experience.

GO FURTHER

Books

Goodman, B. and Clemow, R. (2010) *Nursing and Collaborative Practice: A Guide to Interprofessional Learning and Working*, 2nd edn. Exeter: Learning Matters. A clear exploration of how different professionals can work effectively together.

Thomas, J., Pollard, K. and Sellman, D. (2014) *Interprofessional Working in Health and Social Care: Professional Perspectives*, 2nd edn. Basingstoke: Palgrave Macmillan. A very useful text carefully outlining differing professional perspectives.

SAGE journal articles

Go to https://study.sagepub.com/essentialnursing2e for free online journal articles for this chapter. If you are using the interactive ebook, simply click on the book icon in the margin to go straight to the resource.

FURTHER
READING:
JOURNAL
ARTICLES

Milton, C. (2012) 'Ethical implications and interprofessional education', *Nursing Science Quarterly*, 25(4): 313–15. An interesting article questioning the potential ethical implications for nursing practice.

Nordentoft, H. (2008) 'Changes in emotion work at interdisciplinary conferences following clinical supervision in a palliative outpatient ward', *Qualitative Health Research*, 18(7): 913–27. This article considers the positive impact of clinical supervision on nursing 'emotion work'.

Other journal articles

Cooper, H. and Spencer-Dawe, D. (2006) 'Involving service users in interprofessional education: Narrowing the gap between theory and practice', *Journal of Interprofessional Care*, 20(6): 603–17. A study which investigates whether interprofessional education is more effective when it is co-facilitated by service users.

Hurlock-Chorostecki, C., Van Soeren, M., MacMillan, K., Sidani, S., Donald, F. and Reeves, S. (2016) 'A qualitative study of nurse practitioner promotion of interprofessional care across institutional settings: Perspectives from different healthcare professionals', *International Journal of Nursing Sciences*, 3: 2–10. This study explores nurse strategies used to improve interprofessional working. This may help students to understand which attributes to aspire to once qualified.

Makic, M. and Wald, H. (2017) 'Achieving improved patient outcomes through interprofessional teams', *Journal of interprofessional Education & Practice*, 8: 91–94. This article explores ways of overcoming barriers in interprofessional team working.

Pfaff, K., Baxter, P., Jack, S. and Ploeg, J. (2014) 'Exploring new graduate nurse confidence in interprofessional collaboration: A mixed methods study', *International Journal of Nursing Studies*, 51: 1142–1152. Confidence is needed for interprofessional collaboration. This study explores ways and interventions that enhance & develop confidence in newly qualified nurses. This may help students understand some of the strategies they see in practice.

Weblinks

FURTHER
READING:
WEBLINKS

www.caipe.org.uk – this UK-based website for the Centre for the Advancement of Interprofessional Education (CAIPE) provides access to a variety of resources to help with the promotion of interprofessional learning. It also has areas for both students and qualified staff membership and access.

www.who.int/hrh/resources/framework_action/en – the Framework for Action on Interprofessional Education and Collaborative Practice highlights the current status of interprofessional collaboration around the world and identifies the mechanisms that shape successful collaborative teamwork.

https://healthsciences.creighton.edu/interprofessional-education/center-interprofessional-practice-education-research-ciper/ipe-tools – links to a number of interprofessional resources such as videos, case studies and an algorithm to help with team reasoning.

www.faculty.londondeanery.ac.uk/e-learning/interprofessional-education – the London Deanery website offers a range of open access modules. One module focuses on interprofessional learning in the clinical context, considering the policies and contexts of interprofessional practice as well as how one can design and implement interprofessional learning activities aimed at promoting interprofessional teamwork.

www.scie.org.uk/publications/elearning/ipiac – the interprofessional and interagency collaboration (IPIAC) section of the Social Care Institute for Excellence's website contains freely available e-learning resources such as audio, video and interactive activities to assist in exploring the nature of interprofessional and interagency collaboration and improving collaborative practice.

Go to https://study.sagepub.com/essentialnursing2e for weblinks related to this chapter. If you are using the interactive ebook, simply click on the book icon in the margin to go straight to the resource.

Video links

VIDEO
LINKS

Have a break from the text and go to https://study.sagepub.com/essentialnursing2e for useful videos related to this chapter. If you are using the interactive ebook, simply click on the lightbulb icon in the margin to go straight to the resource.

ACE YOUR ASSESSMENT

ONLINE
QUIZZES

Review what you have learned by visiting the book's online resources at: https://study.sagepub.com/essential nursing2e If using your interactive ebook, just click on the icon in the margin to go straight there.

- Test yourself with multiple-choice and short-answer questions.
- Revise key terms with the interactive flash cards.

REFERENCES

Arslanian-Engoren, C. (1995) 'Lived experiences of CNSs who collaborate with physicians: A phenomenological study', *Clinical Nurse Specialist*, 9: 68–74.

British Association of Social Workers (2012) The Code of Ethics for Social Work: Statement of Principles. Available at: http://cdn.basw.co.uk/upload/basw_112315-7.pdf (accessed 10 March 2015).

Brown, L., Tucker, C. and Domokos, T. (2003) 'Evaluating the impact of integrated health and social care teams on older people living in the community', *Health & Social Care in the Community*, 11(2): 85–94.

Chartered Society of Physiotherapy (2011) Code of Professional Values and Behaviour. Available at: www.cot.co.uk/sites/default/files/publications/public/Code-of-Ethics2010.pdf (accessed 10 March 2015).

College of Occupational Therapists (CoT) (2015) *Code of Ethics and Professional Conduct*. London CoT. Available at: www.cot.co.uk/sites/default/files/publications/public/CODE-OF-ETHICS-2015.pdf (accessed 10 April 2017).

Collin, K., Valleala, U., Herranen, S., Viinkaninen, S. and Paloniemi, S. (2011) 'Interprofessional collaboration during ward rounds in an emergency and infection department'. Paper presented at the Critical Perspectives on Professional Learning Conference. Available at: www.leeds.ac.uk/medicine/meu/events/pll11-docs/Collin.pdf (accessed 18 February 2015).

Department of Health and Home Office (2003) *The Victoria Climbie Inquiry: Report of an Inquiry by Lord Laming*. London: The Stationery Office.

Elston, S. and Holloway, I. (2001) 'The impact of recent primary care reforms in the UK on interprofessional working in primary care centres', *Journal of Interprofessional Care*, 15(1): 19–27.

Francis, R. (2010) *Independent Inquiry into Care Provided by Mid Staffordshire NHS Foundation Trust*. January 2005–March 2009, Volume I. London: The Stationery Office.

General Medical Council (GMC) (2013) Good Medical Practice. Available at: www.gmc-uk.org/guidance/good_medical_practice.asp (accessed 10 March 2015).

General Pharmaceutical Council (GPC) (2012) Standards of Conduct, Ethics and Performance. Available at: www.pharmacyregulation.org/sites/default/files/standards_of_conduct_ethics_and_performance_july_2014.pdf (accessed 10 March 2015).

Health and Care Professions Council (HCPC) (2013a) *Standards of Proficiency: Dietitians*. London: HCPC. Available at: www.hpc-uk.org/assets/documents/1000050CStandards_of_Proficiency_Dietitians.pdf (accessed 10 April 2017).

Health and Care Professions Council (2013b) *Standards of Proficiency: Physiotherapists*. London: HCPC. Available at: www.hcpc-uk.org/assets/documents/10000DBCStandards_of_Proficiency_Physiotherapists.pdf (accessed 10 April 2017).

Health and Care Professions Council (2013c) *Standards of Proficiency: Occupational Therapists*. London: HCPC. Available at: www.hpc-uk.org/assets/documents/10000512Standards_of_Proficiency_Occupational_Therapists.pdf (accessed 10 April 2017).

Health and Care Professions Council (2013d) *Standards of Proficiency: Radiographers*. London: HCPC. Available at: www.hpc-uk.org/assets/documents/10000DBDStandards_of_Proficiency_Radiographers.pdf (accessed 10 April 2017).

Health and Care Professions Council (2014a) *Standards of Proficiency: Paramedics*. London: HCPC. Available at: www.hpc-uk.org/assets/documents/1000051CStandards_of_Proficiency_Paramedics.pdf (accessed 10 April 2017).

Health and Care Professions Council (2014b) *Standards of Proficiency: Speech and Language Therapists*. London: HCPC. Available at: www.hpc-uk.org/assets/documents/10000529Standards_of_Proficiency_SLTs.pdf (accessed 10 April 2017).

Health and Care Professions Council (2015) *Standards of Proficiency: Practitioner Psychologists*. London: HCPC. Available at: www.hpc-uk.org/assets/documents/10002963sop_practitioner_psychologists.pdf (accessed 10 April 2017).

Health and Care Professions Council (2017) *Standards of Proficiency: Social Workers in England*. London: HCPC. Available at: www.hpc-uk.org/assets/documents/10003b08standardsofproficiency-socialworkersinengland.pdf (accessed 10 April 2017).

Kvarnstrom, S. (2008) 'Difficulties in collaboration: A critical incident study of interprofessional healthcare teamwork', *Journal of Interprofessional Care*, 22(2): 191–203.

Lewy, L. (2010) 'The complexities of interprofessional learning/working: Has the agenda lost its way?' *Health Education Journal*, 69(1): 4–12.

McCray, J. (2003) 'Interprofessional practice and learning disability nursing', *British Journal of Nursing*, 12(22): 1335–44.

Maslin-Prothero, S. and Bennion, A. (2010) 'Integrated team working: A literature review', *International Journal of Integrated Care*, 10: e043. Available at: www.ncbi.nlm.nih.gov/pmc/articles/PMC2883237 (accessed 18 February 2015).

Miller, K., Reeves, S., Zwarenstein, M., Beales, J.D., Kenaszchuk, C. and Conn, L.G. (2008) 'Nursing emotion work and interprofessional collaboration in general internal medicine wards: A qualitative study', *Journal of Advanced Nursing*, 64(4): 332–43.

Nursing and Midwifery Council (NMC) (2015) *The Code: Professional Standards of Practice and Behaviour for Nurses and Midwives*. London: NMC.

Reeves, S., Russell, A., Zwarenstein, M., Kenaszchuk, C., Conn, L.G., Doran, D., et al. (2007) 'Structuring communication relationships for interprofessional teamwork (SCRIPT): A Canadian initiative aimed at improving patient-centred care', *Journal of Interprofessional Care*, 21(1): 111–14.

Rushmer, R. (2005) 'Blurred boundaries damage interprofessional working', *Nurse Researcher*, 12(3): 74–84.

San Martín-Rodríguez, L., Beaulieu, M., D'Amour, D. and Ferrada-Videla, M. (2005) 'The determinants of successful collaboration: A review of theoretical and empirical studies', *Journal of Interprofessional Care*, 19(S1): 132–47.

Society of Radiographers (2013) Code of Professional Conduct. Available at: www.sor.org/learning/document-library/code-professional-conduct (accessed 10 March 2015).

Xyrichis, A. and Lowton, K. (2008) 'What fosters or prevents interprofessional teamworking in primary and community care?' *International Journal of Nursing Studies*, 45: 140–53.

INTRODUCTION TO THE PSYCHOLOGICAL CONTEXT OF NURSING

JANET RAMJEET

--- **THIS CHAPTER COVERS** ---

- Why psychology is applicable to nursing
- Understanding psychology and psychological approaches

- Communication
- The psychological impact of attitude

> " I'm 17 and diabetic. When they told me I had diabetes last year I thought there was no way I could inject myself with insulin and that I'd have to give up playing football. So I was really angry when I saw Helen, the diabetes practice nurse, but she was OK – in fact, she was great! She listened to me and taught me about injections and professional footballers with diabetes. I can talk to my mum but with Helen, well, I can tell her how I am really feeling.
>
> Jason, patient "

> " When I was told that psychology was part of the curriculum I thought it was just for mental health nurses – I didn't think it was relevant to me. Then I saw the way that qualified nurses motivated patients who were physically ill and I realised it was a hugely important part of my nursing too.
>
> Lara, adult health nursing student "

Visit https://study.sagepub.com/essentialnursing2e to access a wealth of online resources for this chapter – watch out for the margin icons throughout the chapter. If you are using the interactive eBook, simply click on the margin icon to go straight to the resource.

INTRODUCTION

Do you think it is straightforward to help a young person manage their diabetes? Is it simply about showing them how to inject insulin and giving dietary advice, or is there more to nursing interventions than that? Recognising that Jason may be feeling angry about his diagnosis and managing this is an integral part of his care. Psychological knowledge is required to underpin nursing skills and this chapter will provide the basis for this, as well as emphasising the importance of psychological care in all fields of nursing.

WHY PSYCHOLOGY IS APPLICABLE TO NURSING

Reasons why psychology is not just applicable to nursing but integral to all of the care that a nurse provides are clearly demonstrated in case study 36.1.

CASE STUDY 36.1: SUZIE [HOSPITAL]

Suzie is a specialist stoma nurse. When she gives information to new patients, she tailors the information she gives while observing and assessing the patient's understanding, level of engagement and enthusiasm, and disengagement or distress, as she shows the patient how to attach the bag to their skin around the stoma. A knowledge of psychology helps Suzie to recognise, understand and manage the behaviours being demonstrated by the patient. Suzie will match what she is saying with the use of specific verbal and non-verbal contact to maximise the patient's **receptivity**.

Reflect on the case of Suzie and any experiences you may have had when working with a nurse who demonstrated similar skills:

- Do you think that observing, interpreting and understanding all of the skills (the practical and the psychological ones) being demonstrated by a nurse is made more difficult because they can be very subtle?
- Is it easier to learn a practical skill, such as taking a temperature, than it is to build a **rapport** with a patient?

ACTIVITY 36.1: CRITICAL THINKING

While reading the next section in the chapter, think about how the ideas, theories and examples fit in with your role as a nurse. Critically consider why you feel a theory or a number of theories are most relevant to your practice.

UNDERSTANDING PSYCHOLOGY AND PSYCHOLOGICAL APPROACHES

Psychologists study the individual (self-awareness, coping strategies), two-person relationships (dyads) and small groups, including the family. Psychology provides both explanations and treatment for psychological problems and so involves much more than the application of common sense. Health psychology gives explanations for psychological health and its maintenance.

Psychology has developed over the centuries from the clinical experience and research of a large number of theorists who examined the reasons for behaviour from very different and often competing perspectives. Psychologists have used various types of research methods to develop their theories, including case studies, observation of behaviour and laboratory experiments.

Psychology can be defined simply by five main approaches:

- psychoanalytical
- behaviourist
- humanist
- cognitive (and cognitive developmental)
- biological.

Each of these will be considered in further detail.

I feel that psychology is relevant to nursing because every nurse needs to have knowledge about how certain circumstances can affect people. This helps them care for their patients better.

Hannah Boyd, adult nursing student

Psychology is integral to nursing. From being able to read people (staff, patients and members of the public) and situations, to reading the mood of your patient as depression can impede recovery, and lastly being self-resilient.

Laura Grimley, adult nursing student

Psychology is important as it enables us to understand how our patients feel, why they may behave the way they do and it helps us to understand their attitudes. This enables us to support them to deal with their illnesses, conditions or problems in an understanding, effective way. Some psychological problems lead to physical illnesses, therefore it is important to have a sound knowledge of psychological theories.

Julie Davis, LD nursing student

Psychoanalytical approach

This approach began with the work of Sigmund Freud (1856–1939) and others, including Carl Jung (1875–1961). Essentially, it identifies the unconscious part of the mind, how it is partly controlled by the individual and how, for example, early traumatic childhood experiences are repressed and then revealed in psychological problems in adulthood. This approach was developed from the clinical experience of psychologists and is used today in therapies such as cognitive analytic therapy and group therapy for people with psychological problems.

Behaviourist approach

The behaviourist or behavioural approach, as a contrast to the psychoanalytical, provides explanations for specific behaviours by studying how animals learn and then generalising this to human behaviour. Ivan Pavlov (1849–1936), a Russian physiologist, and B.F. Skinner (1904–90) undertook laboratory-based research to develop their respective theories on learning, which are now used to treat psychological problems. These behavioural treatments are used to treat phobias (because phobias can be unlearned) and are used in cognitive behaviour therapy (CBT) for depression and anxiety.

Humanistic approach

This approach was identified by Abraham Maslow (1908–70) as 'the third force' in psychology, as it was a response to the earlier theories. These focused on either the unconscious mind or on behaviour, but – and this is very important in nursing – did not look at the whole person (holistic approach) and their potential for personal growth. Carl Rogers (1902–87) was a major humanistic theorist who, over 40 years ago, developed the concept of self and how the person's sense of themselves can be influenced by their upbringing.

CASE STUDY 36.2: SARAH

Sarah is a businesswoman who perceives herself to be unsuccessful. However, the external reality, and the perception of others, is that she is excellent at her job. This discrepancy between her **self-perception** and the perceptions of the people around her is related to her self-image. Her distorted **self-image** may have developed in childhood when her parents offered her love only when she behaved well, rather than giving her **unconditional positive regard**.

Rogers suggests that unconditional positive regard and acceptance are important to use in psychological therapy, so the person is not being judged and feels supported; they are therefore more likely to develop trust in the therapeutic relationship and talk honestly about their problems.

ANSWER:
CASE STUDY 36.2

• How would this approach be beneficial for Sarah?

Genuineness is also an important quality in both the humanistic approach and in nursing, as patients need to be able to feel safe to share their feelings (Rogers, 1970). A trusting relationship is a further important element to establish between nurses and patients, so being genuine, non-judgemental and empathic, and giving unconditional positive regard and acceptance, are fundamental qualities for nurses to develop.

CASE STUDY 36.3: COPPER AND ALISE [COMMUNITY]

Copper's 8-year-old daughter, Alise, is morbidly obese. Copper tells you that he and Alise eat a healthy diet and he follows good nutritional advice.

- How can you incorporate trust skills into your professional approach with him and Alise?
- How can you remain open-minded, listen carefully to what you are being told and then evaluate the evidence?
- What questions could you ask about the food Copper feeds Alise to get an accurate understanding?

Cognitive approach

The cognitive approach encompasses thinking, perception and memory, and can be used to explain diverse situations such as why people adopt health behaviours (such as exercise, eating a healthy diet or going to the doctor when they have a serious symptom) and why people become anxious and depressed.

Beck (1976) identified negative thoughts about the self as integral to the development of a person's depression. He developed cognitive behaviour therapy (CBT), which involves challenging the thinking of a depressed person by getting them to undertake behavioural tasks that contradict their negative thoughts about themselves, so lifting their depressed mood. Health-compromising (unhealthy) behaviours can be addressed using the transtheoretical model (Table 36.1), which is designed to support individuals to change unhealthy behaviours such as smoking or being overweight.

An individual does not necessarily move straight from one stage to the next; they can slip back, jump a stage or remain in, for example, contemplation for a period of time. There is also the possibility of relapse, and sometimes individuals need to progress through the stages more than once. The importance of this theory is that it recognises that the way the individual thinks about changing their unhealthy behaviour (stages 1–3) is the trigger to the behaviour change. Health professionals need to match the content of the information they give to the individual's stage of change in order to maximise the chances of success. This also demonstrates that thinking, emotions and behaviour interrelate and influence each other.

Table 36.1 Transtheoretical model including the Stages of Change

Stage	Patient thoughts
1 – Pre-contemplation	Not even thinking about stopping smoking and may believe smoking has no health effects
2 – Contemplation	'I think I want to stop smoking but I am stressed and now is not the right time for me'
3 – Preparation	'I want to stop smoking and am going to start next month before I go on holiday'
4 – Action	Reduces or completely stops their smoking behaviour
5 – Maintenance	Continues to stop smoking

Source: Prochaska and DiClemente (1984)

Cognitive developmental approach

The cognitive developmental approach is used to examine the development of intelligent behaviour. Jean Piaget (1896–1980) was one of the key theorists to explain a child's intellectual and moral development as they progress from early childhood to adolescence (Upton, 2011). He observed his own children to help develop his sequential four-stage theory. For example, the first two years after birth (Piaget's sensory stage) are where the child learns to distinguish himself from the world around him by playing and experimenting with toys and objects. This is followed by the pre-operational stage (2–7 years), within which, at about 2 years of age, there is egocentric thinking, which is an inability to see the world from others' perspectives. Thus, the irate toddler demanding 'I want a drink now!' in the middle of a shopping trip to a furniture store is demonstrating egocentric behaviour and not actually being naughty. Associated behaviours include a difficulty in sharing toys and an inability to conserve objects (an understanding that substances remain the same even when their shape is altered). So, for example, if milk is poured from a tall glass into a short, wide one, the child observing this would say there was more milk in the tall glass even though the amount of milk has not changed.

The concrete operational stage (7–11 years) is, according to Atkinson et al. (2000), the period when the child learns to:

1. conserve objects
2. think logically
3. gain an understanding of reversibility (7 + 8 = 15 and 15 − 8 = 7)
4. understand numbers (around age 6)
5. understand mass (age 7)
6. understand weight (age 9).

The formal operational stage of 11 years and onwards is the last stage of development and signifies the ability to demonstrate hypothetical and abstract thinking.

ACTIVITY 36.2: REFLECTION

Reflect on this conversation between an adult and a 7-year-old child named Britney:

Adult: 'Do you know why you are named Britney?' (meaning she must have been named after Britney Spears)

Child: 'Yes. Because that is what my mummy calls me.'

The child demonstrates an inability to 'decentre', according to Piaget, which means Britney is still centred on herself and her own world (egocentric), whereas the adult has assumed Britney would understand her meaning and did not recognise the ambiguity of the question she was asking.

- How does knowledge of child development, such as this, improve the way you may communicate with a child?

There exist both criticism of Piaget and competing theories of child development, including that of Lev Vygotsky (1896–1934), who emphasised that social interaction and communication are the key factors which enable cognitive development. Essentially, the work of all of these theorists provides explanations for how children begin to understand and interact with the world in which they live. The development of a baby's brain and nervous system from conception is crucial to cognitive and motor development. Motor behaviours occur in sequence, so sitting up will occur before the baby learns to crawl or bottom-shuffle, after which they will learn to pull themselves up and walk. The age at which they complete these tasks can be accelerated or delayed by the type of environment in which they live. So, an unstimulating environment with no play and interaction with the carer will have a delaying effect on a child's development. This demonstrates that there is an interaction between biological (nature) and environmental (nurture) factors in child development.

For nurses, knowledge of childhood development is crucial to their understanding of children's behaviour, particularly when they are unwell or part of a family unit in which a parent, grandparent or sibling is ill. In all situations, in order to deliver holistic care it is important to communicate effectively with all those involved, so an understanding of cognitive development is crucial.

Biological approach

Biological explanations (neurological and hormonal, for example) provide the reasons for and treatment of psychological problems such as schizophrenia and depression. In patients who are depressed, low levels of a neurotransmitter substance called serotonin, which has a role in the regulation of mood, have been found. Anti-depressant medication has been developed to increase serotonin levels, thus reducing depression. Such medication can be used together with CBT to enable someone to maximise the benefit of CBT, as the latter involves active participation, which may be difficult when a patient is experiencing the slow thinking and behaviour associated with depression due to low levels of serotonin.

Psychology and the patient

It is important to understand the underpinning theories that explain behaviour, as their diversity represents the complexity of psychology as a science and the reason why it is intriguing and challenging. All the approaches mentioned here are relevant to the care you will deliver to patients. Mental health nurses call on theories from all approaches to maximise the effectiveness of their care, and behaviourist, humanistic and cognitive explanations are all important to child and learning disability nursing. The humanistic approach provides key guidance to all nurses on attitudes and how to approach patients. A crucial element of holistic nursing care is for patients to be given respect, not judged, and treated as individuals rather than as a medical diagnosis. The ability to do this is based on an understanding of psychology.

Surprisingly, even in the twenty-first century, there is still a belief that psychology is only applicable to people with mental health problems when, as we have seen, it is relevant and useful to all. However, health psychology provides scientific theories and application to practice that can be utilised for all contexts of health. Health psychology is devoted to understanding the psychological influences behind how people stay healthy, why they become ill and how they respond when they do get ill (Taylor, 2015). It includes areas such as social support, coping and health behaviour. Julie's scenario demonstrates how a physical illness (urinary tract infection, UTI) may affect mood and behaviour.

This is an example of a nursing student identifying a change in behaviour in a patient who is at risk of harm (untreated UTI). She communicates her concern to her practice educator and the practice educator utilises her accountability and leadership skills to work with the student to identify the possible reasons for the change. Communication, accountability and leadership skills are core to the development of the practice of nursing.

> As a student learning disabilities nurse I have used a psychological approach in many of my clinical placements. Through getting to know my patient and their history and behaviours I could help adapt my care plan to best meet their needs. In one instance a patient with challenging behaviour became very agitated and exhibited new behaviours. Discussing this with my practice educator we decided to do a urine test and discovered the patient had a UTI. A psychological understanding of my patient gave me the insight to see that her behaviour was challenging but different for her and this enabled me to meet her health needs effectively.
>
> **Julie Davis, LD nursing student**

ACTIVITY 36.3: REFLECTION [HOSPITAL]

Richard is 52 years old, does not exercise, is a heavy smoker, is 30 kg overweight and arrives at A&E with severe chest pain. It is suspected that he is having a myocardial infarction (a heart attack) and requires emergency medical treatment.

- When would you choose to talk with him about strategies to promote his health?

Taylor (2015) describes the 'teachable moment', which means that there is a particular time when a person is more receptive to health advice than others. So, in Richard's case, it would be inappropriate to give health advice when he is in severe pain: advice should be given after this, when the patient has a little residual discomfort and a recent memory of the event. Giving advice at a later stage may mean that the person is less likely to act on it, although **pragmatically**, as in Richard's case, it may be the only opportunity to do so.

COMMUNICATION

Information-giving is not simply telling the patient everything you know about their disease or its treatment. It is about planning what you are going to say by identifying the key facts necessary for the patient to understand using language that is free of jargon, medical terms and abbreviations, using appropriate images and symbols to enhance spoken and written information.

The short-term memory lasts less than 15 seconds and has a capacity of five to seven items (Miller, 1956, in Atkinson et al., 2000), but there are a number of facts that patients need to know, and often patients are very anxious and so likely to remember fewer than the minimum number of five items. If it is possible to link material together (chunking) and repeat it (rehearsal), this will aid the retention of material, as will following it up with written information. Always remember that written information needs to be easy to read, succinct and an accurate representation of the key points, available in all languages commonly spoken in the local area.

Primacy and recency

It is not just the content of what you say that matters; so does the order in which you give information. Ley (1979) studied how medical information is best retained by patients and identifies the primacy effect as important. In other words, the first things you say will be more likely to be remembered than the later things, even if they are not the key points that you wish a patient to remember. Therefore, provide the important information first, use simple language, repeat the important information and be specific and clear.

The next piece of information most likely to be retained is the last thing you say (recency). So it is worth repeating the important information at the end of a conversation. New information which is sandwiched in the middle of a conversation is less likely to be retained, so do not include important facts there. An evaluation undertaken by a community-based diabetes specialist nurse to determine why patients did not bring their own records to appointments as requested (Haylock and Ramjeet, 2012) found that the information about bringing their records to appointments was placed in the middle section of the information letter they received. It needed to be moved to the beginning and repeated at least once.

Application to practice - but this has to remain a secret between us...

Primacy and recency do not just apply to communication: they can also be used to influence first impressions (Atkinson et al., 2000). So, for example, if you are starting on a placement and feeling nervous about how you will be received, make sure you arrive promptly and dress appropriately for the area in which you are working. You will create a positive first impression without saying a word. Once you start communicating, you will reinforce the initial favourable impression if you use appropriate verbal behaviour. If you think you have not performed well, then your chance to fix this comes via the recency effect. Spending time towards the end of the shift asking questions and demonstrating your interest, professionalism and enthusiasm will go some of the way to removing any small hitches experienced earlier.

Information and locus of control

Continuing to think about your performance in your nursing programme, having a sense of personal control over your studies may or may not be very important to you. Some nursing students value information about the programme they are studying on, including the dates for placements and theory, as it is really helpful for them to know this in order to manage their family, social life and other commitments. Others do not see this information as important, and prefer to deal with issues as they arise.

Rotter (1966) describes this as a person's 'locus of control', which can be either:

1. Internal – 'I take control of things that are happening in my life' – so a sense of personal control over their studies would be valued;

OR

2. External – 'I go with the flow, let things happen and with a bit of luck and praying to God, things will work out fine' – so a sense of personal control over their studies would not be important.

It is important to understand that when patients are admitted to hospital they may feel a loss of control, particularly if they have an internal locus of control. They are in a strange environment where they do not know the routine and are therefore dependent on staff to give them information about the ward and what will be happening to them. Therefore, giving the patient and their family relevant information is key to reducing their anxiety and fear.

Health locus of control

Wallston et al. (1978) developed a health locus of control, where an internal locus meant taking responsibility for your own health and an external locus meant thinking that all illness is due to chance or bad luck. Those who had an external locus gave all the responsibility to powerful others such as doctors and took a passive role in their health. This theory can be used to explain the behaviour of a patient who will not stop smoking despite having breathing problems, who says: 'it's OK, my GP will sort this out' or 'Everyone is going to die of something!'

Family, community and social support

The family and friends of patients have an important role to play in supporting their care and adherence to treatment both at home and in hospital. Social support can be defined as information leading the subject to believe that he is cared for, loved, esteemed and a member of a network of mutual obligations (Cobb, 1976), whilst Cohen and Wills (1985) describe it as having two components:

1. Structure: social network (people and pets)
2. Function: resources provided by the network (practical and emotional support).

So, for example, when you visit a patient in their home, you may also meet their family and will find out more about the size of their social network. The component described by Cohen and Wills (1985) as 'function' can be important in the long-term care of patients. Examples of function would include one or more of the patient's social network providing physical help, for example for a person who has a learning disability, or providing companionship and someone to talk to for an older person who has limited mobility and does not leave their house. It is very easy to assume that the presence of one or more people in a social network indicates that they provide social support to the patient. However, never make this assumption, as it may not be the case.

Social support has been identified as an important resource in combating stress (Cobb, 1976; Cohen and Wills, 1985). The onset of illness is a potential stressor, especially if the illness becomes long-term. This is when it is key to ask a patient what support they receive, particularly if they are struggling to cope.

Just ticking a box indicating that the patient has a wife, husband, partner or another family member around does not address whether they are receiving any social support. The husband that you perceive is the patient's main support may also be disabled, or there may be other reasons why they are unable to offer any help. This is especially relevant to patients with long-term conditions – such as chronic depression or rheumatoid arthritis, for example – because they may require both emotional and practical support and may be receiving neither.

As a community nurse or volunteer, for example, you may become part of the person's social network whilst undertaking your role in their care.

Functional support, according to Barth et al. (2012), includes support that is:

- financial
- appraisal (helping someone to re-examine a stressful situation)
- informational

as well as practical and emotional.

WHAT'S THE EVIDENCE?

Haylock, C. and Ramjeet, J. (2012) 'Service evaluation of hand-held records to improve diabetes self-care', *Journal of Diabetic Nursing*, 16(8): 316-24.

In this study, Haylock and Ramjeet (2012) found that patients who remembered their hand-held records at primary care appointments identified informational social support from their spouses (prompting) as the reason for this. As community care is an integral part of the NHS, it is vital that nurses understand the role of family, neighbours, volunteers and charities in the social network of the patient.

FURTHER
READING:
DIABETES
SELF-CARE

Reflection

- Reflect on your understanding of the role of family and friends when someone has a serious illness.
- Does having a large social network mean that the patient receives more support than someone with a small network?
- Now read the article and consider how you could act on the findings.

Implications of a lack of social support

A systematic review and meta-analysis by Barth et al. (2010) found that a lack of social support from their social network (family and friends) had a negative effect on mortality in patients with coronary heart disease. However, the authors suggest that this lack of support could be amended by the individual having contact with other cardiac patients who could share their experiences and information and offer emotional support. What is very interesting about this study is that it is another example of how psychological factors have an influence on physical health. The saying 'healthy body, healthy mind' should perhaps be reversed: 'healthy mind, healthy body'.

Role models

Think back to the story of Suzie, the specialist stoma nurse, at the start of this chapter (case study 34.1). She clearly demonstrates that nursing is both an art and a science. The knowledge she gained by studying textbooks and research articles (science) underpinned her nursing practice, the care she delivered to patients (art). The senior nurses you will work with in practice will set similarly high standards of care. You need to observe them and then try to imitate their behaviours (for example, how they listen to and assess patients).

There will be some nurses whom you will always remember: they will make a positive impression on you either because of an extraordinary incident that you witnessed or because they are consistently outstanding.

ACTIVITY 36.4: REFLECTION [HOSPITAL]

I remember a young theatre sister who was excellent at her job.

When confronted with an angry consultant surgeon who was throwing surgical instruments around the operating theatre, she told the junior nurses – including me – who were scurrying around picking them up, 'Stop, Mr Todd will pick up the instruments himself'.

He did!

This demonstrated her courage in standing up to an irate and badly behaved senior surgeon and directing him to deal with the consequences of his own ill-tempered behaviour. This was in the days when doctors' decisions were not challenged by nurses, so that is why it is so memorable for me.

- Think about the person you will select as a role model in nursing.
- What attributes do they possess that you would like to attain?

Role models in nursing frequently demonstrate the art of nursing – behaviour that nursing students need to observe, imitate and learn to use. These behaviours include practical expertise coupled with expert knowledge, effective interpersonal skills and the humanity and skills required to advocate for patients. The concept of modelling developed from the work of social learning theorists, specifically Albert Bandura (1925–present). Bandura et al. (1961) demonstrated the negative effect of violent role models on children's socialisation processes when they observed and imitated the violent behaviour of adults who were being aggressive towards a large doll.

THE PSYCHOLOGICAL IMPACT OF ATTITUDE

'That nursing student has a poor attitude' is a phrase that conjures up a picture of someone who looks miserable, gives hostile or disinterested verbal responses and exhibits body language suggesting they would rather be somewhere else. As is demonstrated in Figure 36.1, this provides a clue that attitudes are composed of behaviour and emotion but also, importantly, how a person thinks. This applies not only to nursing students, but to patients too!

Usually, there is a consistency within an attitude which means that the thoughts, emotions and behaviour match each other.

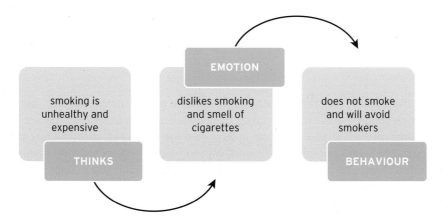

Figure 36.1   Attitudes composed of behaviour and emotion

Patients will demonstrate their attitudes to reducing or giving up health-compromising behaviours such as smoking. If a patient recognises that smoking contributed to their heart attack, they may be persuaded to reduce their smoking behaviour; this, however, may cause cognitive dissonance (Festinger, 1957), which is, in essence, the existence of two conflicting thoughts:

1. I need a cigarette.
2. If I smoke I will have another heart attack.

The fact that the thoughts are conflicting will hopefully result in the patient re-establishing consistency by:

- concluding that smoking is catastrophic for their health (thinking)
- therefore feeling happy (emotions) about reducing their health risk
- and stopping smoking (behaviour).

Ensuring you deliver effective care

Throughout the chapter so far, the application of psychology, with its focus on the mind and behaviour, has been stressed as a way to aid you to deliver effective care. Ensuring your care is patient-centred is fundamental within this.

When the care delivered is not effective

The enquiry report into the Mid Staffordshire NHS Foundation Trust's failures in the delivery of effective patient care (2005–9) highlighted many examples of poor nursing care. Underpinning this was a lack of recognition of patients as individuals and the fact that their needs were not prioritised. The report makes it clear that the failure to give effective physical care was mirrored by the absence of any psychological skills used in the delivery of care. Using good psychological skills alongside the delivery of physical care is an important tool in preventing poor nursing care.

Ion and Lauder (2015) recommend that adult nurses need to develop skills in the psychological care of people who are physically ill. It is evident that ignoring a patient's bewilderment and distress can only be detrimental to their care and treatment.

You can easily incorporate seven essential psychological skills into your practice (see Table 36.2).

WHAT'S THE EVIDENCE?

Jinks, A.M., Cotton, A., Murphy, P. and Kirton, J. (2013) 'Nursing students' attitudes toward patient-centred care in the United Kingdom', *Journal of Nursing Education and Practice*, 13(12): 116–24.

According to Jinks et al. (2013), male nurses, students younger than 20 and child field nursing students achieve the highest scores for positive attitudes.

The authors suggest that caring skills are not inbuilt but can be learned in nursing education by keeping a reflective diary, as a record of your key experiences with patients throughout your programme.

- Reflect on your experiences so far during your programme. Have your caring skills been improved?
- Now read the article and consider how the study applies to you.

WEBLINK:
JINKS ET AL.
(2013)

The bio-psychosocial model in health psychology emphasises the importance of biological, psychological and social causes of health and illness (Taylor, 2015). However, this can be difficult to accomplish in practice as, when a patient presents with either a mental health or a physical need, the priority is to identify the presenting problem and treat it, usually with medication – thereby using a biological approach. This was clearly evident in Activity 36.3, in the care of Richard.

The use of psychology may, at first, appear superfluous to this process. So, there needs to be a clear way of incorporating it, enabling nurses to use psychological skills as part of their practice from the very first day that they work with patients and other health professionals.

Table 36.2 identifies seven core psychological skills that can be used with patients, their family or friends and all of the staff you encounter on a daily basis. They have been developed in collaboration with a senior hospital pharmacist, as twenty-first-century healthcare demands effective multidisciplinary working. The core skills are based on a range of psychological theories (including humanistic and behavioural) and the acronym PERFORM has been used to identify them.

Table 36.2   The components of PERFORM

PERFORM

P	Patient's preferred name (what they wish to be called)
E	Eye contact (maintain appropriate eye contact with patient and family)
R	Respect (always be respectful of the patient, their family and other health professionals)
F	Facial expression (interested, professional and appropriately reflecting the situation)
O	Open-minded (use information from the patient and other sources, but do not judge or make instant decisions without accurate, objective and verifiable information)
R	Recall what the patient says by listening carefully while also observing their non-verbal behaviour for further information
M	Manage yourself (always behave professionally: your distress, tiredness, frustration, etc. must never be vented on a patient, their family, other health professionals or support staff)

Source: Ramjeet and Ramjeet (2014)

Using PERFORM in your practice

1.   Preferred name

It takes less than a minute to ask someone what they like to be called. By doing this, you are affirming them as a person and beginning the process of recognising them as an individual. You need then to ensure that you remember and use their preferred name in future interactions.

2.   Eye contact

This is a key non-verbal behaviour (Argyle, 1983). Looking into someone's eyes denotes your interest in them, as well as giving you the opportunity to begin to assess their mood (anxiety, sadness, happiness) and thinking (interested, distracted).

3.   Respectful

Showing respect is part of accepting a person as an individual. This is demonstrated by the friendly, even tone that you use to speak to them, by using their name and by demonstrating interest in and knowledge of them. This means that, wherever possible, you should find out some information about the patient prior to engaging with them. Again, this will only take a few minutes and you will then be fully prepared.

4.   Facial expression

It is important to control your facial expression, as it indicates to the patient your attitude towards them. Looking interested, smiling or looking concerned in the right circumstances are all appropriate; boredom, a lack of interest or judgemental expressions are unprofessional and never acceptable. Practice is needed to control non-verbal behaviour, so ensure you are always conscious of your expression.

5.   Open-minded

This is related to being non-judgemental and means that you listen to or read information carefully and never pre-judge a situation by forming an initial, inaccurate impression, such as 'as the patient is older and confused, they must have dementia'. There are situations in which you may need to make quick decisions based on the evidence that you have thus far, but always be prepared to revisit and revise your decision in light of further information from the patient and other sources. This may mean admitting to yourself and others that your initial impression was incorrect. In this way, you avoid distorting any information you receive at a later time to fit your original impression.

6.   Recall by listening carefully

Listen to what the patient is saying. They are telling you things that they think are important, so listen to and remember them.

7.   Manage yourself

Being a nurse includes managing your emotions when you are at work, demonstrating emotional intelligence. Simply, this means that difficulties outside work are not expressed as preoccupation or irritability at work. Similarly, when dealing with a patient whom you find 'difficult', you should not vent your frustration at the patient, other patients or members of staff. You need to develop strategies for dealing with daily stress and difficulties so that the patient and their needs remain your focus, rather than meeting your own needs.

It is also possible to use PERFORM as a personal baseline of behaviour, enabling you to rate yourself at the end of the day, which can prompt you to reflect on the reasons why you were unable to perform a particular skill consistently (see Table 36.3). It could also be useful to ask your practice educator to use PERFORM and give you feedback.

CASE STUDY 36.4: POPPY [HOSPITAL]

Poppy is a nursing student on her second placement in a medical ward and was told by the sister to take a drink to a patient in a side room. She was not given any further information. When she opened the door, she saw a man in bed with severe burns to his face and chest. His skin looked like a log of

(Continued)

wood that had burned on an open fire and was blackened, blistered and flaky. Poppy was shocked, but managed to stop her jaw from dropping.

The patient's wife was sitting next to the bed with other relatives, and said to Poppy: 'It's all right for you, nurse, you see this sort of thing every day, but this is my husband. I am struggling to cope!'

This comment was miles from the truth of the situation and not how Poppy was feeling, but she managed to compose herself and replied, 'Yes, it must be really difficult for you.' Poppy did not say how shocked she was as a result of having been unaware of the patient's condition when she entered the room and never having seen severe burns before.

Poppy's actions were correct. Despite the lack of information from the sister, she did not have permission to share her feelings of shock with the patient and his wife. This would have been meeting her own need to express her feelings, rather than meeting those of the patient.

- What could Poppy do to prevent a similar incident occurring in the future?
- How would using PERFORM have helped Poppy in this situation?

Table 36.3 Scoring system for PERFORM

Perform	Score	Scoring grid: Never = 0 Sometimes = 1 Always = 2 Maximum score = 14
Preferred name		
Eye contact		
Respect		
Facial expression		
Open mind		
Recall		
Manage self		
Total		

ANSWER:
CASE STUDY 36.4

It is crucial that PERFORM is used in partnership with the care being delivered – for example, when:

- admitting a young child for an operation
- building a relationship with a new patient who has a learning disability
- visiting a young person who is chronically depressed
- undertaking temperature, pulse and respiration observations on an adult patient.

PERFORM needs to be used simultaneously with, not afterwards or instead of, nursing actions. This ensures the patient is provided with the core physical care they require (for example, hydration, nourishment, pain assessment and management; being kept clean and comfortable; being helped to use the toilet). However, remember that, in an emergency, life-saving actions always take priority.

ACTIVITY 36.5: PERFORM

Use PERFORM to examine your skills in communication. Use with up to 10 different people involved in healthcare (patients, relatives, community or hospital staff).

Each time you complete your score on a person, number them (person 1-10) and then take a few minutes to make notes on the other side of the paper to identify anything that is affecting your score (your skills, patient factors, the environment, etc.). Try to do this every time with as much detail as possible.

When completed, gather all your scores and notes together. This is your data.

Read through your notes several times to carefully examine the factors that have affected your score. You could use different colour highlighter pen for factors that reoccur the most.

Examine them critically and, for example, consider whether your skills improve as you become more experienced at using PERFORM (Do you score lower on person 1 than person 10, for example?) What steps can you take to change the factors that you have highlighted?

CONCLUSION

This chapter has applied psychological theory to practice so you will be able to understand and use it from the beginning of your nursing career. Psychology provides underpinning theory for human behaviours and, as a nurse, you will be engaging with all types of human behaviour on a daily basis, from patients, their relatives, staff and other nursing students. Understanding why people behave in the way they do helps you know how to react and engage with them appropriately. It will also help you understand your own behaviour and how you manage difficult times during your nursing programme – because there will be difficult times!

Social support plays a crucial role in the wellbeing not only of patients, but of us all. Ensure you use this effectively in times of stress by confiding in someone whom you can trust. Listening to someone else discussing the issue that is affecting you will provide perspective on your problem and the act of sharing your concern will give you emotional support.

To help you apply psychological skills, make sure you use PERFORM. It is specifically written to provide you with clear guidance on how to engage professionally and humanely with patients and staff, so you can lead the way in communicating with, caring for and managing students.

CHAPTER SUMMARY

- There are a number of different approaches in psychology.
- Psychology is applicable to all fields of nursing and every patient interaction.
- An understanding of child development will help you communicate appropriately with children of all ages, and will also assist communication with adults who have a learning disability.
- Health psychology helps us to understand how people manage their health and illness.
- Social support plays a crucial role in the care of patients with long-term conditions.
- Nurses must ensure they always impart information effectively to patients.
- Using PERFORM can help you to apply and measure seven core psychological skills.
- Accountability, communication, leadership and coordination of care are key nursing standards that are enhanced by using psychology in nursing care.

—————————— **CRITICAL REFLECTION** ——————————

Holistic care

This chapter has discussed the use of psychology by nurses in all fields of nursing. It has demonstrated that it is important to use psychology not only with patients and their families in order to deliver holistic care, but also with other healthcare staff.

- Reflect on a patient whom you have nursed recently and identify how your knowledge of psychology enabled you to deliver holistic, patient-centred care.
- What skills do you need to develop further?

——————————————— **GO FURTHER** ———————————————

Books

Gross, R. (2015) *The Science of Mind and Behaviour*, 7th edn. London: Hodder & Stoughton. This is a core British psychology text that contains everything you need to understand in terms of theory and information relating to all aspects of psychology.

Taylor, S. (2015) *Health Psychology*, 9th edn. Boston: McGraw-Hill. This is an interesting and comprehensive health psychology text written by an academic who undertakes health psychology research. It covers aspects of health psychology such as social support and coping in greater detail than other texts and clearly applies health psychology to healthcare scenarios.

SAGE journal articles

FURTHER
READING:
JOURNAL
ARTICLES

Go to https://study.sagepub.com/essentialnursing2e for free online journal articles for this chapter. If you are using the interactive ebook, simply click on the book icon in the margin to go straight to the resource.

Reader, T., Gillespie, A. and Mannell, J. (2014) 'Patient neglect in 21st century health-care institutions: A community health psychology perspective', *Journal of Health Psychology*, 19(1): 137-48. This article reviews the concept of patient neglect and the role of community health psychology in understanding its occurrence. A community health psychology perspective shows that the wider symbolic, material and relational aspects of care are crucial to understanding why patient neglect occurs and outlining new solutions.

Skerrett, K. (2010) 'Extending family nursing: Concepts from positive psychology', *Journal of Family Nursing*, 16(4): 487-502. This article identifies how positive psychology can be an important extension to the knowledge base of family nursing. Positive psychology focuses on optimal functioning and is an ideal complement to the strengths-based orientation of family nursing. Suggestions are given for ways to apply concepts from positive psychology to family nursing practice, research and education.

Other journal articles

Currid, T. (2012) 'Meeting the psychological needs of the physically ill', *Nursing Times*, 108(46): 22-5. A well-written review article with a wide range of useful references considering an important area in psychology and nursing.

Weblinks

Go to https://study.sagepub.com/essentialnursing2e for weblinks related to this chapter. If you are using the interactive ebook, simply click on the book icon in the margin to go straight to the resource.

FURTHER READING: WEBLINKS

www.bps.org.uk – the website of the British Psychological Society, which provides information relating to conferences and publications.

www.apa.org – the website of the American Psychological Association. Provides information on research and topics such as depression, anger and anxiety.

www.simplypsychology.org – the Simply Psychology website provides clear explanations of different theories in psychology.

http://psychology.about.com – provides information and a range of resources designed for those wanting to learn more about psychology.

Video links

Have a break from the text and go to https://study.sagepub.com/essentialnursing2e for useful videos related to this chapter. If you are using the interactive ebook, simply click on the lightbulb icon in the margin to go straight to the resource.

VIDEO LINKS

ACE YOUR ASSESSMENT

Review what you have learned by visiting the book's online resources at: https://study.sagepub.com/essentialnursing2e If using your interactive ebook, just click on the icon in the margin to go straight there.

ONLINE QUIZZES

- Test yourself with multiple-choice and short-answer questions.
- Revise key terms with the interactive flash cards.

REFERENCES

Atkinson, R.L., Atkinson, R.C., Smith, E.E., Bem, D.J. and Nolen-Hoeksema, S. (2000) *Hilgard's Introduction to Psychology*, 13th edn. Orlando, FL: Harcourt College Publishers.

Argyle, M. (1983) *The Psychology of Interpersonal Behaviour*, 4th edn. Harmondsworth: Penguin.

Bandura, A., Ross, D. and Ross, S.A. (1961) 'Transmission of aggression through imitation of aggressive models', *Journal of Abnormal and Social Psychology*, 63: 575–82.

Barth, J., Schneider, S. and von Känel, R. (2010) 'Lack of social support in the etiology and the prognosis of coronary heart disease: A systematic review and meta-analysis', *Psychosomatic Medicine*, 72(3): 229–38.

Beck, A. (1976) *Cognitive Therapy and the Emotional Disorder*. New York: International Universities Press.

Cobb, S. (1976) 'Social support as a moderator of life stress', *Psychosomatic Medicine*, 38: 300–14.

Cohen, S. and Wills, T. (1985) 'Stress, social support and the buffering hypothesis', *Psychological Bulletin*, 98(2): 310–57.

Festinger, L. (1957) *A Theory of Cognitive Dissonance*. Stanford, CA: Stanford University Press.

Haylock, C. and Ramjeet, J. (2012) 'Service evaluation of hand-held records to improve diabetes self-care', *Journal of Diabetic Nursing*, 16(8): 316–24.

Ion, R.M. and Lauder, W. (2015) 'Willis and the generic turn in nursing', *Nurse Education Today*, 35(7): 841–2.

Jinks, A.M., Cotton, A., Murphy, P. and Kirton, J. (2013) 'Nursing students' attitudes toward patient-centred care in the United Kingdom', *Journal of Nursing Education and Practice*, 13(12): 116–24.

Ley, P. (1979) 'Memory for medical information', *British Journal of Social and Clinical Psychology*, 18(2): 245–55.

Prochaska, J.O. and DiClemente, C.C. (1984) *The Transtheoretical Approach: Crossing Traditional Boundaries of Therapy*. Homeward, IL: Dow Jones Irwin.

Ramjeet, J. and Ramjeet, S.J. (2014) PERFORM: 7 core psychological skills. Unpublished manuscript.

Rogers, C.R. (1970) *On Becoming a Person: A Therapist's View of Psychotherapy*. Boston, MA: Houghton Mifflin.

Rotter, J.B. (1966) 'Generalised expectancies for the internal versus external control of reinforcement', *Psychological Monographs*, 90: 1–28.

Taylor, S. (2015) *Health Psychology*, 9th edn. Boston, MA: McGraw-Hill.

Upton, P. (2011) *Developmental Psychology*. Exeter: Learning Matters.

Wallston, K.A., Wallston, B.S. and de Vellis, R. (1978) 'Development of the multidimensional health locus of control (MHLC) scale', *Health Education Monographs*, 6: 160–70.

INTRODUCTION TO THE SOCIOLOGICAL CONTEXT OF NURSING

37

RUTH NORTHWAY

- What is sociology and why should we study it?

- Understanding key sociological perspectives – family, poverty, disability and stigma

> " My name is Jamal, I am 13 years old and I enjoy listening to music and playing computer games. Like most teenagers I like being with my friends, but this can be difficult as I use an electric wheelchair. Even though I can use it without assistance, sometimes I can't get to places my friends want to go to and, even if I can, I'm not always able to get in because of steps. This is really frustrating as I just want to do things that other teenagers do.
>
> **Jamal, patient** "

> " My name is Gareth; I am studying to be a mental health nurse and I have recently completed a community nursing placement. I don't know what I was expecting but I was surprised by the degree to which where someone lives has an effect on their health and how families are so different in terms of how they live. It's really made me think about how so many things influence both our physical and mental health.
>
> **Gareth, MH nursing student** "

INTRODUCTION

Sociology is a relatively new addition to nursing courses and there has been debate as to whether this is a positive development. Nonetheless, it is positive to note that the importance of the social sciences is again recognised within the new *Standards* for *Registered Nurse Education* (NMC, 2018). This chapter will therefore provide you with an introduction to sociology and, more importantly, also help you to understand its relevance to nursing practice in all fields. To achieve this, some key sociological perspectives will be introduced, since considering differing views can help you to develop your critical thinking skills. The relevance of sociology to your nursing practice will then be considered through an exploration of poverty, the family, disability and stigma.

WHAT IS SOCIOLOGY AND WHY SHOULD WE STUDY IT?

At a basic level, sociology is concerned with understanding the social world, the systems and structures that operate within society and how people within societies interact at a variety of different levels. Just as physical scientists study the physical world through a structured, scientific approach, so for sociologists the social world is their laboratory and social life is studied in a structured way to identify causes, effects, reasons and explanations.

One area that sociologists have studied is education, and you may come across people who argue that since we have all attended school, we all understand schools: so why do we need sociology? However, are all schools the same? Do they provide all children with an equal chance of a 'good' education, and what *is* a 'good' education? What impact does education have on individuals, communities and society in general? These issues, however, are not ones we often consider as we assume that we understand education. Sometimes we take our social world for granted and we lose the ability to look at it in a critical manner: it is too familiar. What sociology offers is not knowledge based on the experience of one person, but a body of knowledge that has been built up through the systematic research of many sociologists (Fulcher and Scott, 2011). It helps to make 'the ordinary extraordinary' and to reveal the sometimes hidden reasons as to why people behave in the way they do (Allan et al., 2016: 2).

Understanding someone's culture and sociological beliefs can be helpful when planning their care and understanding their beliefs and wishes for the future. Also, societal beliefs shape how individuals live and, by conforming to these ideals, help people to fit into society and be accepted by the community they live in.

Michelle Hill, NQ RNLD

A knowledge of sociology helps to understand the basics of public health and where provisions are given, e.g. help to quit services in a low social economic area.

Laura Grimley, adult nursing student

ACTIVITY 37.1: REFLECTION

Think about an aspect of social life that we take for granted (such as the media, healthcare or employment):

- What do you think are the main questions we should ask if we want to understand it better? Try to identify some 'what', 'why' and 'how' questions.

ANSWER:
ACTIVITY 37.1

Relevance to nursing practice

In 1994, a key paper by Keith Sharp, a lecturer in sociology, was published in the *Journal of Advanced Nursing* in which he urged 'caution' about the inclusion of sociology within nursing programmes. He argued that nurses were concerned primarily with knowing 'how to' perform tasks, whereas sociologists were concerned with theoretical knowledge (knowing 'that'), and, therefore, while sociological knowledge would not impair the performance of nurses, it was not essential. His second argument was that sociology does not provide a single view of how to understand social life and therefore does not offer a useful basis for nursing action. Finally, he noted that students of sociology are expected to question and challenge the assumptions that underpin it: nurses, he suggested, are not expected to adopt such a critical approach.

In response, Sam Porter (1995) argued that Sharp presented a view of nurses as being able only to 'do', rather than being able to question 'why', thus reinforcing the view of nurses as doctors' hand-maidens. Porter also argued that nurses work in complex situations, and therefore explanations that can accommodate such complexity are needed. The differing views and insights offered by sociology provide a range of explanations and nurses need to assess their relevance to the situations in which they find themselves: sociology is thus helpful to nurses and nursing.

While Sharp (1994) suggested that critical thinking may not be required of nurses, change only occurs if existing practices are questioned, and sociology offers us different ways of examining aspects of social life, including nursing practice. Differing explanations can be frustrating if you want to know who is 'right', but looking at different positions can help you to better understand other people's views while also developing your own values and beliefs. Pinikahana (2003), while acknowledging the debate between Sharp and Porter, suggests that what is needed is sociology *applied to* nursing, rather than theoretical sociology. She argues that an understanding of sociology can help us to better under-stand patients' behaviour as well as their psycho-social needs, and this is important if we are to provide holistic and humanitarian nursing care. Keep this in mind when you read Rachel's case study (37.1).

CASE STUDY 37.1: RACHEL

Rachel lives with her husband and two children in a town in the south of England. The family moved there three years ago when Mark, her husband, had to either take redundancy or move with his firm. Two years earlier, Rachel had given up her job as a teacher following the birth of their child, Tom, who suffered **anoxia** during his birth, leaving him with severe physical and intellectual disabilities. The family felt they had to move when Mark's firm moved as they were reliant on his wage, but this meant moving away from their supportive parents.

(Continued)

Six months ago, Mark again learned that he was being made redundant, but this time with no possibility of re-employment. Rachel then found that she was pregnant. Around the same time, Mark started to become depressed as he couldn't find a job and the family were beginning to have financial worries.

Recently, Rachel's mother (who lives in the north of England) has been in hospital following a stroke. Rachel has been telephoned by her brother (who lives close to their mother) to say that the hospital wishes to discharge their mother, but either someone will need to move in to care for her or she will have to move into residential care. He says he cannot help due to his work, so he has told the ward staff that Rachel will help. Rachel feels torn: she can't leave Tom in Mark's care, as he is now so depressed that he rarely gets up before lunch.

- Can you identify the social factors affecting Rachel and her family?

ANSWER:
CASE STUDY 37.1

Rachel's story highlights a number of social factors that affect not only her and her family, but many other individuals and their families. Examples of these are unemployment, disability, family relations

Table 37.1 Examples of sociological theories/perspectives

Sociological theory/ perspective	Key features
Functionalism	• Society can be understood as similar to a biological organism in which systems and structures work together • It is important that social structures and systems work together to maintain the functioning of society • These systems and structures include the family, education, religion and employment • It is important that people conform to rules and cultural expectations so that society functions effectively
Symbolic interactionism	• Human behaviour uses symbols and attaches meaning to these symbols • One form of symbol is language • Meaning emerges from our interaction with others and the meaning we attribute to certain symbols
Marxism	• People need systems to maintain their survival and the arrangements made for this determine other aspects of their lives • Conflicts arise between workers and owners: the owners profit from the labour of the workers • Conflict is necessary to bring about change
Post-structuralism	• Language is viewed as a powerful means of control but it is difficult to separate our ideas from the language we use to express them • There is a focus on how we talk with each other and make sense of the world – this is referred to as 'discourse' • Knowledge is viewed as a means of control
Feminism	• Feminism is a collection of approaches that have both similarities and differences • Traditionally, sociology has been written from a male perspective and this has marginalised the experiences of women • Many theories have accepted the subordinate role of women as 'natural' • Feminism places women's experiences as central and is concerned with explaining gender divisions within society

and the role of carers, all of which sociology can help us to better understand, and so in turn better understand how they affect the lives of those we support.

Sociological perspectives

A key characteristic of sociology is that it encompasses a range of different theoretical perspectives, each of which offers different ways of explaining and understanding the social world. Some of these perspectives and their key features are set out in Table 37.1.

Fulcher and Scott (2011) note that there is no single theory to which all sociologists subscribe; instead, each theory has its supporters and those who argue against it. Each theorist has tended to focus on certain key areas, and so no single theory provides a full explanation of the social world. Furthermore, any theory can only be judged in terms of the extent to which it helps us understand what is happening in everyday life. When reading through the sections within this chapter which relate to different theories, try to bear this in mind and think about how the theory might help you understand the world around you, and in particular the contexts in which nurses work.

ACTIVITY 37.2: REFLECTION

Take one of the perspectives identified in Table 37.1 and try to identify how it might help us to examine the contexts in which nurses work. For example, you might think about symbolic interactionism and consider how people respond to us as nurses because (in some settings) we wear uniforms.

ANSWER:
ACTIVITY 37.2

UNDERSTANDING KEY SOCIOLOGICAL PERSPECTIVES - FAMILY, POVERTY, DISABILITY AND STIGMA

In this chapter, it is only possible to explore a few key concepts and how they are understood through different sociological perspectives. Here, the family, poverty, disability and stigma will be explored.

The family

As has already been mentioned, a functionalist view of society focuses on the function(s) that various social institutions play in maintaining society. The family is one such 'institution', and functionalists would see its role as being to maintain the population (through reproduction) and to raise and socialise children. Historically, the image often presented by functionalists was one of harmony and mutual support, but during the 1970s and 1980s, feminist theory challenged this view (Giddens and Sutton, 2013). Attention was drawn to unequal power relations within the family and the ways in which some members benefited more than others. One example is the way in which women were/are expected to take on caring roles that are often unpaid (think back to case study 37.1). During the 1970s and 1980s, there was also an increased awareness that the family is not a safe environment for everyone: domestic violence and child abuse can have serious consequences for family members.

Until relatively recently, a family was often considered to comprise a married couple (man and woman) with children. However, family composition differs between countries and cultures and over time. Within the UK, we have seen an increase in divorce rates and remarriages over recent decades, leading to what has been termed 'reconstituted families', whereby a couple marry and bring together children from two previous relationships to form a new family. Other changes include single-parent families, gay and lesbian couples raising children and surrogacy becoming more common. People often move away from their home area for work, and this, coupled with increased life expectancy, means that older relatives may be living with little local family support should they become frail.

Families may be very diverse and our view of a family may be very different from the lived realities of some of the people whom we work with and support. However, whether working in a hospital or community setting, whatever our field of practice, all nurses will be involved not only in working with patients but also in working with them in the context of their families. It is important that we do not make assumptions or negative judgements based on our own experiences and values. By encouraging us to question things we take for granted, sociology can help us to identify and challenge our assumptions, and also to see other people's perspectives.

Poverty

Poverty can be a difficult concept to define, but two main approaches are usually discussed: absolute and relative poverty. Absolute poverty relates to whether or not people have sufficient resources (such as shelter, food, clothing) to maintain physical health. It is linked to the concept of subsistence (Giddens and Sutton, 2013), and those lacking these resources are deemed to live in absolute poverty. The basics for subsistence are viewed as being the same for all individuals of equivalent age and build, wherever in the world they live (Giddens and Sutton, 2013); in many developing countries, people lack such resources and live in absolute poverty. While the same may not be true for most developed countries, evidence of great inequalities exists. Relative poverty, therefore, is culturally defined and refers to situations in which people lack the resources to enjoy what is considered essential to a reasonable standard of living within that society. This means that what is considered 'essential' will vary from place to place and over time.

Poverty has been included in this chapter as the links between poverty and ill health have long been discussed.

WHAT'S THE EVIDENCE?

Reflect on the findings of the three reports in Table 37.2 (Black, Acheson and Marmot), in relation to the patients you have been involved in caring for. Are you able to identify any differences that support the findings of the reports?

Table 37.2 Care reports and their findings

Report	Findings
The Black Report (1980): *Inequalities in Health*	• Differences in mortality rates between social classes, with those in social classes 4 and 5 (lower-income, unskilled workers) more likely to die at a young age • Even though there was a decrease in infant mortality rates during the 1960s and 1970s, the difference in rates between those in social classes 4 and 5 combined and those in social classes 1 and 2 (higher income, professional) combined, increased • Inequalities in the use of health services (particularly preventative services) evident, with those in social classes 4 and 5 less likely to access healthcare • Poverty, working conditions and deprivation cause inequalities in health

Report	Findings
The Acheson Report (1998): *Independent Inquiry into Inequalities in Health*	• While mortality rates had fallen for all groups over the previous 20 years, the difference between the top and bottom social classes increased • Noted growing evidence of social class differences in relation to many common diseases, including coronary heart disease, stroke, lung cancer and respiratory disease • Substantially more people in the 'lower' social classes were noted to have self-reported long-standing illnesses • In 1960 the % of the population living below 50% of average income was 10%, but by 1995 this had grown to 17% • Noted the complex nature of inequalities: characteristics such as gender, race and disability also exert an influence
The Marmot Report (2010): *Fair Society, Healthy Lives: A Review of Health Inequalities in England*	• People living in the poorest neighbourhoods die on average seven years earlier than those in more affluent areas • On average, those living in poorer areas spend 17 more years of their lives living with disabling conditions • A complex range of factors affect health, including housing, education, income and disability • Health inequalities are largely preventable: action is required across a range of areas, such as employment, income, education and housing

Understanding the links between poverty and health inequalities can help nurses to target their interventions more effectively. For example, it may be important to focus particularly on those with low incomes to encourage them to have preventative health checks. In addition, the need for nurses to engage with others in broader activities, such as campaigning for better housing and education, can be seen.

Disability

ACTIVITY 37.3: REFLECTION

Before reading any further, write down what you understand by the term 'disability'.

Historically, disability has often been viewed in terms of an 'individual' or 'medical' model, whereby disability is perceived as an illness and disabled people as being 'sick' and in need of a 'cure'. One sociologist who explored the 'sick role' is Talcott Parsons (1902–79). Taking a functionalist perspective, Parsons saw sickness and ill health as dysfunctional to society and therefore in need of elimination. Accordingly, he argued that those who take on the sick role are afforded two rights, but also have to accept two responsibilities. The responsibilities are as follows:

• They must obtain medical confirmation of their 'illness' and comply with medical instructions to get better.
• They must view being 'ill' as undesirable and want to get better.

The rights of those taking on the sick role are as follows:

- Once medically diagnosed, they are relieved of all responsibilities and social expectations.
- They are not held responsible for their 'illness'.

While this may be appropriate for a short-term illness, where being told to rest for a few days and having someone else take on your responsibilities can be good, it is not so appropriate when it is applied to what may be a lifelong condition. For example, if you are disabled, is it reasonable to view your condition as undesirable and for others not to expect you to achieve anything? Nonetheless, the influence of this view of disability can be seen within current society, where medical assessment is required in order to claim some welfare benefits and to be 'excused' from the responsibility to seek employment. Consider also how people refer to someone 'suffering' from disability, when in fact many disabled people live full and rewarding lives.

Challenging such a view, the Disability Movement, including some disabled sociologists, proposed an alternative view of disability, termed the 'social' model of disability. This approach argues that rather than being unable to do things (due to their disability), people with impairments (whether mental, physical or sensory) are disabled by a range of barriers that prevent or limit their full participation in society (see Oliver (1996) for further information).

CASE STUDY 37.2: LISA

At handover, a ward sister informs her staff team that they are expecting a new admission. She adds that the medical notes say the woman 'suffers from Down's syndrome'. One member of staff says she once nursed someone with Down's syndrome and that they were really difficult. Another says she wouldn't know where to start in terms of providing care and hopes a carer is coming to look after her. The sister also admits she doesn't have much experience in this area and thinks they should put the patient in a side room on her own. Having undertaken a placement working with people with learning disabilities, Helen (a first-year nursing student) asks whether she can do the admission as she needs to develop her communication skills.

When Lisa Barton later arrives, with her sister, they are met by Helen and taken to the side room. Helen chats with Lisa and discovers her fears and concerns about the procedure and about her life, as well as her likes and dislikes. Lisa lives independently, although her sister supports her with some things. She works as a carer in a residential home for older people and doesn't like missing work to come to hospital. She also says that she likes going out with her friends, reading and listening to music. She asks why she has been put in a room on her own - she had hoped to be able to talk with other patients.

- What assumptions did the ward staff hold about Lisa before she arrived, and on what did they base these assumptions?
- How might these assumptions impact on the way in which they provide nursing care for Lisa?
- What could be done to try and prevent such situations from occurring?

ANSWER:
CASE STUDY 37.2

For example, someone is not disabled by the fact that they need to use a wheelchair but rather as a consequence of buildings being built with stairs rather than with ramps and lifts. Whereas the individual or medical model of disability locates the 'problem' of disability within the individual, the social model argues that the 'problem' lies within socially created barriers that disable people. The focus for change therefore becomes the barriers rather than the person.

The social model of disability has been criticised by some authors. For example, Crow (1996) argued that it underplays the impact impairments may have on disabled people, such as pain and low energy levels, and how these effects can themselves limit participation. She argues for a 'renewed' social model that recognises these effects and which therefore more accurately reflects the reality of the daily lives of many disabled people.

Stigma

Erving Goffman, whose book *Stigma* was published in 1963, highlighted how, as human beings, we all categorise other people according to the characteristics that we deem to be 'normal' for people within these categories. This means that when we meet someone belonging to a specific category or group, we have some idea of how to interact with them. For example, you probably have some idea of what to expect and how to behave when you meet a ward sister, even if you have not met them personally before. These expectations are often based on stereotypes, but they enable us to function socially, as they help to prepare us for new situations. However, in some situations we meet people who are different in some way to what we would view as being 'normal' for someone within their category, and often these differences are judged negatively. This then leads to negative judgements being made about the person. The negative characteristic(s) are referred to as 'stigma', which Goffman (1963: 13) defines as 'an attribute that is deeply discrediting'. He makes the point, however, that stigma is only relevant in terms of how it influences the relationship between one person and others: the characteristic itself is neither positive nor negative. For example, think back to Lisa's case study (37.2). Down's syndrome (her 'stigma') was viewed negatively by some staff, but not by Helen.

I work in mental health nursing and many of those that experience mental health problems have experienced prejudices during their life, including the prejudice of having mental health problems. The care provided to those with mental health problems should be non-judgemental, but it can be difficult and if you're working with individuals with many different values and opinions to your own then you may unknowingly react in a way that could be perceived to be prejudiced. To have an awareness of your own values and beliefs and preconceptions can help to give you a better understanding of how you may react in situations that can be challenging to you. It is of the upmost importance as a nurse that you treat those you're working with equally and fairly and this cannot be done unless you have some insight into your own preconceptions – often, these preconceptions can be misplaced or stem from information that is inaccurate. This is something that students and newly qualified nurses need to be aware of so those in your care can feel they are receiving a fair and equal service that is compassionate and understanding of what can be a very stressful experience for them.

Samantha Vanes, NQ RNMH

Goffman (1963) further distinguishes between characteristics that are discredited (they are immediately evident) and those that are discreditable (the individual is aware of them but may or may not disclose them to others because of concerns about how others will react). Examples of discreditable characteristics and how they may impact on someone's health and healthcare are provided in Table 37.3.

Table 37.3   Examples of how 'discreditable' characteristics may impact on people's health

'Discreditable' characteristic	Potential impact on health or healthcare
James is a young man diagnosed with type 1 diabetes, but he doesn't want to tell his friends as he worries they will see him as different and not want to be friends with him. He wants to fit in with his peer group	James does not stick to his diet when he is out with friends and plays lengthy games of football without checking his blood sugars. He has a hypoglycaemic attack while with his friends but because he has not told them about his condition they do not know what to do. As well as posing an acute risk to his health, such behaviour over a period of time would place him at risk of long-term complications of diabetes
Sally is a young woman with mild learning disabilities who lives at home with her partner and their young son. Both Sally and her partner attended special schools but between them they manage to cope with day-to-day life. Their son is currently unwell and Sally has brought him into hospital but she doesn't want to tell the staff that she cannot read in case they report her to social services and her child is taken away	On leaving hospital, she is given medication for her son and is told there is a leaflet which tells her what to do with it. No one checks her understanding of what is required and, as a consequence, her son ends up being readmitted due to the effects of taking too much medication. Social services are then informed by the staff of concerns they have regarding her ability to care for her child
Simon, a 36-year-old man, is acutely ill and his wife feels that he needs to attend the local A&E department. However, ten years ago he was a frequent visitor to this department when he was regularly taking illegal drugs. He subsequently went through a rehabilitation programme and has been clean for five years. His wife is unaware of this history and he is worried that if he goes to the emergency department, staff may recognise him and his wife will find out	It is obvious that if Simon is acutely ill then he is likely to need assessment and possibly treatment as a matter of urgency: delays could have a sudden and serious impact on his health. If he does attend the emergency department but does not disclose this aspect of his medical history, then there is a risk that important factors relevant to his current problems may be overlooked
Ms Emily Lucas is a 73-year-old retired school teacher who has lived in a small village all of her life. Recently, she has noticed that she is getting very forgetful, particularly about things such as what she needs to buy when she arrives at the local shop. She recently turned up at church on Saturday for a service that only takes place on Sunday. Despite being aware of this problem, she does not want to seek advice in case anyone suggests that she is not capable of living alone	If this loss of memory persists and support is not provided, Ms Lucas may place herself at risk. For example, she may either forget to take important medication or take too much. She may fail to turn off electrical equipment and perhaps find herself away from home without knowing where she is or how she got there

People may therefore keep certain 'differences' secret, fearing the consequences of disclosure, and this in turn may have a negative impact on their health. As nurses, it is important to be alert to this possibility and to use our assessment skills sensitively so that patients get the support they require. Some fears of disclosure may prove to be well founded, as disclosure is sometimes met with negative reactions, even amongst health professionals. Think, for example, of how someone might be judged if the words 'substance misuse' appear on their notes. If you read such a description before you met the person, what would your thoughts be? Negative assumptions can occur due to our preconceptions and prejudices, but an understanding of sociology can help us to identify and challenge these assumptions.

People to whom stigmatising 'labels' are applied are often seen as homogenous groups, and their individual differences in terms of (for example) abilities, achievements, relationships and support needs are overlooked. Instead, a group identity is conferred and this is usually negative, being associated with characteristics such as danger, untrustworthiness and unpredictable behaviour. This is the negative side of stereotypes: while they can sometimes be helpful, as they help us to predict what may happen in certain circumstances, they can also lead us to make assumptions based on prejudice rather than on personal experience of interacting with individuals.

Apply what you have learned in this chapter around attitudes and prejudices by reading Jasmine's case study, at https://study.sagepub.com/essentialnursing2e.

CASE STUDY:
JASMINE

CONCLUSION

At a basic level, sociology is concerned with understanding the social world, the systems and structures that operate within society and how people within societies interact at a variety of different levels. A key characteristic of sociology is that it encompasses a range of different theoretical perspectives, each of which offers different ways of explaining and understanding the social world.

What sociology offers to nursing is not knowledge based on the experience of one person, but a body of knowledge that has been built up through the systematic research of many sociologists.

The differing views and insights offered by sociology provide a range of explanations and nurses need to assess their relevance to the situations in which they find themselves. Sociology provides information which can help us to better understand patients' behaviour as well as their psycho-social needs, and it is important if we are to provide holistic and humanitarian nursing care.

CHAPTER SUMMARY

- Sociology enables us to understand the social world.
- There is value in nursing students studying sociology, so they can apply this to their practice.
- Different sociological perspectives offer us alternative ways of understanding.
- Sociology can help to challenge our assumptions and develop our critical thinking skills.
- Clear links exist between sociological views and the development of nursing practice.
- By encouraging us to question things we take for granted, sociology can help us to see other people's perspectives.
- An understanding of sociological concepts such as the family, poverty, disability and stigma enables us to deliver effective and holistic nursing care.

CRITICAL REFLECTION

Holistic care

Think of a patient or family that you have been involved in caring for recently. Try to identify how an understanding of sociology might have provided you with different perspectives concerning their situation. How could you have used this information to enhance the holistic care you provided?

GO FURTHER

Books

Allan, H., Traynor, M., Kelly, D. and Smith, P. (2016) *Understanding Sociology in Nursing*. London: SAGE. This book aims to enable nurses to understand how sociology can assist with better understanding the individuals and families with whom they work and the factors that impact on their practice.
Goodman, B. (2015) *Psychology and Sociology in Nursing*, 2nd edn. London: SAGE. A text specifically aimed at nursing students working in all fields of practice.

Journal articles

Pinikahana, J. (2003) 'Role of sociology within the nursing enterprise: Some reflections on the unfinished debate', *Nursing and Health Sciences*, 5: 175–80. A review of the literature on the relevance of sociology to nursing, exploring some of the arguments for and against sociology in nurse education.

Porter, S. (1995) 'Sociology and the nursing curriculum: A defence', *Journal of Advanced Nursing*, 21: 1130–5. A response to Sharp's argument that sociology cannot provide a knowledge base for nursing, reasserting the appropriateness of including sociology within a nursing curriculum.

Sharp, K. (1994) 'Sociology and the nursing curriculum: A note of caution', *Journal of Advanced Nursing*, 20: 391–5. An assessment of the relevance of sociology to the nursing curriculum, which concludes that it cannot in principle provide a knowledge base for action-orientated conduct such as nursing work.

Weblinks

FIND OUT MORE!

Go to https://study.sagepub.com/essentialnursing2e for weblinks related to this chapter. If you are using the interactive ebook, simply click on the book icon in the margin to go straight to the resource.

FURTHER READING: WEBLINKS

www.sochealth.co.uk/public-health-and-wellbeing/poverty-and-inequality/the-black-report-1980 – a link to the Black Report, which explores inequalities in health.

www.archive.official-documents.co.uk/document/doh/ih/part1b.htm – a link to the Acheson Report regarding inequalities in health.

www.instituteofhealthequity.org/resources-reports/fair-society-healthy-lives-the-marmot-review/fair-society-healthy-lives-full-report-pdf.pdf – a link to the Marmot Report on inequalities in health in England.

www.britsoc.co.uk/about – the website of the medical sociology study group within the British Sociological Association.

www.esrc.ac.uk/research – the website of the Economic and Social Research Council, where you can access information regarding current and recent research relating to social aspects of health and society.

http://webarchive.nationalarchives.gov.uk/20160704145749/http://www.improvinghealthandlives.org.uk/projects/particularhealthproblems – provides a range of research that presents evidence of the health inequalities experienced by people with learning disabilities.

Video links

VIDEO LINKS

Have a break from the text and go to https://study.sagepub.com/essentialnursing2e for useful videos related to this chapter. If you are using the interactive ebook, simply click on the lightbulb icon in the margin to go straight to the resource.

ACE YOUR ASSESSMENT

ONLINE QUIZZES

Review what you have learned by visiting the book's online resources at: https://study.sagepub.com/essentialnursing2e If using your interactive ebook, just click on the icon in the margin to go straight there.

- Test yourself with multiple-choice and short-answer questions.
- Revise key terms with the interactive flash cards.

REFERENCES

Acheson, D. (1998) *Independent Inquiry into Inequalities in Health*. London: HMSO. Available at: www. archive.official-documents.co.uk/document/doh/ih/part1b.htm (accessed 25 June 2014).

Allan, H., Traynor, M., Kelly, D. and Smith, P. (2016) *Understanding Sociology in Nursing*. London: SAGE.

Black, D. (1980) *Black Report: Inequalities in Health*. London: DHSS.

Crow, L. (1996) 'Including all our lives: Renewing the social model of disability', in C. Barnes and G. Mercer (eds), *Exploring the Divide: Illness and Disability*. Leeds: The Disability Press. pp. 55–73.

Fulcher, J. and Scott, J. (2011) *Sociology*. Oxford: Oxford University Press.

Giddens, A. and Sutton, P.W. (2013) *Sociology*, 7th edn. Cambridge: Polity Press.

Goffman, E. (1963) *Stigma*. Harmondsworth: Penguin.

Marmot, M. (2010) Fair Society, Healthy Lives (Marmot Review). Available at: www. instituteofhealthequity.org/resources-reports/fair-society-healthy-lives-the-marmot-review (accessed 16 May 2017).

Nursing and Midwifery Council (NMC) (2018) *Standards for Registered Nurse Education*. London: NMC.

Oliver, M. (1996) *Understanding Disability: From Theory to Practice*. Basingstoke: Macmillan.

Pinikahana, J. (2003) 'Role of sociology within the nursing enterprise: Some reflections on the unfinished debate', *Nursing and Health Sciences*, 5: 175–80.

Porter, S. (1995) 'Sociology and the nursing curriculum: A defence', *Journal of Advanced Nursing*, 21: 1130–5.

Sharp, K. (1994) 'Sociology and the nursing curriculum: A note of caution', *Journal of Advanced Nursing*, 20: 391–5.

INTRODUCTION TO PUBLIC HEALTH

CHARLENE LOBO

THIS CHAPTER COVERS

- What is public health?
- Why public health is important
- Inequalities in health

- Public health policy
- Public health practice in nursing

> " It is really difficult to get my children to eat any vegetables, but since the school started the allotment project, our children are really interested. The health visitor has managed to get the same project set up for our mum's group and now we all do it together – it is so much fun. We now not only eat more healthily, the exercise is also doing us good.
>
> **Charita, mother** "

> " I take a public health approach to practice by making sure that I work in partnership with all the members of staff involved in patients' care to make sure that the patients have the best experience they possibility can. I believe that this is a good thing because it helps provide holistic care for the patient.
>
> **Hannah Boyd, adult nursing student** "

> " A public health approach to practice is a good thing because it educates people about their own health needs, it raises awareness of what they can do to help themselves and it informs them where help is available to them. If people become more responsible and knowledgeable about their health this will lead to less demand on resources, with more resources being used for preventative care rather than reactive care, and lead to a healthier lifestyle for them.
>
> **Julie Davis, LD nursing student** "

Visit https://study.sagepub.com/essentialnursing2e to access a wealth of online resources for this chapter – watch out for the margin icons throughout the chapter. If you are using the interactive eBook, simply click on the margin icon to go straight to the resource.

INTRODUCTION

Public health takes a broad perspective on health with a focus on populations, considering what causes their ill health and how it can be improved, or how people can be prevented from becoming ill in the first instance. For some patients, ill health is caused by their living and working environments. Therefore, nurses should not just be working reactively, treating the illnesses, but should work proactively – preventing the occurrence of these illnesses in the first place. It could be argued that patients have a right to expect all nurses to advocate for them to improve the conditions in which they live and work so that they do not become ill. This chapter will explore what is meant by public health and, specifically, the role of nurses in the promotion of public health.

WHAT IS PUBLIC HEALTH?

ACTIVITY 38.1: REFLECTION

Before reading this chapter any further, take a few minutes to write down what you think public health means.

Public health is a field of practice that tackles health needs at a population level as opposed to an individual level, which is where most nurses usually focus their practice. In their day-to-day care of patients, nurses identify problems and deliver care that optimises health. However, this focus at an individual level may not encompass the broader remits of health which might impact on the people for whom you care. It could be argued that many nurses work so hard downstream, saving people from drowning, that they fail to look upstream to see why people are falling in the water in the first place! For example, we know that good nutrition is important for wound healing, and most nurses will promote this as part of their patient care. However, it is not only their lack of knowledge of good nutrition that may prevent people from achieving a healed wound, but a combination of other factors, such as access to affordable healthy food options, impaired mobility or social isolation.

Nurses often do not recognise or address the wider determinants of health in their patient care, making public health a marginalised area of practice for nursing. However, the growing public health challenges make it imperative that all nurses play a more active role in tackling the root causes of ill health (RCN, 2012).

Understanding the history of public health provides insights that can help to consider the position of public health today. Table 38.1 presents a summary of the evolution of public health, based on the work of Flemming (2012: 34), demonstrating how the underpinning philosophies of the times impacted on the scope of public health practice.

This historical perspective enables us to see that public health started with improved sanitation and social reform, and that responsibility for public health lay with local authorities. Public health grew in importance at the turn of the century, after the industrial revolution, as it became evident that the poor health of the workforce was having a significant impact on productivity. The health of the population was enhanced through improving the environmental conditions in which people live and instituting laws that protect the public from harm. With scientific advances and the emergence of

Table 38.1   Historical perspectives of public health (PH)

Time period	Public health perspective
1700–1880	The Industrial Revolution created the urbanisation of cities, with poor housing, sanitation and water, resulting in major epidemics of diseases such as cholera, typhoid and tuberculosis in the mid-nineteenth century. Many believed the miasma theory: that illness and disease were brought about by foul smells and poor atmosphere. This influenced the work of Florence Nightingale, who focused her work on hygiene and identified five essential points in securing health in houses: pure air, pure water, efficient drainage, cleanliness and light. The Industrial Revolution heralded many social and environmental reforms resulting from the Public Health Act of 1849
1880–1910	The development of germ theory and bacteriology became a major influence in the late nineteenth century, with the recognition that specific organisms cause specific diseases. Health boards were developed to provide guidance and aid to local authorities in developing their services, which covered sanitation, refuse collection, water supply, etc. Within the health services, the antiseptic and aseptic techniques, hand-washing and the use of carbolic acid were beginning to become popular practice in hospitals and contributed to improved health outcomes for the general population
1910–60	In the early part of the twentieth century, infectious diseases remained a major cause of death, but biomedical advances in vaccinations and antibiotics, the formation of the National Health Service and the expansion (and professional education) of health professions contributed to a strong **medical model** of health
1960–75	The medical model continued to dominate the health service, with advances in treatments and medical technologies. The early 1960s saw the emergence of conditions associated with lifestyle, such as hypertension, stroke and type 2 diabetes. Health education began to play an important role in dealing with these 'lifestyle diseases'
1975–80	Deaths due to lifestyle diseases were increasing and a seminal piece of research by Michael Marmot, commonly known today as the Whitehall Study, demonstrated a correlation between health, social status and the wider determinants of health. Despite this, health policy focus remained very strongly on health education and personal responsibility for health
1980–90	This era is known as New Public Health. It has been strongly influenced by the World Health Organization, and the main focus of public health has been the importance of socioeconomic and political influences on health and the resulting inequalities in health. The emergence of HIV/AIDS, lifestyle diseases and the management of long-term conditions led to increased strategies focusing on primary care and health promotion
2000–current	We are now in an era of 'ecological public health', which has seen an increase in infectious disease, a heightened burden of chronic illness on individuals and health services, and an appreciation of the impact of globalisation on health. There is a recognition that public health needs to find a stronger ecologically and environmentally sustainable strategy. Cost-effectiveness is a key driver, and multi-disciplinary (different professionals working together) and **multi-sectoral** (different organisations working together) strategies remain central to managing the health complexities of the twenty-first century

the National Health Service, public health developed a strong medical focus and health was achieved primarily through curative measures. However, we can now see that curative measures are inadequate to ensure the health of a population.

Today, the main causes of premature death come from lifestyle diseases and illnesses, so there is an impetus to focus on avoiding ill health and minimising the complications of existing conditions through promoting health. It has also become clear that there is a social gradient in the experience of health; this means that those worse off in society experience poorer health, often caused by the wider determinants of health. There is therefore a second impetus for nurses to focus on the wider socio-political agenda to improve the health of the people they care for.

ACTIVITY 38.2: CRITICAL THINKING

What does it mean to focus on the socio-political agenda? Such a focus is demonstrated by the 'Jamie's School Dinners' initiative. In 2005, British chef Jamie Oliver fronted a television series called 'Jamie's School Dinners' in which he highlighted the poor quality of school dinners. As a result, he began a major campaign to improve school dinners in British schools, which was very successful and continues to influence current school meal practices.

- Should school dinners and children's healthy diets be a concern for nurses in their role as patient advocates?
- What do you think nurses could do?

It is possible to relate such initiatives to nursing practice. Nurses in all fields of practice are aware of the increasing trends of obesity and type 2 diabetes, especially in the developed world. Where is the nursing voice, as the largest group of health professionals, to campaign for healthier diets? Nurses, and especially school nurses, could have played a very important role in joining Jamie's campaign. The nursing voice could do much to influence better food labelling and a reduction in salt and sugar in processed foods.

This is an example of where nurses could work 'upstream', using their political strength to put pressure on government to change policy and working on the wider socio-political agenda to improve health.

ACTIVITY 38.3: REFLECTION

Some nurses claim that they were drawn to nursing to provide care, not to be politicised. However, as has been identified within this chapter so far, health *is* a political issue.

- Reflect on your experience so far as a nursing student and consider whether you can observe inequalities in health and do nothing about them.

Definitions of public health

> Public health is the science and art of preventing disease, prolonging life and promoting health through the organized efforts of society. (Acheson, 1988: 1)

This is the most common definition of public health used and has been proposed by the World Health Organization (WHO, 2011). It was originally put forward by Winslow in 1920, was adapted by Acheson in 1988, and still holds true today. There are a number of very important concepts within this definition. First, it defines public health as a science and an art; in this way it not only puts public health within the medical and scientific domain but also includes the art of building social, therapeutic and multi-sectoral relationships important to public health practice. The second important concept is that public health is not only about reducing mortality, but also about improving quality of life and promoting health. Lastly, the notion of 'organized efforts of society' means that public health is the responsibility of everyone: governments, public, private and voluntary organisations. We all need to work together to improve health.

This definition involves activities that aim to provide conditions in which people can be healthy and focus on entire populations, not on individual patients or diseases. Thus, public health is concerned with the total system – not only with the eradication of a particular disease but also with identifying the major causes of illnesses and preventing them from occurring. According to the WHO (2014), the three main public health functions are:

- assessment and monitoring of the health of communities and populations at risk to identify health problems and priorities
- the formulation of public policies designed to solve identified local and national health problems and priorities
- to ensure that all populations have access to appropriate and cost-effective care, including health promotion and disease prevention services.

This definition is supported in the UK by the Faculty of Public Health (2010) and used in the public health policy *Healthy Lives, Healthy People* (DH, 2010). It highlights three domains of public health:

- health improvement
- health protection
- health services.

The domains are expressed diagrammatically in Figure 38.1, and enable us to think about the boundaries of practice in public health.

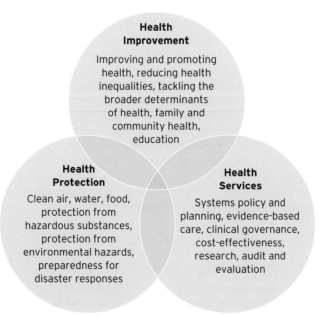

Figure 38.1   The domains of public health

Nursing practice tends to work primarily within the domain of healthcare services, providing evidence-based care, research, audit and evaluation. Nurses need to work more in the other domains, considering how they might contribute to health improvement, promoting health, reducing inequalities in health and influencing government policy that protects people's health.

ACTIVITY 38.4: LEADERSHIP

Will is a 4-year-old boy admitted for the second time this winter with acute exacerbation of asthma. He lives in local authority housing with his parents and two other siblings: Joshua, 7, who also has asthma, and Jasmin, 2, who has severe eczema. Their mum complains that the flat they live in is very damp, but she has asked to move with little success.

As a nurse, how could you exercise your public health role in this situation?

- What service could you provide?
- How might you promote their health in the future?
- How might you protect their health in the future?

WHY IS PUBLIC HEALTH IMPORTANT?

As has been outlined, historically the main cause of death in populations was infectious disease, which responded well to the medical and curative approaches to health. However, this focus on maintaining the health of populations can no longer meet the challenges of the twenty-first century, primarily due to the escalating costs of healthcare. This is for a number of reasons:

- Technological advances are continual and the resulting cost of diagnostic and therapeutic interventions constitutes a major expense in health service provision. It is possible to maintain life today in ways that were unimaginable even two decades ago.
- Demographic changes have implications for healthcare demand. People are living much longer with increasing levels of morbidity, and therefore greater levels of health and social care are needed.
- There are changes in disease patterns. For example, when the health service was first established, people tended to die from infectious diseases which responded relatively easily to curative measures. However, today the major cause of death is lifestyle diseases, requiring a very different and more complex approach to health. We need to consider how we might change the health service from an illness-focused system to an illness-prevention system.
- There is increasing demand and patient expectation. The internet has been a major factor in this debate. People have quick and easy access to information, and although this information may not always be appropriate or accurate, it does influence people's expectations and demands relating to what they believe to be the right treatment for them.

Working within learning disability services, I see many health inequalities for the people I support. There are still ongoing issues with physical access in many health settings. Although they may have put in ramps to enable access to the building, they haven't allowed for the extra room required inside the building to manoeuvre around when the individual is a wheelchair user. I have also encountered several incidents of diagnostic overshadowing, whereby health conditions have been attributed to someone's learning disability or diagnosis. For example, someone I supported was given antibiotics for a urine infection without any examination.

Michelle Hill, NQ RNLD

- In addition to the increased cost of ill health, there are increasing inequalities in health. This is discussed in more detail in the next section, but health inequalities, where poor people experience poor health, are gaining increasing significance and contradict the notion of a fair and just society that underpins the constitution of the NHS. Tackling inequalities in health requires a different approach, one that puts a strong emphasis on preventing ill health and looks for solutions to ill health in the environmental and socio-economic domains that contribute to it in the first place.

INEQUALITIES IN HEALTH

Inequalities in health have been gaining greater importance in the public health landscape over the past few decades. As the public health movement grows towards a more ecological and ethical value base, so inequalities in health are taking a more central role on the public health agenda. Health inequalities are about avoidable, unjust differences in the health experience between different societal groups (Whitehead and Dahlgren, 2006), as is clearly identified in the Marmot Review:

> The Marmot Review states there are gaps of up to 7 years in life expectancy between the richest and poorest neighbourhoods, and up to 17 years in disability-free life expectancy… It also highlights wide variation within areas; for instance in London, in one ward in Kensington and Chelsea, a man now has a life expectancy of 88 years, compared with 71 years in Tottenham Green, one of the capital's poorer wards. Low income and deprivation are particularly associated with higher levels of obesity, smoking, mental illness and harms arising from drug and alcohol misuse. (DH, 2010: 15)

Over the past few decades, valid research has emerged that attributes these inequities predominantly to the social and economic conditions in which people live (Black, 1980; Acheson, 1998; Marmot, 2010). This means that the poorer you are, the worse your health experience is, as the poorest in society tend to be most exposed to health risks through exposure to unhealthy environments.

I cared for one patient that had a history of alcohol and drug abuse and as a result of this some of the members of staff treated him a bit differently from the other patients and did not show him as much empathy. As a result of this I was more drawn to this patient and I think that I helped make his stay a bit more positive by cheering him up and being there if he wanted to talk. I did not think I cared for him any differently than the other patients, I just gave him the dignity and respect he deserved.

Hannah Boyd, adult nursing student

Although the issue of inequalities in health is complex, there is a strong body of theory (Marmot, 2010; Wilkinson and Pickett, 2009) that seems to identify three main causal pathways:

- Early childhood experiences affect future health.
- Income, education and position in the social hierarchy have direct impacts on health.
- People with social capital and who have strong 'social connectedness' have lower mortality and are less likely to experience ill health.

These causal pathways suggest that the answer to reducing these health inequalities lies in working with groups and communities to tackle the wider determinants of health, incorporating the basic principles of public health practice.

Nurses see these inequalities in health on an everyday basis. Because of the presence of inequalities in health, it follows that nurses will care for a higher proportion of people who experience an unfair disparity in health outcomes. To abide by their code of conduct (NMC, 2015), all nurses should incorporate the principles of public health practice in the everyday care they provide to their patients.

WHAT'S THE EVIDENCE?

FURTHER
READING:
HOW HEALTHY
ARE WE?

Acheson, D. (1998) *Independent Inquiry into Inequalities in Health*. London: HMSO; Buck, D. (2011) How Healthy Are We? Available at: www.kingsfund.org.uk/topics/public-health/how-healthy-are-we; Marmot, M. (2010) Fair Society, Healthy Lives: The Marmot Review. Available at: www.ucl.ac.uk/marmotreview.

In 1998, Sir Donald Acheson produced a report, commissioned by the Labour government, on the evidence of inequalities in health. He presented a range of research that supported the emerging theories on the disparity of health experience between those of higher and lower social status. This report had a significant and wide-ranging impact on much of the subsequent policy output from the Labour government of the time. In 2009, Sir Michael Marmot was commissioned by the government to conduct a review of health inequalities in England, and his report, Fair Society, Healthy Lives, makes compelling reading. He states that differences in healthcare matter, as do differences in lifestyle, but the key determinants of inequality in health lie in the circumstances in which people are born, grow, live, work and age. More recently, David Buck (2011) produced an excellent commentary which explores some of the evidence on inequalities in health and raises some interesting insights regarding possible solutions.

What inequalities in health can you identify by reflecting on your experience of caring for patients?

- What suggestions would you make to reduce these inequalities?
- Now read any of the above reports and see whether your solutions are similar to those recommended.

PUBLIC HEALTH POLICY

Government policy plays an important role in providing direction for healthcare provision and significantly impacts on public health practice in relation to the nurse's role.

Much public health policy in the UK has evolved as a result of initiatives from the World Health Organization (WHO). The WHO, as part of the United Nations, leads on global health, setting standards and guidelines, highlighting areas for research, monitoring health trends and helping countries that might face serious health challenges to work towards better health (WHO, 2014). One of the most influential documents and developments in public health policy is the WHO Declaration of Alma-Ata (1978), which articulated the concept of 'Health for All by 2000'. The key messages were:

- The original definition of health was 'a state of complete physical, mental and social wellbeing and not merely the absence of disease or infirmity' and a human right.

- Health inequality brought about due to socio-economic reasons is unacceptable.
- Economic and social development are not only important for good health, but good health is also important for economic and social development.
- People have a right to participate in the planning of their care.
- Governments have a responsibility for the health of their people, and a key target was 'health for all by 2000'.
- Primary healthcare must take centre stage in helping to achieve these targets.

It is clear that these targets have not been met, but the principles of this declaration still hold and underlie much public health policy in the UK today.

UK policy

Within the UK, central government at Westminster decides what happens in England, with Wales, Scotland and Northern Ireland having their own parliamentary systems. These produce strategic plans for their own nations, but still acknowledge central government policy and guidance.

The key document currently influencing public health within all nations of the UK is the White Paper *Healthy Lives, Healthy People: Our Strategy for Public Health in England* (DH, 2010). The foreword by Andrew Lansley, the then Minister for Health, describes the state of health in the UK:

> Britain is now the most obese nation in Europe. We have among the worst rates of sexually transmitted infections recorded, a relatively large population of problem drug users and rising levels of harm from alcohol. Smoking alone claims over 80,000 lives every year. Experts estimate that tackling poor mental health could reduce our overall disease burden by nearly a quarter. Health inequalities between rich and poor have been getting progressively worse. We still live in a country where the wealthy can expect to live longer than the poor. (DH, 2010: 2)

This policy document sets out the government's vision for how it will respond to the major public health challenges of the twenty-first century – such as smoking, obesity, alcohol abuse – through a redefined public health service. It was followed by the Health and Social Care Act 2012, which radically reformed the way healthcare is commissioned and, in England, moved the function of public health from the NHS to local authorities. All health-promotion activities remain NHS roles in Wales, Scotland and Northern Ireland, but in England a new body, Public Health England, was established in 2013 to provide strategic leadership, support and health protection.

Public Health England represents an integrated, national public health service, with public health teams sitting within local authorities to place health at the heart of public services. This move reflects the pre-1974 NHS, when many of the community health services were under local authority control. Public Health England has the overall remit to protect and improve the nation's health and improve inequalities. The main directories within Public Health England are:

- emergencies
- health and wellbeing resources
- health protection data and knowledge gateway
- public health regional and local teams.

This organisation is an important resource for nurses to use in exercising their public health role.

ACTIVITY 38.5: REFLECTION

What do you think are the main public health challenges that face your nation? Which health challenges should all health professionals, and especially you as a nurse, attempt to improve in practice?

PUBLIC HEALTH PRACTICE IN NURSING

The aim of public health practice in nursing is to focus on care upstream, and therefore reduce the amount of downstream work in each of the domains of public health, as outlined above. This is done by:

- trying to understand health conditions in a population: what is making people sick, and why? (Diseases and their determinants, distribution, risk factors, etc.)
- trying to determine how we ameliorate these conditions and how we prevent them
- considering ways in which we treat conditions when we cannot prevent them.

We will now explore the nurse's role in public health, focusing on these key areas of practice.

Trying to understand health conditions in a population

The aim of this practice is to try to understand the needs of the people, whether it is a group, community or population.

The first step is to examine the overall profile of the people for whom you care. Who are they? What is their health like? How does this compare to other people in other areas? This is the function of the Joint Strategic Needs Assessment (JSNA). The JSNA is a high-level analysis of the health of the population. It is developed between local public health teams and the local authorities and tells you about the health of people in your area, and is available through local council or neighbourhood statistics websites. Public Health England (2013) has information on a range of indicators from all over the country which can be used to compare the health of different populations.

ACTIVITY 38.6: REFLECTIVE PRACTICE

You and your practice educator Glyn, a community mental health nurse, are working with a patient who has schizophrenia:

- What are the wider implications of your practice?
- How big a problem is this in your area?
- What are the **root causes** of the problem?
- How might you combine resources, and who with, to tackle the problem?

> I had been dealing with an unpopular patient in A&E who had multiple admissions over many days. This patient had poor hygiene and therefore was creating a negative impact in the environment for other patients. After many attempts with staff to address this aspect of this patient's care, given that this department doesn't often deal with this, I was able to get a member of staff to help me assist addressing this patient's hygiene needs. This resulted in a positive mood in the patient, removing the unpopular label and a positive environment for patients.
>
> Laura Grimley, adult nursing student

Trying to determine how we improve these conditions

Public health is about the wider environment in which we live and the opportunities we have: it's about prevention rather than cure. Health improvement is concerned with positively influencing the factors that promote health in populations and reducing unfair variations between communities in terms of health outcomes. Areas such as tobacco control, smoking cessation, physical activity promotion, healthy eating and obesity prevention would all be expected to feature as desirable health outcomes. However, educational attainment, fulfilling work and affordable housing are also factors that impact on health outcomes. The wider environment's influence on health requires policy interventions to be increasingly evidence-based and also preventative, focusing on the root cause of ill health rather than just simply treating the consequences of its development. This supports the argument that nurses need to think beyond the remit of the NHS and work in partnership with other organisations and disciplines in order to create positive environments for health.

Social (wider) determinants of health

Health education or campaigns alone are not, however, enough to change everyone's behaviour. Lifestyle choices are greatly influenced by people's living, working, financial and social circumstances. Where a person lives, whether they have work, how much money they have and the social support networks available to them are all vital factors influencing risks to their health. Even wider determinants of health include the availability of food, access to health services, climate change and environmental pollutants. Health promotion involves addressing the so-called inequalities in health in these circumstances. Having healthy public policies and strategic plans in place can enable people, through social change, to make healthier choices. The ban on smoking in public not only protects non-smokers from passive smoking, it also enables smokers to avoid the pressure to smoke and to consider quitting. Vouchers for healthy food for low-income mothers, traffic regulations, free condoms for sex workers and needle-exchange programmes for drug addicts are further examples of national and local strategic policies designed to address inequalities.

The contribution of social and economic factors to health outcomes is the driving force underpinning the transfer of public health to local government. The local authorities at both county and district levels oversee the delivery of a number of services and set the local direction in important areas such as leisure, transport, environmental health, housing, economic regeneration and development, all of which directly impact on the health outcomes of residents. Nurses need to consider how they might influence and engage in the development of such services. Deprivation is strongly linked to poor health outcomes. We also know that people from lower socio-economic classes are more likely to smoke and find it harder to give up compared to those from higher classes.

ACTIVITY 38.7: REFLECTIVE PRACTICE

You and your practice educator, Maidie, a learning disability nurse, are visiting a patient who has diabetes. The patient has a carer, Jim, who gives her insulin injections, but Jim is struggling to help the patient manage her diet and has asked for support.

- What is your public health response?

Health protection is the area of public health practice that aims to reduce the dangers to health from infections, chemicals and radiation hazards. Public health practitioners ensure that surveillance systems are in place to allow early identification and response to public health threats. They work closely with emergency preparedness, resilience and response agencies, such as the police and the fire and rescue service, to plan and respond to a range of incidents and emergencies that can impact on the health of individuals and communities.

ACTIVITY 38.8: REFLECTIVE PRACTICE

You are working on a children's ward with Padraig, your practice educator, and are about to discharge a premature baby. The mother of this baby is very anxious and worried about the effect of immunisation on such a small baby.

- How will you respond to her anxieties?

How we treat conditions when we cannot prevent them

Public health practice is concerned with improving the equity of provision and quality of health and social care services; it is about getting the most out of the money we spend on health and social care. Services should be provided on a basis of need and using the best evidence to ensure it is effective and cost-effective. Ultimately, NHS and social care prioritisation needs to focus on preventing the use of expensive hospital and care services; this can be done by investing in programmes and services designed to keep people independent, active and following a healthy lifestyle.

Apply your understanding of treating conditions you cannot prevent by reading Adrianne's case study, at https://study.sagepub.com/essentialnursing2e.

CASE STUDY:
ADRIANNE

ACTIVITY 38.9: REFLECTION

Many nurses feel that they don't have enough time to care, and so engaging in the wider public health agenda is an unrealistic aspiration:

- If this is the case, how will we ever change?
- Do you think that nurses have a right to choose how it is most effective to use their time to produce the best patient outcomes?

CONCLUSION

All nurses work in public health, to a lesser or greater extent depending on where they work, the type of work they do and the position they hold. Nurses need to move their focus from the individual to the population perspective, consider how the broader determinants of health might impact on a patient's health and know what and whom they can work with to improve outcomes for patients.

If nurses are to be true advocates for their patients, they need to play a strong role in the political arena and use their strength in numbers to work together to campaign to improve the environment in which their patients live. There is an urgent requirement to move from the prevailing dominant medical model of illness to a social model of wellness (DH, 2014) as the current model will make healthcare unaffordable.

CHAPTER SUMMARY

- The health of the nation has changed over the past century and there is a need for a different approach to maintaining the health of populations.
- Public health is very wide-reaching and encompasses promoting health, protecting health and treating illness. However, most health resources are spent on the latter and there needs to be a stronger shift towards promoting health.
- Public health is about having a stronger focus on the population perspective.
- Nurses need to understand the wider determinants of health in order to widen their health-promotion practice.
- Public health is about working across organisations and disciplines to improve health outcomes.
- There needs to be much more focus on reducing the widening health inequalities between rich and poor.
- Working in public health requires advocacy, communication and negotiation skills to influence policy.

CRITICAL REFLECTION

Holistic care

This chapter has highlighted the importance of public health in providing holistic care for your patient. Review the chapter and note down all the instances where you think applying public health practice will help meet the patient's physical, psychological, social, economic and spiritual needs. Think of a variety of different patients across the fields, not just within your own field. You may find it helpful to make a list and refer back to it next time you are in practice, and then write your own reflection after your practice experience.

GO FURTHER

Books

Linsley, P., Kane, R. and Owen, S. (2011) *Nursing for Public Health: Promotion, Principles and Practice.* Oxford: Oxford University Press. This is a very accessible text that comprehensively addresses public health from a nursing perspective. A strong theoretical base underpins practice perspectives supported by a range of case studies and discussion points, which greatly enhances the understanding of proposed concepts.

Wilkinson, R. and Pickett, K. (2010) *The Spirit Level: Why Equality is Better for Everyone.* London: Penguin. This book is compelling reading about the evidence on inequalities in health and the impact of income inequality on health. It makes a powerful moral argument for a fairer society and will help you think critically about your role as a nurse.

Journal articles

Glasper, A. (2014) 'The nursing and midwifery contribution to public health', *British Journal of Nursing,* 22(15): 900-1. Glasper explains nursing and midwifery's public health contribution to UK health policy. This is a very accessible article that identifies the different government public health initiatives and the roles nurses can play.

Hogg, R., Ritchie, D., de Kok, B., Wood, C. and Huby, G. (2013) 'Parenting support for families with young children: A public health, user-focused study undertaken in a semi-rural area of Scotland', *Journal of Clinical Nursing,* 22(7-8): 1140-50. This article describes a range of public health interventions to provide support to parents of young children. It is helpful in demonstrating multi-disciplinary and multi-sectoral working in public health.

Long, J.D., Boswell, C., Rogers, T.J., Littlefield, L.A., Estep, G., Shriver, B.J., et al. (2013) 'Effectiveness of cell phones and mypyramidtracker.gov to estimate fruit and vegetable intake', *Applied Nursing Research,* 26(1): 17-23. This research study demonstrates an effective intervention for one of the major public health challenges on healthy eating. It is helpful as it demonstrates effective, innovative responses to the government public health agenda.

Weblinks

FURTHER
READING:
WEBLINKS

Go to https://study.sagepub.com/essentialnursing2e for weblinks related to this chapter. If you are using the interactive ebook, simply click on the book icon in the margin to go straight to the resource.

www.equalitytrust.org.uk - this site includes excellent resources that explain the evidence of inequalities in health and signposts further resources for intervention planning.

www.nice.org.uk - operating within the domains of public health and public health practice, a wealth of information on public health guidance and best practice interventions in a range of topics is provided on the National Institute for Health and Care Excellence website.

www.gov.uk/government/organisations/public-health-england – the government's Public Health England website covers a whole range of information related to public health. It is important for you to access this site so that you are aware of the range of public health work that is covered in the UK and the information available to health professionals.

http://fingertips.phe.org.uk/profile/health-profiles – this site is part of Public Health England and holds the health profiles of all local authorities in England. It is useful for you to look at to gain insight into what the health of your community is like and how it compares to other areas.

www.gov.uk/government/collections/developing-the-public-health-contribution-of-nurses-and-midwives-tools-and-models – another site which is part of Public Health England and offers a range of information and guidance on the nursing contribution to public health.

www.fph.org.uk – the Faculty of Public Health is an organisation that sets the standards for specialist public health practitioners. It is a particularly useful site as it produces critiques of government health policy. It also offers access to the *Journal of Public Health*.

─────────────────── **ACE YOUR ASSESSMENT** ───────────────────

Review what you have learned by visiting the book's online resources at: https://study.sagepub.com/essential nursing2e If using your interactive ebook, just click on the icon in the margin to go straight there.

ONLINE
QUIZZES

- Test yourself with multiple-choice and short-answer questions.
- Revise key terms with the interactive flash cards.

REFERENCES

Acheson, D. (1988) *Public Health in England: The Report of the Committee of Inquiry into the Future Development of the Public Health Function*. London: HMSO.

Acheson, D. (1998) *Independent Inquiry into Inequalities in Health*. London: HMSO. Available at: www.archive.official-documents.co.uk/document/doh/ih/part1b.htm (accessed 25 June 2014).

Black, D. (1980) *Black Report: Inequalities in Health*. London: DHSS.

Buck, D. (2011) How Healthy Are We? Available at: www.kingsfund.org.uk/topics/public-health/how-healthy-are-we (accessed 20 July 2014).

Department of Health (DH) (2010) *Healthy Lives, Healthy People: Our Strategy for Public Health in England*. London: HMSO.

Department of Health (2014) Wellbeing: Why it Matters to Health Policy. Available at: www.gov.uk/government/uploads/system/uploads/attachment_data/file/277566/Narrative__January_2014_.pdf (accessed 20 July 2014).

Faculty of Public Health (FPH) (2010) What is Public Health? Available at: www.fph.org.uk/what_is_public_health (accessed 20 July 2014).

Flemming, L. (2012) 'History and development of public health', in L. Flemming and E. Parker (eds), *Introduction to Public Health*, 2nd edn. Sydney, NSW: Elsevier.

Marmot, M. (2010) Fair Society, Healthy Lives (The Marmot Review). Available at: www.ucl.ac.uk/marmotreview (accessed 20 July 2014).

Nursing and Midwifery Council (NMC) (2015) *The Code: Professional Standards of Practice and Behaviour for Nurses and Midwives*. London: NMC.

Public Health England (PHE) (2013) *Nursing and Midwifery Contribution to Public Health: Improving Health and Wellbeing*. London: PHE. Available at: www.gov.uk/government/uploads/system/uploads/attachment_data/file/210100/NMR_final.pdf (accessed 20 July 2014).

Royal College of Nursing (RCN) (2012) *Going Upstream: Nursing's Contribution to Public Health*. London: RCN.

Whitehead, M. and Dahlgren, G. (2006) Concepts and Principles for Tackling Social Inequities in Health: Levelling up – Part 1. Available at: www.euro.who.int/__data/assets/pdf_file/0010/74737/E89383.pdf (accessed 20 July 2014).

Wilkinson, R. and Pickett, K. (2009) The Spirit Level: Why equality is better for everyone. Available at: www.dur.ac.uk/resources/wolfson.institute/events/Wilkinson372010.pdf (accessed 10 March 2015).

Winslow, C. (1920) 'The untilled fields of public health', *Science*, 51(1306): 23–33.

World Health Organization (WHO) (1978) The Declaration of Alma-Ata. International Conference on Primary Health Care, Alma-Ata, USSR, 6–12 September. Available at: www.who.int/publications/almaata_declaration_en.pdf (accessed 10 March 2015).

World Health Organization (2011) Strengthening Public Health Capacities and Services in Europe: A framework for action. Available at: www.euro.who.int/__data/assets/pdf_file/0011/134300/09E_Strengthening PublicHealthFramework_110452_eng.pdf (accessed 20 July 2014).

World Health Organization (2014) Glossary of Globalization, Trade and Health. Available at: www.who.int/trade/glossary/story076/en/ (accessed 20 July 2014).

INTRODUCTION TO HEALTH POLICY AND THE POLITICAL CONTEXT OF NURSING

SIOBHAN MCCULLOUGH

THIS CHAPTER COVERS

- Health policy, politics and the political context of nursing

- The impact of health policy devolution in the UK
- UK health policy themes

> " As an American citizen, every time I visit the UK I marvel at its wonderful healthcare system. Yes, there is always talk in the media about problems and the politicians like to 'tinker' with it, but the NHS has to be one of the best ideas in the history of the world.
>
> **Oscar B. Hades, American tourist** "

> " It is my first week at university and I have just checked my timetable, and noticed I have lectures on politics and health policy and a visit to the Northern Ireland Assembly. I am surprised because I did not think nurses need to know about politics. However, in our first lecture when it was explained why it is relevant to me as a nursing student, I understood! I am now really looking forward to the visit to the Assembly and the whole class are busy preparing questions to ask our elected representatives.
>
> **Tara, first-year child nursing student** "

Visit https://study.sagepub.com/essentialnursing2e to access a wealth of online resources for this chapter – watch out for the margin icons throughout the chapter. If you are using the interactive eBook, simply click on the margin icon to go straight to the resource.

INTRODUCTION

'There isn't a magic money tree that we can shake that suddenly provides for everything that people want.' (Sparrow et al., 2017)

96% drop in EU nurses registering to work in Britain since Brexit vote. (Siddique, 2017)

The above were headline news in *The Guardian* newspaper, capturing some of the reasons why it is important for you to understand the relationship between nursing, health policy and the political context of care, in the United Kingdom's National Health Service (NHS). The first headline relates to Prime Minister Theresa May's response during a general election special edition of BBC's *Question Time*, when a nurse asked how it could be fair to earn the same wage in 2017 as she did in 2009, in light of the job nurses do. This refers to the 1 per cent cap on annual public sector pay since the 2010 general election, which has resulted in a decrease in salary, due to inflation. The second headline relates to one of the consequences of the 2016 UK referendum vote to exit the European Union, which has led to an apparent reluctance amongst EU nurses to seek employment in Britain. This is in the context of a pre-existing shortage of 30,000 nurses in England alone (Siddique, 2017). It is important to look beyond the headlines, however, because behind the headlines lie many complex arguments. Thus, understanding the political, economic and social context of these arguments helps you to critically reflect on health policy theoretically and professionally, and to view nursing within an informed political context, which will enable you to advocate for people in your care.

To assist you to develop your knowledge, this chapter will identify a number of health policy issues, including the 'shift' from acute hospital-based care to community care, the quality of nursing care, devolution and the Francis Report (Mid Staffordshire NHS Foundation Trust Public Inquiry, 2013).

HEALTH POLICY, POLITICS AND THE POLITICAL CONTEXT OF NURSING

As Tara highlighted at the start of the chapter, many nursing students (and registered nurses) perceive politics and nursing to be incompatible, so therefore irrelevant to them. This may be because politics involves making choices about scarce resources, which is at odds with the notion of care and nursing practice guided by altruism. Alternatively, it may be that nurses are uninterested in politics because it is largely absent from the nursing curriculum, and thus nurses have not been socialised or taught to be politically aware. As a result, nursing students often report that they find politics boring, difficult to understand or complex. However, as they progress through their degree programme and beyond, many students begin to realise that politics affects them intrinsically – not just as nursing students but also as citizens – and come to realise how important it is to understand the political context of care and to also influence it. Furthermore, the standards for education and training (and the standards of proficiency) (NMC, 2015, 2017) reflect the need to implicitly understand the contemporary health and social care agenda and to achieve student empowerment.

WHAT'S THE EVIDENCE?

WEBLINK:
NICE

Ball, J.E., Griffiths, P., Rafferty, A.M., Lindqvist, R., Murrells, T. and Tishelman, C. (2016) 'A cross-sectional study of "care left undone" on nursing shifts in hospitals', *Journal of Advanced Nursing*, 72(9): 2086-97; NHS Improvement (2016) Safe Staffing for Adult Inpatients in Acute Care. Available at: https://improvement.nhs.uk/resources/safe-staffing-improvement-resources-adult-inpatient-acute-care; NICE (2014)

Safe Staffing for Nursing in Adult Inpatient Wards in Acute Hospitals. Available at: www.nice.org.uk/Guidance/SG1.

In a Swedish study based in acute care hospitals, Ball et al. (2016) considered how the number of nurses providing care related to 'care left undone' (or missed care), and if lesser registered nurse numbers contributed to poorer care quality and thus adversely influenced patient outcomes.

Until relatively recently, little evidence existed about hospital nurse staffing levels' impact on the outcomes of care. However, there is growing evidence internationally that in hospitals where nurses care for fewer patients, better outcomes in patient mortality and nurses' job satisfaction are achieved. This study adds to this evidence. NICE (2014) published guidance on safe staffing. However, in June 2015 NICE suspended work on the safe staffing programme, as this was to be taken forward by the newly formed NHS Improvement, in conjunction with NHS England. In June 2015, NICE had been developing safe staffing evidence reviews in four areas, which had not progressed through the full development process. NICE did however decide to release these reviews.

- Reflect on your experiences of placement areas in terms of staffing levels, particularly in acute care settings and how this affects you as a nursing student.
- What influence do you feel nurse staffing levels have on patient care, registered nurses' job satisfaction and the support you receive to facilitate your learning?
- Read the Ball et al. (2016) study and see if it reflects your own experiences in practice.
- Read the NICE (2014) and NHS Improvement (2016) guidelines and reflect on your observation and experiences of patient–nurse ratios in practice.

Adopting a political perspective and becoming politically aware do not mean you have to become active in political party politics. However, it will provide you with some of the tools to enable you to reflect critically on practice, and support you to deliver care which is holistic, compassionate and person-centred (Kitson et al., 2013). Contemporary examples of political issues which affect nurses include: the removal of student nurse bursaries in England, the impact of NHS funding, the political debate relating to the impact of the UK exit from the EU and the current cap on public sector pay.

The World Health Organization's definition of health as 'a state of complete physical, mental and social well-being and not merely the absence of disease or infirmity' (WHO, 1948) is a holistic and positive view of health, which reflects the philosophy underpinning nursing. Accepting this definition broadens the topic of health to include politics, economics, social and environmental processes. This can help you begin to understand how nurses are well positioned to help address health inequalities, poverty and social justice issues.

ACTIVITY 39.1: CRITICAL THINKING

Construct a timeline of the main policy developments within healthcare, over the past 30 years. The following documents will help you to do this:

- Nuffield Trust (n.d) The History of NHS Reform. Available at: http://nhstimeline.nuffieldtrust.org.uk
- English Heritage (n.d.) Back to the Community: Disability equality, rights and inclusion. Available at: www.english-heritage.org.uk/discover/people-and-places/disability-history/1945-to-the-present-day/back-to-the-community

Can you identify any themes within the policy developments you have placed on your timeline?

WEBLINK:
NUFFIELD
TRUST

ANSWER:
ACTIVITY 39.1

Considering how nursing has developed professionally and what it means to become a registered nurse gives you some insight into what policy-making involves. Nursing evolved from early religious and military roots, and this journey was punctuated by developments in many areas, including professional registration, a code of practice, educational degree status, standards for education and practice, quality of care issues and an evidence-based focus. These developments were often the result of pressure from both inside and outside nursing, and they took place in a political context.

A useful way of beginning to think about nursing in a political context is to consider Chaffee et al.'s (2012) definition of politics as the process of influencing the allocation of scarce resources. Health policy-making takes place in a political context because those developing policy are accountable for resources and for policy formulation, implementation, outcomes and the evaluation of that policy. Politics is inextricably linked to the development of health policy and 'health policy is often seen as a party political football' (Baggott, 2015: 21).

Although health policy-making is often referred to as a rational process, with a number of clear-cut stages, the reality is more complicated than this, with many factors influencing the progress of policy. Thus, there are a myriad of influences affecting the processes of health policy formulation and implementation. This happens within a political context, whereby political parties try to influence and persuade electors to vote for them, by offering to be the party who will change aspects of healthcare (and other policies), within the UK. As we have already outlined, however, nurses, in the UK and internationally, often do not engage with politics or health policy to any significant degree and thus they tend to exert limited influence in this arena. However, if you are armed with knowledge and understanding of health policy, this could enable you to engage more fruitfully and critically in the political arena.

The reasons for this are complex, but it seems nurses have tended to regard themselves as less intellectual and therefore less influential than other professions. Thus, in general, nurses do not expect their opinions to be valued and do not value political involvement. Furthermore, political content in nurse education programmes tends to be minimal or absent, so it is little wonder nurses perceive politics as complicated and hard to understand and find policy content abstract

It is important to be politically aware as government ideologies, budgets and policies directly impact our working environment. It is important to be aware of the guidelines they produce and the impact these have on the services we provide. We can also influence policy and laws by being politically active and making governments aware of the needs of our service and the good it has also done.

Julie Davis, LD nursing student

Being politically aware can be advantageous to gaining awareness or support for services or projects. It can help with positive changes.

Laura Grimley, adult nursing student

and intangible. Returning again to the development of the nursing profession, nursing has historically been seen as 'women's work', and so is under-resourced and under-analysed, which then leads to internal ambiguity (Davies, 2004). This means that the status and legitimacy of the nurse may be questioned, resulting in nurses not being regarded as equal partners in the policy arena (Davies, 2004).

THE IMPACT OF HEALTH POLICY DEVOLUTION IN THE UK

Adopting a political perspective involves an understanding of the national and international political context. Westminster politics has tended to dominate the UK political landscape and, since 1945, governments have usually been single-party majority governments of either the Labour or Conservative party. This is due to the first past the post electoral system. The 2010 general election was thus politically significant, having resulted in the creation of a Conservative/Liberal Democrat coalition government. The 2015 general election resulted in a Conservative government, with a small and precarious majority of only 12 seats. The snap election called by Theresa May in 2017, ostensibly to provide the Conservative government with a greater mandate to undertake the complex UK exit from the EU negotiations, lead instead to a hung parliament. This meant no party had an overall majority of seats with which to form a government. Thus, the Conservative party, which had the largest number of seats (317), formed a minority government with the support of Northern Ireland's Democratic Unionist Party (DUP), who had won 10 seats. This was not quite the mandate Theresa May had anticipated and her minority government is currently experiencing a torturous journey through the Brexit negotiations. It is also important to bear in mind that English health policy often seems to be portrayed as NHS health policy – an incorrect portrayal, because health policy differs within the four countries that make up the UK. This view may have come about because England has the largest population and English health policy emanates from the Westminster parliament, and so is subject to much greater media scrutiny and public discussion.

In 1999, the Labour government devolved some powers to Northern Ireland, Scotland and Wales, giving them authority over areas such as health, while retaining power over the economy and defence. Before then, NHS reforms had been applied similarly across all of the nations that form the UK, although there were some differences in structure – which became more pronounced after devolution. An excellent example of policy difference is prescription charges: prescriptions are free in all nations except England. There has, however, also been convergence in health policy across the four nations, particularly in efforts to reduce health inequalities. In Northern Ireland, ongoing political problems and suspensions of the Northern Ireland Assembly have resulted in limited health policy development for much of the post-devolution period.

UK HEALTH POLICY THEMES

Political parties hold a set of values and beliefs called an ideology, which will contribute to the formation of their policies (see Table 39.1). Of course, other factors will contribute to policy formation, including global events, economic issues, professional influences, media influence, lobby groups and public and patient pressure groups, all in a bid to increase the party's electoral success. UK political parties are also broad churches, with members holding a range of views across the political spectrum.

ACTIVITY 39.2: LEADERSHIP

The four nations of the UK have some divergent and some convergent health policy approaches, particularly since devolution in 1999.

Access each country's health department website and identify the policies relating to health inequalities:

WEBLINK:
HEALTH
POLICIES

- Department of Health (Northern Ireland): www.health-ni.gov.uk
- Department of Health (Wales): http://wales.gov.uk/topics/health/?lang=en
- Department of Health (Scotland): www.scotland.gov.uk/Topics/Health
- Department of Health (England): www.dh.gov.uk

List these policies according to nation and compare their approach to health inequalities.

Table 39.1   Socialist and conservative ideology

Socialism	Conservativism
Collective action	Individual action
State ownership	Private property
Equality – is natural	Equality – being unequal is natural
Economy – state control	Economy – primacy of free market and capitalism
Social ownership of means of production	Privatisation of services
Social justice	Strong on law and order

ANSWER:
ACTIVITY 39.2

From the 1940s to the 1970s, the two dominant post-war parties (Labour and Conservative) were ideologically similar in many ways, and this resulted in a broad consensus in policy terms. This was termed **Butskellism**, and was underpinned by a **Keynesian economic** approach, which focused on the belief that the state should play a significant role in the marketplace, to stimulate economic growth and stability through taxation and interest rates and by investing in infrastructure. Awareness of the ideology of a political party can help you understand their health (and other) policies, particularly as they affect you and the patients you care for. Political ideology is often characterised on a continuum from left to right wing (see Figure 39.1).

Left wing _____ **Right wing**

Communism   Socialism   Liberalism   Conservatism   Fascism

Figure 39.1   Political continuum

Political ideology tends to be fluid and changes over time, as was evident in the 1970s onwards, when the Conservative party diverged sharply from the Keynesian consensus, leading to a political movement called 'the New Right'. Ideologically, this advocated the importance of the **free market**, private property and freedom of the individual (Baggott, 2015). In the 1990s, the Labour party adopted the 'Third Way' under the leadership of Tony Blair, as it sought to rebrand itself as 'New Labour'. Interestingly, within the Third Way it is possible to see similar beliefs and values to those of the preceding Conservative government, for example in the support of the free market, privatisation and tight control of public expenditure.

No metaphor was successfully applied to effectively describe the coalition government's (2010–15) ideology, but key characteristics included deficit reduction, privatisation, austerity measures involving a reduction in public spending and 'rolling back the state'. The Conservative government from 2015 has broadly continued in the same vein, despite a change of prime minister in 2016, following the result of the EU referendum vote, when Theresa May replaced David Cameron. So far, 'Mayism' has not emerged as a coherent ideology and it appears to contradict the Conservative 2017 election manifesto, claiming to reject untrammelled free markets, whilst at the same time seeking to pare down the role and size of the state.

ACTIVITY 39.3: LEADERSHIP

Imagine that the UK general election is fast approaching and the largest Westminster political parties – Labour, Conservative, Liberal Democrats and the Scottish National Party – are setting out their manifestos:

- List their main health and social care policies. To help with this, use Khomami, N., Torpey, P., Carrilho da Graca, D. and Holder, J. (2017) 'Who should I vote for? The UK election manifestos compared', *The Guardian*. Available at: www.theguardian.com/politics/ng-interactive/2017/may/19/who-should-i-vote-for-the-uk-election-manifestos-compared.

WEBLINK: GENERAL ELECTIONS

ANSWER: ACTIVITY 39.3

The development of healthcare

In order to place current UK healthcare policy in a political context, you need to understand the historical development of healthcare and the welfare state. This development is linked to the extent to which the state accepts responsibility for the health and welfare of its citizens, which is determined by a range of complex factors, including historical and political events, public expectations, philanthropy, the media, pressure groups, political party ideology and professional organisations. State responsibility for health and welfare gradually increased in the UK in the early twentieth century, and it was a central aspect of the new welfare state in 1948. However, the scope of state responsibility since 1948 has not remained static and it fluctuates depending on the ideology of the current government and the wider economy. This was seen rather spectacularly in the 1980s during the Conservative government of Margaret Thatcher and more recently following the many changes to the NHS, including the insidious attempts at privatisation and repair of the global financial crash. Thus, understanding this context helps you appreciate how political and economic events impact on health and welfare policy.

How visible are nurses in health policy?

Historically, in comparison to doctors, nurses have not achieved either the same level of political representation or been successful in influencing health policy. There is broad agreement that the nursing profession in the UK has never managed to translate its large numbers into a powerful political or professional voice. This was evident when, in the interwar period, nurses failed to gain representation on government health policy bodies and were only included in the late 1930s due to the necessity of wartime planning in the emergency medical services. The expectation seems to be that nurses would accommodate whatever arrangements were made; this acquiescence was evident in the drafting of NHS legislation, where there was little evidence of pressure from nursing organisations (Rafferty, 1992). Nursing's invisibility was also apparent in the midst of the many challenges faced by the NHS in the 1980s, with nurses paying little attention to the social, political and economic factors shaping their practice (Salvage, 1985). This situation has not changed: nurses remain sadly invisible at all levels of political activity, especially the national policy level (Klein, 2013).

A brief review of politics and health policy in the UK since the 1980s

Health policy is influenced by, amongst other things, the economic context of the country. Thus, public-sector spending increases at times of strong economic growth, and it may decline at times of low economic growth. This was evident during the global oil crisis of the 1970s, the economic downturn in the 1980s and the 2008 economic recession. The focus of this section is the English Westminster parliament.

As previously noted, following the Second World War, the two main political parties (Conservative and Labour) broadly agreed on how to manage the economy. Political and policy consensus between the two main parties then began to diverge during the 1970s. This divergence was most evident at the end of that decade in the 'New Right' ideology of the newly elected Conservative government (1979–97) led by Margaret Thatcher. The 'New Right' principles translated into economic policies favouring a smaller state, economic monetarism, the free market and privatisation, and all these principles were evident in the Conservative government's health policies in the 1990s, particularly the introduction of a quasi-market – the so-called internal market.

A Labour government was elected in 1997 (to 2010) with a landslide parliamentary majority of 179 – the largest Labour majority ever. The Labour party's ideology at this time, termed the 'Third Way', was an attempt to navigate a way through the politics of the left and right and it was often viewed as a disjointed collection of initiatives, rather than a coherent set of policies. The Third Way's main values were greater equality, social justice, the value of the community, personal responsibility, public/private partnerships, balanced budgets and an increase in the role of the state. In terms of health policy, the 1997 Labour government initially adopted the previous Conservative government's policies, but serious lapses in patient care related to chronic underfunding led to a large injection of cash from 2000 to 2010, under The NHS Plan. The internal market was replaced by primary care groups (PCGs) and private finance initiatives (PFIs) were used to fund expensive hospital building projects – creating an increasing role for the private sector.

In 2010, no political party gained a majority of seats in the Westminster general election; thus the Conservative and Liberal Democrat parties agreed to form a coalition government, led by David Cameron. This has been referred to as 'partnership politics' and it meant both parties had to fuse ideologically, although the Conservative party's ideology and principles were much more dominant. This ideology espoused free-market ideas, centring on the idea of the Big Society and small government and state; social responsibility not state control; decentralisation; deficit reduction; and public-sector spending cuts.

The short-lived Conservative government of David Cameron (2015–16) was scuppered in June 2016, when the UK voted narrowly in a referendum to leave the European Union. David Cameron bequeathed to the new Conservative Prime Minister Theresa May an NHS which was underfunded, required to make significant cuts, and an NHS tasked with seeking out ever more ways to improve service delivery. The NHS had to try to manage ever growing demand for services, with rationing, resultant increases in waiting times, ever higher thresholds for treatment, plummeting staff morale and staff shortages. Yet the 2017 general election contained very little substantial discussion about the NHS or health policy. At this point, it is helpful to remind ourselves that the NHS still remains fundamentally an equitable, just and value-for-money entity and it commands enormous public support.

Health policy themes

Health policy does not take place in a vacuum and each new government inherits the NHS left behind by the previous government. A number of consistent UK health policy themes have emerged since the 1980s, and successive governments have tended to continue with these, while adding their own ideological twist. A brief overview of some themes of English health policy will now be provided. Some of these can be seen reflected in aspects of health policy in the other UK nations.

The NHS as a marketplace and funding the NHS

The first consistent theme is the notion of the NHS as a marketplace, which will respond to market principles and be motivated by incentives (e.g. competition) to improve efficiency and effectiveness. This theme emerged when a shortfall in NHS funding in the second half of the 1980s led to a crisis whereby the supply of services was unable to meet the demand. This resulted in a review of the future of the NHS chaired by Margaret Thatcher, and the outcome was the NHS and Community Care Act 1990. A central idea here was the creation of an internal market, which would mimic the operation of the free commercial markets, but within services that were to remain largely state-financed. This would create conditions for competition between hospitals and other service providers through separating purchaser and provider responsibilities and establishing new organisations called 'self-governing trusts'. It also opened the way for private providers. GPs were involved as GP fund-holders, purchasing care directly from NHS trusts, and the notion was that money would follow the patient and thus providers had an incentive to treat more patients.

In 1997, the newly elected Labour government stated it was rejecting the internal market, although it appeared to reinvent it: it maintained the purchaser–provider split and abolished GP fund-holding but extended its principles to all family doctors and community nurses through the creation of primary care groups, later primary care trusts (PCTs). Thus, a primary care-led NHS evolved, with GPs remaining gatekeepers to the rest of the healthcare system. The aim was to create a patient-led NHS, with patients able to choose from a more diverse range of providers from the public and private sectors (Ham, 2009).

The 2010–15 coalition government's controversial Health and Social Care Act 2012 had a very rocky passage through parliament and it enshrined a much greater level of private sector delivery of NHS care. It introduced an economic regulator called 'Monitor' to regulate NHS Foundation Trusts and not-for-profit and private organisations. PCTs were replaced by clinical commissioning groups (CCGs), which were GP-led. They commission, or buy, most of the services funded by the NHS. NHS trusts were reconfigured as foundation trusts and some bodies, including strategic health authorities, were abolished. NHS funding since 2010 is increasing at a much slower growth rate (1.1%) than historical trends and this is worryingly far below the long-term average increases of around 4 per cent a year, since 1948 (The King's Fund, 2017). This has placed increasing pressure on the NHS because demand for services has continued to grow and many NHS providers are reporting significant financial deficits. Concerns have been raised that eradicating these deficits will lead to brutal service reduction and bed closures. Worryingly, some NHS funding has to come from cuts to public health and the devolution of powers to local areas has led to concerns about accountability.

Management and performance

Another consistent theme is a focus on the management and performance of the NHS. This began in the 1980s with the introduction of general management, marking what was termed the beginning of the NHS's managerial revolution (Klein, 2013). A focus on efficiency initiatives and performance indicators followed, thus allowing a comparison of services across regions. This has made the NHS a more self-aware organisation with greater visibility of its activities, so its performance is open to public scrutiny. However, in 2016 concerns about accountability were raised following the devolution of NHS powers to local areas, such as local councils.

Community care

Community care has been another important and enduring theme in health policy. The creation of the NHS in 1948 left the acute hospital sector better resourced and more powerful than the community care sector. This meant community care was a relatively neglected sector until the 1960s, when the deinstitutionalisation policy and scandals in long-stay hospitals led to the closure of a number of large institutions, including psychiatric hospitals. This prompted a re-examination of community care, and the NHS and Community Care Act 1990 was a seminal attempt to address this. The policy emerging from this act aimed to enable people to remain living at home or in a homely setting, with local authorities playing the lead role in the provision of care. Technological advances in hospital-based care have given this impetus: hospital stays are now much shorter, and there is an expectation that most types of ongoing care, both physical and psychological, can move into a community setting and many models of care delivery in the community are developing.

In mental health, due to deinstitutionalisation, there has been a substantial decrease in hospital beds over the past few decades; this means that if a patient is in a crisis situation requiring hospitalisation, it may be difficult to access a hospital bed. From a learning disability perspective, deinstitutionalisation means moving people from 'institutional environments' into their own homes, which could be shared flats, hostels or the family home. According to Baggott (2015), however, there is evidence that this has led to social isolation and poor access to healthcare. A recent scandal in 2012 involving the abuse of patients at Winterbourne View (a private hospital for those with a learning disability) highlights that much work is required to ensure the provision of appropriate nursing and social care. Despite these developments, community care policy remains somewhat vague and nebulous. Furthermore, because it straddles health and social care – where the criteria for access to each differ – patients often find navigating these processes very complex. Despite the many challenges, it is important to recognise that these types of changes have also brought many opportunities and have had a positive influence on the human rights of people with learning disabilities, such as the change from 'patient' status to 'tenant' or 'home owner', from recipient of 'care' to 'employer' of care staff.

Primary care

The next theme, primary care, developed alongside community care. Primary care can be defined as the care received at the first point of contact with (and the route into) the NHS. This consists of a wide range of services, including GPs. The introduction of GP fund-holding in the 1990s meant GPs were able to increase their involvement in primary care, which shifted the balance of power towards GPs rather than hospital consultants and acute care (Klein, 2013). Initially, the aim was to place greater emphasis on health promotion and disease prevention and provide greater patient choice. This was to be delivered through the work of GPs and facilitated via GP contracts. However, this has led to an increase in the workload of GPs and led David Cameron to promise greater patient accessibility to GPs by additional investment and extending GP surgery opening hours. Conversely, there is now a significant shortage of GPs because this additional investment is not reaching GP practices, many GPs are choosing to work shorter hours and there is ever growing patient demand. Despite this, NHS England's Five Year Forward View (2014) has proposed that GPs may combine with nurses, other community health professionals, hospital specialists and other health and social care workers, to develop innovative models of care delivery. One of the aims of the Five Year Forward View (2014) is also to break down barriers in how care is provided and to try to integrate primary and acute care.

'One-nation NHS'

The final theme is the drive to ensure a 'one-nation NHS' providing the same standards of service for everyone. This was to be achieved through the creation of a plethora of regulatory bodies, National Service Frameworks (NSFs) and a range of agencies, including the National Institute for Health and Care Excellence (NICE), the Healthcare Commission which is now the Care Quality Commission (CQC) and Health Improvement. The CQC controls and regulates service providers and ensures they provide similar care standards in hospitals and primary care. Performance is assessed here using efficiency, health improvement, fair access, effective delivery, patient experiences and health outcome measures, setting off an avalanche of target-setting for the NHS (Klein, 2013). Clinical governance was introduced into all trusts, whereby systems were set up for monitoring standards and identifying poor performance. Trusts also had to ensure implementation of the NSF's clinical standards and the NICE recommendations. The aim of tackling inequalities between different areas and different groups was laudable, as was the aim to achieve continuous quality improvement. NHS England's Five Year Forward View (2014) holds that the economic prosperity of Britain depends on significantly upgrading prevention measures and public health. However, there is evidence of some of the difficulties in developing the quality agenda in nursing.

WHAT'S THE EVIDENCE?

Haycock-Stuart, E. and Kean, S. (2012) 'Does nursing leadership affect the quality of care in the community setting?' *Journal of Nursing Management*, 20(3): 372-81.

Haycock-Stuart and Kean (2012) investigated Scottish community nurses' perceptions and experiences of leadership in an attempt to identify nursing leadership's effects on the quality of care in the community setting.

While political parties place quality issues at the heart of their health policies, this concept is ambiguous in many healthcare settings - the community, for example, where patients are discharged home 'quicker and sicker' and community nursing work is 'invisible', rendering it difficult to assess the quality of care. Haycock-Stuart and Kean's findings identify that apart from the complaints mechanism, quality indicators related to the nurse-patient relationship, mechanisms to monitor patient safety and technical aspects of nursing care in the community are mainly absent. Thus, the authors conclude that a reactive rather than a proactive approach to quality exists here.

- Reflect on your experience of caring for patients. What high-quality care have you been involved in delivering?
- How is this high-quality care measured or evaluated?
- Do you think the patients who received the care you regarded as high-quality would share your view?
- Now read the study and see if you agree with its conclusions.

Health policy and the economy

In 2008, a global banking and financial crisis led to a major UK recession. Following the election of the 2010 coalition government, political debate swiftly shifted to where and by how much public services could be cut. NHS Chief Executive David Nicholson warned that NHS spending would be capped, with efficiency savings of £20 billion to be made by 2015 (Nicholson, 2013). This was at odds with the widely accepted view that the NHS requires a 4 per cent increase in funding each year, to provide services at current levels (Klein, 2013). The result of this has now become evident in the NHS (and beyond), and in your practice placements you may be aware of problems related to bed shortages and the necessity to very closely monitor patient flow. It may be that you have witnessed how nurses are required to act as patient advocates due to this and it is vital that all nurses practise holistically, to ensure social justice for all patients in their care.

The Francis Report (2013)

In 2008, despite the existence of a system of healthcare designed to ensure quality, serious concerns emerged about care in the Mid Staffordshire Foundation Trust.

On 6 February 2013, Robert Francis QC published his long-awaited report, a public inquiry into the scandal of poor care in Stafford Hospital, Staffordshire between 2005 and 2009. It cost £13 million (up to November 2013) and the documentation ran to one million pages.

Sadly, the Francis Report illustrates how, despite care standards set by a plethora of regulatory authorities and professional bodies, the quality of patient care can deteriorate to such a level that it can directly contribute to the morbidity and mortality of large numbers of patients. The findings from this report have rocked the NHS to its core and all professions and layers of the NHS hierarchy have lessons to learn from it. The warning signs, such as high mortality rates and very poor standards of care, initially failed to trigger an investigation. Abysmal lapses in the standards of nursing care included patients being left lying in urine and faeces or left sitting on commodes for hours, food and drink left out of patients' reach, patient falls concealed from relatives, atrocious hygiene standards, call bells unanswered and staff callousness. Francis found that the reasons why care was poor included an understaffing of nurses, an inappropriate skill mix, leadership failure and an endemic bullying and negative culture in the Trust. Staff and patient concerns were ignored, despite Mid Staffordshire nurse Helene Donnelly raising concerns, and senior management had a greater focus on balancing the books than on the quality of care.

Francis made 290 recommendations, which centred on:

- shared common values
- maintaining fundamental standards
- openness
- transparency and candour
- compassionate, caring, committed nursing
- strong patient-centred healthcare leadership
- accurate, useful and relevant information
- culture change, which was not dependent on government.

Mid Staffordshire nurse whistleblower Helene Donnelly was a key witness in the subsequent public inquiry and Helene demonstrated the need to act when patient safety was jeopardised. However, Helene's experiences also demonstrated the difficulties nurses encounter during and after whistle-blowing. A range of interventions followed, with the NMC (2015), for example, highlighting that whistleblowing was a way of raising concerns and enhancing workplace accountability. When a concern is raised in this context, there are a number of criteria to fulfil for the concern to qualify as whistleblowing and in this situation the person who is blowing the whistle has legal protection (NMC, 2015).

In 2015, the Secretary of State for Health, Jeremy Hunt, launched Sir Robert Francis's follow-up report on the progress made on implementing the Francis recommendations and on whistleblowing. Hunt said good progress had been made, such as setting up the MyNHS website in England, to enhance transparency about staffing levels, and the incidence of falls and hospital-acquired infections. However, Hunt suggested that the NHS had not made fast enough progress in creating a transparent, no-blame learning culture, in which staff felt supported to speak out about patient care concerns. Thus, changes were necessary and the principles and programme of action set out by Francis in this report were all accepted in principle by the government. These included appointing one staff member in each trust as a 'freedom to speak up guardian' and enshrining rights to speak up, in staff contracts.

CASE STUDY 39.1: FREYA

Freya, from Northern Ireland, is 45 and lives with her 75-year-old mother, Joan. They are very close and do everything together. Freya has a learning disability, but manages to cope with daily life with constant support and guidance from her mother. One of their favourite pastimes is taking long walks along the coast near their home.

On returning from a walk one Friday evening, Freya's mother complained of feeling unwell, with a severe headache and speech problems. They called for an ambulance and by the time they arrived at the local Accident and Emergency (A&E) department, Freya's mother's symptoms had worsened. Joan was admitted to an observation ward attached to A&E, because there were no beds available anywhere else in the hospital.

Although Freya found the whole experience very confusing and was extremely distressed and tearful, the staff did not identify that she had learning difficulties. Freya could not understand what was happening to her mother but didn't feel able to ask any questions because all the staff seemed too busy to talk to her. One of the nurses did mutter 'Your mum has had a stroke', but no one explained to Freya exactly what this meant. Freya did not know what she should do, so decided it was best just to sit quietly next to her mother's bed.

Over the next four hours, Freya's mother's level of consciousness deteriorated and her speech became less coherent. However, because the staff were very busy, her condition was only monitored every two hours and her deterioration went unnoticed.

Just after 11 pm, a nurse said to Freya, in a very cold and rude manner, 'What are you doing here? Please leave'. Feeling very upset, Freya thought it best to leave, but was unsure how to get out of the hospital, let alone get home. Luckily, at that very moment, her mother's best friend Dora arrived; she arranged to take Freya to her house, because she knew Freya could not look after herself. When Freya said goodbye to her mother, it was the last time she ever spoke to her. When she returned at 2 pm the next day, she was distraught to find that her mother was deeply unconscious and that her continuing deterioration had not been acted on. Joan died the next day, without regaining consciousness.

- Did the nursing staff treat Freya in an acceptable manner, with the compassion she deserved?
- Should the staff have identified Freya's learning disability and met her needs?
- If you were the nurse caring for Freya's mother, what would you have done?

> There was a young boy who came onto the ward from A&E very late one night and his mother and grandmother were over the moon at the care that had been provided (family-centred approach) and said there was too much negativity in the newspapers about the NHS and thanked myself and my practice educator for what we had done, as well as the other staff that had been involved as everyone had worked so hard to ensure everything that could be done was.
>
> Siân Hunter, child nursing student

CASE STUDY 39.2: JOAN

Joan is a 75-year-old woman from Northern Ireland, whose husband died five years previously. Joan lives with her 45-year-old daughter Freya, who has a learning disability. They both enjoy taking long walks along the coast.

On returning from a walk one Friday evening, Joan complained of feeling unwell, with a severe headache and speech problems. At 7 pm, when they arrived at the local A&E department, Joan's symptoms had worsened. She was admitted onto an observation ward attached to A&E, because there were no beds available in the hospital.

Although Joan's level of consciousness seemed to be deteriorating and her speech was becoming less coherent (both of these developments are serious causes for concern), her condition was only monitored every two hours. When Freya left her mother at 11 pm, Joan was just able to respond, but by the time Freya returned at 2 pm on the Saturday Joan was deeply unconscious. This deterioration had not been acted on by the staff, although they had continued to record her neurological observations every two hours. Joan did not regain consciousness and died on the Sunday.

- Joan's care highlights some of the problems experienced by patients when they visit A&E. Identify these problems and reflect on how they could have been prevented.
- What national standards should have guided Joan's treatment and care?

NHS England's Five Year Forward View (2014) recognised that urgent and emergency care (UEC) was under severe pressure, and aims to redesign UEC to integrate a range of available services, to ensure people get the right care in the right place. This includes smaller hospitals forming partnerships with other hospitals and partnering with specialist hospitals. So, existing trauma and specialist stroke networks will be built on and five urgent specialist services will be delivered as part of a network approach: these are hyper acute stroke, emergency vascular, major trauma, paediatric intensive care and STEMI heart attack. The aim is that all patients will receive a consistent standard of treatment, seven days a week, regardless of where they live.

The NHS remains very popular

The NHS is politically prominent because it is both the largest employer in Europe and a large consumer of public expenditure. The values underpinning it in 1948 remain unchanged but the world has changed considerably. The proportion of the UK gross domestic product (GDP) consumed by the NHS has increased from 3.4 per cent to 8.5 per cent in the past 50 years, which compares unfavourably internationally (many EU countries spend more), and it is also unclear how future expenditure increases will be funded (Appleby, 2017). NHS costs are escalating due to demographic changes, life-style issues, an increase in long-term conditions, increasing medical technology, ambitious clinical staff and increasing patient expectation (Nicholson, 2013). The NHS touches the lives of every UK citizen from birth to death and its popularity has remained consistently high. For those benefiting from the services of the NHS, despite recent concerns and problems, it occupies a unique and well-loved position in the welfare state – as highlighted by Oscar in the patient voice at the start of the chapter – and patients are generally very happy with the care they receive.

Many of the service users I have worked with have viewed the NHS in a positive way and have valued that service and level of care that they have received. I have worked with individuals that have come into hospital that have been experiencing poor mental health and have expressed that just being able to get the opportunity to be listened to has helped them in their recovery. To me this is important as it is showing the values of the NHS and its staff being delivered in the clinical setting.

Samantha Vanes, NQ RNMH

ACTIVITY 39.4: REFLECTION

Reflect on the comments throughout this chapter, urging nurses to become more politically aware and even active:

- Do you agree with this argument?
- Record your current answer to the question above, and at the end of your nursing programme answer the question again.
- Is your answer still the same? If not, why not?

ANSWER:
ACTIVITY 39.4

CONCLUSION

Many nurses perceive politics and nursing to be incompatible and therefore irrelevant to them. This may be because politics involves making choices about scarce resources, which is at odds with the notion of nursing practice. However, health policy and the political context of nursing are inextricably interwoven, and if nurses are to achieve meaningful policy involvement they need to become more politically aware and active. This will hopefully lead to a more politically engaged profession, whose members are better equipped to meaningfully contribute to health policy.

Adopting a political perspective and becoming politically aware does not mean you have to become involved in party politics, but that you understand how to influence health and other types of policy. This knowledge will provide you with some of the tools which enable you to reflect critically on practice, supporting you to deliver care which is holistic, compassionate and person-centred.

It is important to remember that although English health policy often seems to be portrayed as NHS health policy, this is an incorrect portrayal, because health policy differs within the four nations that make up the UK.

The ability of the NHS to provide effective and high-quality healthcare throughout the entire UK is frequently challenged. There have been some recent high-profile failings, from which all members of the healthcare professions must learn. Despite this, however, the NHS touches the lives of every UK citizen from birth to death, its popularity remains consistently high and it is a respected and indeed revered element of the welfare state.

CHAPTER SUMMARY

This chapter has:

- defined politics and health policy
- identified nursing's general lack of engagement in health policy
- outlined the importance of education to ensure nurses develop political awareness
- discussed how political ideology influences health policy
- outlined how devolution affects health policy
- identified a range of health policy themes.

CRITICAL REFLECTION

Holistic care

This chapter has illustrated the importance of viewing health policy in a political context – which includes a broad analysis of health policy – when providing holistic care for your patient:

- Think about a patient you have cared for recently within any setting and identify how any aspect of health policy in your country has influenced your ability to care holistically for this patient, meeting their wider physical, emotional, social, economic and spiritual needs.
- Would there be any difference if you were caring for a patient from another field of nursing?
- Make a note of your thoughts. Refer back to this next time you care for a patient and then write your own reflection on your experience.

GO FURTHER

Books

Baggott, R. (2015) *Understanding Health Policy*, 2nd edn. Bristol: Policy Press. This book comprehensively discusses health policy in England and, to a lesser extent, the three other UK countries and internationally.

Traynor, M. (2013) *Nursing in Context: Policy, Politics, Profession*. Houndmills: Palgrave Macmillan. This book provides a comprehensive insight into the development of nursing professionally and educationally and examines health policy related to nursing.

SAGE journal article

FURTHER
READING:
JOURNAL
ARTICLES

Go to https://study.sagepub.com/essentialnursing2e for free online journal articles for this chapter. If you are using the interactive ebook, simply click on the book icon in the margin to go straight to the resource.

Hewison, A. (2008) 'Evidence-based policy: Implications for nursing and policy involvement', *Policy, Politics and Nursing Practice*, 9(4): 288-98. This article argues that while some nurses are involved in health policy development, they tend to be at a senior level. Nurses need to develop policy literacy early in their careers, during educational programmes.

Other journal articles

Alpers, R.R., Brown, G., Jarrell, K. and Wotring, R. (2009) 'Teaching politics to nursing students: An innovative project', *Teaching and Learning in Nursing*, 4: 104–5. This article demonstrates that nurses can gain the skills to influence health policy by engaging in educational programmes, which include political content and political projects.

Ball, J.E., Griffiths, P., Rafferty, A.M., Lindqvist, R, Murrells, T and Tishelman, C. (2016) 'A cross-sectional study of "care left undone" on nursing shifts in hospitals', *Journal of Advanced Nursing*, 72(9): 2086–97. This article provides further evidence in support of increased nurse staffing levels.

Weblinks

Go to https://study.sagepub.com/essentialnursing2e for weblinks related to this chapter. If you are using the interactive ebook, simply click on the book icon in the margin to go straight to the resource.

FURTHER
READING:
WEBLINKS

www.kingsfund.org.uk/blog/2016/01/how-does-nhs-spending-compare-health-spending-internationally – discusses NHS funding and compares it internationally.

www.health.org.uk/sites/health/files/TheFourHealthSystemsOfTheUKHowDoTheyCompare_fullversion.pdf – a discussion of the funding and performance of healthcare systems, in all four UK nations.

www.kingsfund.org.uk/publications/health-policy-under-coalition-government – a discussion of the coalition government's (2010–15) health policy.

www.nhs.uk/NHSEngland/keogh-review/Documents/UECR.Ph1Report.FV.pdf – the findings of Professor Keogh's (NHS England) review of urgent and emergency care.

www.kingsfund.org.uk/health-care-explained – identifies some of the key health-related trends for the next 20 years, including population changes and technology advances.

ACE YOUR ASSESSMENT

Review what you have learned by visiting the book's online resources at: https://study.sagepub.com/essential nursing2e If using your interactive ebook, just click on the icon in the margin to go straight there.

ONLINE
QUIZZES

- Test yourself with multiple-choice and short-answer questions.
- Revise key terms with the interactive flash cards.

REFERENCES

Appleby, J. (2017) *How does NHS Spending Compare with Health Spending Internationally?* London: The Kings Fund. Available at: www.kingsfund.org.uk/blog/2016/01/how-does-nhs-spending-compare-health-spending-internationally (accessed 25 July 2017).

Baggott, R. (2015) *Understanding Health Policy*, 2nd edn. Bristol: Policy Press.

Ball, J.E., Griffiths, P., Rafferty, A.M., Lindqvist, R., Murrells, T. and Tishelman, C. (2016) 'A cross-sectional study of "care left undone" on nursing shifts in hospitals', *Journal of Advanced Nursing*, 72(9): 2086–97.

Chaffee, M.W., Mason, D.J. and Leavitt, J.K. (2012) 'A framework for action in policy and politics', in D.J. Mason, J.K. Leavitt and M.W. Chaffee (eds), *Policy and Politics in Nursing and Healthcare*, 6th edn. St Louis, MO: Elsevier Saunders.

Davies, C. (2004) 'Political leadership and the politics of nursing', *Journal of Nursing Management*, 12: 253–41.

English Heritage (n.d.) Back to the Community: Disability equality, rights and inclusion. Available at: www.english-heritage.org.uk/discover/people-and-places/disability-history/1945-to-the-present-day/back-to-the-community (accessed 20 July 2017).

Ham, C. (2009) *Health Policy in Britain*, 5th edn. Houndmills: Palgrave Macmillan.

Haycock-Stuart, E. and Kean, S. (2012) 'Does nursing leadership affect the quality of care in the community setting?' *Journal of Nursing Management*, 20(3): 372–81.

Khomami, N., Torpey, P., Carrilho da Graca, D. and Holder, J. (2017) 'Who should I vote for? The UK election manifestos compared', *The Guardian*. Available at: www.theguardian.com/politics/ng-interactive/2017/may/19/who-should-i-vote-for-the-uk-election-manifestos-compared (accessed 14 December 2017).

King's Fund, The (2017) The NHS Budget and how it has Changed. Available at: www.kingsfund.org.uk/projects/nhs-in-a-nutshell/nhs-budget (accessed 27 July 2017).

Kitson, A., Marshall, A., Bassett, K. and Zeitz, K. (2013) 'What are the core elements of patient-centred care? A narrative review and synthesis of the literature from health policy, medicine and nursing', *Journal of Advanced Nursing*, 69(1): 4–15.

Klein, R. (2013) *The New Politics of the NHS: From Creation to Reinvention*, 7th edn. Oxford: Radcliffe Publishing.

Mid Staffordshire NHS Foundation Trust Public Inquiry (2013) The Francis Report. Chaired by Robert Francis QC. Available at: www.midstaffspublicinquiry.com/report (accessed 1 July 2017).

National Institute for Health and Care Excellence (NICE) (2014) Safe Staffing for Nursing in Adult Inpatient Wards in Acute Hospitals. Available at: www.nice.org.uk/Guidance/SG1 (accessed 20 July 2017).

NHS England (2014) Five Year Forward View. Available at: www.england.nhs.uk/five-year-forward-view (accessed 25 July 2017).

NHS Improvement (2016) Safe Staffing for Adult Inpatients in Acute Care. Available at: https://improvement.nhs.uk/resources/safe-staffing-improvement-resources-adult-inpatient-acute-care

Nicholson, D. (2013) Interview, *The Today Programme*, BBC Radio 4, 11 July.

Nuffield Trust (n.d) The History of NHS Reform. Available at: http://nhstimeline.nuffieldtrust.org.uk (accessed 10 March 2015).

Nursing and Midwifery Council (NMC) (2015) *Raising Concerns: Guidance for Nurses and Midwives*. London: NMC. Available at: www.nmc.org.uk/standards/guidance/raising-concerns-guidance-for-nurses-and-midwives (accessed 28 July 2017).

Nursing and Midwifery Council (2017) *Consultation on Education Framework: Standards for Education and Training*. London: NMC. Available at: www.nmc.org.uk/education/education-consultation/framework (accessed 25 July 2017).

Rafferty, A.M. (1992) 'Nursing policy and the nationalization of nursing: The representation of "crisis" and the "crisis" of representation', in J. Robinson, A. Gray and R. Elkan (eds), *Policy Issues in Nursing*. Milton Keynes: Open University Press.

Salvage, J. (1985) *The Politics of Nursing*. London: Heinemann.

Siddique, H. (2017) '96% drop in EU nurses registering to work in Britain since Brexit vote', *The Guardian*, 12 June. Available at: www.theguardian.com/society/2017/jun/12/96-drop-in-eu-nurses-registering-to-work-in-britain-since-brexit-vote (accessed 30 July 2017).

Sparrow, A., Phipps, C. and Rawlinson, K. (2017) 'Question Time leaders' special: May under fire over NHS and education – as it happened', *The Guardian*, 2 June. Available at: www.theguardian.com/politics/live/2017/jun/02/general-election-2017-immigration-target-david-davis-question-time-politics-live (accessed 30 July 2017).

World Health Organization (WHO) (1948) Preamble to the Constitution of the World Health Organization as adopted by the International Health Conference, New York, 19–22 June, 1946; signed on 22 July 1946 by the representatives of 61 States (Official Records of the World Health Organization, no. 2, p. 100) and entered into force on 7 April 1948. Available at: www.who.int/about/definition/en/print.html (accessed 20 January 2014).

INTRODUCTION TO THE GLOBAL CONTEXT OF NURSING

CATHERINE DELVES-YATES

--- **THIS CHAPTER COVERS** ---

- The global role of the nurse
- Differences and similarities in healthcare systems and patients' health beliefs across countries and cultures

- The importance of cultural competence in nursing care
- International placements and learning opportunities

"

My name is Fondip. I am 5 and live in Buea, a town in Cameroon, West Africa. My mum took me to the health centre as I have been feeling poorly with a fever for nearly a week and haven't been able to play football. We saw Sam, the nurse – he was great! He says I have malaria and gave my mum some tablets to make me better. But the best bit was that Sam gave me a bar of chocolate, because I was so brave – and it is just for me, not for sharing with my sisters!

Fondip, patient

"

"

I've always dreamed about living and working in Australia. When I had the opportunity to go on an elective placement, I went to see what mental health nursing was like on the other side of the world.

Arranging my placement was time-consuming but what I got from the experience was priceless. I learned so much about patient care and was surprised by how much I already knew and could apply to practice. This did wonders for my confidence! I gained more from the experience than I could ever have imagined and even came home with a job offer!

Fiona I'Anson, MH nursing student

"

Visit https://study.sagepub.com/essentialnursing2e to access a wealth of online resources for this chapter – watch out for the margin icons throughout the chapter. If you are using the interactive eBook, simply click on the margin icon to go straight to the resource.

INTRODUCTION

Is your experience of nursing a patient similar to that of a nursing student 6,000 miles away? Would you and a nurse in another country care for a patient in the same way and agree that the same aspects of care were important? Could you care for a patient in a country where healthcare resources are scarce? The patient voice above outlines how patients worldwide value the reassurance and comfort that good nursing care brings, and, as Fiona's comment shows, much can be gained from an experience of nursing in another country.

Nursing care is truly global, with the ability to transcend international boundaries. Although concepts of the nurse, the care they provide and the resources available may differ, the value of the nurse as a provider of healthcare is common to all countries.

This chapter introduces the global context of nursing. Differences within the role of the nurse worldwide and the topic of health beliefs are highlighted, with the importance of culturally sensitive care identified, no matter where a patient is cared for. Discussion within the chapter encourages you to think about undertaking an international placement and some important factors that need considering are identified.

THE GLOBAL ROLE OF THE NURSE

There are 19.3 million nurses and midwives worldwide. If this figure is considered in relation to the number of people within a population, ratios vary from a high of 75 nurses per 10,000 people in Europe to a low of 11 nurses per 10,000 people in Africa (WHO, 2016).

Within the developing world, there are high rates of disease and birth and the numbers of nurses are low. In these areas, nurses frequently work with minimal resources, healthcare equipment and medication are often unavailable and access to other healthcare professionals is limited. Unlike in the UK, the nursing fields of mental health, learning disability and child nursing tend not to exist as specialisms, and in many countries – not just developing ones – midwifery care is not a specialism but an aspect of all nurses' roles. A nurse can be called upon to care for an adult with a chronic illness, a child who is critically ill with cholera or a woman experiencing complications in labour, or to offer advice on sanitation and the hygiene practices of street food vendors.

The low number of nurses and high disease and birth rates in developing countries contrast with the situation in the developed world, where there is a higher number of nurses and significantly lower rates of disease and birth. Considering the UK specifically as a developed country, access to healthcare is an unremarkable aspect of daily life which, in general, remains free at the point of use. It is possible to consult a doctor 24 hours a day if necessary, healthcare is available in the community for those in need, vaccination programmes are freely provided and in an emergency it is possible to summon an ambulance with a telephone call. Throughout the developed world, there are a variety of differing healthcare systems, some funded by taxation, others depending on individuals taking out health insurance. These all act as a 'safety net' to ensure that the most disadvantaged in society have access to healthcare, although it has to be remembered that this approach does not remove all health inequalities. For those experiencing ill health in a developing country, there is frequently no such safety net. If the example of Cameroon is considered, there is no national health service and generally patients have to pay before they receive care or medication, both of which are expensive. The nearest doctor can be more than a day's walk away and walking may be the only option for travel. The only support within the community for those in need is provided by family members. In a dire emergency, the only way to get an acutely sick patient to hospital may be in the back of a truck or by carrying them on a homemade stretcher. Although the health needs of the population are great, in comparison to the situation in the UK, healthcare professionals are scarce (see Table 40.1).

Table 40.1   Healthcare professionals per 10,000 population

Country	Nurses/midwives/doctors
Cameroon	5.2
The UK	116.1

Source: WHO (2016)

DIFFERENCES AND SIMILARITIES IN HEALTHCARE SYSTEMS AND PATIENTS' HEALTH BELIEFS ACROSS COUNTRIES AND CULTURES

In many developing countries, nurses frequently work in remote settings. They could be the only formally qualified healthcare provider for many miles, and even those working within a hospital may not have continuous medical support, as doctors frequently cover more than one hospital or health centre. The nurse may well have to deal with emergencies without support from any other healthcare professionals: at worst, medical equipment and medication may not be available and the provision of clean water and electricity can be unreliable. While the treatment of ill health can be limited, programmes to promote health may well be non-existent and living conditions can be challenging, even to those who are fit and healthy.

Looking at recent events in Africa, it is clear to see why British nurses are so sought after. We have access to training where we learn hand-washing and have access to PPE. As nursing students we have access to equipment and can carry out procedures that aren't available in developing countries.

Laura Grimley, adult nursing student

As many developing countries have a long history of traditional medicine, the local hospital may not be the first place patients visit when they are sick. This is not just because they may be a considerable distance away from it, but also because traditional practitioners offering cures for major and minor ailments alike are often chosen in preference to the western medicine on offer at a local hospital (Labhardt et al., 2010).

Nurses practising in developed countries function within a very different environment to those practising in developing countries. In many developing countries, the care provided for patients with learning disabilities or mental health problems is poor and the behaviour they sometimes demonstrate can be considered to be a result of the individual being possessed by evil spirits. This clearly contrasts with the situation in many developed countries, where nurses are specifically educated to have the skills required to care for patients with a learning disability or mental health needs, and work as part of a wider healthcare team with a range of specialist skills. Most nurses working in developed countries have daily contact with their healthcare team and team members are easily available to offer advice and discuss treatment plans. If a patient's condition deteriorates, assistance can quickly be obtained. While there are always exceptions – poverty and populations with poor access to healthcare can exist even in developed countries – medical equipment and medication are usually easy to obtain, health-promotion programmes commence at birth and continue throughout the lifespan, and the vast majority of patients live in housing unlikely to make them ill.

CASE STUDY 40.1: NOMSA

Nomsa is 25 and has two children, of 3 years and 18 months, who have had three episodes of diarrhoea in the last two months. She is worried that germs in the water from the village water hole might be causing her children to become ill.

- What simple measure could you advise Nomsa to undertake before her family drink the water?

Similarities and differences

While there are differences in the role of the nurse in developing and developed countries, the core nursing values of care, compassion, competence, communication, courage and commitment remain steadfast (DH, 2012). Nurses occupy a unique position within the healthcare delivery system of any country, working with patients at every stage of their lives, constantly putting their patients first and doing their utmost to provide effective care in every situation.

I think that both my experience of nursing and that of a nursing student in a developing country will be similar in that we will both get the experience of meeting some amazing people and learning so much from them.

Hannah Boyd, adult nursing student

Health beliefs

In the UK, healthcare delivered by the NHS is almost exclusively based on western medicine. While there is some complementary medicine available on the NHS, such as osteopathy for back pain and acupuncture for arthritis, this is only made available following the provision of scientific evidence of its effectiveness, thus actually enabling it to fulfil the definition of western medicine.

For patients, however, scientific proof of effectiveness may not be important. Past experience of a treatment working or a belief in its effectiveness handed down from previous generations can result in particular treatments being valued. Thus, a patient's health beliefs, the personal beliefs they have regarding how illness can be prevented or treated, may reflect what seem to be opposing ideologies; some beliefs may be based on past experience and long-held beliefs, others on scientific evidence. So, it is possible to believe that sitting on cold ground will cause haemorrhoids – a belief without any scientific basis – while also believing that antibiotics are ineffective in the treatment of colds – a belief based on science: colds are caused by a virus, so antibiotics will not be effective.

Pluralistic medical societies

Most societies in both developed and developing countries can be viewed as pluralistic, meaning several medical traditions exist and so western medicine is not thought to be the only way to treat illness. The UK, however, is a country where, over the last 300 years, there has been a process of change, where medicine based on past experience and long-held beliefs in, for example, herbalists, folk medicine and astrology has been replaced, almost universally, by western medicine (Helman, 1978).

ACTIVITY 40.1: REFLECTION

- Reflect on your health beliefs, those of your family and those of the patients for whom you have cared.
- Are the majority of these based on scientific evidence, or past experience and long-held belief or tradition?
- How can you ensure that the care you deliver to a patient always respects their health beliefs?

ANSWER:
ACTIVITY 40.1

When considering approaches to disease, despite the existence of a variety of medical traditions, healthcare professionals – even those practising in developing countries – normally adhere to a western system of healthcare. The danger of this is that a patient's need for other methods of healing is rarely recognised. Such an approach is criticised as being ethnocentric, describing healthcare which is delivered in a form that only takes into account western culture and misunderstands other groups.

However, if disease aetiology is considered in terms of a patient's belief, it becomes clear that for treatment to be effective, the patient must see it as appropriate to the cause.

There is clear logic in this approach and, actually, the exact cause of an illness can be irrelevant. For example, a patient who believes they are ill because they have broken a rule will not be completely cured by antibiotics. The mind is extremely powerful and in order to effectively treat a patient's 'dis-ease', their belief must be addressed before their body can be effectively treated.

As a nurse, it is important to avoid blindly adhering to an ethnocentric view and instead to assess any illness from the patient's perspective, whether the patient shares your culture or not. Never discount the merits of others' beliefs. Although you may feel safe in supporting western medical beliefs with scientific results, not everything can yet be explained.

Healthcare needs of refugees and asylum seekers

One out of every 122 people across the globe is either a refugee, internally displaced or seeking asylum, with approximately half of these people being children under 18 years old. At the end of 2016, the UK hosted nearly 119,000 refugees and 46,784 asylum seekers (UNHCR, 2017).

Refugees and asylum seekers are amongst the most vulnerable groups in society. They represent a wide range of differing cultures, languages and backgrounds, with each individual having personal experiences which may include fleeing war, torture or sexual violence. Their healthcare needs can be complex and, possibly, urgent. Language and cultural barriers may hinder access to care and impede an awareness of what is available. Whilst as individuals they have a wide range of differing physical and psychological health needs, as a group it is possible to describe a number of needs that are frequently encountered (see Figure 40.1).

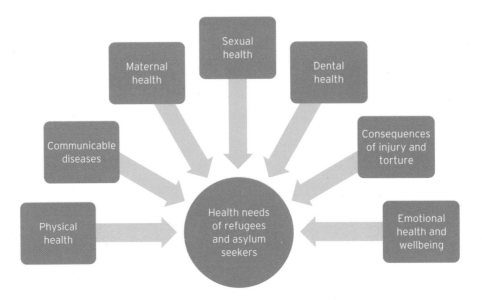

Figure 40.1   Health needs of refugees and asylum seekers

Source: Adapted from Cromer (2016: 17)

ACTIVITY 40.2: CRITICAL THINKING

Consider the health needs of refugees and asylum seekers and make a list of the core nursing values which need to be paramount in the care you deliver.

THE IMPORTANCE OF CULTURAL COMPETENCE IN NURSING CARE

Good nursing care is transcultural, taking account of the patient as an individual. A patient's culture is another aspect of their uniqueness, which, along with other information, a nurse needs to understand in order to provide effective care (Leininger, 1985).

As nurses, we have our own cultural backgrounds and are socialised into the culture of our profession (Spector, 1979). We develop nursing beliefs, practices, habits, likes, dislikes, norms and rituals, all of which comprise a nursing culture. We learn to speak a unique language (nursing terminology) and our understanding and beliefs relating to health and illness differ greatly from those of non-nurses. However, it is an impossible challenge for nurses to meet a patient's needs, as defined by the patient, if they are unable to understand differing health beliefs.

It is crucial to treat a patient as a unique individual with an existence outside the care setting. Effective nursing care takes account of all beliefs regarding health and illness, adapting the approach to one which will meet the patient's specific needs.

While there are helpful transcultural nursing models, for example Sunrise Enabler (Leininger, 2002), some encourage placing patients in boxes determined by their culture, race and ethnicity. But no two individuals are identical, even if they do share the same culture, race and ethnicity.

It is important to remember that what a patient is thinking may well be very different from your thoughts, and that other providers of healthcare involving non-western medicine both exist and can be fundamental in a patient's recovery.

CASE STUDY 40.2: MABOH

Maboh is 31, lives in a rural village in the Southwest Province of Cameroon, West Africa and relies on care delivered by his parents for feeding, washing and moving. He communicates using simple words and gestures. Maboh often has epileptic fits, which his parents treat by holding his head above a pit latrine (open toilet) as is the local practice; the aroma from the ammonia is thought to act like 'smelling salts', helping to 'bring him round'.

- How could you encourage Maboh's parents to treat his fits in a way that maximises his, and their, safety?

When working in a care home we ensured the needs of a Muslim patient were met with understanding and care. We ensured her personal care was given only by female carers and when she passed away the rituals and customs of her religion and culture were adhered to.

Julie Davis, LD nursing student

Culturally competent care in practice

Practising culturally competent care involves identifying and understanding first your own views and beliefs and then those of the patient, without resorting to stereotypes. In the same way that you find out other information from a patient, ask them about their health beliefs. You need to know all the facts before you can provide good nursing care. When practising in this manner, it becomes clear that it is not necessary to travel to faraway places to encounter cultural differences – the challenge of integrating differing beliefs is present in every patient encounter.

INTERNATIONAL PLACEMENTS AND LEARNING OPPORTUNITIES

It may be possible that your university will allow students to participate in an international placement during their course. However, as an international placement is not necessary for the course award, for most programmes it will not be organised or funded by your university. This may make it sound daunting, but don't be put off: as Fiona mentioned in the student voice at the start of the chapter, all of the time spent arranging a placement really is worth it. Students identify international placements as positive experiences, enabling them to:

- grow personally and professionally due to increased cultural sensitivity (Grant and McKenna, 2003)
- increase their awareness and acceptance of other cultures (Rivzi and Walsh, 1998)
- care more effectively for multicultural populations (Inglis et al., 2000)
- reflect on personal belief systems (Jones et al., 1998)
- compare healthcare systems and practices to re-evaluate their own (Scholes and Moore, 2000)
- identify health inequalities across the globe (Button et al., 2005).

Many nursing courses include an **elective placement**, an ideal opportunity to consider experiencing nursing abroad.

Think carefully...

The idea of experiencing nursing in any country can be exciting, but think about it carefully. If you choose to go to a developing country rather than a developed one, it is likely that you will encounter much more austere conditions than those you are used to. While this brings a fantastic opportunity to experience diverse cultures, differing healthcare provision and practices, it will need thorough planning.

The first person to talk to is your lecturer. You may be able to take part in a project that already exists between your university and a healthcare organisation in another country. You will also need to consider what you wish to achieve from this experience and link this to the learning on your course, and you must have the support of your university before you go. Considering the impact of your visit on your host is of utmost importance. While you are undertaking the placement as a learning experience, the relationship cannot be one-sided. You need to ensure that your visit will be as positive for your host as it is for you.

CASE STUDY:
THEO

Apply your understanding of international placements by reading Theo's case study, at https://study.sagepub.com/essentialnursing2e.

If you decide to undertake an international placement, you must understand any risks involved.

FURTHER READING:
MORGAN
(2012)

WHAT'S THE EVIDENCE?

Morgan, D. (2012) 'Student nurse perceptions of risk in relation to international placements: A phenomenological study', *Nurse Education Today*, 32: 956-60.

Morgan (2012) identifies the risks perceived by nursing students when undertaking an international placement:

- Reflect on the risks you would perceive when planning an international placement.
- How could you reduce these risks?
- Now read the article and consider whether your concerns were the same as the students'.

CHECK YOUR
ANSWERS!

ANSWER:
WHAT'S THE
EVIDENCE?

Your health and safety

Health and safety must be considered as paramount. The Foreign and Commonwealth Office (FCO) offers advice on travel, safety, assistance and living abroad and is an excellent place to start your investigation of a country you wish to visit.

To make the most of your experience, you must be supervised by an appropriate individual. Throughout your international placement, you are still bound by a professional code, have a duty to act responsibly and ethically at all times and must not become involved in care where you are unsupervised or for which you have not been trained.

ACTIVITY 40.3: CRITICAL THINKING

- What information should you familiarise yourself with before you leave for an international placement?
- Which sources would you need to consult in order to ascertain this information?

ANSWER:
ACTIVITY 40.3

Communication

Think carefully about arranging a placement in a country where you are unable to speak the language. If you are unable to talk with the patients, providing appropriate and effective care is going to be hugely problematic, even if you have access to a translator.

During your experience, in addition to any other written work you may be required to complete, maintain a daily reflective diary. This will assist you to carefully consider your experiences, both while you are there and when you return home. After your placement, consider how you can share your experiences. You may wish to do a presentation for other students, or maybe develop an aspect of your experience by using it as the focus for your dissertation.

Experience of nursing in another country not only offers an understanding of a differing approach to patient care; more importantly, it also provides the experience of immersion in a different culture. Such experiences develop insight into your own views and beliefs, an understanding of cultural differences and nursing reflexivity.

CONCLUSION

Nursing care is truly global, with the ability to transcend international boundaries. Although the concepts of the nurse, the care they provide and the resources available may differ, the value of the nurse as a provider of healthcare is common to all countries.

While there are differences between the role of the nurse in a developing and a developed country, the core nursing values of care, compassion, competence, communication, courage and commitment remain steadfast.

Good nursing care in any setting within any country is transcultural, taking account of the patient as an individual. A patient's culture is another aspect of their uniqueness which, along with other information, a nurse needs to understand in order to provide effective care. It is not necessary to travel to faraway places to encounter cultural differences: the challenge of integrating differing beliefs is present in every patient encounter.

The idea of experiencing nursing in any country can be exciting and much can be gained, but think about it carefully. If you choose to go to a developing country rather than a developed one, it is likely that you will encounter much more austere conditions than you are used to. While this brings a fantastic opportunity to experience diverse cultures and differing healthcare provision and practices, it will need thorough planning.

CHAPTER SUMMARY

- Nursing, in any country worldwide, has more similarities than differences.
- All nurses share a specific body of knowledge and skills which they implement within the confines of their specific environment to provide effective patient care.
- Patient care must always be culturally competent.
- Patients have a wide range of health beliefs that need to be considered to ensure the care they receive is acceptable.
- It is not necessary to travel to faraway places to encounter cultural differences; the challenge of integrating differing beliefs is present in every patient encounter.
- Refugees and asylum seekers are amongst the most vulnerable groups in society who have a wide range of healthcare needs.
- An international placement requires careful planning, but will greatly improve your nursing knowledge.

CRITICAL REFLECTION

Holistic care

This chapter has highlighted the importance of cultural competence when providing holistic care for your patient.

- Think about a patient you have cared for recently and make a list of how caring for them with an understanding of their culture can help meet their wider physical, emotional, social, economic and spiritual needs.
- Would there be any difference if you were caring for a patient from another field of nursing?
- Make a note of your thoughts and refer back to it next time you care for a patient, and then write your own reflection on your experience.

GO FURTHER

Books

Dawood, R. (2012) *Travellers' Health: How to Stay Healthy Abroad*, 5th edn. Oxford: Oxford University Press. An outstanding reference book for those who want advice on staying healthy while travelling.

Leininger, M. (1991) *Culture, Care, Diversity and Universality: A Theory of Nursing*. New York: National League for Nursing Press. A comprehensive overview of the importance of the cultural dimension of care.

SAGE journal articles

FURTHER
READING:
JOURNAL
ARTICLES

Go to https://study.sagepub.com/essentialnursing2e for free online journal articles for this chapter. If you are using the interactive ebook, simply click on the book icon in the margin to go straight to the resource.

Mkandawire-Valhum, L. and Doering, J. (2012) 'Study abroad as a tool for promoting cultural safety in nursing education', *Journal of Transcultural Nursing*, 23(1): 82–9. Available at: http://tcn.sagepub.com/content/23/1/82. How an experience of nursing abroad can enable the development of an understanding of how communities address their own health problems.

Other journal articles

Clark, J. (2010) 'Student experiences in the real world of nursing: Starting out – I was shocked, then inspired by visit to Indian Mission Hospital', *Nursing Standard*, 25(10): 29. An insightful account of a student's experience on an international placement.

Coatsworth, K.Hurley, J. and Miller-Kosser, K. (2017) 'A phenomenological study of student nurses volunteering in Nepal: Have their experiences altered their understanding of nursing?, Collegian, 24: 339–44.

Levine, M. (2009) 'Transforming experiences: Nurse education and international immersion programmes', *Journal of Professional Nursing*, 25: 156–69. The views of nursing students who participated in an international placement.

Weblinks

Go to https://study.sagepub.com/essentialnursing2e for weblinks related to this chapter. If you are using the interactive ebook, simply click on the book icon in the margin to go straight to the resource.

FURTHER
READING:
WEBLINKS

www.tcns.org – the website of the Transcultural Nursing Society, which seeks to provide nurses with the knowledge required to ensure cultural competence in practice, education, research and administration.

www.fco.gov.uk – the Foreign and Commonwealth Office (FCO) website offers a wealth of advice on travel, safety, assistance and living abroad.

www.masta.org – provides travel advice and travel clinics plus a free, personalised brief on staying healthy during your travels.

www.who.int – the World Health Organization (WHO) website offers advice on international travel including risks, precautions and vaccination requirements.

www.nmc-uk.org – the Nursing and Midwifery Council (NMC) website outlines the standards for nurses that must be maintained, no matter where you are providing care.

www.icn.ch – the International Council of Nurses website, which aims to promote quality nursing care and sound health policies globally.

Video links

Have a break from the text and go to https://study.sagepub.com/essentialnursing2e for useful videos related to this chapter. If you are using the interactive ebook, simply click on the lightbulb icon in the margin to go straight to the resource.

VIDEO
LINKS

ACE YOUR ASSESSMENT

Review what you have learned by visiting the book's online resources at: https://study.sagepub.com/essential nursing2e If using your interactive ebook, just click on the icon in the margin to go straight there.

ONLINE
QUIZZES

- Test yourself with multiple-choice and short-answer questions.
- Revise key terms with the interactive flash cards.

REFERENCES

Button, L., Green, B., Tengnah, C., Johansson, I. and Baker, C. (2005) 'The impact of international placements on nurses' personal and professional lives: Literature review', *Journal of Advanced Nursing*, 50: 315–24.

Cromer, K. (2016) Health Needs Assessment: Refugees and asylum seekers in Calderdale. Available at: www.calderdale.gov.uk/v2/sites/default/files/refugees-asylum-seekers-hna.pdf (accessed 1 July 2017).

Department of Health (DH) (2012) *Compassion in Practice*. London: DH.

Grant, E. and McKenna, L. (2003) 'International clinical placements for undergraduate students', *Journal of Clinical Nursing*, 12: 529–35.

Helman, C. (1978) 'Feed a cold, starve a fever', *Culture, Medicine and Psychiatry*, 2: 107–37.

Inglis, A., Rolls, C. and Kristy, S. (2000) 'The impact on attitudes towards cultural difference of participation in a health focused study abroad program', *Contemporary Nurse*, 9: 246–55.

Jones, M., Bond, M. and Mancini, M. (1998) 'Developing a culturally competent workforce: An opportunity for collaboration', *Journal of Professional Nursing*, 14: 280–7.

Labhardt, N.D., Aboa, S.M., Manga, E., Bensing, J.M. and Langewitz, W. (2010) 'Bridging the gap: How traditional healers interact with their patients – A comparative study in Cameroon', *Tropical Medicine and International Health*, 15(9): 1099–108.

Leininger, M.M. (1985) 'Transcultural care diversity and universality: A theory of nursing', *Nursing and Healthcare*, 6(4): 209–12.

Leininger, M.M. (2002) Sunrise Enabler. Available at: www.tcns.org/files/sunrisenew2.ppt (accessed 25 June 2014).

Morgan, D. (2012) 'Student nurse perceptions of risk in relation to international placements: A phenomenological study', *Nurse Education Today*, 32: 956–60.

Rivzi, F. and Walsh, L. (1998) 'Difference, globalisation and the internationalisation of the curriculum', *Australian Universities Review*, 41: 7–11.

Scholes, J. and Moore, D. (2000) 'Clinical exchange: One model to achieve culturally sensitive care', *Nursing Inquiry*, 7: 61–71.

Spector, R.E. (1979) *Cultural Diversity in Health and Illness*. New York: Appleton Century Crofts.

United Nations High Commissioner for Refugees (UNHCR) (2017) Global Trends: Forced displacement in 2016. Available at: www.unhcr.org/statistics/unhcrstats/5943e8a34/global-trends-forced-displacement-2016.html (accessed 1 July 2017).

World Health Organization (2016) *World Health Statistics Report*. Geneva: WHO.

GLOSSARY

Abrasions superficial skin damage.

Accessory muscles additional muscles used to assist breathing during times when the body needs to process extra energy, during exercise, stress or an asthma attack, for example.

Accountable to ensure any actions and care are to the highest possible standard and be able to give a reason or explanation for any actions undertaken or care delivered.

Acronym a word formed from or based on the letters or syllables of other words.

Activities of daily living the activities we undertake every day to remain independent.

Acute a disease with rapid onset or lasting for a short time or the immediate post-injury healing processes.

Ad hoc a solution designed for a specific problem or task.

Adhesion attachment to another surface.

Adjunct additional and supplementary part.

Adjuvant therapy treatment that is given in addition to the main or initial treatment.

Advance Decision (or Advance Directive or Living Will) a statement made by a competent individual refusing specified treatment should she or he lack capacity in the future.

Advocating to speak or act in support of.

Aetiology the cause, set of causes or manner of causation of a disease or condition.

Affective domain the manner in which we deal with things emotionally, such as feelings, values and attitudes.

Algorithms a process or set of rules to be followed in calculations or other problem-solving operations.

Altruism being unselfish; selflessness.

Amyotrophic lateral sclerosis (ALS) also known as motor neurone disease (MND), and Lou Gehrig's disease, is a specific disease which causes the death of neurons controlling muscles.

Analgesia medication given to control pain.

Analgesic pain-relieving medication.

Analytical applying logical reasoning.

Aneroid operates by the effect of air.

Anonymise to remove the name and any other identifying features.

Anoxia inadequate oxygen levels in the body's tissues.

Anticoagulation therapy administering regular drugs that reduce the body's ability to form clots.

Appraise to assess.

Arrhythmia irregular heartbeat.

Arteriovenous fistula a surgically formed connection between an artery and a vein, normally created for haemodialysis, a treatment for patients with renal failure.

Asphyxiate suffocate.

Aspiration to remove by suction.

Assertive outreach teams community teams which focus on those with mental health issues, who might otherwise need a hospital admission. These teams have small caseloads and provide intensive support.

Assess Plan Implement Evaluate (APIE) an established tool to help assess, plan and deliver care which requires a meta-paradigm to determine what should be included within the assessment.

Autonomy the freedom to make binding decisions, within the scope of practice that are based on professional ethics, expertise and clinical knowledge.

Avoidance coping   this is an approach which involves withdrawing from a situation which is found to be stressful. Whilst this may be helpful in the short term it does not enable the skills to be developed to effectively deal with the experience encountered.

Bacterial flora   micro-organisms that live normally within the gut.

Balance of probabilities   this refers to the obligation imposed upon a claimant to demonstrate that his or her claim is more likely to be true than not.

Battery (or Trespass to the Person)   the touching of a competent patient without his or her consent. Unlike negligence, harm does not necessarily have to be caused to establish battery.

Benchmark standard   a standard by which something may be judged. This is usually a standard of good practice and set by best evidence in the arena.

Benchmarking   a measurement of quality by comparison with similar services. Benchmarking determines what improvements are required in services by analysing how others who offer similar services are able to offer higher quality and then uses this information to improve quality.

Best practice   the most effective nursing care required to address an individual's specific nursing needs/problems.

Bipolar disorder   a mental condition marked by alternating periods of elation and depression.

Bottom-up   where the need for change is communicated upwards.

Butskellism   the consensus related to policy issues between the Conservative and Labour parties from the 1950s to the 1970s. The term is an amalgamation of R.A. Butler and Hugh Gaitskell's names; they were the chancellors of the two parties during part of this time.

C. difficile (Clostridium difficile)   a bacteria that is capable of producing a toxin that can result in diarrhoea. The bacteria produces spores that survive in the environment for long periods of time and can be passed from one patient to another, resulting in outbreaks of diarrhoea.

Candour   truthfulness and sincerity.

Cannulae   thin tubes inserted into a vein or body cavity to administer medication or drain off fluid.

Capacity (or Competence)   the ability of an individual to make one's own decisions.

Cardiac arrest   when the heart abruptly stops generating an effective beat.

Cardiovascular status   effectiveness of heart and circulatory system functioning.

Care   to look after with kindness and regard.

Care Quality Commission   an English government body which checks whether hospitals, care homes, GPs, dentists and services in the home meet national standards. Other countries of the UK have bodies with a similar function, such as The Regulation and Quality Improvement Authority (RQIA) in Northern Ireland.

Case study research   a research methodology where a study is based on the analysis of one or more cases or histories.

Catatonia   a state of apparent unresponsiveness to external stimuli in a person who is apparently awake.

Causal   making something happen.

Cause of action   a specific legal claim (such as negligence, defamation, or breach of contract) for which a claimant seeks compensation from the court.

Chlorhexidine   a common disinfectant used in health and dental care. It can be applied to the skin as a wash or in hand hygiene products to reduce the number of bacteria present. It is commonly used in surgical scrub solutions and as a skin wash for decolonisation of patients who carry MRSA or prior to surgical procedures.

Chronological   arranged in order of time.

Claimant   a person who brings a civil action in a court of law and makes a claim against the defendant.

Clinical guidelines   principles giving practical guidance, allowing for professional initiative.

Clinical interventions   the actions undertaken by healthcare professionals to improve a patient's condition.

Clinical outcome   clinical relates to the observation and treatment of patients and outcome is the consequence of that treatment.

Coagulation disorder   when the body is unable to control blood clotting.

Coalition government   created when two political parties merge temporarily to enable the formation of a government.

Coercion   to compel an individual to undertake an action.

Cognitive   the mental processes of perception, memory, judgement and reasoning.

Cognitive domain   this refers to knowledge and the development of intellectual skills.

Collaborative   to work in association with, to co-operate.

Collegiate   working in partnership.

Common Law (or Case Law)   the law developed by judges through the decisions of cases.

Community   used to refer to care delivered outside a general or acute hospital setting.

Compensation   the financial award made to those who have established that they have been the victims of battery or negligence.

Competence   refers to the overarching set of knowledge, skills and attitudes required to practice safely and effectively without direct supervision.

Complementary medicine   treatments which are often based on a holistic view of the patient, used in conjunction with and not as alternatives to western medicine.

Comprehensive   the principle that a wide range of welfare services should be available to everyone.

Compromised   to be impaired.

Concepts   these are general ideas about single things which can be defined.

Concordance   following medical advice or planned treatment.

Concordant   if two things are concordant then they are in agreement or consistent with each other.

Concordantly   following medical advice.

Confidentiality   this relates to the expectation of patients that their medical details will be shared only with those who have a legitimate right to this information.

Consent   this refers to the agreement of a patient to undergo treatment. To be valid consent, the patient must be competent and fully informed, and should not be subject to any duress or undue influence.

Consequentialist   the morality of an action is judged according to how good or bad its consequences are.

Consolidation   a region of lung tissue that has filled with liquid.

Contact precautions   this is a term commonly used in association with standard precautions and isolation precautions. It implies that precautions (e.g. gloves and aprons) are required to prevent the spread of micro-organisms as a result of contamination in the patient environment.

Contemporaneous   at the same time.

Contemporary   up-to-date current approaches.

Contentious   an issue where controversy or disagreement exists.

Context   the setting.

Contextual drivers   factors that contribute to defining the need for change.

Contusions   bruises.

Convergence   come together, become more similar.

COPD   chronic obstructive pulmonary disease, a common lung disease which makes it difficult to breathe.

Coping mechanisms are how stress is managed, adapted to or acted upon.

Core body temperature the temperature of structures deep within the body.

Core mission statement a declaration of central beliefs held by a group.

Counselling helping individuals to adjust to or cope with personal problems by enabling them to discover for themselves the potential solution within a supported environment.

Crisis intervention teams home treatment community teams, which are an alternative to inpatient care for people experiencing an acute mental health crisis.

Critical analysis the ability to show in your writing how the evidence you have considered and evaluated in preparing for your written work has informed or challenged your understanding of the issues under discussion and can (or cannot) be applied to the nursing care of a given individual/patient group.

Critical appraisal judging the quality of research evidence in a systematic way.

Culture the attitudes and values which inform an individual, group or society.

Cyanosis blue or purple colouration of the skin, usually seen around the lips or fingers/toes, usually due to low levels of oxygen in the blood.

Data analysis finding patterns in research data and establishing their significance.

Deep vein thrombosis a blood clot in one of the deep veins in the body (often in the legs).

Defecation to pass faeces from the bowels.

Defendant a person against whom an action is brought in a court of law.

Deficit reduction when government expenditure exceeds income, this is termed a deficit; government economic policy is currently focused on reducing this.

Deinstitutionalisation this is when long-stay institutions such as large mental health or learning disability hospitals close and are replaced by some type of care provision outside institutions. It has been an ongoing policy since the 1960s and accepts the argument that large institutions negatively impact on health.

Delegation the passing of authority and responsibility for specific tasks to another. A nurse or midwife should only delegate an aspect of care to a person who has had appropriate training and whom they deem competent to perform the task.

Demographic an analysis of the structure of a population.

Dessication to dry.

Developed countries a term used to describe relatively rich countries such as America, Germany, the UK, France, Japan, Spain and South Korea.

Developed world a term used to describe relatively rich countries such as America, Germany, the UK, France, Japan, Spain and South Korea.

Developing countries a term used to describe the relatively poor and underdeveloped nations of Asia, Africa and Latin America.

Developing world a term used to describe the relatively poor and underdeveloped nations of Asia, Africa and Latin America.

Devolution the transfer of certain powers from a central (Westminster) to a subordinate level (Northern Ireland, Scotland and Wales).

Diabetes several diseases, with the most common (diabetes mellitus) caused by an insufficiency of insulin resulting in excess sugar in the blood and urine.

Diabetologist a specialist in diabetes.

Diastole the period of time when the heart relaxes and refills with blood following contraction.

Diastolic blood pressure the pressure when your heart is resting.

Dietetic assessment an in-depth review of a patient's nutritional requirements and actual intake.

Dilate become wider, larger or more open.

Disease aetiology the cause of a disease.

Dispositional control a tendency to sort things out for oneself.

Dissertation a formal and extended essay based upon the author's primary or secondary research, often a requirement for an academic qualification.

Domains areas of activity.

Downstream working reactively treating ill health.

Drivers influences for change.

Duchenne Muscular Dystrophy a condition which causes muscle weakness. It is a genetic condition which starts in childhood and usually only affects boys, but girls can carry the Duchenne gene.

Duty of care a legal obligation to ensure that others are not foreseeably harmed by one's actions.

Dysfunction impaired or abnormal functioning.

Dysmenorrhea pain during menstruation.

Early intervention teams community mental health teams, targeted at 14–35-year-olds with first presentation of psychotic symptoms.

Economic monetarism the policy of controlling an economic system by increasing or decreasing the money supply.

Egalitarian believing in or based on the principle that all people are equal and deserve equal rights and opportunities.

Egocentric self-centred.

Elective planned and pre-arranged.

Elective placement a placement in a clinical environment of a student's choice.

Electrolytes the smallest of chemicals that are important for cells in the body to function properly.

Embodied expressed or personified.

Emergence the process of coming into existence.

Empower/empowering/empowerment to give an individual the power to take decisions in matters relating to themselves.

Endocrinologist a specialist in endocrine conditions.

Endogenous from within an organism, tissue or cell. Usually applies to the origin of a micro-organism or infection. Endogenous causes arise from the patient themselves and not as a result of cross-infection.

Endorphins naturally occurring pain-relieving hormones in the body.

Enteral by way of the intestine (rather than given, for example, directly into the blood).

Equitable the principle that welfare services should be available to everyone, in the same way.

Erythema redness of the skin.

Ethnocentrism belief in the superiority of one's own cultural group and a corresponding misunderstanding of other such groups.

Evidence the knowledge and information we use to help us to make effective decisions, not just for nursing but in all the decisions we make in life.

EWSS/PEWS Early Warning Scoring System and Paediatric Early Warning System, tools which help to assess and determine early warning scores to identify deterioration of patient conditions.

Exogenous from outside an organism, tissue or cell.

Expectorate/expectorating to cough up phlegm/sputum.

Extended family a family unit comprising not only a couple and their children but other relatives, such as grandparents, aunts and uncles.

Extravasation leakage of fluid into the tissues around infusion sites.

Extubation the removal of artificial breathing support, usually mechanical ventilation.

Exudate fluid such as pus or clear fluid which leaks out of blood vessels into nearby tissues or out of the body.

Faecal–oral route one way that infection can be transmitted. Small particles excreted in the faeces must enter the mouth of the next victim. Includes infections such as norovirus and C. difficile. Placing hands in the mouth after contact with a contaminated (not visibly) environment are usually the way that this occurs.

Fibrin a fibrous, non-globular protein involved in clotting.

Field-specific specialised, applicable to only one field of nursing.

Fields of nursing practice the different areas nurses in the UK can specialise within – mental health, child, learning disability and adult, each being named after the patients which nurses in these fields care for most frequently.

First past the post this relates to a voting system in which the winner (a political party) needs to receive more votes than anyone else.

Fissure a linear crack in the skin that may extend from the epidermis into the dermis.

Fitness to practise the skills, knowledge and character to practise your profession safely and effectively, thus being suitable to be on the NMC register without restriction.

Flaccid soft and limp.

Formative assessment assessments which provide you and your lecturers with feedback on your progress but do not count towards your academic award.

Fraser competent is a term used to describe a child under 16 who is considered to be of sufficient age and understanding to be competent to receive contraceptive advice without parental knowledge or consent.

Free market where economic activity takes place and is not controlled by government.

Fresher's Week week of activities designed specifically to welcome first-year students to university.

Gait manner of walking.

Generic general, applicable to any field of nursing.

Genre a type or style.

Genuineness being yourself rather than presenting a false persona.

Gerontologist studies the processes of growing old.

Glasgow Coma Scale (GCS) a neurological scale that aims to provide a reliable and objective way to record the conscious state of a patient.

Global relating to the whole world.

Good character describes an individual's conduct, behaviour and attitude.

Good health to be capable of safe and effective practice without supervision.

Gross domestic product (GDP) a country's total income.

Gynecomastia benign enlargement of breast tissue.

Haemorrhoids dilation of a vein around the anus, often called piles.

Health beliefs the personal beliefs a patient has regarding how illness can be prevented and treated.

Health coaching a process that facilitates healthy, sustainable behaviour change by challenging a patient to develop their inner wisdom, identify their values, and transform their goals into action.

Health inequalities can be defined as differences in health status between different population groups. For example, differences in mortality rates between people from different social classes.

Hemiplegia the paralysis of the arm, leg and trunk on the same side of the body. This can be right or left-sided in nature. This may be identified at birth or may be caused by illness or injury.

Hierarchical a system in which members of an organisation or society are ranked according to perceived status or authority.

Hierarchy of evidence a list of different types of evidence that are ranked in order of strength.

Histamine a substance manufactured by the body involved in immune responses.

Holistic considering all aspects of a person, their physical, psychological, social, emotional, intellectual and spiritual needs.

Homeostasis the tendency of a bodily system to ensure internal stability.

Hydrated maintaining sufficient water for bodily needs.

Hyper-extend bending a bodily joint beyond its normal range of motion.

Hypertension high blood pressure.

Hypotension low blood pressure.

Hypothesis a proposed explanation made on the basis of limited evidence as a starting point for further investigation.

Hypothetical a provisional explanation.

Hypovolaemia decreased fluid volume in the body.

Ideological based upon a certain way of thinking, a view of how the world should be.

Ideologies the sets of beliefs and values patients hold.

Ideology a collection of ideas which reflect the needs and aspirations of a particular social group or setting.

Immunosuppression a reduced immune response.

In situ a Latin phrase which means in position.

Inception the initial setting up of an organisation

Independence not relying upon others.

Independent mental capacity advocate (IMCA) a person whose role it is to help incapacitated people who face important decisions about serious medical treatment and/or change of residence and/or detention.

Integrated care combined with that of other healthcare professionals.

Integrity sound, unimpaired, in perfect condition.

Interdisciplinary involving more than one group of health professionals – nurses, doctors and physiotherapists for example.

Intermittent self-catheterization a procedure performed by a patient to empty their bladder on an ad hoc basis by inserting a urinary catheter into the urethra.

Intermittently occurring at irregular intervals.

Internal market this is a pseudo-market which mimics how the free market operates. It creates the conditions for competition between hospitals and other service providers, through the separation of purchaser and provider responsibilities.

Interplay the dynamic relationship between two or more concepts, including how they act or react towards one another.

Interprofessional the dynamic relationship between two or more professional groups.

Interprofessional learning occasions when two or more professionals learn with, from and about each other.

Interstitial fluid tissue fluid, a solution that bathes and surrounds the cells in the body.

Interwoven joined together.

Intra-abdominal within the abdomen.

Intravenous (IV) the infusion of liquid substances directly into a vein.

Ischaemia a restriction of blood supply to the tissues which causes damage.

Ischaemic   lack of blood.

Keynesian economics was an approach developed by the British economist John Maynard Keynes in the 1930s in an attempt to understand the Great Depression.

Klebsiella spp   a common family of bacteria that have the potential to be multi-resistant and are commonly found in high-dependency areas such as ITUs.

Korotkoff sounds the sounds listened to when recording blood pressure.

Lactic acid   a chemical compound that plays a role in numerous bodily processes.

Laterally   related to the side.

Learning outcome the knowledge you should gain from completing the work you are undertaking.

Legislate   make legal.

Legislation   law making.

Liability   an obligation or responsibility, the dereliction of which may lead to legal action.

Licensed   all medications are licensed only to be used in a specific way.

Liverpool Care Pathway (LCP) palliative care options for patients in the last hours or days of life in the UK (apart from Wales). It was developed to ensure that patients receive quality end-of-life care.

Long-term   lasts for months or years.

Lymphoedema   localized fluid retention and tissue swelling caused by a compromised lymphatic system.

Mandible   lower jaw bone.

Manifestos   declarations of policies and objectives produced by political parties, usually prior to an election.

Mastication   chewing.

Maxilla   upper jaw bone.

Meatal   an opening or passage.

Medical model   this is an approach to health that is functional and illness-orientated.

Meta-analysis   a research methodology where several similar but separate studies are analysed in order to learn more about their significance.

Metacognition   awareness and understanding of one's own thought processes.

Meta-paradigm   a group of statements that identify a phenomenon drawn from a series of philosophical beliefs.

Metabolic rate   the rate at which a body burns calories.

Methodology   a system used in research.

Micturition   urination.

Mixed methods research   in simple and general terms, using both qualitative and quantitative research approaches to answer a research question.

Models of nursing   an outline framework or blueprint which emanates from a collation of philosophical views and from contemporary evidence. May be a meta-paradigm or may include greater tested empirical evidence within a more specific area of focus. A model helps to steer the delivery of nursing, by enabling a team to share a common direction.

Modules   units of learning which make up a course.

Morbidity   a diseased state, disability or ill health which can have any cause.

Mortality   number of deaths in a given time or place.

MRSA   meticillin-resistant *Staphylococcus aureus* – a bacteria. A member of the Staphylococcus aureus family that is resistant to the antibiotic meticillin and is frequently responsible for difficult-to-treat infections.

Mucosa   the lining of the mouth, lips, nostrils.

Mucous membrane   a layer of tissue lining an area of the body which comes into contact with air.

Multi-disciplinary team a varying number of professionals working towards the same objective.

Multi-sectoral different organisations (usually government departments) working together. For example, public health, environment agency, nursing and education.

Myocardial infarction (MI) death of heart muscle tissue. Commonly known as a heart attack.

Named nurse a specific nurse responsible for overseeing the organisation and management of all aspects of a patient's care.

Nasogastric reaching or supplying the stomach via the nose.

Nasogastric (NG) tube a narrow bore tube passed into the stomach via the nose.

National Institute for Health and Care Excellence (NICE) an organisation set up to produce authoritative national guidance on the use of new and existing technologies.

National Service Frameworks (NSFs) national standards and models for services, which establish quality requirements for care. These are based on the best available evidence of treatment and services. They include mental health, coronary heart disease, cancer, older people, diabetes, children, renal services, long-term neurological conditions, chronic obstructive pulmonary disease and stroke.

Negligence this occurs where there has been a breach in the standard of care, leading to reasonably foreseeable harm.

Neonate a baby in the first 28 days after birth.

Neuropathy damage to the peripheral nervous system.

NMC register to work as a nurse in the UK you must be on the register of nurses and midwives held by the NMC.

Non-compliant not following professional advice.

Non-institutional caring for patients within an individual setting rather than communally, such as in a hospital.

Non-invasive not penetrating the body.

Noradrenaline a naturally occurring hormone and neurotransmitter.

Normally distributed a statistical term describing a frequency distribution, such as weight. When plotted on a graph a group of individuals will produce a curve similar in shape to a bell, where the weight of most of them will be grouped within a relatively small range and only a minority will fall outside this central cluster.

Norovirus a highly infectious infection caused by a virus which results in diarrhoea and vomiting. It is particularly problematic in hospitals, schools and cruise ships and frequently causes outbreaks of infection in staff and patients.

Nurse prescribing registered nurses with an additional qualification are able to prescribe drugs from a specified list.

Nursing and Midwifery Council (NMC) the nursing and midwifery regulator for the UK who sets the standards that nurses and midwives must meet in their working lives, ensures that nursing students and student midwives have the right education at the start and throughout their career and keeps a register of all nurses and midwives in the UK.

Nursing reflexivity nursing with an understanding of yourself: your values, attitudes, beliefs and the impact this has on the care you provide.

Objective based on facts.

Oliguria low urine output.

Opioid an opioid is any chemical that acts on the brain, resembling morphine or other opiates in its pharmacological effects.

Organic material a general term that includes dirt and soiling, which in healthcare can include blood, body fluids and excreta.

Package of care an individually designed range of support and heathcare services to meet a patient's needs.

Palliative care the World Health Organization defines this as an approach that improves the quality of life of service users and their families facing the problems associated with life-threatening illness, through the prevention and relief of suffering by means of early identification and impeccable assessment and treatment of pain and other problems, physical, psychosocial and spiritual.

Palpate   examine an organ medically, by feel.

Parameters   a characteristic, feature or measurable factor that defines a particular system.

Paranoia   a false belief that people are trying to harm you. Obsessively anxious about something or unreasonably suspicious of other people, their thoughts or motives.

Paraphimosis   the foreskin becomes trapped behind the glans penis and cannot be returned to its normal position.

Partnership   to work with a patient, as equals, towards the same goal.

Patient   a person receiving or registered to receive medical treatment, also referred to as 'client', 'service user' or 'person with a learning disability'. More important is to refer to the patient by their preferred name and in their preferred manner.

Patient Advice and Liaison Service   a confidential service that provides advice and support for patients.

Patient group directives (PGD)   specific written instructions for the supply and administration of a licensed named medicine to specific groups of patients.

Patient scenarios   situations based upon real-life patient experiences and stories.

Patient-specific directives (PSD)   instructions written on a prescription form which provide instructions for the supply and administration of a licensed named medicine to an individual patient.

PEG (Percutaneous endoscopic gastrostomy) tube   a percutaneous endoscopic gastrostomy (PEG) is a medical procedure where a PEG tube is passed into a patient's stomach through the abdominal wall, normally to provide a way to feed the patient.

Perfusion   supply of blood.

Peripheral arterial disease   a condition in which a build-up of fatty deposits in the arteries restricts blood supply to leg muscles.

Peripheral vascular disease   disease of the arteries and veins located outside the heart and brain where they become partially or completely blocked.

Permeable   allows liquids or gases to pass through it.

Personhood   attributes possessed by human beings that make them a person.

Pervasive   to extend through the whole, to permeate.

Phagocytosis   the process by which a cell engulfs a solid particle.

Pharynx   the throat.

Philanthropy   this relates to benevolence and generosity.

Philosophy   a theory or belief which can act as a guiding principle for behaviour.

Phlebitis   inflammation of a vein.

Physiological   being in accord with or characteristic of the normal functioning of a living organism.

Placement   healthcare areas nursing students attend to be involved in patient care during their course (also called practice experience).

Pluralistic   more than one.

Pneumothorax   presence of air in the pleural cavity surrounding the lungs, causing pain and difficulty in breathing.

Portfolios   a collection of evidence to support professional and personal learning and development (may also include formal assessment evidence).

Post-partum   following child birth.

Practice   the wide range of activities nurses undertake when caring for patients.

Practice educator   a nurse on the NMC register who, following successful completion of an

NMC-approved preparation course, is entered on a local register and is eligible to supervise and assess students in a practice setting.

Practice supervisor a suitably qualified professional who will support a student, ensuring the care they provide is safe and effective.

Pragmatically practically, in a manner that is convenient.

Praxis of nursing a process by which nursing is carried out or practised.

Pressure ulceration a type of injury caused when the skin is placed under pressure.

Pre–assessment clinic usually a nurse-led clinic where it is determined whether patient is physically fit enough to have treatment (such as surgery and an anaesthetic).

Privatisation to sell off services previously held in public ownership to the private sector.

Proactive action behaviour which anticipates situations rather than responds after they have occurred.

Professionally socialised acting with an identity within accepted norms for the identified professional group.

Protocols detailed descriptions of the steps taken to deliver care or treatment to a patient.

Psychomotor domain this relates to physical movement, coordination and the use of motor skills.

Pulmonary embolism (PE) a clot in the main artery of the lung or one of its branches.

PVI third-sector settings health and social care services delivered by private, voluntary or independent sector organisations.

Pyrexic feverish, having a high temperature.

Qualitative research in simple and general terms, research that generates answers in the form of words.

Quality of life an individual's assessment of their wellbeing, considering a physical, psychological, social, emotional, intellectual and spiritual perspective.

Quantitative research in simple and general terms, research that generates answers in the form of numbers.

Randomised controlled trial (RCT) a study in which a number of similar people are randomly assigned to two (or more) groups to test a drug or treatment.

Rapport connection, emotional bond.

Reagents a substance used in chemical analysis.

Receptivity able to relate to ideas.

Reflection a process that allows us to critically review our personal experiences and learn from them.

Reflective practice the reviewing of care by questioning how and why decisions are made and care provided in order to facilitate better practice.

Registered nurse a person registered as a nurse with the Nursing and Midwifery Council, who can be further defined as: 'a professional person achieving a competent standard of practice at first cycle level following successful completion of an approved academic and practical course. The nurse is a safe, caring, and competent decision maker willing to accept personal and professional accountability for his or her actions and continuous learning. The nurse practices within a statutory framework and code of ethics delivering nursing practice (care) that is appropriately based on research, evidence and critical thinking that effectively responds to the needs of individual clients (patients) and diverse populations (European Tuning project).

Regulatory body a public or government agency responsible for setting standards.

Reification depersonalisation.

Repressed unconsciously forgotten.

Research a systematic and trustworthy way of finding answers to questions.

Rheumatoid arthritis an autoimmune disease that results in a chronic, systemic inflammatory disorder.

Role-models people whose character and behaviour you would like to imitate.

Rolling back the state where the scope of state responsibility does not remain static.

Root causes the fundamental factors that led to the outcome or effect being considered.

Safeguard to protect individuals from the risk of harm or abuse.

SBAR Situation Background Assess Record, an established tool which helps to assess, plan and deliver care to patients and requires a meta-paradigm to determine what should be included within the assessment.

Sclera the white of the eyes.

Secondary supplemental, not the primary condition.

Secular not concerned with religion.

Self-determination the process by which a person controls their own life.

Self-efficacy belief in one's own abilities.

Self-esteem opinion of oneself.

Self-image an individual's view of themself.

Self-perception the way an individual perceives themselves.

Seminal work work which may be older, but the message remains pertinent today and therefore has never been superseded.

Sequential following a sequence.

Serotonin a neurotransmitter chemical.

Setting the environment care is delivered in: this may be in a hospital, in the community, in a patient's home or in a medical centre, for example.

'Sharp' a term for devices used in patient care with sharp points or edges that can puncture or cut skin.

Sickle cell anaemia a genetic blood disorder in which red blood cells develop abnormally.

Skin integrity condition of the skin.

Skin turgor the skin's ability to change shape and return to normal elasticity.

Smegma a combination of exfoliated epithelial cells, skin oils and moisture that occurs in both male and female genitalia.

SOAPIER Subjective Objective Assessment Planning Implement Evaluate Re-assessment, an established tool to assess, plan and deliver care to clients which requires a meta-paradigm to determine what should be included within the assessment.

Social capital the networks of relationships among people who live and work in a particular society.

Social gradient the distribution of health outcomes that closely correlates to social status.

Social networking sites e.g. Facebook, Twitter, blogs, instant messaging sites.

Socialisation the way in which we become aware of society and our relationships with others.

Socialised have acquired the specialised knowledge, skills, attitudes and values of a group.

Socio-political social and political aspect.

Somatogenic a disease process having its origin in the body due to external forces. Contrasts with psychogenic, where the origin of the disease or illness is in the mind.

Sphygmomanometer a device used to measure blood pressure.

Standard of care this refers to the actions of a reasonably competent professional practising under the same or similar circumstances.

Statutory the law enacted by Parliament and which takes precedence over the common law if the latter is in conflict with it.

Statutory body a public or government agency with the authority to check that the activities of organisations or individuals are legal.

Steroid therapy medication given to improve a large number of conditions.

Stethoscope a medical device used to listen to sounds.

Stigmatising to attach a negative label to an individual or group of people.

Stoma any artificial opening usually leading to the surface of the body, e.g. abdominal surface.

Subjectivity perspective, experiences, feelings, beliefs, desires, etc. that depend upon situation, perception, experience, expectation and personal or cultural understanding. The opposite to objectivity, which is based on facts.

Summative assessments those that have to be passed in order for you to progress on the course and complete it successfully.

Supporting the act of assisting a patient to meet their needs, be these physical, social, emotional, intellectual or spiritual.

Survey a means of investigating the opinions or experience of (a group of people) by asking them questions.

Synthesis/Synthesise putting ideas together and drawing conclusions from them.

System drivers factors influencing the delivery of care to be more effective.

Systematic methodical.

Systematic review a research methodology which sums up all the best available research on a specific subject.

Systemic spread throughout the entire body.

Systole contraction of the heart.

Systolic blood pressure the amount of pressure exerted on the blood vessels when a heart contracts (beats).

Tachycardia fast heart rate.

Therapeutic interventions activities undertaken to maintain or improve someone's health and wellbeing.

Therapeutic relationships refer to the relationship between a healthcare professional and a patient. This describes how they interact with each other in order to produce beneficial change for the patient.

Top-down where the need for change is communicated downwards.

Topical of or applied to a definite or localised area of the body.

Topical application a medication applied to the skin.

Torsion twisting.

Traditional medicine applies knowledge and practices frequently handed down from previous generations, whether or not they can be explained, to prevent, diagnose and eliminate physical, mental or social imbalances.

Transcultural embracing all cultures.

Unconditional positive regard consistent respect even when people exhibit behaviours you do not like.

Universalism the principle that welfare services should be publicly funded and available to all, on the basis of need.

Upstream working on the root causes of ill health. Looking at how policy and service delivery can be influenced to improve health.

Validate check or prove validity or truth.

Venepuncture taking blood.

Welfare state where the government takes lead responsibility for providing a range of services for its citizens that can include education, social care services, housing and health.

Western medicine an approach taught in a classical curriculum that is said to be based upon scientific evidence.

Wha–nau often translated as 'family', but its meaning is more complex than this, as it includes emotional, physical and spiritual dimensions. It is a multi-layered, flexible and dynamic concept that is based upon a Maori worldview where the values, histories and traditions of ancestors are adapted for the contemporary world.

White Paper documents produced by the government which set out the details of future policy.

Wider determinants of health these are social and political factors, such as people's living and working conditions, education, political and economic policies, that shape and influence the health outcomes of people.

Wound bed the base of a wound.

INDEX